Expediting Drug and Biologics Development

A Strategic Approach

Third Edition

Expediting Drug and Biologics Development

A Strategic Approach
Third Edition

Steven E. Linberg, Ph.D.

PAREXEL International Corporation
Waltham, MA
Publishers

Expediting Drug and Biologics Development

A Strategic Approach
Third Edition

by
Steven E. Linberg, Ph.D.

Production: Joanna White

PAREXEL International Corporation
200 West Street
Waltham, Massachusetts 02154 USA
800-856-2556, x2200/610-565-2622

ISBN Number: 1-882615-76-X

PREFACE

I am greatly indebted to the contributors to this Third Edition. Everyone was very gracious in agreeing to participate, and all know that their hard work has once again gone to support pediatric research at the Children's Center, Johns Hopkins University Hospital. The work that was pioneered there by John M. Freeman, MD, now at least partially retired, has been an inspiration to me and countless others. Interested parties might want to visit http://www.neuro.jhmi.edu/Epilepsy/Peds/. I only wish we could do more for them.

At some time during the compilation of the Third Edition it became clear that the subtitle of the book, *A Strategic Approach*, might be a bit misleading or confusing. The intended use of the word "strategy" might not be as obvious as originally hoped. In this usage, the strategy is to plan carefully and execute aggressively while focused on the target. It is as simple as that, and different from "strategy" as used in other contexts. This book is not about regulatory strategies in drug development, and for any confusion, I apologize. The intent here was to be more down-to-earth and focus on efficient operations. The contributors to this text are all operations people, with rare exception, as you will gather from their chapters. They actually do the work.

While many of the chapter topics remain the same from the earlier editions, many of the authors have changed to provide different perspectives. Additionally, there are a few new chapters in this edition that help to more fully address the overall development process.

Finally, I owe a debt of gratitude to Mark Mathieu and his wonderful team at PAREXEL for putting up with me for 10 years and three editions. I have learned a lot and grown from the association.

Steven E. Linberg

CONTRIBUTORS

Paul A. Andrews, Ph.D.
Assistant Vice President, Toxicology
ImClone Systems Incorporated

David Bernstein, Ph. D.
Principal Consultant
Bernstein CMC Regulatory Consulting

Steven A. Biedenbach, M.S.
President
Biedenbach & Stein, Inc.

Michele D. Bronson, Ph. D.
Director, Regulatory Affairs—Oncology
Chiron Corporation

Gus Cicala
Chief Executive Officer
Project Assistants, Inc.

Steven C. Cohen
Senior Vice President
Executive Communications Group
Division of E.C.G., Inc.

Matthew R. Dauphin, M.S.
Clinical Scientist
Shire Development Inc.

Wei Dong M.D., Ph.D.
Senior Epidemiologist
Genentech, Inc.

Janet C. Donnelly, CIP
Director
Chesapeake Research Review, Inc.

Angela Fleming
Sr. Quality Assurance Specialist
MedImmune Inc.

Diana Fordyce, Ph.D., R.A.C.
Principal Regulatory Affairs Scientist
Cato Research Ltd.

Paul W. Goebel, Jr. CIP
President
Paul W. Goebel Consulting, Inc.

Steven Hirschfeld, M.D., Ph.D.
Capt. USPHS
Office of Cellular, Tissue and Gene Therapy
Center for Biologics Evaluation and Research
Food and Drug Administration

Christine Kochi, Pharm.D.
Senior Manager, Medical Writing
Biogen Idec, Inc.

Antonis Koutsoukos, Ph.D.
Associate Director, Biostatistics
Amgen

Carolyn M. Laurençot, Ph.D.
National Cancer Institute

Steven E. Linberg, Ph.D.
Managing Director, Treasurer
Chiesi Pharmaceuticals Inc.

Walker A. Long, M.D.
Vice President Clinical
Atherogenics, Inc.

James Matcham, M.Sc., C.Stat.
Associate Director,
Biostatistical Scientist
Amgen

Louis A. Morris, Ph.D.
President
Louis A. Morris & Associates, Inc.

Craig Ostroff, Pharm.D., R.Ph.
Associate Director and Liaison
Global Regulatory Affairs
Schering-Plough

Natalia Owen, M.S., C.C.R.A.
Clinical Research Manager
RS Medical

Leo Pavliv, R.Ph., M.B.A.
Vice President, Operations
Cumberland Pharmaceuticals

Stephen A. Raymond, Ph.D.
Chief Scientific Officer and Quality Officer
PHT Corporation

Peg Regan
President & CEO
PharmaPros Corporation

Denis Roy, Ph.D.
Senior Director, Nonclinical Safety Development
Cato Research Ltd.

Deborah I. Scott, M.I.M., R.A.C.
Principal
Avanti Research, Inc.

Bill Shipman, M.B.A.
Senior Director, Information Systems Technology
NPS Pharmaceuticals

Beverley Smith
Global Head of Clinical Quality Assurance
Amgen

Janice M. Soreth, M.D.
Director, Division of Anti-Infective Drug Products
Center for Drug Evaluation and Research
Food & Drug Administration

Bao-Van Tran, M.S.
Senior Clinical Scientist
Shire Development Inc.

Stephen P. Truocchio, M.S., R.A.C.
Associate Director, Regulatory Submissions
Otsuka Maryland Research Institute, Inc.

Hugh N. Tucker, Ph.D., F.A.C.N., C.N.S
Vice President, Global Regulatory and
Scientific Affairs
Bristol-Myers Squibb Mead Johnson Nutritionals

Christine Ver Straate
Vice President, Clinical Programs
PharmaPros Corporation

Michael J. Vivion, Ph.D.
Vice President, Executive Communications Group
Division of E.C.G., Inc.

Karl Whitney, Ph.D., R.A.C.
Program Manager
RTI International

Steven Wilkinson, M.S.
Wilkinson Consulting

Andrea Wright
Supervisory Regulatory Project Manager
Office of Cellular, Tissue and Gene Therapy
Center for Biologics Evaluation and Research
Food and Drug Administration

CONTENTS

Chapter 1. Beginning at the Destination: A Corporate Culture 1

Chapter 2. Project Management and Pharmaceutical Development 7

Chapter 3. Integration of CMC into Drug Development: Avoiding the Common Delays 17

Chapter 4. Nonclinical Development 25

Chapter 5. Clinical Development Plans: Target Product Profile 45

Chapter 6. Information Systems in Support of Pharmaceutical Development 51

Chapter 7. Title 21 CFR Part 11 61

Chapter 8. Format and Content of the Common Technical Document (CTD) 67

Chapter 9. Streamlining the Drug Development and Approval Process 93

Chapter 10. Meeting with the FDA 103

Chapter 11. The Investigational New Drug Application 109

Chapter 12. The Investigator's Brochure 125

Chapter 13. The Phases of Clinical Development 129

Chapter 14. Clinical Trials Enrolling Children 145

Chapter 15. Clinical Study Reports 155

Chapter 16. Standard Data Presentations 163

Chapter 17. Analysis Plans 183

Chapter 18. Data Capture 193

Chapter 19. The Clinical Protocol 217

Chapter 20. Informed Consent and IRB Review 231

Chapter 21. Clinical Trial Operations 239

Chapter 22. Clinical Monitoring 245

Chapter 23. An Integrated Approach to Data Management 259

Chapter 24. Evaluation of Safety During Clinical Drug Development 267

Chapter 25. Developing a Risk Minimization Action Plan 279

Chapter 26. Assembling and Filing the Common Technical Document 289

Chapter 27. The FDA Marketing Application Review Process 299

Chapter 28. Preparing for FDA Inspection 309

Chapter 29. Preparing for an FDA Advisory Committee Meeting 317

Chapter 30. Post-Marketing Safety Assessment 327

CHAPTER 1

Beginning at the Destination: A Corporate Culture

By Steven E. Linberg, Ph.D.

The ultimate goal of the pharmaceutical (drugs and biologics) development process is to improve the standard of health care by providing new or improved therapies for the prevention and treatment of illnesses. While this is certainly a worthy and altruistic goal, the practical development of pharmaceuticals is a complicated, costly and time-consuming process. According to the most recent *PAREXEL's Pharmaceutical R&D Statistical Sourcebook*, numerous surveys now estimate that the average cost of developing one successful pharmaceutical product is above $800 million (including the cost of failed products). Estimated development costs for one successful product, exclusive of failures (we should all be so lucky), still run in the hundreds-of-million dollar range. The time involved from the conception of the product to final marketing averages about 11 years, depending on the specific development and testing obstacles.

The fruits of these labors and investments can be great, however, particularly for the first products within a class to obtain marketing approval. With some notable recent exceptions, the financial rewards of subsequent "me-too" products often diminish progressively with the timing of their market entry and the number of competitors already on the market. Typically, getting to the market quickly and ahead of the competition is critical. Intelligence and efficiency are the keys to getting there.

While there are many notable exceptions to the "first to market" rule, "second to market" products must possess some notable improvements over the innovator to overcome the leader's position. For "second to market" products, the focus of the development effort should be differentiating, or adding value beyond that of the innovator product, and on reaching the market as quickly as possible (other competitive products will also likely be in the development process). The added value may include benefits such as a more convenient dosing regimen, better safety profile, improved effectiveness, better patient acceptance, among others. Regardless of the competitive environment, however, speed should be the goal in any product's development. The more crowded the market is, the tougher it will be to penetrate, no matter what a product's benefits may be.

The single most critical stage in pharmaceutical development is the clinical testing phase. The purpose of clinical development is to provide the "substantial evidence" of a product's safety and effectiveness in humans, which the FDA requires before it will approve the product for marketing. One measure of a clinical program's success is the speed and efficiency of the subsequent review and approval of the corresponding new drug application (NDA) or biologic license application (BLA). A product's approval is dependent upon the proper, successful implementation of a well-designed product (e.g., dosage form), assays, and nonclinical (formerly referred to as preclinical) and clinical development programs. As such, the entire development process must be designed and implemented with the goal of a successful NDA/BLA submission in mind. While this may seem simple and logical, the amount of time and planning necessary in doing so is extensive.

The major factors in the clinical development process are related to safety, effectiveness, cost, and time. When a product first reaches the clinical development stage, its safety in human populations has only been theorized based on nonclinical testing. Given the unknown safety profile of the investigational compound, the potential benefits to be gained from exposing research subjects to the product must outweigh the risks. If an acceptable benefit-to-risk ratio exists, the demand for efficiency would dictate that the fewest possible subjects be exposed to the experimental product for the minimum length of time necessary to obtain sufficient data to support the drug's safety and effectiveness. Therefore, the development team has a responsibility not only to the subjects, but also to the company to ensure that the clinical data from every trial will significantly expand the knowledge base of the product in a meaningful way and that the trial will meet its predetermined objectives. However, development teams cannot fall into the trap of cutting corners in an attempt to reduce the amount of time and money needed to properly conduct the clinical trials. The price of a hurried submission to please management or investors may well be an unnecessarily extended review and/or the disapproval of the product. Needless to say, there is a delicate balance to be maintained between the various, and sometimes conflicting, goals.

Taking these issues into account, the general interests of all involved must be to conduct the clinical development process in the safest, most efficient, and most economical manner possible. This text will present a general philosophy forged by experience in conducting clinical development programs with these issues in mind.

> "Experience is the hardest kind of teacher. It gives you the test first, and the lesson afterwards."

> —Anonymous

This text's ultimate goal is to assist pharmaceutical developers in conducting safe, efficient, and cost-effective clinical programs that lead to the rapid submission and approval of marketing applications.

Intended Readership This book is designed to provide important information not only for those individuals "in the trenches" of pharmaceutical development, but also to their managers, who must understand the process at least as well. Today, clinical development is undertaken and conducted by more than just employees of traditional pharmaceutical companies, and includes related groups, such as contract research organizations (CROs). Large numbers of products, and in particular many with orphan status, are being developed by small biotech companies and "non-industry" groups, such as activist-oriented health organizations and academic institutions. The motivation driving these two types of groups— industry professionals and those in the "public sector" —are not vastly different, despite public perceptions. Ultimately, both groups want to provide better health care. Regardless of whether profits will go to stockholders, the government, or charitable foundations, these groups must maintain their professional approach given the high stakes and the potential gains to be made in health care.

International Regulations In contrast to clinical research in general, the clinical development process for pharmaceuticals is highly regulated. Given the experimental nature of new products and the lack of safety information, the public must be protected from exposure to potentially dangerous substances. The U.S. Food and Drug Administration (FDA) has been empowered to regulate the development and marketing of new pharmaceuticals. With the public health at stake, the FDA's scientific research standards are both reasonable and universally applicable.

Serious and life-threatening illnesses for which there is a need to develop new therapies as quickly as possible present a particular challenge. The pressing need for new therapeutic alternatives all too often feeds the temptation to cut comers in the process. As a general rule, however, this is not a wise path, and is taken less often by those who are familiar with the consequences. Essentially, the FDA's regulations and guidelines were developed for very sound reasons. While some may view following such regulations and guidelines to the letter as unnecessary in some cases, no one can argue that it does not foster good science.

Title 21 of the Code of Federal Regulations (21 CFR) contains a tremendous amount of information for the clinical developer, as do the numerous guidelines published by both the FDA and the International Conference on Harmonization (ICH). Successfully meeting these regulations and guidelines forms a sound scientific basis for approval, and anyone in the "business" of obtaining approval for new drugs or biologics should incorporate this information into their plan from the very beginning. The importance of periodic compliance checks of company programs against published guidelines and regulations, and early and frequent consultation with the relevant FDA reviewing division, cannot be over-emphasized. This is particularly important when a non-standard approach is attempted or if it has been some time since the FDA reviewed a product within the same therapeutic class. Science marches on. FDA personnel change positions or move on over time. In all cases, the FDA reviewer is the audience that must be convinced that the sponsor did all that was scientifically appropriate and medically required. Developing new products without a clear understanding of what the customer—the FDA reviewer—wants is in most cases a costly and significant mistake.

As is true in any other endeavor, proper planning is paramount. Of particular note are the elements of "adequate and well-controlled" trials for use in support of an application (as described in 21 CFR Part 314.126). These elements are essential to the successful conduct of clinical trials and, as such, have been thoroughly incorporated into the procedures specified in this book. Given the enormous expense of clinical development and the risks to which research subjects are exposed, there is simply no excuse for not conducting a clean, safe trial that has a high likelihood of producing usable results.

Philosophy of This Text The previous discussion about the nature of clinical development provides an appropriate preamble to a discussion about the philosophy of this book: Deciding where you, the sponsor or developer, want and need to be at the end of the process before actually beginning in earnest. The ability to plan for the final product—a successful

NDA/BLA—enables one to focus all of his or her resources on the task at hand, thereby minimizing unnecessary effort. Focus is extremely important, as the example below illustrates.

Consider that you, the developer, wisely decide to incorporate a particular data presentation described in the FDA's *Guideline for the Format and Content of the Clinical and Statistical Sections of an Application* into your NDA/BLA (i.e., an old, but solid, guidance). Such a section might provide the demographics of the study population, an analysis of dose-response characteristics, or a display of adverse events and occurrence rates. Individual scientists working for too many sponsors will present this information differently in the final reports of each for the various clinical trials. Then, when the integrated summaries are being prepared for the NDA/BLA, this information must be painstakingly manipulated in some manner to allow for the desired common presentations. Work that was completed once must be re-addressed unnecessarily.

There is a different, much easier, and less costly way of obtaining standard presentations in this example. At the outset, the sponsor should realize that integrated summaries of safety and effectiveness will be needed for the NDA/BLA (21 CFR 314.50). In addition, the sponsor should know that the FDA will not only review each study in isolation, but will also compare similar information across all studies included in an NDA/BLA. Therefore, it is ideal if the presentations in each clinical trial report follow the same format and include the same general content that will ultimately be presented in the NDA/BLA. In this way, the sponsor will present similar information across all studies in a similar manner, all of which will aid an FDA reviewer in comparing studies and facilitate the integration of data from different studies into the integrated summaries. Programming the various analyses and presentations can be minimized if a serious attempt is made to standardize the data presentations. Along the same lines, if the sponsor has decided that a particular data presentation will be included in the NDA/BLA and that this presentation will be incorporated into the format and content of each study's final report, the case report forms should be designed to capture this information and the protocols should contain the mechanisms to generate these data. The result is a streamlined process through which all information vital to a successful NDA/BLA submission is collected.

The Clinical Development Plan Before a developer immerses himself or herself too deeply into planning and conducting an individual clinical trial, however, it is a good idea to consider all of the different trials that must be conducted to obtain the information necessary for product approval. An effective starting point is a draft of the "ideal" package insert (PI) for the compound in question. Here again, published guidance from the FDA can help in such areas as planning for adequate dose-response information, long-term effectiveness, and age or pharmaceutical interactions. Ultimately, each of the clinical statements in the draft PI must be supported by the data. The statements in the draft PI can then be annotated to the sections/pages of the clinical development plan, and later the NDA/BLA, to identify individual trials that will specifically address each stated claim. While the draft PI's content will undoubtedly change over time to reflect the actual data as they become available, there is comfort in knowing that all information "suggested" by the FDA and identified by the sponsor as part of the marketing profile will be addressed in the planned clinical program.

Anticipating the Data Analysis The planned methods for clinical data analysis should be considered in the early stages of the trial, before the protocol is written. Anyone who has been in the position of having collected the data without first consulting a statistician has heard statements such as, "Well, the design you used does not easily lend itself to analysis," or "If only you had done things this way." Hearing such statements after data collection is simply devastating. The best time to consult with a statistician is during the development of the trial objectives and prior to the point at which a study design is adopted. It is astounding to see the many ways that a knowledgeable statistician can increase a trial's power and decrease the number of subjects (and money) needed through slight alterations in study design. Few people realize, for example, that if the situation permits, a good crossover design can decrease the number of subjects significantly, depending upon intra- versus inter-subject variability, compared to a parallel-group design, given the same power requirements. True, crossover designs are not appropriate in every circumstance, but the point is that an experienced statistician, when consulted at an early stage in the study design process, can significantly improve the chance that the trial objectives will be attained.

While working on study design issues, it is wise to consider the manner in which the data should ultimately be presented in the tables and figures included in an NDA/BLA. Given this information, a statistician can arrange to have the analysis and the anticipated data presentations programmed while the trial is being conducted. The first set of data to arrive from the clinical site can be used to test the programming. In this way, when all of the data are in and the quality of the data is assured, the results of planned analyses will be available much more quickly (sometimes in a few days) than would otherwise be possible. If planned properly, this may account for 95% or more of the total programming effort, pending any unforeseen, last-minute analyses. Again, the emphasis is on efficiency and cost-effectiveness. Senior management in industry is not accustomed to sitting back and patiently waiting for the data. Patients in need of the new therapy should also not have to wait any more than is absolutely necessary. When the data are in, everyone wants the results as soon as possible. There is no reason why the results should not be readily available, particularly since there may be so much riding on the results in terms of resource allocation or future trial designs.

Case Report Forms as a Protocol Template Another important aspect of protocol development is the drafting of a set of case report forms (CRFs). While these data-collection tools have been paper-based traditionally, electronic data capture methods are rapidly gaining favor for a variety of reasons. The philosophy of what and how much data to capture remains the same, however. The exact data to be collected must be established in the planned data presentations (e.g., demography, effectiveness or safety data). Once the necessary data are known, user-friendly CRFs can be drafted with both the data-entry personnel and study-site personnel in mind. The meticulous design of CRFs can reduce data discrepancies, facilitate data entry, and generally streamline the entire data collection and entry process. The draft CRFs should also be used to dictate the content of the protocol's procedures section, rather than the reverse. Drafting the CRFs after the protocol is finished will undoubtedly lead to problems at some point, and may necessitate late changes in the protocol to accommodate oversights. Planning the analyses, identifying the needed data, creating efficient CRFs, and drafting the protocol are best handled in a sequential manner. A graphic presentation of this "reverse engineered" process is presented in the exhibit below.

Clinical Trial Planning and Execution

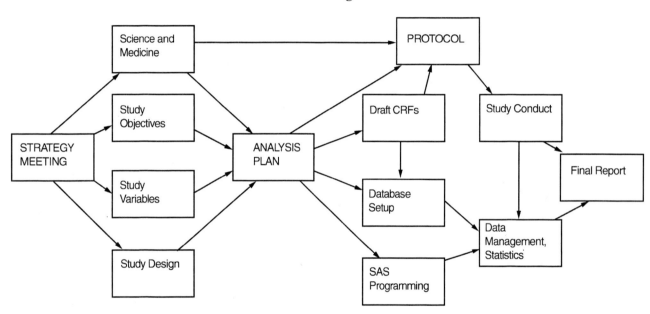

Coordination with Product Development One must not forget that the active entity's development (e.g., manufacturing, characterization and stability of the new drug or biologic) progresses in conjunction with, but just slightly ahead of, clinical trials. Having to repeat clinical trials due to dramatic changes in the dosage form is inexcusable. Activities in each of these disciplines must progress in a fully synchronized fashion as determined by proper advance planning, project management and, most importantly, frequent interdisciplinary communication. Although press releases seem to highlight only the progress of clinical trials, there would be no clinical trials without clinical trial material.

The Forest and the Trees The clinical development process can be analogized to the concept of the forest and the trees. The meticulous pharmaceutical developer must know every tree, but must, at all times, know just exactly where each particular tree and all others fit within the forest. When pharmaceutical development is conducted properly, it can be a smooth, efficient and relatively economical process. When it is not, things can get ugly. Those who regularly attend FDA advisory committee meetings have seen many examples of both situations. Ultimately, proper planning is the key. Execution adds the finishing touches. Planning at the outset, with the end goal constantly in sharp focus, is the most efficient way to ensure clinical success and advance the standard of medical care.

How to Use This Book It should be clear that pharmaceutical development is a delicate process that has many potential pitfalls. The entire clinical process involves a complete cycle of thought from planning the NDA/BLA, planning the report, planning the analysis, designing CRFs, writing the protocol, conducting the trial, writing the report, and finally writing and submitting the NDA/BLA (see exhibit below).

For this reason, this text's chapters appear in a sequence consistent with the recommended progression of thought processes rather than the traditional approach of protocol first, report last. The knowledge of how each element of the clinical development process relates to the successful NDA/BLA submission will maximize the likelihood that the process will be rewarded to the fullest extent possible. This book should be used in the same way. No chapter is to be considered in isolation, but rather in view of the chapters preceding and following it.

As a final note, please remember that, as "there is more than one way to skin a cat," there are many ways to achieve the goals discussed within this book without following the exact format and content of the examples presented. While the examples presented have been shown to work and have resulted in FDA approval, other formats and contents will obviously also work.

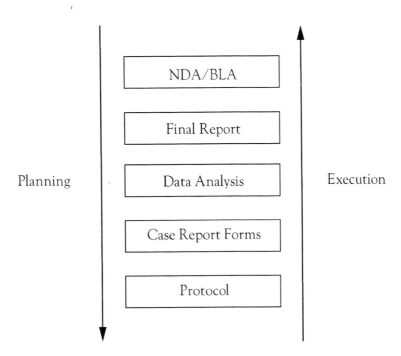

CHAPTER 2

Project Management and Pharmaceutical Development

By Gus Cicala

"Being busy does not always mean real work. The object of all work is production or accomplishment and to either of these ends there must be forethought, system, planning, intelligence, and honest purpose, as well as perspiration. Seeming to do is not doing"

- Thomas Alva Edison

Project management delivers the promise of an on-time, on-budget delivery of a unique deliverable according to specification. The concept was first introduced in the early 1950s by contractors for the U.S. Department of Defense, which found project management practices to be a useful means of accelerating the development of new weapons during the early days of the Cold War.

Why are project management concepts and practices useful to the goal of expediting drug and biologics development? Since project management promises on-time, on-budget delivery, the corollary of this idea implies that, without project management, we should not expect projects to finish on time and on budget. By using project management practices for the development of new drugs, we are following a deliberate approach to predict, manage, and control a budget and schedule. Given that human beings have not mastered the art of accurately predicting the future, most project predictions will be wrong. Even employing project management to assist in predicting the launch dates for new product launches, the best we can do is to improve our predictions. This is especially true for drug and biologics development projects that rely on several unpredictable factors that affect key performance indicators, such as schedule and budget:

- The inability to control patient registration for clinical trials
- The uncertain completion and outcome of the FDA's (and similar regulatory agencies in other countries) review of an NDA or BLA
- The unpredictability of clinical outcomes that can present significant challenges to schedule predictions

Successful project management ensures a more reliable means of successfully launching new compounds into the marketplace—on time, on budget, and within the specifications of the label.

This chapter explores how and why project management concepts and practices are useful in expediting drug and biologics development. Project management is useful to any business application that attempts to build a unique outcome that has never been done exactly the same way before. Examples include a new computer system for tracking customer orders, a 40-story building in the center of town, a new type of laundry detergent, and the development of a new drug. It is not that these things have never been developed before, but more a matter that they typically have not been developed in quite the same way each time.

What is a Methodology?

Let's start with a deeper investigation of methodologies—what they are, and how a project management methodology is used on a typical clinical development project.

A methodology is an integrated, cohesive, well-documented set of repeatable processes that provide for quality deliverables through the consistent execution of practices that have been proven to work. Methodologies are usually developed in organizations that are tired of "reinventing the wheel." Processes that have been successful are documented and shared across the organization. Methodologies often include the following: document templates, such as sample design reports; procedures, such as detailed approaches for producing a data model; forms, such as requests for system enhancements; and work plans, such as Microsoft Project work plan templates.

Expediting Drug and Biologics Development

In summary, a methodology:
- Defines repeatable processes
- Instills quality into service-based processes
- Removes creativity from processes that should not be creative
- Provides a floor-not a ceiling
- Organizes project tasks in the work plan
- Forms the foundation for continuous improvement

How should a Project Manager Use Methodology? Methodology is the project manager's primary means of ensuring quality in a project. It supplies the project manager and the entire project team with a "cookbook" for performing the tasks in the project plan.

While project management is consistent from project to project, methodologies tend to vary. The project manager needs to determine whether the organization has a methodology for the specific type of project to be managed.

Samples of Methodologies Methodologies are used to develop the outputs of a project. Some examples of methodologies include: the construction of a single family home; project management; the development of a new drug; and the management of the process of publication and regulatory submissions to the FDA

The 'Horizontal' versus the 'Vertical' Methodologies Required to Successfully Develop and Deliver a New Drug to Market

Many drug developers view the development of new drug as the embodiment of the scientific processes required to develop that drug. While it is true that these processes are extremely important to the success of the project, they are not project management. The project manager's responsibilities include both the on-time, on-budget delivery of the new product and the delivery of that product within specifications.

The project manager can rely on two distinct and separate process groups to define and manage the drug development effort:
- The "Horizontal" Process: The project management methodology is the overarching set of business controls that the project manager utilizes to define and control project outcomes according to schedule and budget.
- The "Vertical" process: The drug development methodology that defines the steps that need to be followed in order to order to achieve the desired outcomes of the project (i.e., "the label" or claims that the drugmaker will ultimately be required to prove to obtain FDA approval).

The core project management processes, or "horizontal methodology," can be organized into three distinct process groups:

Definition and Planning Processes: This stage of the project management process illustrates the steps that need to be followed before a project starts to ensure that the proper definition and planning steps are completed and to increase the chances that the project will be delivered on time and on budget.

Execution and Control Processes: This stage of the project management process illustrates the steps that need to be followed when the project is underway in order to understand if the project is going according to plan at each stage of the project.

Close-out Processes: This stage of the project management process illustrates the steps that need to be followed when the project is completed in order to ensure that the outputs of the project are properly transitioned to the teams that will be responsible for the life cycle of the product.

The exhibit below provides a sample of the processes that define how a new drug is brought from "concept to market," and details the processes involved in researching and developing a new drug.

The "Vertical" methodology illustrated below is a sample of a generic methodology for drug development. Many of this book's chapters will explore the finer details involved in a drug development methodology.

So how does the project manager combine the vertical and horizontal processes into a successful approach to managing the project? To answer this question, we must take a closer look at each of the three stages of project management.

The Definition and Planning Stage of Project Management

Generate the Project Charter A project charter is a document that is intended to formally define the initial project

The "Vertical Methodology" - Sample Drug Development Processes

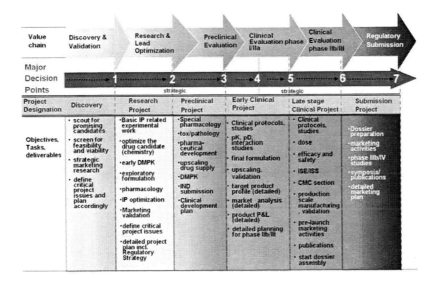

concept in specific terms that make the "scope" of the project clear to all involved. So if we understand the definition of "scope," we are well on our way to understanding what basic elements need to go into a project charter.

Think of project scope as a series of questions about a project with a series of answers to those questions (as can best be developed before a project begins). For a project to achieve an on-time and on-budget completion according to specifications, the elements of scope are defined to direct a project towards a successful outcome. If we anticipate the types of questions that any business will want answered about a project, we can begin to see the major sections that a project charter document should cover:

- "Why"-Answers to the question, "Why are we doing this project?" are typically found in a section called "Goals and Objectives." These goals and objectives should encapsulate the measurable outcomes that will define the success of the project.
- "How"- Answers to the question, "How will we do this project?" are typically found in the section called "Approach." The approach will be based on the "vertical methodology" to be followed in order to produce the project deliverables.
- "What"- Answers to the question, "What are the expected deliverable(s) from this project?" are typically found in the section called Deliverables Guidelines.
- "When"- Answers to the question, "When will the project start and finish?" are typically found in the section called Estimated Schedule, which is usually a summary-level view of the project schedule.
- "How much"- Answers to the question, "What will it cost to perform this project?" are typically found in the section called Estimated Business Investment.
- "What can go wrong"- Answers to the question, "Can anything go wrong to threaten the success of this project?" are typically found in the section called Risk Management.
- "What don't we know"- Answers to the question, "Are there unknowns in this project that need to be addressed?" are typically found in the section called Assumptions.

Targeted Product Information (TPI) Section of the Project Charter In the world of drug development, the project charter is typically referred to as the "Target Product Profile" document, or "Targeted Product Information" document. This section of the project charter document is important because the FDA has specific regulations for drug labeling. The "Target Product Profile," or simply "the label," established the scope or medical "claims" that will ultimately be reviewed and, ideally approved, by the FDA.

The FDA's labeling regulations (21 CFR 201.56 and 201.57) describe the specific regulatory requirements for the content and format of labeling for human prescription drugs, such as:

- Description
- Clinical Pharmacology

- Indications and Usage
- Contraindications
- Warnings
- Precautions
- Adverse Reactions
- Drug Abuse and Dependence
- Overdosage
- Dosage and Administration
- How Supplied
- Animal Pharmacology and/or Animal Toxicology (if necessary)
- Clinical Studies/References (if necessary)

The TPI should be treated as a supplement to the other sections of the project charter that are covered above. The TPI is not a substitute for this other, pertinent project scoping information, however (see chapter on TPI elsewhere in this text).

Plan and Organize the Project A good way to look at project planning is to view this process as a series of connected logical questions that can be used to develop the initial project schedule and budget.

- Review "What" is to be built - The project deliverables (or TPI) in the project charter should provide a clear roadmap of the outputs of the project. It is these outputs that ultimately will drive the "vertical methodology" that should be used to develop the tasks that are necessssary to perform the project and build the deliverables.
- Define what actions need to happen to build the deliverables: The Work Breakdown Structure (WBS) is a logical grouping of high-level tasks, activity groups, detailed tasks, tasks, and sub-tasks that define the overall approach to completing the project.

Many methodologies are accompanied by suggested work plans that have been built based upon the WBS used on previous successful projects employing the work plan. These work plan templates are a valuable source of information that the project manager can use in building an initial project work plan.

A word of caution: The work plan templates that accompany methodologies can sometimes contain hundreds, or even thousands, of pre-defined tasks. It is important that you validate these work plan templates since it is tempting to think that a plan that incorporates that level of detail must be right.

Since every project is unique, it is important that the project manager involve the project team early in determining which tasks are right for your particular project. These details are best worked out in a facilitated session with the key project team members who have the requisite knowledge to ensure that the right WBS is built to start the project.

In addition to the WBS from previous projects, the body of FDA regulations provides significant guidance regarding what needs to happen for a new drug to be successfully launched in the United States.

Once the basic tasks of the "vertical methodology" are added (drug development activities), the plan is completed by adding "horizontal methodology," the project management activities, and any key milestones that will be used to report on the highest visability events that are of interest to the stakeholders. These milestones will be the key to simplifying management reporting (see section on communications management below).

- Decide "who" will staff the project: Once the WBS is defined, it is possible to develop a resource assignment plan based upon the skills that are needed to perform the tasks.

In many organizations, the project manager does not have the authority to specify the exact persons that will be necessary to perform the work. The initial work plan may contain generic skill types, such as "clinical data analyst" or "medical writer," to which the manager will assign specific individuals in each of the skill centers.

- Estimate "how long"—Work estimates

Before you start estimating the labor for each task in the plan, the next step is to decide if the WBS contains sufficient detail (or too little detail). How do you know? A plan with three phases that each contains 1,000 hours is not sufficient detail. However, if you loaded every step in a procedure into your work plan, that would probably be too much detail (e.g. a plan that contains 3,000 tasks, each one hour of effort).

So what is the difference between a methodology procedure step and a task? Tasks are estimated, scheduled, and have resources assigned. You wouldn't want to go through all that effort for a procedure step. It's simply not worth it. What we need are some estimating rules of thumb for determining the right amount of detail. The "Rule of 80" is one way to test whether the WBS contains enough detail. In the book *Productivity Management*, Donald Plummer states the Rule of 80 as follows, "The 80-hour rule stipulates that you break a project into tasks of 80 hours or less, each of which must result in a tangible product or deliverable."

- Decide "in which order"- To get an idea of the overall project schedule, it is vitally important to have a grasp of the order in which tasks must be performed. For example, a clinical study must be designed before a study can start.

Once the WBS is defined and the tasks have been sequenced, it is possible to depict the initial project schedule in what is known as a "Gant Chart," which provides a visual representation of the tasks, how they are scheduled and how they depend upon one another. Most project management tools will provide a view that contains this visual representation of project schedule information.

Sample Gantt from Microsoft Project

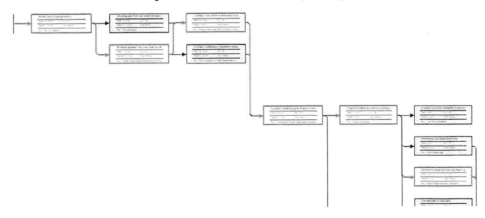

Something called the "Network Activity Diagram" can also be drawn at this point in the project planning process. This diagram is a means of visually depicting the sequence of events that results from defining the WBS, and then assigning successor/predecessor relationships between the tasks in the WBS.

Sample Network Activity Diagram

The network activity diagram is the foundation for determining how long the project will take from start to finish, known as "the critical path."

Just as the longest pole in the tent defines the overall height of the tent, the critical path is the longest path through the network based upon task duration, which defines the shortest amount of time in which the project can be completed

This technique for determining how long a project will take is also referred to as the "Critical Path Method," or CPM. The technique is sometimes coupled with a technique called PERT (Program Evaluation, and Review Technique), a project management planning process in which the probable schedule is evaluated based on three scenarios—a best-case, expected-case, and worst-case scenario. The most probable schedule may be stated in terms of scenarios that are designed to determine the duration of a task, its start date, or its finish date.

- Is the project schedule realistic? To build a project that will meet its stated objectives, it is important to ensure that the resources required to staff the project are available during the time frames in which their tasks will be scheduled. This exercise is often referred to as "load-leveling." The process requires that the labor demands stated in the project plan can be staffed from the limited resource capacity of the organization. This exercise often requires that a project plan be considered in light of all other projects that are placing demands upon a common pool of shared resources.

A project plan that does not consider the availability of the resources required to perform the project is a project plan that is destined to miss its deadline.

- How much will the project cost?—Once the project is scheduled and the resources necessary to perform the work are known, it is possible to derive a time-phased project budget, primarily based on the cost of internal resources, external resources, and material resources.

Scope, Quality, Risk and Communication Management Plans In addition to the basic project schedule and budget, it is important that the project manager develop specific written plans for how scope will be managed, how risk will be managed, how quality will be assured, and how and when communications will be disseminated.

The Execution and Control Stage of Project Management

Once the project charter is completed and the project plans are developed, the project typically is ready to begin. Most projects begin with a project kick-off meeting to introduce key players, review the project charter, and communicate the project plans.

Once the project starts, the project manager's primary responsibility is to establish and maintain control of the project. While the attributes of an effective project manager are addressed below, let's first look at what it means to be in control.

Project control means that the project manager is actively spending time managing the project using the project plan. As a result, the project manager knows where the overall project stands during the project's execution. A project manager who is actively managing the plan will always know where he/she stands in relation to the original approved project plan.

Track Status Before the project manager starts to track progress, it is important that there be a snapshot of the original project plan. This concept is often referred to as "the baseline." The baseline is captured so that the project manager has a stake in the ground by which to measure progress as the project begins. It is one of the final steps before the project starts. The baseline is the foundation for reporting the "plan vs. actual," which is so fundamental in gauging whether a project is on course.

Tracking project progress is often referred to as "collecting actuals." As the name implies, it is simply the process of gathering progress information from all project resources on a regular basis. Tracking progress presents the project manager with the first step towards validating the estimated work effort for the planned tasks. As a result, the project manager has a vehicle for continuing to keep accountability to the plan with the entire team. If the team members know that you intend to measure their progress against their estimates, the entire team will share a commitment to the estimates.

In cultural terms, many organizations are not prepared for the requirements posed by the project manager who wants to track progress on a regular basis. Since the project manager is often not the personnel manager for all of the resources, resistance to the idea of tracking may present a problem. The project manager needs to consider how realistic it is to institute a tracking process in an organization that is not ready for it.

Perform Risk Management A risk is any potential threat to the overall success of the project. The subject of risk is first addressed during the definition process, since this stage of the project presents an opportunity for deciding how threats to success will be dealt with.

What can you do about risk? The approach to dealing with risk is generally broken down into five major processes:
- Identifying risk
- Assigning probability factors
- Determining the impact
- Selecting unacceptable Risks
- Development of contingency plans.

Methodologies help the risk manager by providing the project manager with a checklist to help assess risk.

Conduct Variance and Root Cause Analysis Once a project manager collects the facts necessary to determine a project's actual progress, he/she must then compare the original plan to current progress to see if any variances to plan are occurring. Variance analysis is the process of identifying and understanding differences between current progress against the initial baseline estimates for a project work plan. Obviously, variance analysis is an important aspect of project control because it highlights potential and/or developing trouble spots in a work plan.

One of the overriding questions that variance analysis addresses is whether the project can still be completed on schedule. Among the key indicators in determining this is the total remaining work for the entire project.

Questions that variance analysis should be able to answer including the following:
- Can the remaining work be completed by the end date?
- Do estimates need to be adjusted based on current variance trends?
- Are resources arriving as scheduled?
- Are schedule bottlenecks preventing tasks from starting and completing as planned?
- Which tasks or resources require additional attention to get back on course?

In reality, project managers should expect variances and be prepared to explain both the causes of those variances and the actions required to get the project back on course. The project variances form the foundation of the measurable key performance indicators that are typically reported in the project status report.

Before the project manager can revise the plan, there are often project stakeholders who must approve the revised strategy. In such situations, a project manager is often forced to make trade-offs:
- A cheaper resource can help the project remain within budget, but the work estimates may increase due to the less costly resource's lack of experience.
- A scope reduction may help, but that probably means sacrificing some of the objectives to stay within schedule and budget.
- Adding lead (overlapping tasks) increases the risk of missing the schedule.

The unfortunate reality is that serious oversights in the project charter, or plan, can significantly reduce the chances of completing the plan according to all of its original expectations, and sometimes leads to a project's cancellation.

Control and Manage Scope Effective scope management makes two important assumptions:
1. The project manager has clearly defined the project scope. A sound approach to change control highlights the importance of the Project Charter document, specifically how it defines project completion criteria.
2. Strict scope management also requires adherence to the deliverables acceptance procedure. Change requestors must also be willing to acknowledge that their request is out of scope.

Even when these two assumptions are valid, scope management requires a tenacious approach on the part of the project manager. Project managers sometimes become overly concerned with client satisfaction when they are asked to make "free" scope changes. To prevent this from happening, a scope change control procedure should be developed as part of the initial project plan and should be communicated during the project kick-off.

Manage Communications Project communications comprise a key component of the project manager's role. The constant setting, re-setting, and managing of expectations is critical for both the project team members as well as the project stakeholders.

The initial project communications plan should define the types of communications and the frequency of those communications. The project status report is a regular project management deliverable and, as such, its structure should be communicated and outlined in the initial project communications plan.

Besides the regular "push" of project communications, there are many tools on the market today that can assist the project manager in publishing information to a central database to make information available "on demand" from web-based applications.

For example, drug development projects can be grouped by therapeutic area to show a summary of all clinical trials within each therapeutic area.

Summary of Projects by Therapeutic Area

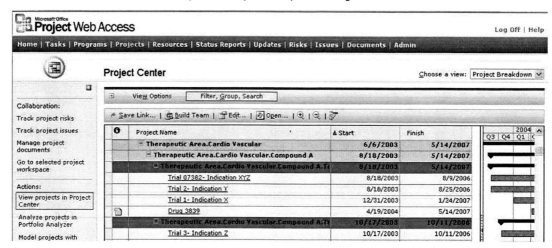

Project information can also be summarized to show how key skill areas are being demanded across the organization. By summarizing all project plans against a central resource pool, it is possible to develop a roll-up of resource skill areas into a resource breakdown structure (RBS).

Summary of Resource Demands by RBS

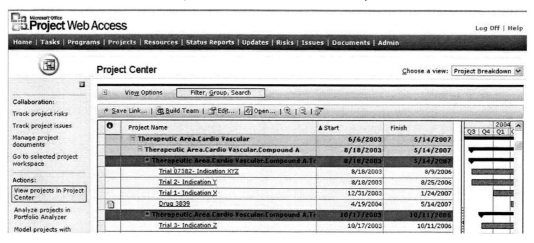

The preceding summary views provide a brief overview of what is possible with EPM technology.

The Close-out Stage of Project Management

Complete Project Transition Once all scheduled tasks in the project are completed and the product is approved, the project manager should perform an orderly close-out of the project. Close-out activities should actually be the final tasks in the project plan and may include activities such as archiving project documents, collecting final project key performance indicators, developing a final status report(s), conducting a final steering committee meeting, and transitioning product information to the commercial organization (sales, marketing, manufacturing).

Ensure Continuous Improvement To ensure that the organization learns from mistakes and builds on now-tested ideas and methods, it is a good idea to capture close-out information. This occurs most commonly via a lessons learned check list, which is a brief walk-through of the project management process.

A Sample Project Management Methodology

For an organization to standardize its approach to project management, it is a good idea to have a roadmap of what a project manager will need in undertaking all of the necessary steps to manage a project. The following exhibit shows an example of project management "horizontal methodology" that is commercially available for purchase on an "off the shelf" basis and that can then be modified to an organization's needs.

Sample Components of a Project Management Methodology

Stage	Document	No.	Class	Audience	Signoff By
Initiation	Handover form	32	C2	Deliverer manager	None
	Project binder	51	C1	PM	None
	Classification worksheet	53	C1	PM, deliverer manager	None, but reviewed by deliverer manager
	Scope definition checklist	54	C1	PM, customer approver, CPM, deliverer manager	None
	Project charter	01	C2	Customer approver, CPM, deliverer manager	PM, customer approver, deliverer manager
	Satisfaction criteria	04	Policy	PM, customer approver, deliverer manager	PM, customer approver
Planning	Work breakdown structure	07	C1	PM	None
	Activity definition	10	C5	PM, executing team member	None directly. Approval with Proj. Plan
	Assumptions checklist	03	C2	PM	None directly. Approval with Proj. Plan
	Constraints checklist	02	C2	PM	None directly. Approval with Proj. Plan
	Cost estimate worksheet	12	C2	PM, deliverer manager	PM, deliverer manager
	Cost management plan	13	C4	PM, deliverer manager, customer approver (T&M)	PM, deliverer manager, customer approver (T&M)
	Schedule management plan	11	C4	PM, customer approver, CPM, deliverer manager	PM, customer approver, deliverer manager
	Staffing requirements form	56	C2	Deliverer manager	None
	Scope management plan	05	C3	Customer approver, deliverer manager	PM, customer approver, deliverer manager
	Risk assessment checklist	16	C1	PM, deliverer manager	None directly. Approval with Proj. Plan
	Risk management plan	17	C4	PM, customer approver, deliverer manager	PM, customer approver, deliverer manager
	Communications management plan	15	C5	PM, CPM, team members	PM, customer approver
	Quality management plan	55	C4	PM, CPM, project team	PM, customer approver, deliverer manager
	Project plan	14	C1	PM, deliverer manager, customer approver, CPM	PM, deliverer manager, customer approver
Execution	Time sheet	24	Policy	PM	None
	Corrective actions checklist	23	C1	PM, team members	None
	Scope change request form	19	C1	Customer approver, PM	Customer approver
	Deliverable review form	52	C3	PM, team members	Team members
	Formal acceptance signoff form	21	C2	Customer approver, PM. (Deliverer mgr.→project)	Customer approver, PM
	Status report	25	C1	Customer approver, CPM, deliverer manager	None

Attributes of the Successful Project Manager

In addition to having a methodology, project charter, and the other concepts and tools discussed above, it is equally important for a company to staff project management positions with the types of people that are that can successfully manage a project. Since project management is really the process of managing a series of business controls, the skills required to ensure the success of these business controls is really quite broad. The project manager that has an appropriate balance of the attributes discussed below has really attained a set of skills that are of great value within an organization and that have significant applicability to many other parts of a business organization.

The Take Charge Attitude Many organizations do not have a project management process that is so clearly defined that a project manager knows exactly what he or she is and is not supposed to do after being appointed as a project manager. We have all heard the phrase, "it's easier to ask for forgiveness than it is to ask for permission." Many project managers find that this attitude is necessary to establish their leadership on a project.

Ability to Make Effective Trade-offs To achieve the expected project outcomes, the project manager is often faced with the realization that things are not always going to go according to plan. In a real-world project, the most common trade-offs are often referred to as the "Iron Triangle"—scope, schedule and resource.

Comfortable Operating in the "Gray area" Given the uncertainty that is project management, the project manager is often faced with problems that may not have been encountered before, may not have been anticipated, and may not have clear cut solutions. These situations are often compounded by lines of authority that may not be clear, organizational policies that do not support an expeditious resolution, and stakeholders that expect these problems to go away quickly. Often, the alternatives are not black and white. Therefore, an ability to operate in the gray area is critical.

Not Afraid to Be the Lone Dissenter and Point Out Unpopular Risk Project management can be lonely. The project manager knows all too well that the project team members and stakeholders may not understand how project management is supposed to work. Since project management occurs in a world of uncertainty, things do not always go according to plan and there is almost always a risk of failure.

All too often, the project manager is the bearer of bad news that is always unwelcome. It can be tempting to downplay or avoid delivering bad news, and if often takes courage to deliver the facts as they are. It also takes time to investigate alternatives and present options for mitigating the unpleasant implications of bad news.

Communicate Effectively, with an Understanding of the Biases of the Audience Because many project managers have "Type A" personalities, communications are too often thought of as the transmission of information. While it is important that a project manager effectively transmit the project's key performance indicators on a regular basis, it is equally important that the right information be transmitted. This information can only be learned by turning off the transmitter long enough to receive the information required to build effective project communications.

There are three keys to effective communication: listen, listen, and listen. People will tell you what they need if you take the time to hear what they are trying to say. Poor listening skills often are the symptom of people being so focused on their own agenda that they do not listen long enough to hear what others are trying to say.

People-oriented Interpersonal Skills The effective project manager understands that successful project outcomes depend on the individual actions of the people on the team and those who support and manage the team. A project manager who instills the team with a "two heads are better than one" attitude generally will be more successful than one who espouses a "there are two ways to do it: my way or the wrong way" approach. Necessary people skills include the concept of fairness, openness, effective conflict resolution, respect, honesty, coaching and team support.

Commitment to Quality The project manager is responsible for the project's success. It is the project manager's commitment to quality that will drive the team to deliver what is expected. Since it is the "vertical" methodology that describes how the project will produce a quality outcome, it is the project manager who must ensure that the processes are followed and that each task in the project is completed by following the correct approach.

Ability to Think Analytically Project managers are frequently faced with unanticipated changes—schedules change, market conditions change, team members change jobs, commitments to funding change, and pipeline priorities change. Responding to change requires solid problem-solving skills that are based on an ability to think analytically.

To think analytically, one must have a solid grasp of the details and not take things for granted. Before a problem can be solved, the root cause must be understood. Analysis of the available information leads to knowledge. An understanding of that knowledge is gained by applying good judgment. Generating reasonable alternatives requires an understanding of the current situation so that the choice of possible actions is built upon a good prediction of likely outcomes.

A repeatable and measured approach to problem-solving will lead to a rich set of alternatives that leads to the selection of the best options.

References

1) Effective Project Management: How to Plan, Manage, and Deliver Projects on Time and Within Budget. Robert K. Wysocki, Robert Beck, David B. Crane. Publisher: John Wiley & Sons. 1995.

2) Strategic Planning for Project Management Using a Project Management Maturity Model Harold Kerzner. Publisher: John Wiley & Sons. 2001.

3) Pharmaceutical Project Management. Tony Kennedy. Publisher: Marcel Dekker. 1997.

4) Total Project Management: Strategies and Tactics for the Healthcare Industries. Roger Dabbah. Publisher: Interpharm Press. 1993.

5) National Committee for Clinical Laboratory Standards. Methods for Dilution Antimicrobial Susceptibility Tests for Bacteria that Grow Aerobically - 4th Edition; Approved Standard NCCLS Document M7-A4, Vol 17, No. 2, NCCLS, Wayne, PA, January, 1997.

6) National Committee for Clinical Laboratory Standards. Methods for Antimicrobial Susceptibility Testing of Anaerobic Bacteria - 3rd Edition; Approved Standard NCCLS Document M11-A4, vol 17, No. 22, NCCLS, Wayne, PA, December 1997.

7) National Committee for Clinical Laboratory Standards. Performance Standards for Antimicrobial Disk Susceptibility Tests - Sixth Edition; Approved Standard NCCLS Document M2-A6, vol 17, No. 1, NCCLS, Wayne, PA, January, 1997.

Endnotes

(i) From "Project Management using Microsoft Project 2003", (c)2003 Project Assistants, Inc.

(ii) From "PMG Overview and Implementation Manual" (c)2004. Westwind Consulting

CHAPTER 3

The Integration of CMC into Drug Development: Avoiding the Common Delays

By David Bernstein, Ph. D.

Chemistry, manufacturing and controls (CMC) activities include the active pharmaceutical ingredient's (API) synthesis, pre-formulation and formulation development, analytical methods development, and the preparation of the clinical trial material (CTM) to be used in clinical trials (frequently referred to as the study drug or test article, and as investigational medicinal product in the EU). Typically, CMC activities are focused on providing investigational new drugs for clinical use, although in some cases the technical activities can be used to define toxicological formulations as well. CMC activities are predominantly sequential since the API is necessary to begin formulation development, analytical tools are necessary since they are the criteria for selecting formulations for further study, and viable and stable experimental formulations must be developed and evaluated prior to actual CTM manufacturing. Most pre-formulation studies designed to characterize the chemical, physical and mechanical properties of an API should be conducted in parallel. However, some pre-formulation studies are best conducted sequentially, since the data from one study can fine-tune the specific investigations that follow. The final, and most visible, activity in the overall sequence is the preparation (manufacturing, packaging, labeling, testing and releasing) of CTM.

Most readers probably are familiar with any number of anecdotal examples of development projects that have had delays due to CMC issues. Some of these delays are due to scientific and technical problems encountered during early CMC development. These problems have various root causes, including poor and inadequate planning, insufficient communication, false starts, errors in judgment, and attempts to shortcut CMC activities by circumventing key pre-formulation or formulation studies. These issues are exacerbated when unrealistically short timelines are designed by those who are not responsible for actually conducting the necessary CMC activities.

Time constraints in delivering a new product to the clinic are endemic in the pharmaceutical and biotech industry. Financial constraints are endemic to the smaller, emerging companies who may not have any products on the market. Many of the newer and smaller companies are naïve to FDA requirements or good scientific approaches to early CMC development. When any (or sometimes all) of these factors guide CMC development, experience has shown that problems will arise. Many of these issues result in delays in drug development programs. Most of these issues, however, can be identified, anticipated, and avoided. All of the common reasons for delays can be avoided or minimized by simply applying time-honored and good scientific practices into R&D efforts. Adopting philosophies attributed to other industries (e.g., "Just Do It" [Nike] and "Do It Right the First Time" [TQM, total quality management]) are the keys to success). The adaptation of such philosophies within the pharmaceutical industry will involve the following key concepts in CMC activities:

- Have a CMC development plan
- Never allow the API to be rate limiting
- Learn where the CMC minefields are located
- Know your compound
- Know your dosage form
- The IND CMC section is just the tip of the iceberg
- Plan for Success
- Adopt Smart Development Practices

The CMC Development Plan The CMC development plan defines the interdisciplinary approach to be used for API synthesis, pre-formulation, formulation development, analytical methods development, and the preparation of the CTM.

Expediting Drug and Biologics Development

As can be appreciated, these disciplines are inter-related, and some activities depend on completion of activities in another area. The general approach is similar for any therapeutic area, and is specific to the API synthesis technique (e.g., small molecule synthesis, fermentation or genetic engineered materials), the dosage form, and delivery system (oral solid, IV or topical). The development plan's creation should begin when a compound is elevated to clinical candidate status. At that time, little is known about the API's physical or chemical properties that will impact drug product performance, although visionary organizations will have selected the compound based on multi-disciplinary criteria optimization, including pharmaceutics characteristics that will not inhibit "developability." Therefore, few specifics will chart the course.

For example, the aqueous solution stability of a parenteral drug candidate is not known. Therefore, we cannot predict if the investigational drug product will be a ready-made solution or a lyophilized dosage form that will require reconstitution by a pharmacist at the clinical site. The CMC development plan should briefly outline the path for either option: (1) if the pre-formulation studies indicate that the API is both soluble over the biologically relevant pH range and stable in typical injectable vehicles (e.g., water for injection, saline solution), a solution dosage form will be prepared; or (2) if not, the focus will be on a lyophilized dosage form.

Since a lyophilized dosage form involves additional excipients (a cryoprotectant and bulking agents are needed for the freeze drying process) and a more elaborate manufacturing process (several steps each requiring the identification of critical process parameters), projected timelines will need to reflect the increased complexity of this dosage form. A similar scenario is often encountered in solid dosage forms: the simplest approach for rapid entry into the clinic may appear to be a powder in a bottle, or a powder in a capsule. The former requires favorable solubility and inconsequential taste characteristics that can be avoided by the latter. However, if the API does not wet, it will not dissolve in the gastrointestinal tract if it is contained in an unformulated capsule. It should be obvious that the determination of the key physical and chemical characteristics is a prerequisite to the formulation approach. If the dose is very small (e.g., 1 to 5 mg), a granulation manufacturing process may be necessary to ensure homogeneity in processing and dosing. Granulation, like lyophilization, involves more process parameters and additional studies to define the appropriate process parameters even for the first Phase 1 CTM.

The CMC development plan outlines the parallel and sequential activities that are conducted within the CMC departments or external contractors. For example, early stage, small-scale synthesis of the API is necessary to "fuel" the development of analytical techniques ("tools") and for the first evaluation of pre-formulation characteristics. Subsequently, larger amounts of API will be needed for formulation development, and perhaps toxicology studies. "Pre-formulation" means prior to formulation. During pre-formulation, the API's physical, chemical, mechanical and microbiological characteristics are evaluated to identify the properties that often can suggest where problems will be encountered. Some view pre-formulation as an exercise to identify the properties that can facilitate prototype formulation development; others view it as problem-avoidance. With either viewpoint, an intelligent pre-formulation program facilitates formulation development.

Typically, several small-scale formulation variations are developed and placed in a screening stability program. After sufficient data have been obtained (usually two to five data points and over one to three months), one formulation and manufacturing process is selected for clinical manufacturing (and a second is identified as a backup). During this same timeframe, the clinical protocol requirements that impact CMC are elucidated so that the appropriate packaging configurations and labeling text can be likewise identified, sourced and prepared under current good manufacturing practices (cGMP) standards. The entire clinical supply chain ends with a quality assurance (QA) review of all documentation, the submission of the CMC section of the investigational new drug application (IND), a formal CTM release, and the establishment of procedures for the shipping and distribution of the test article to clinical sites. The entire process is depicted in the exhibit below.

The CMC development plan also takes into account the requirements of its ultimate customers. The primary customers of API production are toxicology, analytical R&D, and formulation development. The primary customer of formulation development is CTM manufacturing and eventually the clinical/medical team and ultimately the subject or patient. As the CMC development plan is being created, the specifications and complexities of the clinical program and the CTM that will "fuel" clinical research are not yet known. Likewise, the complexity of the clinical supply operation and the resulting time and financial costs are not yet known and cannot be predicted. However, the general process, communication pathways, and the general approach can be defined with reasonable accuracy by those having substantial experience in these areas.

Never Allow API or CTM to be Rate Limiting (or Always Make More) Cars, airplanes and pharmaceutical development run on fuel. Gasoline for automobiles is plentiful, and gas stations are conveniently located, cars are equipped with gas gauges and warning lights. In the worst-case scenario (i.e., you inadvertently run out of gas), there is

Inter-Relationships Among CMC Activities Enabling An IND

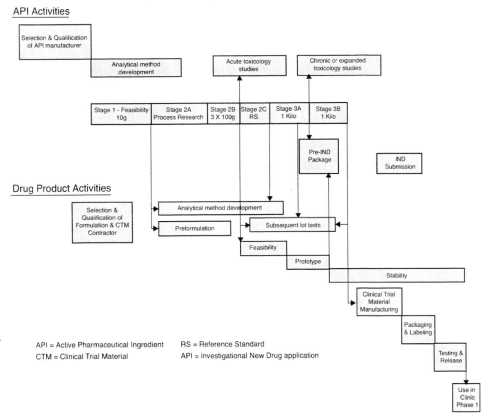

always AAA. Federal Aviation Administration (FAA) rules require a pilot to carry a quantity of fuel that will keep a plane airborne for at least 45 minutes longer than the projected flight time. Since aviation fuel weighs about six pounds per gallon and the weight of the fuel contributes to the costs to fly a plane, there is a balance between flying with a full tank (i.e., a "heavy" aircraft) and a minimal amount. In contrast to the car analogy, however, running out of fuel while airborne can be catastrophic.

The "fuel" in pharmaceutical development is the API and CTM. As shown in the exhibit above, early API synthesis begins with gram scale amounts, and proceeds in well-defined stages to larger and larger amounts. The increase in batch size is usually dependent on equipment availability, the percentage yield of the process, what is known about the efficiency of the process, and the projected needs (grams or kilograms) for the toxicology and CMC programs. Early in development, toxicology requirements usually are predominate, especially for IND-enabling toxicology studies. Toxicology study requirements are calculated using a mathematical multiple of factors, such as the number of days involved, the number of doses per day, the number of animals to be used, and the dose escalation amounts in mg/kg. If there are modifications to any of these factors (as would be the case if the FDA wanted additional numbers of animals), additional amounts of API would be required.

Take, for example, a hypothetical toxicology study involving a dose escalation from 0.25 mg/kg to 32 mg/kg in a geometric progression (0.25, 0.5, 1, 2, 4, 16 and 32). If the highest dose does not exhibit dose-limiting toxicology, a higher dose of 64 mg/kg will be proposed. Obviously, the 64 mg/kg dose essentially requires a doubling of the total amount of API required to conduct the entire study.

The "always make more" principle is also applicable to the drug product program. If the API is limited in early development, fewer prototypes can be developed and studied. Or smaller batches will have to do. The latter restriction cannot address any scale-up concerns; the former restriction limits your choices and chances for success.

CTM (both manufacturing and packaging) is usually designed to meet the requirements of a specific clinical protocol. If the clinical protocol is changed once the cascade of CMC activities leading to the CTM begins, it is very possible, and quite probable, that insufficient clinical supplies would be available. Assume, for example, that a preliminary estimate indicates that 100 patients in both an active and placebo group will be needed to demonstrate that the validity of a clinical hypothesis, and that the CMC team plans to respond to that CTM requirement. Subsequently, additional information suggests that 100 patients per regimen will be insufficient to power the study, but that 150 patients per group will be acceptable. Obviously, if CTM is limited at this point, another batch might have to be prepared. In many cases, there may not be adequate API to immediately make another batch. "Always make more" is a philosophy not unlike an insurance policy. You hope you won't need it, but you know know it's there in case you do.

Learn Where the Minefields Are CMC drug development is strewn with minefields. These include physical and chemical characteristics that limit solubility, that negatively influence stability, that promote crystalline changes in the molecule, or that interact with excipients, to name just a few. Minefields are also present when physical characteristics of the API change as a result of scale-up and render some or all of the early formulation work obsolete. Minefields occur when scale-up of the API results in a new or higher level of impurities than what was tested in toxicology studies. Minefields arise when unanticipated changes occur to the API or drug product as the result of storage, temperature changes, or time.

Two illustrations may provide relevant examples here. In the exhibit above, API stage 2A "process research" is intended to define acceptable process parameters for the manufacture of the API. Manufacturing of the API occurs in distinct steps, beginning with starting materials and proceeding through a number of sequential chemical reactions and ending with the isolation of the API, purification and final processing (e.g., drying or milling). Process research involves numerous small-scale experiments designed to determine a rough range of process parameters (e.g., reaction times, temperatures, pressures, molar equivalents, purification solvents, drying times and temperatures) for each reaction step. Many of these parameters will not be critical—that is, the parameters will not impact the quality of the end product. However, several parameters will be critical and will impact the ability of the entire sequence of chemical changes to result in the desired end product. In this way, we define an envelope of acceptable process parameters that can yield an acceptable product. It is important to note that this is not a process optimization exercise; it is a systematic exploration into what works and what does not. A reaction temperature that is too low may not allow the chemical reaction to proceed smoothly or rapidly; too high a temperature may result in high amounts of impurities. At the early stages of development, all that is needed is a workable range. Usually, a DOE (design of experiment) approach allows multiple parameters to be studied concurrently so that a change's effect in one input parameter can be linked to the overall effect of an output characteristic, such as an impurity profile.

On the drug product side, formulation development is fraught with its own minefields. These depend on the dosage form and delivery system and represent potential manufacturing issues. Most pharmaceutical professionals have learned (some theoretically, some the hard way) that pre-formulation work can identify the large majority of problem areas. This systematic screening of an APE's characteristics is discussed in detail in the section below.

Know Your Compound Given the pharmaceutical industry's history of formulation problems, wouldn't it be nice to have a predictive tool that could identify the potential and real formulation challenges in advance? The branch of pharmaceutics and the discipline of pre-formulation are as close as we have come to developing the ideal tool.

The pharmaceutics studies that should be undertaken for APIs should provide the following elements:

- pH-solubility profile across the biologically relevant pH range
- pH-stability in solution
- particle size determination
- micromeritics (flow properties, density, compressibility)
- thermal analysis by differential scanning calorimetry (DSC)
- permeability assessment by octanol/water partition coefficient and log P
- particulate dissolution
- drug excipient compatibility
- UV spectrum for assay method development
- microscopy
- solubility enhancement by use of surfactants or particle size reduction
- solid state stability
- hygroscopicity
- water content (potentiometric titration, loss on drying and thermo-gravimetric analysis (TGA)
- solid state and solution photostability
- intrinsic dissolution
- surface area
- polymorphism
- sensitivity to oxygen

This list is not exhaustive and, as the discussions below indicate, some tests may not have equal applicability for all dosage forms.

The pH-solubility profile has applicability in both oral solid dosage forms and injectable dosage forms, but for different reasons. In an oral dosage form, bioavailability is a function of the sequential processes of disintegration, dissolution, absorption and distribution. The solubility of the API in the gastrointestinal (GI) tract, coupled with the knowledge of the absorption window (where the drug is absorbed), will permit an evaluation of whether or not the drug should be administered on an empty stomach (where the pH is 4-6) or with a meal (where the pH of the stomach is 1-2). For an intravenous (IV) solution dosage form, knowledge of where on the pH scale the API is soluble (and stable) permits the selection of the appropriate buffer ingredients and quantities. This knowledge also provides early warnings of possible bio-pharmaceutical problems resulting from solubility. For example, if the API is only soluble (and stable) below pH 3, a formulation can be designed to keep the IV solution at pH 3, although the implications and outcome when the solution is injected into a vein (where the microenvironment of the blood is at pH 7) should be determined.

Unfortunately, there is no way to determine what the minefields are for any specific compound in advance. Conducting all the prudent studies to identify and locate these minefields is the best insurance policy there is.

Know Your Dosage Form The science, technology and regulatory requirements for most dosage forms are well known. Each dosage form has its own unique degree of difficulty that should be considered early in development. Some of the issues for several common dosage forms are depicted in the exhibit below.

Degree of Difficulty of Pharmaceutical Dosage Forms

(degree of difficulty in ascending order)

Dosage Form	Comments and challenges
oral solution	API must be soluble and stable; taste; microbial concerns
IV solution	API must be soluble and stable; sterility and pyrogenicity; oxygen and light sensitivity; filter compatibility; aseptic processing
IV lyophilized	API, cryoprotectants and fillers must be compatible; lyophilization cycle needs to be evaluated
oral immediate release solid	knowledge of API characteristics that impact drug product performance; in vitro availability (dissolution method and specification; homogeneity
oral sustained-release solid	controls and consistency of release mechanism; multi-point dissolution methodology
topical cream or transdermal patch	drug release from the vehicle; homogeneity
Nasal solution spray	container-closure integral to drug product efficacy; device performance tests; many additional unique control tests; difficulty making formulation, process or container changes after phase 1
MDI (metered dose inhaler, containing a solution for inhalation)	same as nasal spray; strict control of particle size

---

The IND CMC Section is Just the Tip of the Iceberg The FDA has emphasized that the US Pharmacopeia's (USP) standards and drug monographs represent the minimum standards for the control of drug substances and drug products. The scope of cGMP in Title 21-Code of Federal Regulations, Part 211.1 (21 CFR 211.1) states that, "The regulations in this part contain the minimum current good manufacturing practices for preparation of drug products for administration to humans or animals." In 21 CFR 312.23, the FDA uses less than a single page to identify and describe the information to be included in the IND's CMC section. Further, the FDA's November 1995 *Guidance for Industry: Content and Format of Investigational New Drug Applications (INDs) for Phase 1 Studies of Drugs, Including Well-Characterized, Therapeutic Biotechnology-Derived Drugs* indicates that summaries of the CMC information are preferable to full reports and that the information submitted should emphasize those characteristics that may have an impact on safety of the human subjects. The recent EU CTA IMPD (European Union Clinical Trial Authorisation Investigational Medicinal Product Dossier) guidance indicates that the CTA should include summaries (France's guidance indicates that the entire CTA should be limited to 200 pages). All these regulatory expectations have been sometimes interpreted by regulated industry as follows: "Why do I need to do more? The FDA only wants the minimum."

At the IND stage, the overriding focus of regulatory scientists is understandably subject safety. There is also a recognition that the CMC database is a constantly changing landscape in which changes to scale, specifications, analytical methodology, formulations, packaging components, etc., are made with regularity as development proceeds. Therefore, although government regulators may need only a portion of the scientific database, the clinical study sponsor needs much more information to accomplish its goals from a good science perspective. While the FDA focuses most intently on subject safety at this stage, the focus of the forward-thinking development company also includes proceeding through drug development as rapidly as possible while minimizing risks and potential hurdles.

Since the risk of CMC-related delays in drug development rises with the amount of information that is NOT known, the common sense approach is to develop a comprehensive database on your candidate compound. Obviously, this internal database will be more extensive than that required by FDA. Again, the reason is simply that the FDA and the pharmaceutical firm have completely different objectives and uses for the same database.

Plan for Success Most pharmaceutical management personnel will probably think to themselves, "we plan for success." In truth, however, few practice the core concepts crucial for success. Success can be defined as advancing into clinical development only those compounds that have a high probability of reaching Phase 3, that are easily studied clinically with defined endpoints, and that have an economically desirable potential market share (we are not including the screening INDs, in which several candidates are taken to humans to select the best one for further study). Success may also include having a compound with "developability" or that has an effect on "drugable" biological targets.

Given the resources involved in the drug development process, the prevailing philosophy in the pharmaceutical industry, today more than ever, is to "kill" the bad compounds fast. By extension, this philosophy can lead to a strategy of not conducting any unnecessary studies, since the odds are that the compound may not make it through the development gauntlet. This translates to a CMC mandate to "do the minimum" until proof-of-concept Phase 2 studies show that the candidate compound meets its objectives. This strategy has often resulted in CMC problems, which have cascaded to clinical study delays, an inability to interpret clinical data, an inability to reproduce the API impurity profile, or an inability to demonstrate drug product consistency and consistent clinical efficacy.

The CMC development process adopted within the generic drug industry represents an alternative approach for new drug development. Generic drugs do not require safety or efficacy studies; studies to establish safety and efficacy have already been conducted by the innovator. The focus of an application for a generic drug product is the CMC database and, specifically, a company's ability to produce a drug product that is bioequivalent to the innovator. In other words, the development of a generic drug product focuses not on "if" but "when." Generic product development begins with the pre-formulation activities as depicted in the CMC activities exhibit above, since the API is typically available from a variety of API contractors. Although one might think that the disclosure of the qualitative ingredients of the generic product (in the package insert or the PDR) would eliminate many studies, the generic development laboratory must still determine the grade (e.g., hydrous or anhydrous, large or small particle size) of each excipient and its quantity. Since the generic API is produced by a different route of synthesis than is the innovator, the innovator and generic API impurity profile may differ. So might physical-mechanical properties, such as particle size, density, and flow, any of which can impact drug product performance. While one might think that specifications for the generic drug product are defined by the innovator and that this aspect of development can be eliminated, it is equally difficult to have to conform with another's specifications as compared to determining your own. The end result of these issues is that generic CMC drug development proceeds rapidly, since most companies follow the systematic procedure depicted in the CMC activities exhibit provided above.

Adopting Smart Development Practices "Smart" development can be defined as using good science, better knowledge and appropriate planning to systematically conduct the activities outlined in the CMC activities exhibit above. We have discussed the value of conducting process research (stage 2A), and how the knowledge of the acceptable envelope of process parameters at small scale can maximize your chances of a successful scale-up. Otherwise it's hit or miss. The multiple "reproducibility" API batches at an increased 10 X scale are intended to demonstrate process capability at a relatively small scale and provide the fuel for toxicology studies and CMC efforts. Ideally, these replicate batches in stage 2B would be made identically and have identical characteristics and impurity profiles; however, there may be circumstances in which the analytical results from the first replicate batch suggest a modification to one or more process parameters. For example, the process research effort might define reaction and purification parameters that yielded an acceptable impurity profile, but the first replicate batch might have a 10-fold higher level of one impurity than the smaller scale batches. If the systematic process research studies had been conducted, it may be easy to identify the variable or conditions that led to increased levels of that impurity and then to modify that variable or condition. But if the process research had not been conducted, you are stuck with the higher impurity level, since you will not know how to address this and the timeline for initiating toxicology studies will be approaching rapidly.

In stage 3, the two scale-up to kilo quantity batches are intended to provide fuel for toxicology and CMC (stage 3A) and CTM in stage 3B. The first of these two batches is intended to confirm that an additional 10 X scale jump yields the same quality material. If it does, then stage 3B, which involves the manufacture of the batch intended for eventual clinical use, can be initiated without delay. Since chemistry is not always linear, there may be a need to fine-tune one or more process parameters, although this will require a risk assessment to ensure that increases in impurity profiles or different physical characteristics do not result from the modifications made.

The drug product's development also benefits from a systematic approach. Here, simultaneous evaluation of the analytical tools needed to assess the adequacy of the ensuing formulations and the evaluation of the physical/chemical characteristics of the API begin this process.

Often, the analytical method for the API can be adapted for use in the early pre-formulation and formulation development investigations. Typically, the assay method developed for the API focuses on quantitation of the API and the separation of the API from the impurities. "Smart" method development includes forced degradation studies. In this case, the method is also selective with respect to potential degradation products. Forced degradation studies allow for the identification of where the degradation products (i.e., due to exposure to heat, light, extremes of pH and oxygen) can be seen on the chromatogram. Thus, during screening stability studies, if a peak appears in the chromatogram, its placement can often identify the cause and permit a rapid elimination of the inherent cause of the instability. In any event, the analytical method is originally developed for a "pure" API and not for the API that is "contaminated" with excipients used in formulation. The drug product analytical method must separate out the API from the excipients themselves and from any degradants due to the formulation or its processing. While the methods used in the early IND stages need not be validated, they must be stability indicating.

Adaptation of the API method to a drug product may be simple or difficult depending on the dosage form. For an IV solution, the typical excipients are usually buffers and saline, perhaps a preservative if a multiple-use product has been designed, or perhaps a sugar as a cryoprotectant if a lyophilized dosage form is required. In this case, it may be relatively easy to adapt the API method.

An equally important tool is the technique that evaluates *in vitro* drug release—the *in vitro* dissolution test that is used for solid, transdermal and topical dosage forms. Dissolution measures the amount of drug released from the dosage form as a function of time. Its ultimate use is as a quality control (QC) test to differentiate "good" from "bad" products. In early development, however, it is used as a criterion for evaluating the adequacy of prototype formulations. The technique requires a knowledge of biopharmaceutics. For topical dosage forms, the pH of the skin (~5.5) suggests that the media used for the test be at that pH. For oral drugs, we must know the site of absorption in the GI tract. For an oral immediate release dosage form, we must have determined the pH-solubility profile so that "sink" conditions can be determined (these ensure that the dissolution test will not be influenced by solubility limitations) and appropriate conditions can be established. The technique is also best used when benchmark or baseline data exist. This is usually obtained by intrinsic dissolution or particulate dissolution studies. In the latter, the dissolution profile of the API, as it is obtained from the API manufacturer, is determined as an unformulated powder or as a powder in a capsule. Particulate dissolution is also studied as a function of particle size (where small, medium, and large "cuts" of the API are studied separately) or as a function of surfactant concentration (this identifies wetting problems and identifies one approach to improving the solubility in the *in vivo* environment).

Other pre-formulation studies provide additional guidance to formulation development. Drug excipient compatibility studies are conducted with binary mixtures of potential excipients to identify incompatibilities. The techniques that have been used include high performance liquid chromatography (HPLC) analysis of purity and degradation products, or DSC. The former emphasizes chemical interactions; the latter can detect physical interactions. One must determine the trade-offs between each technique's sensitivity (there are false positives with DSC), and whether the analytical HPLC tool is available at the time that this test needs to be conducted and the time allotted for a determination (DSC takes days while HPLC may not show interactions for weeks or months even at elevated temperatures.).

Conclusion Everyone in the pharma and biotech industry wants to develop the next blockbuster therapeutic. Whether or not a candidate molecule will be a commercial success is a function of many factors, including unmet medical needs, the indications and labeling for the existing products on the market, and how fast the entire development cycle can be completed. CMC development is only a part of the overall drug development process, albeit an important one. The API provides the fuel for toxicology studies and the balance of the CMC program. CTM provides the fuel for clinical research.

The concepts mentioned here are intended to facilitate the preparation of these fuels, both for internal CMC programs and other external disciplines. Many of these concepts involve incorporating good scientific principles into good management practices. Some of these concepts involve insurance policies, or the conceptualization of "what-if" scenarios, and the ability and preparation to embark on a "plan B" on a moment's notice. Experience has shown that a well-thought-out and systematic plan is the most efficient means to reach the many milestones along the path of drug development.

CHAPTER 4

Nonclinical Development

By Paul A. Andrews, Ph.D., Carolyn Laurençot, Ph.D., and Denis Roy, Ph.D.

Success in the medicinal product development process often is measured by the ability to discover compounds with promising therapeutic effects and, through efficient testing in animals and humans, to learn enough about their properties so these compounds can be used in a manner such that the observed benefits outweigh the potential risks to the patient. From a business perspective in which efficiency is the key to survival, success is most often measured by the ability to reach the destination in the most expeditious manner while using the fewest resources possible without compromising the quality of the essential information gathered along the process. This chapter's goal is to provide an understanding of the key nonclinical elements and concepts that must be addressed and integrated with the overall medicinal product development process to expedite successful clinical testing and marketing approval.

Nonclinical Testing: Introduction and Brief History Nonclinical testing is an integral part of the development of new medicines. The initial nonclinical development stage is a key decision point for determining if a medicinal product (i.e., a drug or biologic) is a suitable candidate to take forward into clinical investigations. The initial goal of a nonclinical program is to provide information about the product's safety and potential efficacy to perform a risk-benefit assessment. If the potential benefits appear to outweigh the potential risks, the product can proceed to the clinical stage of development. In addition, nonclinical pharmacology and toxicology information is required by regulatory agencies not only prior to, but throughout the clinical testing of investigational products. Late-stage toxicology studies provide additional information on the safety of the medicinal product after extended exposure (e.g., carcinogenicity studies) or in special populations (e.g., pregnant animals). Information from these studies is used to determine specific human safety concerns and the product's market potential.

For centuries, exogenous substances, including drugs, have been tested in animals. However, not until the early 20th century was it widely accepted that nonclinical testing for therapeutic activity and safety should be performed on drugs prior to their use in humans. At this time, physicians and scientists recognized the importance of nonclinical testing and, in a discussion on the principles for the rational clinical use of new agents based on pharmacologic studies in animals at the American Medical Association meeting in 1929, it was duly noted that "There is no shortcut from chemical laboratory to clinic, except one that passes too close to the morgue" (Leake, 1929). The requirement for regulatory nonclinical testing is the result of several human health tragedies. Prior to 1938, safety testing in animals was not conducted on drugs or biologics prior to marketing. The elixir of sulfonamide tragedy in 1937, in which 107 people, mostly children, died due to toxicity of the solvent ethylene glycol, prompted the United States Congress to pass the Federal Food, Drug and Cosmetic (FDC) Act of 1938. One of the major provisions of the FDC Act was to mandate the premarket testing of pharmaceuticals for safety in experimental animals. In 1962, federal requirements for nonclinical safety testing became more stringent under the Kefauver-Harris Amendments (to the 1938 FDC Act), which was passed by Congress in response to the thalidomide tragedy. The Kefauver-Harris Amendments required extensive animal pharmacological and toxicological testing before a pharmaceutical could be tested in humans. In addition, this amendment stipulated that the data from these studies must be submitted in an investigational new drug (IND) application for FDA review prior to initiation of the clinical studies.

Nonclinical testing includes *in vitro* (e.g., in cell extracts, cultured cells, or tissue preparations) and *in vivo* studies conducted to determine the pharmacologic and toxicologic profiles of pharmaceutical agents. The nonclinical activities are driven by two major areas of pharmacology—pharmacodynamics (including mechanism of action, biochemical and physiological effects in appropriate animal models, and toxicology studies) and pharmacokinetics.

Pharmacology is the scientific discipline that provides the foundation for medicinal product development and encompasses such fields as chemistry, biochemistry, physiology, anatomy, and medicine. Pharmacology is basically the study of pharmaceuticals and their interaction with living systems (for a review, see Fredholm, 2002). Pharmacologic studies can provide information about the safety, effectiveness and mechanism of action of a new therapeutic.

Pharmacokinetics is defined as what the body does to the pharmaceutical product, and includes the physiological processes of absorption, distribution, metabolism and excretion (ADME). All of these processes can affect the level of the pharmaceutical in the blood and, ultimately, the concentration of the pharmaceutical at the tissues and organs where it elicits an effect. The ADME of the pharmaceutical will be affected by its properties, such as lipid solubility, pKa, salt form, and molecular weight, as well as the properties of the administered product, such as crystal structure, particle size, and excipient content. If a pharmaceutical candidate is not available in sufficient concentrations at the target site due to poor absorption from the gastrointestinal tract, extensive metabolism, or high plasma protein binding, then it will most likely fail to proceed to clinical trials regardless of its *in vitro* potency or specificity. Therefore, the characterization of a compound's ADME properties is a critical early activity in medicinal product development.

Pharmacodynamics is defined as what the pharmaceutical does to the body, and refers to the desirable (therapeutic) and undesirable (toxic) actions of the pharmaceutical in the body. The study of the desirable effects can include direct measures of activity for the desired outcome (e.g., antitumor effect, anti-inflammatory measures, and protection from infection), inhibition of the target, or indirect measures of downstream biological markers believed to correlate with or indicate that the selected target has been "hit." The study of a pharmaceutical's undesirable pharmacodynamic effects on living organisms falls into the field of toxicology.

Toxicology is the science that deals with poisons and their effects on living organisms or systems. In the context of drug development, toxicology is concerned with identifying potential hazards and assessing the risk for their occurrence in humans. Although pharmaceuticals are usually selected for development based on their ability to interact with a specific target and elicit a desirable effect, no pharmaceutical is absolutely specific for the intended therapeutic target. As stated in the 16th century by Paracelsus, the father of pharmacology, "All substances are poison; there is none that is not a poison. The right dose differentiates a poison from a remedy." In nonclinical studies, the margin of safety of a pharmaceutical is determined by comparing the dose that causes the therapeutic effect to the dose that causes toxicity. This ratio of efficacy to toxicity is called the therapeutic index, which is established from nonclinical studies and is used to estimate the potential risks to humans. Therefore, nonclinical studies are undertaken to determine toxicities as well as the potential human benefit of the new pharmaceutical.

Nonclinical Development: A Multidisciplinary Integration During the medicinal product development stages, expertise is required from several interrelated scientific and regulatory disciplines. The successful development of a pharmaceutical candidate critically relies on the close integration of all disciplines involved, including project management, regulatory, clinical, nonclinical, and chemistry and manufacturing expertise.

The development team must also assure that the experts from each discipline work toward a common and compatible goal. Frequently, what might seem to be a simple or minor change for one discipline might turn out to be a major obstacle for another area of expertise. Since the nonclinical plan is driven by the clinical plan, for example, changing the schedule or duration of administration in a planned clinical trial could have a major impact on the design and timing of the nonclinical studies—and, more importantly, on the quantity of test material required to complete the study. Therefore, it is imperative that the relevant disciplines work synchronously with others to minimize the risks of unexpected surprises and to avoid unnecessary detours during the development program.

Formulating a Development Plan Prospective planning is one of the key steps for efficiently leading any large, multiyear project to a successful completion. One of the first steps in initiating a successful development program is the design and preparation of a development plan that integrates the key chemistry and manufacturing, nonclinical, clinical and regulatory activities. Although the plan itself does not constitute a guarantee of success, it maximizes the chances of success while minimizing the chance of unexpected and unnecessary detours. Although there are many commonalities in the types of nonclinical toxicology studies used to support the safety of a new pharmaceutical, there is no one checklist relevant to all products. Before one embarks on a nonclinical program to support the development of a new pharmaceutical, one must construct a plan that carefully lays out the studies that are essential for supporting the clinical development. The plan should include the timing of the studies, the amount of test article needed, the costs involved, the personnel needed to execute the program, a clear understanding of the risks involved in any given approach, and contingencies to address potential adversities. Such a plan will give the nonclinical program direction and focus that, in turn, promotes speed and efficiency. There are at least five general principles for creating a successful nonclinical development plan:

    1. Plan backwards, execute forwards. The overall clinical development plan needs to drive the nonclinical safety assessment plan. Although many issues will not be known with certainty, a develop-

ment team needs to have reasonable ideas of where the product will be situated on the market. Issues that could affect the nonclinical strategy include: the targeted patient population (is it a life-threatening disease or an easily treated condition?), the length of time patients will likely need to take the product (will treatment recur intermittently throughout life?), the timeline for starting longer-duration clinical studies, whether initial trials will be in healthy volunteers or patients, the schedule of administration, the route of administration, the proposed formulation (will new excipients be used? has their safety been established?), and whether the pharmaceutical is expected to have clinical benefit as a monotherapy or will need to be combined with other therapeutics.

2. Risks need to be evaluated in animals before they have the potential to be encountered in humans (in general and within reason). This means that toxicology reports must be available in advance of the anticipated clinical milestone that they support. Understanding these intertwined timelines is critical for avoiding delays in overall development based on nonclinical studies. Risks that must be evaluated in animals before humans are exposed include those related to duration of administration, formulation, impurities or degradants, route and schedule of administration, exposure profiles, and risks to sensitive systems (including developmental and reproductive toxicity). There are numerous caveats to this general principle. For example, although humans should not be exposed to risks related to dosing duration before these risks have been evaluated in appropriate toxicology studies, there are exceptions and limitations. One exception is in the setting of advanced cancer, where it is considered unethical to withdraw treatment in subjects who are responding simply because long-duration animal studies have not been conducted to identify potential hazards. A limitation of this general principle is that the default maximum duration of general toxicology studies is six months in rodents and nine months in nonrodents. However, humans will often need to be treated longer than this to demonstrate or maintain efficacy. One must keep in mind that these durations represent significant portions of the lifespans of the animals (six months is approximately 25% of the rat lifetime), and that significant shorter-term human testing will have occurred by the time trial duration needs to exceed nine months. Another caveat is that the risk of carcinogenicity in rodents is not known until late in development, well after hundreds, if not thousands, of subjects have been exposed in clinical trials. There are also many reasonable instances in which switches in formulation, exposure to new impurities, or changing the route or schedule of administration can be justified in the absence of direct or additional nonclinical data. The principal message is that aggressive clinical plans require aggressive nonclinical plans to provide appropriate assessments of the risks involved.

3. Seek input from "stakeholders." To construct a realistic, robust, and relevant plan, those who will execute the plan, use the data, and regulate the development should ideally contribute to the plan's design. These stakeholders in the plan's outcome include corporate officers, discovery scientists, clinical trial designers, principal investigators, partners in contract research organizations, and regulatory reviewers.

4. Consult published guidances. Today, there is a large and growing collection of regulatory guidelines, journal articles, points-to-consider documents, and position papers that provide information on the expected approaches for supporting the safety of many diverse pharmaceutical products. These include documents from the International Conference on Harmonisation (available on www.fda.gov), the United States Food and Drug Administration (www.fda.gov), and the Committee for Proprietary Medicinal Products (CPMP) within The European Agency for the Evaluation of Medicinal Products (www.emea.eu.int). In addition, redacted FDA review documents for approved products are available and can provide insights on the studies conducted during the development of similar products. One must remember three rules when studying guidance documents, however: (1) just because it is written in a guidance does not mean that it has to be done; (2) just because a study is not specified in a guidance does not mean that it does not have to be conducted; and (3) what was considered necessary for a similar product yesterday may not be either necessary or sufficient for your product today.

5. Concentrate on information flow. The goal of a nonclinical safety plan is not to fill out a checklist of available reports, but to provide information regarding the adverse effects of a pharmaceutical at appropriate junctures in clinical development. To provide a nonclinical plan that is fully integrated into the overall development plan, one must consider who needs the information, what information is needed, when it must be available, and how the information will be obtained. Discovery

scientists (compound selectors) will want nonclinical information so that they can attempt to improve the pharmacokinetic properties and diminish non-mechanism-based toxicities in next-generation compounds. Clinical trials designers will want nonclinical information to aid in designing trials with the best chance of demonstrating efficacy with minimal toxicity. They will want to know the toxicological hazards that have been identified so that these toxicities can be appropriately monitored in the study. Likewise, clinical investigators will need data regarding mechanism of action and proof-of-concept as well as the compound's potential to cause toxicity so that they can best serve the interests of the subjects in their trials. Finally, regulatory reviewers will need the nonclinical information so that they can independently determine product safety.

Drugs: Nonclinical Safety Testing Establishing the safety profile of the substance is the principal goal for nonclinical safety testing for pharmaceuticals. This is best accomplished by obtaining data on the following: dose-response relationship(s); the no-observed-effect level (NOEL), the no-observable-adverse-effect level (NOAEL), and the maximum tolerated dose (MTD) or maximum feasible dose (MFD); target organs and endpoints of toxicity; time-related drug-induced effects (latency); gender-related differences; correlation of systemic or local drug exposure with toxicity; reversibility; and species-specific differences.

The NOAEL is one of the most important values to establish because it is most often used as a starting point for extrapolating a reasonably safe starting dose in initial Phase 1 trials. While there are numerous definitions of NOAEL, for selecting a starting dose the FDA has defined the NOAEL as the highest dose level that does not produce any significant adverse effects. Since there can be different opinions in defining a significant adverse effect, sound scientific judgment should be used when assessing the data. An effect could be considered beneficial (e.g., lowering cholesterol) or be the intended pharmacodynamic effect and thus not considered adverse. Effects that are either statistically significant or biologically significant will need to be considered in the determination of the NOAEL. The NOEL refers to any effect, not just adverse effects. Likewise, MTD has variable definitions depending on context. In short-term studies, the MTD generally means the highest dose level at which no more than 10% of the animals experience serious or life-threatening toxicity. In chronic studies, the MTD can mean the dose that is predicted to produce a minimum toxic effect over the course of a two-year carcinogenicity study. This would be the highest dose that does not produce alterations that would be predicted to alter the animal's normal life span. In this context, a dose causing a 10% decrease in body weight gain would be considered the MTD. In some cases, it might not be possible to define the MTD before technical considerations or physicochemical properties limit the amount of the pharmaceutical that can be delivered. When this occurs, the maximum feasible dose (MFD) will have to be defined and justified. Determining the NOAEL and MTD is important because they set the outer bounds of the dose-response relationship.

Although there is no single testing checklist that fits all pharmaceuticals, there are default approaches that dictate the core battery of studies that should be conducted as well as their timing. This section will deal specifically with the conventional nonclinical toxicology program for most drugs. Since a drug's indication and intended patient population have a bearing on which toxicology studies are required prior to and throughout clinical development, all of the studies described below are not required for every drug. While many of these studies will also be appropriate for biologics, such products have many unique issues (an overview of the nonclinical development of these products is provided in a separate section below).

General Toxicology Testing Requirements As stated above, the nonclinical development plan needs to focus on information flow to the relevant stakeholders in the process. The critical reference for determining when nonclinical information (studies) is expected for regulatory purposes is the ICH guidance entitled, "Nonclinical Safety Studies for the Conduct of Human Clinical Trials for Pharmaceuticals" (M3). The general recommendations for aligning the nonclinical program with clinical development are summarized below.

Studies Expected Prior to Phase 1 Testing: Safety Pharmacology Studies Safety pharmacology studies are designed to assess the adverse effects of a pharmaceutical on the function of vital organ systems, such as the central nervous, cardiovascular and respiratory systems. In contrast to general toxicology studies, which principally investigate the effects of agents on biochemical or anatomical parameters, safety pharmacology studies evaluate the actual functioning of an organ or system.

The ICH S7A (Safety Pharmacology Studies for Human Pharmaceuticals) and S7B (Nonclinical Evaluation of the Potential for Delayed Ventricular Repolarization (QT Interval Prolongation) by Human Pharmaceuticals) guidances present the standard panels of studies expected prior to the first human exposure. Although it is acceptable in some instances to incorporate some of these assessments into toxicology studies, they are often provided as separate studies in small numbers of animals. The standard core battery of expected studies addresses toxicity to the cardiovascular, central nervous, and respiratory systems. In addition to this core battery of *in vivo* studies, the ICH S7B guidance provides a nonclinical testing strategy that addresses the potential for delayed ventricular repolarization and that includes *in vitro* studies. The guidances and other documents should be consulted for more details on safety pharmacology testing strategies.

Genetic Toxicity Genetic toxicity testing involves the use of *in vitro* and *in vivo* tests designed to determine if a compound induces genetic damage directly or indirectly by various mechanisms. These tests typically enable researchers to identify a compound's potential to induce gene mutations, chromosomal damage, or recombination and numerical chromosome changes.

In vitro tests of genetic toxicity (mutagenicity and clastogenicity) as specified in the ICH S2B guidance (Genotoxicity: A Standard Battery for Genotoxicity Testing for Pharmaceuticals) are expected prior to Phase 1 testing. Usually, a reverse mutation assay in bacteria and a chromosome aberration assay in rodent or human lymphocytes are used at this stage of development for *in vitro* genetic toxicity assessment. Positive findings would trigger additional testing. In some indications, positive findings will preclude further development.

Pharmacokinetics and Metabolism Pharmacokinetic and metabolism information can be important in interpreting toxicities and assessing human risks. Knowledge of the systemic exposure to a pharmaceutical and its metabolites can provide a better basis for interspecies comparisons of toxicity than dose alone. Pharmacokinetic similarities between species can provide confidence in extrapolating findings to humans, whereas large differences between animal models can raise concerns about the appropriately safe human dose. Pharmacokinetic data may also suggest modifications in the intended dose, route, or schedule for the clinical trial.

Ideally, systemic exposure and ADME data in animals should be collected prior to human clinical trials. Although not critical for evaluating human safety (since data in humans are not available for comparison), the human data are often available at the end of Phase 1, at which time the comparisons can be made. Pharmacokinetic and metabolism data can also identify potential problems (short or long half-lives, rapid metabolism), and allow comparisons of toxicities in animals based on exposure as measured by concentrations in the blood over time.

Toxicity Studies The principal objectives for the initial toxicity studies are to determine the target tissues for toxicity (hazard identification), the dose response for toxicity, and the reversibility of toxicities so that a safe starting dose and dose escalation scheme can be selected for humans (risk assessment). The nonclinical studies should identify appropriate parameters for the monitoring of safety in the clinic. To identify what toxicities are possibly associated with an agent, animal toxicology experiments should be designed to elicit toxicity. This often requires that animals be given doses to induce toxicities and that are many-fold above those anticipated for use in humans.

Toxicology studies in both a rodent and a nonrodent species are generally necessary to support the intended Phase 1 trial. These studies should be conducted using the route, schedule, and formulation intended for humans. The duration of treatment should match or exceed the duration proposed for the clinical trial. Typically, range-finding studies of increasing duration are conducted so that appropriate doses can be selected for the definitive studies designed to support the Phase 1 trial. These range-finding studies also usually provide preliminary identification of the target organs of toxicity and initial pharmacokinetic data. Therefore, there are often several toxicology studies available in each species prior to the first human trial. Since the duration of dosing in Phase 1 trials usually does not exceed one month, one month is typically the longest duration study necessary for this phase of development.

Endpoints in toxicity studies generally include clinical observations, body weight, food consumption, ophthalmological examinations, electrocardiography (nonrodents only), clinical pathology (hematology, serum chemistry, coagulation, and urinalysis), gross pathology, organ weights, and histopathology.

Studies Expected During Clinical Development: Genetic Toxicity *In vivo* tests of genetic toxicity as specified in the ICH S2B guidance are expected prior to Phase 2 testing. An *in vivo* mouse or rat micronucleus test is the typical test used. Although an *in vivo* test (e.g., micronucleus test) is not required until Phase 2, it can be advantageous to conduct this test and the *in vitro* tests simultaneously before Phase 1 in order to minimize costs.

Toxicity Studies Toxicology studies in rodents and nonrodents will be needed to support the duration of dosing if it lengthens as development proceeds. Typically, the standard durations of animal studies are 2 weeks, 1 month, 3 months, 6 months, 9 months, and 12 months.

Dose selection is critical, as each study should establish the safety profile of the pharmaceutical and, therefore, should ideally identify a NOAEL as well as a toxic dose. Any decision to conduct long-term toxicology studies without adequate shorter-term toxicology data is risky, and should be carefully evaluated. A toxicology study that does not produce an adequate characterization of the safety profile (e.g., doses too high to define a NOAEL or doses too low to define end-organ toxicities) will probably have to be repeated. This will lead to major delays in the program and substantial additional expenses, including test article costs.

Developmental and Reproductive Toxicity To fully assess the potential for developmental and reproductive toxicity, three studies are conducted to cover the period of pre-mating through weaning, and assess the pharmaceutical's effect on libido and sexual function, fertility, embryofetal development, birthing, maternal care, and the growth and development of offspring. These studies have been conventionally called Segment I, II, and III. More recently, the ICH established the different stages of development from stage A to F, with each letter representing a different stage of the reproductive cycle (see ICH S5A guidance, Detection of Toxicity to Reproduction for Medicinal Products). Segment I studies (ICH stage A-B) are known as fertility studies, Segment II studies (ICH stage C-D) are known as developmental toxicity or teratology studies, and Segment III studies (ICH stage C-F) are known as peri-postnatal studies.

In a Segment I study, male and female animals are dosed from pre-mating through implantation (for females), and for up to one complete spermatogenesis cycle (for males). The study assesses maturation of gametes, mating behavior, fertility, pre-implantation stages of the embryo, and implantation. A single Segment I study in rodents (usually rats) is usually sufficient to support medicinal product development. In a Segment II study, animals are dosed during the major period of embryogenesis, which is from the time of implantation to closure of the hard palate. Fetuses are then examined at the end of pregnancy for embryofetal death, altered growth, and structural changes. Studies in rodents and nonrodents (usually rats and rabbits) are expected. In a Segment III study, dams are dosed from the time of implantation through weaning. Assessments include prenatal and postnatal death of offspring, maternal care, altered growth and development, and functional deficits in the offspring, including behavior, maturation (puberty), and reproduction. A study in rodents (usually rats) is typically sufficient, and many studies design variations, including multi-generation studies, are available, and is usually selected based on the safety concerns for the investigational products.

Currently, there are regional differences (European Union, Japan, United States) in the expected timing of developmental and reproductive toxicity (DART) studies (see the ICH M3 guidance). The general approach for pharmaceuticals developed in the United States can be characterized as follows:

- Men may be included in Phase 1 and 2 trials prior to conducting a Segment I fertility study, provided that an evaluation of the pharmaceutical's effect on male reproductive organs has been included in the relevant repeated-dose toxicity studies. A fertility study that includes dosing of males should be completed prior to the initiation of Phase 3 trials that include men.
- Women incapable of bearing children (i.e., permanently sterilized or postmenopausal) may be included in clinical trials without DART studies, provided an evaluation of the pharmaceutical's effect on female reproductive organs has been included in the relevant repeated-dose toxicity studies.
- Women capable of bearing children may be included in early, carefully monitored studies without support from DART studies, provided that appropriate precautions are taken to minimize risk. These precautions include pregnancy testing, use of a highly effective method of birth control, entry into the trial only after a confirmed menstrual period, and continued pregnancy testing and monitoring during the trial. As clinical development proceeds, assessment of female fertility in a Segment I study and of embryo-fetal development in Segment II studies should be completed before women of childbearing potential using birth control are enrolled in Phase 3 trials.
- The pharmaceutical's effect on pre- and post-natal development in a Segment III study should be submitted during development if there is cause for concern. Otherwise, submission at the time of marketing application is adequate.

Special Toxicity Additional targeted nonclinical studies may be needed if nonclinical or clinical findings with the product or related products have indicated special safety concerns. Examples might include studies targeted to address unusual toxicity to a specific tissue or site, such as the kidneys, peripheral nerves, adrenal glands or injection site. The studies would include specialized assessments and are often intended to investigate mechanism.

There is growing interest in harmonizing the expectations for immunotoxicity testing. The FDA had issued a draft 2002 guidance on the topic (Immunotoxicity Evaluation of Investigational Drugs), and the EMEA expects all pharmaceuticals to be screened for immunotoxic potential, as specified in its "Note for Guidance on Repeated Dose Toxicity (CPMP/SWP/1042/99)." These guidances should be studied to determine when and to what extent immunotoxicity testing will be expected for a given product. An ICH guidance on immunotoxicity testing (ICH S8, Immunotoxicity Studies for Human Pharmaceuticals) has reached the draft stage. In addition, phototoxicity testing is appropriate for some pharmaceuticals; both the FDA and EMEA have issued guidances on the topic.

Additional Studies Expected to Support a Marketing Application: Toxicity Studies Chronic toxicology studies in a rodent and a nonrodent species will be needed to support clinical exposure of long duration. The duration of the animal studies should cover the duration of the human exposure up to a maximum of 6 months in rodents and 9 months in nonrodents. Under some circumstances, either a 6-month or a 12-month study in nonrodents might be sufficient or necessary, respectively, to support chronic human exposure.

Carcinogenicity The objectives of carcinogenicity studies are to identify the tumorigenic potential of the drug in animals and its relevance for humans. In carcinogenicity studies, animals are dosed repeatedly (typically daily) for two years because this duration covers their expected life spans. All tissues are then examined microscopically for benign and malignant neoplasias. Selecting the correct doses is a critical decision because of the costs and time involved in carcinogenicity studies. The ICH S1C guidance (Dose Selection for Carcinogenicity Studies of Pharmaceuticals) covers acceptable approaches for selecting the high dose. The FDA's agreement on the overall carcinogenicity study design and dose selection should always be sought through the "special protocol assessment" procedure. At the time of the marketing application, carcinogenicity studies in two rodent species are needed if the medicinal product will be used continuously for at least 6 months or as frequent intermittent therapy, and if the life expectancy of the targeted population is greater than two to three years. Additional recommendations regarding carcinogenicity testing are available in the ICH's S1A guidance document (The Need for Long-term Rodent Carcinogenicity Testing of Pharmaceuticals).

Nonclinical Safety Testing for Biologicals

Different statutes govern the regulation of drug and biologic products in the United States. Whereas both drug and biologic products are subject to the Food, Drug and Cosmetic Act of 1938, biologic products are also regulated by the Public Health Service Act of 1944. The differences in the regulation of drug and biologic products are mainly due to the basic premise that most drug products have a known structure and are chemically synthesized, whereas biologic products are derived from living sources (such as humans, animals, plants, and microorganisms), may not have a completely defined structure, tend to be heat sensitive, and are prone to microbial contamination. According to the federal regulations, a biologic product means "any virus, therapeutic serum, toxin, antitoxin, or analogous product applicable to the prevention, treatment or cure of diseases or injuries of man" (21 CFR 600.3(h)). Biologic products include blood and blood products, monoclonal antibodies, immunotoxins, radioimmunotherapy, therapeutic proteins, preventative and therapeutic vaccines, somatic cell therapy, gene therapy, and banked human tissues (bone, skin, corneas, ligament, and tendon).

Overview of Nonclinical Testing for Biologic Products Until recently, the FDA's Center for Biologics Evaluation and Research (CBER) was responsible for ensuring the safety of all biologic products. With the establishment of the Office of Drug Evaluation VI and the Office of Biotechnology Products in the Center for Drugs Evaluation and Research (CDER) in 2003 (http://www.fda.gov/cder/biologics/), the review of biologic products is now the responsibility of both CBER and CDER. However, the therapeutic biologic products transferred to CDER will continue to be regulated as licensed biologics. Therefore, the principles of nonclinical toxicology testing for biologics discussed in this chapter applies to products regulated by both centers. The objectives for nonclinical studies with biologics are similar to those with drugs—establish "proof of concept" for efficacy, and provide safety information. The ICH S6 guidance entitled, "Preclinical Safety Evaluation of Biotechnology-Derived Pharmaceuticals" provides a general overview of issues relevant to the nonclinical development of biologic products. In addition to safety issues related to the pharmacology of the biologic, safety concerns may also arise from the presence of impurities or contaminants; therefore, it is essential that the biologic product meets specifications for purity, safety (free of adventitious agents), sterility, identity, and potency throughout nonclinical and clinical testing. Comparability testing for each lot of the biologic must be performed to assure that the product used for nonclinical studies meets the same specifications as the product used in the clinical trials.

The types of nonclinical studies recommended for supporting ongoing biological product clinical development and eventually a biologic license application (BLA) are conceptually similar to those discussed previously for drugs, although there are some notable exceptions. Classical genetic toxicity, carcinogenicity and metabolism studies are generally not applicable to most biologics (ICH S6; Cavagnaro 2002) and, therefore, alternative approaches may be employed to address these issues. In addition, certain characteristics of biologic products, such as species specificity and immunogenicity, often preclude the conventional paradigms for toxicity testing of pharmaceuticals (i.e., testing in one rodent and one non-rodent species). There are numerous appropriate avenues for the nonclinical development of biologic products. The unique properties of each product and the availability of crucial resources (e.g., relevant animal models) will dictate which approach is optimal. Therefore, it is essential that the nonclinical plan for each biologic be developed on a case-by-case basis.

Key Principles for the Nonclinical Development of Biologics: Relevant Animal Model The fundamental principle for the nonclinical safety testing of biologics is the use of a relevant animal model. In contrast to drug products, nonclinical testing in one rodent and one non-rodent is not always required for biologics. Rather, testing in two relevant animal models is suggested. If only one or no relevant animal models exists for a biological product, however, testing in only one or no species may be appropriate (ICH S6). The FDA should always be consulted regarding the choice of animal model for the safety studies, and regarding the possibility of a waiver of the requirement for such studies in the absence of a relevant animal model.

A relevant animal model is one in which the product is pharmacologically active due to the expression of the target molecule and for which the target plays a similar physiologic role as the human target. To serve as a more predictive model for human toxicity, the animal model should also display similar tissue distribution patterns for the biologic target as observed in the human. The most relevant animal model may be identified via a comparison of the tissue cross-reactivity of the biologic product in different species, including human tissues. Species that have a similar tissue binding profile and binding affinity compared to human tissues can often serve as relevant animal models for toxicology studies. The animal target's interaction kinetics with the pharmaceutical should be similar to those for the human target. It is essential that the model used be capable of providing information that can aid in risk assessment decisions. The exhibit below outlines relevant criteria in selecting an animal model for nonclinical studies of a biologic. If two relevant species exist, some studies may be required in both species. Conversely, if no relevant animal models exist, the use of relevant transgenic animals expressing the human target or the use of a homologous protein should be considered for safety testing. For example, in support of a Phase 1 gene therapy clinical trial investigating human IL-12 DNA, toxicology studies were conducted in mice using murine IL-12 DNA (Imboden, 2003), since human IL-12 is not active in the mouse. Dose selection for the nonclinical studies should take into account differences in receptor affinity between species. As mentioned, a scientifi-

Species Selection Considerations

Criteria	Comment or Examples
Phamacodynamics, Biological Activity	Receptor presence, homology and distribution; Mechanism of action
Pharmacokinetic, ADME	Comparable kinetics or adequate kinetics versus humans; metabolic and detoxification pathways
Biology, Anatomy, and Physiology	Absence of gallbladder and higher folate endogenous levels in rats; Deficient glucuronidation in cats; Deficient N-acetylation in dogs; Longevity in rodents is shorter than non-rodents and are therefore most suitable for carcinogenicity testing
Historical Databases	Background biological variability in normal animals must be known; Most GLP toxicology laboratories have significant databases for most standard species
Regulatory Requirements	Specific species requirements as per guidance documents and regulatory expectations; Class effects
Economical Considerations	Rodents are fairly inexpensive as compared with dogs and primates; Primates are approximately 10 times more expensive than dogs
Timelines	The time to get animals to the toxicology laboratory is significantly longer for monkeys than dogs; generally not an issue for rodents
Route of Administration	Continuous intravenous administration is more challenging in small rodents like mice and is difficult to perform for very long duration
Test Article Availability	More test article is required for bigger species assuming that there are no major interspecies differences in sensitivity

ADME: Absorption, distribution, metabolism and excretion

cally valid and informative study is expected to identify a substantially toxic dose level as well as the NOAEL. To correctly interpret the toxicological findings observed in non-traditional, but pharmacologically relevant, animal models (if used), it is necessary to include positive and negative controls in the study design as well as to provide extensive baseline data (Serabian, 1999).

Immunogenicity Immunogenicity refers to an exogenous agent's ability to induce an immune response. Since most biologic products are polypeptides, proteins or express protein products (i.e., gene therapy), an immune response can be elicited (in humans and other animal species) that may alter the risk to benefit ratio of the biologic. The need for immunogenicity testing in nonclinical studies is often controversial, since it is expected that human proteins will be recognized as foreign substances in animal models, thereby resulting in immunogenicity. The human protein products would not be expected to trigger an immune response in humans, however. In addition, it is generally accepted that antibody formation in animals does not predict antibody formation in humans. However, there are several notable exceptions, such as with human growth hormone and insulin, in which the appropriate animal model predicted human immune response (Weirda, 2001).

The characterization of the immunogenicity of biologics aids in the interpretation of results from toxicology studies, the assessment of the utility of chronic toxicity studies and, in certain situations, the selection of the appropriate biological product to move forward into the clinic. Several factors contribute to the immunogenicity of a protein therapeutic, including dose, route and duration of administration, dosing regimen, pharmacological properties, overall protein structure, formulation and purity. Therefore, these factors should be considered in designing toxicology studies and evaluating the need for immunogenicity assessment. Types of immunogenicity include hypersensitivity reactions (allergic response) and antibody formation. The selection of an appropriate animal model is dependent upon the type of immunogenicity observed with the product.

Immunogenicity is most often associated with the formation of antibodies rather than T-cell directed responses. Antibodies or immune complexes could inherently cause new toxic events or affect the pharmacological parameters of the biologic product, resulting in an altered toxicity or efficacy profile. Direct toxic effects in the animal model may occur if a homologous protein is tested in the animal with the resultant formation of antibodies that cross-react with the endogenous counterpart. The toxicity profile of the biologic may also be compromised if systemic exposure to the biologic is not maintained, or if toxicity is due to a reaction to a foreign protein (Green, 2000). Antibodies can affect drug exposure by neutralizing the activity of the biologic product, or by altering its clearance or distribution. Therefore, the biologic's true pharmacologic and toxic potential may not be elucidated in nonclinical studies if immunogenicity occurs in the animal studies but not in humans.

Although traditional animal models are not generally predictive of clinical immunogenicity, some animals, particularly nonhuman primates, can be used to investigate the immunogenic potential of biologic products under certain situations (e.g., products in which the protein is highly conserved between species). In addition, several genetically engineered mouse models, and *ex vivo* immunological assays, such as the *ex vivo* T-cell activation assay, can be employed to assess the immunogenicity of biologics (Chirino, 2004). Immunogenicity can be further investigated in nonclinical studies designed to include regimens using immunological adjuvants designed to increase the likelihood of generating an immune response to the biologic product. If antibodies develop in several animal models, the biologic may cause general immunogenicity that could extrapolate to humans (Koren, 2002).

Immunotoxicity Immunotoxicology is the study of the adverse effects of products on the immune system, which include effects such as immunosuppression, immunogenicity, hypersensitivity, autoimmunity and adverse immunostimulation (see 2002 FDA guidance entitled, "Immunotoxicology Evaluation of Investigational New Drugs"). As discussed above, an immunogenic product can alter a biologic's toxicity profile. Immunotoxicity may also result from products that are intended to stimulate or suppress the immune system, or that change the expression of surface antigens on target cells. With such products, animal studies should be implemented to address the potential for autoimmunity. All animal species are not immunologically similar; therefore, a comparison of the structure and function of the human immune system and the immune system of the animal model is necessary for the selection of a relevant animal model for immunotoxicology studies, for designing these studies, and for data interpretation (Haley, 2003).

Product Characterization Safety concerns may arise from the presence of impurities or contaminants in the biological product; therefore, it is essential that the product meet specifications for purity, safety (free of adventitious agents), sterility, identity, and potency throughout nonclinical and clinical testing. The actual tests required for product safety testing depend on the product's source and nature, as well as the method of manufacture. Nonclinical product testing includes the rabbit pyrogen test as part of the purity analysis, the general safety test in guinea pigs and mice (which is performed primarily as a check on the adequacy of the filling procedure of the final containers to ensure that extraneous toxic substances have not been introduced and is not intended as a safety test of the product itself), and *in vitro* or *in vivo* tests for potency, such as animal studies assessing the immunogenicity of vaccines. The product class and the phase of clinical investigations will influence which nonclinical product tests are required. For example, the general safety test is not required for therapeutic DNA plasmid products, therapeutic synthetic peptide products of 40 or fewer amino acids, monoclonal antibody products for *in vivo* use, therapeutic recombinant DNA-derived products, blood products, or cellular therapy products (21 CFR 601.2(a), 21 CFR 610.11(g)). Also, while potency tests are not required for gene therapy products used in Phase 1 clinical trials, the development of these assays should be underway at that point. Product-specific safety concerns may necessitate additional nonclinical product testing, such as the neurovirulence test for live or attenuated vaccines.

Comparability testing for each lot of the biologic must be performed to assure that the product used for nonclinical studies meets the same specifications as the product used in the clinical trials. Manufacturers of biologic products often modify the manufacturing procedure during product development to improve the quality, yield or manufacturing efficiency of their product (FDA Comparability Guidance, 1996). Since biologics are difficult to manufacture consistently, changes in the manufacturing procedure could alter the safety, purity or potency of a biologic product. Comparability studies are conducted to demonstrate that the pre-change and post-change products are highly similar, and that no adverse effects on safety or efficacy resulted from the manufacturing change. Comparability determination can include analytical tests, *in vitro* or *in vivo* biological assays, nonclinical safety studies and clinical studies. Comparability studies in animals may be required to assess the effect of manufacturing process changes on the product's pharmacokinetics, activity, or toxicity, since these parameters cannot be sufficiently evaluated with analytical testing methods (FDA Comparability Guidance, 1996). Nonclinical studies are also used to assess any changes in immunogenicity elicited by the post-change product, since manufacturing changes can alter the structure of the protein product and these alterations may lead to enhanced immunogenicity. The nature of the biologic product, the scope of the manufacturing process change, and the stage of product development must be considered in assessing the degree of testing required to demonstrate comparability.

Product-Specific Nonclinical Issues for Biologics The properties of each specific class of biologic product necessitate that the nonclinical development plan for each biologic be individually tailored. In addition, the clinical indication for which the biologic is intended has a bearing on which studies are required in the nonclinical plan. For example, carcinogenicity testing is not required for oncology agents, but should be considered for immunosuppressant agents, since these agents can be associated with increased cancer risk. The exhibit below identifies some of the nonclinical issues associated with certain classes of biologics. To ensure that the nonclinical plan is sufficient to aid in risk-assessment decisions, it is imperative that the plan be discussed with the FDA prior to the initiation of the studies, preferably in a pre-IND meeting.

Nonclinical Issues Pertinent to Specific Classes of Biologic Products

Product Class	Class-Specific Nonclinical Issues
Monoclonal Antibodies	immunogenicity, stability, tissue cross-reactivity, effector mechanisms
Somatic Cell Therapy	biodistribution, trafficking, and persistence of the cells, ancillary product testing
Gene Therapy	biodistribution, persistence, and genomic integration of the vector, species specificity of the transduced gene, permissiveness for infection by viral vectors, duration and level of gene expression
Recombinant Proteins	immunogenicity, autoimmunity
Therapeutic Vaccines against homologous proteins (i.e., cancer vaccines)	tissue distribution of antigen, autoimmunity, cytokine release, immunogenicity
Preventive Vaccines	enhancement of the intended disease, autoimmunity, tolerance, cytokine release, immunogenicity, protection from disease

Monoclonal Antibody (mAb) Products Nonclinical issues regarding monoclonal antibodies are addressed in the EMEA's 1995 directive entitled, "Production and Quality Control of Monoclonal Antibodies," and the FDA's 1997 guidance document entitled, "Points to Consider in the Manufacturing and Testing of Monoclonal Antibody Products for Human Use." Monoclonal antibody (mAb) products include intact immunoglobulins produced by hybridomas, immunoconjugates, and immunoglobulin fragments and recombinant proteins derived from immunoglobulins, such as chimeric and humanized immunoglobulins, F(ab') and F(ab')^2 fragments, single-chain antibodies, and recombinant immunoglobulin variable regions. Mechanism of action studies for mAbs should include *in vitro* and *in vivo* studies for antibody specificity, affinity, and efficacy. When designing a nonclinical development program, mAb product properties such as immunogenicity, stability, tissue cross-reactivity, and effector mechanisms should be carefully addressed. Prior to Phase 1 testing in humans, the cross-reactivity of a mAb product to a panel of normal human tissues or human cells *in vitro* must be evaluated to determine if the antibody binds to non-target organ tissue (Points to Consider in the Manufacture and Testing of Monoclonal Antibody Products for Human Use, FDA 1997). In addition, the stability of immunoconjugates should be evaluated *in vitro* in pooled human serum at 37°C and *in vivo* in pharmacokinetic studies. Since manufacturing changes often occur in the development of mAb products, further *in vitro* or *in vivo* nonclinical studies may be required to demonstrate comparability between product lots.

Somatic Cell Therapy In the 1998 "Guidance for Human Somatic Cell Therapy and Gene Therapy," the FDA defines somatic cell therapy as "the administration to humans of autologous, allogeneic, or xenogeneic living cells which have been manipulated or processed *ex vivo*." Examples of somatic cell therapies include immunotherapies, such as activated dendritic cells and tumor-infiltrating lymphocytes, and stem-cell reconstitution therapies for use after myeloablative chemotherapy, such as CD34+ hematopoietic stem cells. Due to the strict species specificity of many cellular therapy products, staff in CBER's Office of Cellular, Tissues and Gene Therapies (OCTGT) should be consulted for agreement on nonclinical study designs prior to initiating any studies. An animal model of disease can often be used to study the homologous animal cellular therapy product to provide information on *in vivo* function, survival time, and trafficking of the manipulated cells. Toxicology studies should be conducted in a relevant animal model, and should evaluate distribution, trafficking, and persistence of the cells in addition to the standard toxicity parameters. Depending on the nature of the cellular therapy product, carcinogenicity testing may also be required.

Cellular therapy products are often manufactured using ancillary products. Ancillary products are defined as products used in the manufacture of other products intended for *in vivo* use. Ancillary products include monoclonal antibodies that are used for the purification of other products (*ex vivo* purging of cells to remove tumor cells), and cytokines or growth factors used in the *ex vivo* culturing of cellular therapies. The primary concern with ancillary products is that they could potentially affect the quality (i.e., safety, purity, and potency) of the final therapeutic product. The quality of ancillary products should be characterized in a similar fashion as products intended for *in vivo* administration. Tests for potency will often include *in vitro* or *in vivo* assays that demonstrate that the ancillary product functions as required in the process to manufacture the therapeutic product.

Gene Therapy Gene therapy is defined as any recombinant DNA product used to prevent, treat, diagnose or cure diseases in humans. Gene therapy products can be characterized as either "in vivo" or "ex vivo" products, depending on whether they are directly administered to the patient or are administered as a component of a cellular therapy product. The final formulated gene therapy product should be used in the nonclinical studies. Changing the formulation (e.g., by adding liposomes, altering pH, or adjusting salt concentration) may modify the biodistribution of the product and thereby affect bioactivity or toxicity. In designing nonclinical studies for gene therapy products, factors such as the species specificity of the transduced gene, permissiveness for infection by viral vectors, and comparative physiology should be considered. Bioactivity studies provide the rationale for the introduction of the gene therapy product into human clinical trials. These studies should be designed to determine the duration and level of gene expression, the dose-response relationship, and the optimal route of administration and dosing regimen to be used in the clinical trial. In certain situations, such as with an oncology product, efficacy studies in animal models can be used to support the safety of gene therapy products if the animal is monitored for toxicity endpoints during the efficacy study.

Safety issues of significant concern with gene therapy products include the distribution of the vector from the site of injection and the genomic integration of vector sequences. Biodistribution studies are necessary to determine the distribution and persistence of the vector in non-target organs. Of particular importance is the vector distribution to the germ cells; therefore, testicular and ovarian tissues must be analyzed in nonclinical studies for the presence of the gene therapy product. Other tissues that should be evaluated in the biodistribution study include peripheral blood, tissue at the injection site, highly perfused organs such as brain, liver, kidneys, heart, and spleen, as well as tissues that could be affected due to the route of administration or the toxicity of the transgene. The presence of the vector sequence in tissues can be evaluated via DNA-PCR methodology designed to detect a sequence unique to the product. If vector sequences are observed in non-target tissues, studies should be conducted to determine whether the gene is expressed and/or associated with any toxicity (Pilaro, 1999). Often, the safety and biodistribution of vectors can be evaluated in the same toxicology study. Toxicology testing should obtain information regarding the toxicities related to the vector delivery system and the safety of the expressed gene. Vector persistence, *in vivo* expression of the transgene, identification of the target organs, and the reversibility of toxicities should be determined. As the gene therapy product's clinical development progresses, nonclinical studies must address genetic toxicity, chronic toxicity, and reproductive toxicity to support marketing approval. Factors such as the properties of the vector, the transgene product, the delivery system, and the clinical indication must be considered in the design and implementation of these studies (Frederickson, 2003).

Recombinant Proteins Recombinant proteins include such products as cytokines, growth factors, enzymes, and fusion proteins. As discussed above, the species specificity of certain recombinant protein products (e.g., cytokines) may dictate that the most relevant model for safety assessment is the use of a homologous protein in a relevant species. Of particular concern for recombinant proteins is the immunogenicity of the product due to foreign protein responses or the induction of autoimmunity if the protein cross-reacts with normal tissues. The immunogenicity of the therapeutic protein can be assessed in blood samples collected at relevant times from appropriately designed, repeated-dose toxicology studies. A complete characterization of the antibody response (including titer, neutralizing or non-neutralizing status, effects on clearance, and number of responding animals) generally is necessary to interpret whether antibody formation was affecting pharmacokinetic, pharmacodynamic or toxicologic parameters (ICH S6). This complete characterization requires the development and validation of appropriate immuno- and cell-based assays.

Preventive and Therapeutic Vaccines Regulated by CBER's Office of Vaccine Research and Review, preventive vaccines are a heterogeneous class of agents, including peptides, viral and bacterial vectored products, nucleic acid products, as well as traditional vaccines such as live or attenuated viruses. Nonclinical study requirements will depend on the type of vaccine, route of administration, and patient population. For example, reproductive toxicology studies are required if the vaccine will be used in women of child-bearing potential or pregnant women, since the vaccine may cause fetal infections resulting in fetal abnormalities. Product-specific studies include biodistribution, duration and genomic integration studies for plasmid DNA vaccines, neurovirulence studies for live or attenuated vaccines, and studies evaluating reversion to virulence for attenuated organisms or toxins.

Potential safety concerns associated with vaccines include general systemic toxicity, the enhancement of the targeted disease, the induction of local toxicity, pyrogenicity, adverse immunologic effects such as autoimmunity or sensitization and, in some cases, teratogenic/reproductive effects (CPMP Vaccine Guidance, 1998). In contrast to most other biologic products and drugs, doses evaluated in vaccine nonclinical studies are not scaled on body weight or surface area, but rather on total dose. Vaccine efficacy should be demonstrated in protection studies in which a relevant animal model is challenged with the pathogenic organism after vaccination. Immunogenicity studies are conducted to determine the potency of the vaccine. Additional nonclinical immune function studies should be conducted to determine tolerance, production of immune complexes that can enhance the disease, the release of cytokines that may affect the functions of the immune system, and hypersensitivity reactions (CPMP Vaccine Guidance, 1998).

Unlike preventive vaccines, all therapeutic vaccines are currently regulated by CBER's OCTGT. Therapeutic vaccines can include monoclonal antibodies (anti-idiotype vaccines), peptides, recombinant proteins, cellular therapy and gene therapy. Therefore, the product-specific issues discussed above will also be applicable. Most therapeutic vaccines are designed to target homologous proteins (e.g., cancer vaccines that produce immunity to tumor-associated antigens). Tumor-associated antigens are either expressed solely in tumor tissue or have more prevalent expression in tumor tissue compared to normal tissue. Therefore, it is essential to determine if a vaccine targeting a tumor-associated antigen has the potential to cause autoimmunity to normal tissues. The level of expression of the tumor-associated antigen in a panel of normal human tissues should be evaluated. The autoimmune potential of peptide vaccines should be further assessed by performing a homology search in a protein database to determine the abundance of the peptide amino acid sequence in all known proteins. Depending on the immunogenic properties of the cancer vaccine, it may be prudent to further evaluate the potential for autoimmune-mediated toxicity in relevant animal models.

NONCLINICAL SAFETY TESTING: GENERAL TECHNICAL AND SCIENTIFIC CONSIDERATIONS

The proper design of a toxicology study requires an excellent understanding of the regulatory requirements and expectations, standard good industry practices, and hands-on experience in animal husbandry and study execution. Most toxicology laboratories have extensive experience in conducting different types of nonclinical studies, and are undoubtedly a useful source of information and guidance. Experienced study directors with proper toxicology training are exposed to a wide variety of complex and unusual problems, findings, and challenges, and should, therefore, be involved in all discussions regarding the design of a study protocol. In all cases, the toxicology study design should be customized for the product under development so that scientific, regulatory, and corporate objectives are met.

General Study Design Concepts Ideally, a study design should include at least one control group (some studies may require two control groups—for example, inhalation studies using an air control and a vehicle control group) and three treated groups. The studies ideally should include a full safety assessment, including but not limited to clinical signs and detailed examinations, body weight, food consumption, ophthalmology, electrocardiogram (non-rodents only), clinical pathology (hematology, serum chemistry, coagulation, urinalysis), gross pathology (macroscopic examination and selected organ weights), and histopathology. In addition, the assessment of systemic exposure and its relation to observed toxicities, or lack thereof, is a critical component of any toxicology study. Therefore, toxicokinetic assessments should also be integrated into the study design whenever possible. Accordingly, an appropriate number of satellite animals (rodents) should be used in appropriate groups to assure that blood collection for special analyses (e.g., immunogenicity) or toxicokinetic profile determination will not compromise the safety data. One must also carefully consider adding recovery groups (as a minimum in the control and high dose groups) in pivotal studies to determine the reversibility of the observed toxicities.

Animal safety studies should also comply with Good Laboratory Practice (GLP) regulations (21 CFR part 58). The GLP regulations set forth standards for conducting and reporting nonclinical safety studies used to support or intended to support FDA-regulated clinical research or U.S. marketing approval. The regulations cover corporate organization and personnel, facilities, equipment, testing facilities operation, test and control article documentation, the study protocol, record keeping and reporting, and procedures for disqualifying testing facilities. The purpose of the GLP regulations is to assure the quality and integrity of the nonclinical safety data submitted to regulatory agencies. The GLP regulations were developed to apply to a broad variety of studies, test articles and test systems. In general, any definitive study intended to support the safety of a pharmaceutical should be conducted according to GLP regulations. Such studies include those addressing genetic toxicity, safety pharmacology, general toxicity, reproductive and developmental toxicity, and carcinogenicity. GLP regulations do not apply to all studies, however. For example, GLP compliance may not be required—or even be possible—when disease model systems are employed for testing the safety of gene therapy products. Sponsors should consult the FDA to determine whether certain key studies supporting safety can be conducted without full compliance with GLP provisions

Species Selection As discussed, one of the most important factors in designing a toxicology program is the selection of appropriate animal species—many times referred to as the test system. Indeed, the selection of proper animal species will optimize the usefulness of the safety data generated and improve its predictiveness for effects in humans.

Historically, animal species were selected based on little or no considerations beyond practicality and availability. The selection of species for any toxicology program requires multiple careful considerations before the toxicology program's initiation. The most commonly used rodent and non-rodent species in safety testing are presented in the exhibit below.

Justifications to support the choice of the species used in a toxicology program are now expected, and sponsors are required to provide a scientifically sound rationale supporting the relevancy of the species used. One of the key factors that will determine the relevance of a species is the presence (or absence) of the intended biological effects of the pharmaceutical. In addition, special considerations should be given to the ADME profile (e.g., pharmacokinetic profile and *in vitro* and *in vivo* metabolism) of the product, since the species selected should be as similar as possible to humans. Other criteria, such as animal availability, potential test article requirements (dogs can require approximately three to four times more test article than monkeys assuming a similar safety profile), physiology and biology (rats do not have a gall bladder), availability of historical databases and expertise for that species (limited number of laboratories can conduct primate reproductive studies), regulatory requirements, costs (monkeys are more expensive than dogs), and route of administration (continuous intravenous infusion is not easy in mice) should all be considered in the selection process. Ultimately, the species selected should be the ones with a relevant biological activity and a comparable ADME profile to humans while fulfilling regulatory requirements and practical, corporate and technical considerations.

Dose Level Selection A scientifically valid toxicology study ideally should establish a high dose level at which toxicity is observed in animals so that these potential human toxicities may be carefully monitored or avoided in clinical trials. Establishing a low dose at which no toxicity is observed is typically required for most indications. Doses should be high enough to induce toxicity, unless limitations restrict the achievable doses in these studies (e.g., dose volume, solubility). Generally, dose levels for pivotal repeated-dose toxicology studies are selected based on the results of acute and dose range-finding toxicology studies. Ideally, the study design should include at least one control group and three treated groups.

Common Animal Species Used in Nonclinical Safety Testing

Type	Species	Commonly Used Strain	Comments
Rodents	Mice	BALB/c, CD-1, C57BL/6	Limited blood volume, size is limiting for instrumentation, low test article needs, good historical databases
	Rats	Sprague-Dawley	Good size, good historical databases, easy instrumentation, higher test article need as compared to mouse
	Hamsters	Golden Syrian	Good size, good historical databases, easy instrumentation, aggressive nature
	Guinea-Pigs	Hartley	Good historical databases
Non-rodents	Rabbits	New-Zealand	Blood volume not limiting, species typically used for reproductive toxicology studies and/or vaccine safey assessment
	Cats	Variable	Excellent for neurology studies, special housing and handling, GLP facilities with experience are limited, good suppliers are limited and supply is heterogeneous
	Mini-Pigs	Yucatan	Size allow easy instrumentation including devices, good model for dermal product, test article need is major, animal availability is limited, GLP facilities with experience are limited
	Dogs	Beagle	Blood volume not limiting, size allow easy instrumentation including devices, test article need is major
	Monkeys	Marmoset	Small size require less test article, easy to handle, animal availability is limited, seasonal breeding pattern can be a problem, GLP facilities with experience are limited, small size limit blood sampling
		Cynomolgus	Blood volume not limiting, size allow easy instrumentation including devices, animal availability can be limited, special handling and housing requirements, availability of sexually mature animals is limited
		Rhesus	
	Pigs	Yorkshire	Blood volume not limiting, size allow easy instrumentation including devices, test article need is major, GLP facilities with experience are limited

Accordingly, the initial toxicology program should be designed to provide the required key information on the pharmaceutical's safety profile and allow the projection of appropriate dose levels for subsequent repeated-dose toxicology studies.

Pre-established dose levels based on multiples of the expected efficacious clinical dose is usually a sub-optimal approach. This approach carries the risk of testing doses that will not support later clinical needs in cases in which higher doses than anticipated are needed. It also carries the risk of providing little information on potential toxicities and the steepness of the dose response if toxicity is not achieved. This then leads to problems in designing appropriate monitoring procedures and dose escalation schemes.

Route of Administration The route of administration must be selected carefully based on multiple considerations, including physicochemical properties, pharmacokinetics, pharmacodynamics, intended therapeutic use, technical practicality, marketability, and patient compliance. The route of administration selected for the toxicology program should be similar to the proposed route for the clinical investigations. The failure to consider the route of administration in a toxicology program carefully can lead to serious problems as the program progresses. For example, the route of administration will significantly affect the amount of test article that is required. Continuous intravenous infusion studies require substantially more test article than studies that involve the administration of the same dose by intravenous bolus (due to the dead volumes in the pumps, reservoirs, and tubing).

Extrapolating Doses Between Species A critical step in assessing human risk is the extrapolation of doses associated with hazards in animals to humans. A common misconception is that, when doses are normalized to body weight (i.e., expressed in mg/kg), a given dose will generate an equivalent effect across species. For the majority of systemically administered small molecules, this is not true. Like many biologic parameters, equivalent doses are related by a power equation in which dose = a(body weight)^b. Doses of small-molecule therapeutics administered systemically to animals are usually assumed to scale well between species when the exponent b=0.67, which also defines the relationship of body surface area (m^2) to body weight. Therefore, a dose expressed in mg/m^2 is believed to have reasonably equivalent effects across species of widely varying size. The physiologic reasons for this relationship are complex and beyond the scope of this chapter (West 1999, Gilooly 2001, Darveau 2002). The FDA guidance entitled, "Estimating the Maximum Safe Starting Dose in Initial Clinical Trials for Therapeutics in Adult Healthy Volunteers" also explains the basis for interspecies dose extrapolation. This guidance also provides the standard factors for converting doses between different species.

The exhibit below identifies the factors for converting doses between different species. Note that while these dose conversion factors work well for small molecules, they may not be appropriate for extrapolating doses of biologics or locally administered products (e.g., topical products or products administered to compartments such as the CNS or the eye).

Equivalent Dose Conversion Factors

Factors for converting doses expressed in mg/kg from one species to an approximate equi-effect dose expressed in mg/kg in a second species. The calculation assumes equi-effect doses scale approximately according to (body weight), which defines the relationship of body surface area to body weight, and that there are no major differences in metabolism, protein binding, bioavailability (if oral), or routes of administration between the two species. The factors in the table were derived from the factors for converting mg/kg doses to doses based on body surface area (mg/m2) in each species as listed in the FDA guidance entitled, "Estimating the Maximum Safe Starting Dose in Initial Clinical Trials for Therapeutics in Adult Healthy Volunteers." These conversion factors are: mouse, 3; rat, 6; rabbit and monkey, 12; dog, 20, human, 37. For example, a 10 mg/kg/day in mice is 30 mg/m2 whereas a 10 mg/kg/day dose in dogs is 200 mg/m2. The dog-equivalent to a 10 mg/kg mouse dose is 1.5 mg/kg.

Species	Mouse	Rat	Rabbit	Monkey	Dog	Human
Body Weight (kg)	0.02	0.15	3	3	12	60
Mouse	1	0.25	0.25	0.25	0.15	0.08
Rat	2	1	0.5	0.5	0.30	0.16
Rabbit	4	2	1	1	0.60	0.33
Monkey	4	2	1	1	0.60	0.33
Dog	7	3.3	1.7	1.7	1	0.5
Human	12	6.1	3	3	2	1

Dose Volumes and Good Practices The most common mistake in toxicology testing is the use of an inappropriate dose volume to administer the product in animals, especially in less-experienced laboratories. Readers are strongly recommended to refer to several publications (Derelanko MJ, 2001; Hull RM, 1995, Roy D, 2004, Diehl KH, 2001) on the subject before making decisions on dose volumes. As a rule of thumb, the selected dose volume should never compromise the study's scientific integrity. When the physicochemical properties of a test article dictate that the maximum feasible dose (i.e., maximal biocompatible concentration given at the maximal recommended dose volume) will be reached before significant toxicity is achieved, the maximum feasible dose should not be exceeded.

Establishing Timelines Developing timelines for toxicology studies requires an understanding of the different phases of each study. As depicted in the exhibit below, the in-life (dosing) phase of each study (represented by the solid area) only represents a fraction of the overall timeline. Indeed, pre-study activities which include the contractual agreement, protocol writing/finalization, and animal ordering must be completed prior to animals being brought into the testing facility. Once the animals arrive at the facility, there is a rest period during which the animals are allowed to acclimate to their new environment and recover from the stresses of transportation, transfer and manipulations. Another major component of the time involved in conducting a study is the in-life portion, which usually is the time used to identify a study. For example, a three-month toxicology study is one where animals are typically treated for three consecutive months (total duration of the dosing). Once the in-life portion of a study has been completed, the samples generated need to be processed and analyzed, the data compiled and a report written. The amount of time required to complete this part of a toxicology study is often underestimated and can cause confusion in project timelines. Ten to 12 weeks is the typical time required by most GLP toxicology laboratories to generate a report. From the end of the in-life phase where animals are euthanized and tissues collected for histopathology examination, at least four to six weeks are generally required for getting an assessment from the pathology laboratory. During this time, tissues are processed, fixed, trimmed, embedded, cut, mounted on slides, stained, and covered before they can be reviewed by a pathologist. Adding some quality control process, or any need to re-cut or reprocess some tissues for a few animals, can extend those timelines. With a typical rodent study design including 20 animals per sex per group times 4 groups at approximately 60 tissues each (total of 9600 tissues), one can easily appreciate the amount of work involved in reading the slides and annotating the findings.

Pharmacokinetic sample analysis and reporting can also be time intensive and delay the overall report if not carefully scheduled. The rest of the time required for reporting is study director authoring, quality assurance review, scientific review, and non-technical review.

Study Timelines

Time Scale (Weeks/Months)

Pre-Study	Acclimation	In-Life	Reporting
·Test Article ·Protocol ·Contract ·Animal Supply	·Rats: 1-2 wks ·Dogs: 4 wks ·Monkeys: 4-6 wks	·Treatment ·Clinical Signs ·Body Weight ·Food Consumption ·Ophthalmology ·Clinical Pathology ·Toxicokinetics ·Cardiovascular (ECG) ·Necropsy ·Histopathology	·TK Analysis ·Clinical Pathology ·Histopathology ·Recovery ·Data Compilation ·Data Analysis ·Quality Assurance

Typical Cost Estimates The toxicology program usually consumes most of the initial financial resources allocated for nonclinical development of a product candidate. Most companies therefore have a great interest in obtaining precise external cost estimates for their toxicology program. External costs are the costs associated with subcontracting the toxicology study to a GLP-compliant contract research organization (CRO). Study costs can vary greatly depending on the animal species, the route of administration, the duration of treatment, the laboratory selected, and the economic situation of the laboratory or of the CRO market. Differences in study costs between toxicology CROs should be expected even for an identical study design. Reputation, experience, quality, timeliness, professionalism, financial status, sophistication of instrumentation, and company organization are all contributing factors that will lead to appreciable cost variations between CROs. Additional costs should also be expected when specific or specialized analyses such as special stains, histopathological examinations, or clinical chemistry parameters, specific cardiovascular assessments, or toxicokinetic analyses and modeling are requested.

Reporting cost estimates for toxicology studies is of uncertain value as the costs can become outdated in a relatively short period of time, depending on the nuances of the marketplace. The cost estimates outlined in this chapter nonetheless provide a good reflection of the actual market and can be used to estimate the projected toxicology program costs. The exhibit below presents cost estimates and typical durations for report generation for most toxicology studies generally conducted for most products. These estimates may vary greatly depending on the study design, the species selected, the type and nature of the analyses conducted during the study, and the toxicology CRO selected. In addition, the cost estimates provided do not include test article costs, analytical method development and validation, toxicokinetic sample assessment and modeling, special histopathology assessment and/or tissue collection, special clinical pathology, satellite groups for toxicokinetics, recovery groups, or modified study designs.

Outsourcing Safety Studies For many companies, the technical and regulatory requirements relating to the conduct of nonclinical safety studies will require the use of external laboratories. Such laboratories will allow a company to produce valid nonclinical safety information to support applications to regulatory agencies for advancing the medicinal product to clinical trials. The selection of laboratories that will be responsible for conducting pivotal portions of the tox-

Estimated External Costs for Representative Nonclinical Safety Studies

Study Type	Approximate External Costs[a] (US $)			Approximate Duration[b] (weeks)
SINGLE DOSE AND RANGE-FINDING	Rats	Dogs	Monkeys	
Single Dose	6,000-25,000	20,000-50,000	20,000-70,000	10 to 12
Combined Single and 7-day Repeat Dose	20,000-80,000	40,000-90,000	80,000-120,000	10 to 12
Combined Single and 10-day Repeat Dose	35,000-67,000	45,000-75,000	85,000-125,000	10 to 12
REPEAT-DOSE TOXICOLOGY	Rats	Dogs	Monkeys	
7-day Repeat Dose	20,000-35,000	34,000-70,000	55,000-75,000	14 to 16
14-Day Repeat-Dose	40,000-115,000	90,000-130,000	100,000-190,000	14 to 16
28-Day Repeat-Dose	70,000-150,000	100,000-225,000	300,000-500,000	16 to 18
3-Month Repeat-Dose	110,000-270,000	200,000-300,000	450,000-700,000	30 to 34
6-Month Repeat-Dose	215,000-350,000	450,000-500,000	550,000-800,000	40 to 44
9-Month Repeat-Dose	275,000-375,000	250,000-500,000	600,000-1,000,000	52 to 56
12-Month Repeat-Dose	400,000-550,000	500,000-650,000	800,000-1,200,000	68 to 74
GENETIC TOXICOLOGY				
Ames Test	5,000-10,000			8 to 12
In vitro Chromosomal Aberration Assay	10,000-35,000			12 to 16
In vivo Micronucleus Test (mice/rats)	10,000-30,000			12 to 16
REPRODUCTIVE TOXICOLOGY	Mice / Rats		Rabbits	
Fertility Study: Rats	75,000-160,000		-	20 to 24
Range Finding Developmental Toxicity	30,000-50,000		40,000-60,000	12 to 16
Developmental Toxicity	60,000-145,000		125,000-175,000	16 to 24
Peri- and Post-Natal /Multigeneration	155,000-250,000		-	22 to 42

a   Cost may vary greatly depending on study design, the species selected, and the Contract Research Organization. Costs do not include test article costs, analytical method development and validation, toxicokinetic sample assessment and modeling, special histopathology assessment and/or tissue collection, or special clinical pathology.

b   Approximate duration represents the total duration starting from the initiation of treatment up to the completion of an audited draft report.

icology program usually necessitates much focused attention, but is often an area that is readily neglected, especially when staff is overburdened with other tasks. The exhibit below outlines criteria for selecting a toxicology CRO.

SUMMARY: THE FINE BALANCE BETWEEN SOUND SCIENCE, REGULATORY EXPECTATIONS, AND CORPORATE OBJECTIVES

Nonclinical programs are complex and a complete integration of multiple disciplines, including chemistry, manufacturing and controls (CMC), clinical, regulatory, corporate, legal, and project management, is required in order to successfully implement the program.

Overall, the toxicology program needs to support the proposed clinical trials from Phase 1 to a marketing application. Indeed, it is critical to understand that the toxicology program will likely not be efficient or successful if the clinical approach contemplated has not been clearly defined (i.e., targeted population, route of administration, dosing regimen, treatment duration, and development timeline). This does not imply that a fully defined clinical protocol needs to be in place before initiating the toxicology program, but rather that the critical components are known or at least estimated so that the toxicology program can be tailor-made for the clinical approach.

Another component that needs to be considered when designing a toxicology program is the corporate objectives of the company. Nonclinical program strategists often hear that, even though they have provided the most scientifically sound toxicology program for their product, the project will not be viable for the company if it is time or cost intensive. Obviously, from a corporate perspective, the toxicology program should be short and inexpensive, but of sufficient quality and informational content so that safety can be thoroughly addressed and that no major questions are raised either internally or by the regulatory agencies. Therefore, one of the biggest challenges for the toxicologist is trying to find the

Criteria for Selecting Toxicology CROs

Criteria	Comments
Expertise	Make sure the laboratory has the experience to conduct the type of studies requested. Relying solely on corporate brochures or assurances is not a reliable method.
Responsiveness	The laboratory should be able to respond to your requests and be reachable when needed. Important delays in returning calls or for providing information on a study are good indicators of potential responsiveness problems.
Organization	The level of organization in a toxicology laboratory usually greatly reflects the level of organization in your study.
Staff Qualification and Experience	Study Directors, technical staff and experts involved in the conduct of the study should be qualified (training records, education). Unqualified personnel invariably lead to problems in studies. At an initial visit, the people that you meet are most likely not going to be the people conducting your study.
Localization / Accessibility	The laboratory should be accessible. Time zone differences complicate communication and require more intensive management and traveling.
Costs / Timelines	Costs vary greatly between different laboratories for the same design. Decisions made strictly based on costs are discouraged, as it is not by itself a reliable decision making criterion.
Species Availability	The laboratory should not only have access to the appropriate species selected for your program but should also have significant experience working with them.
Reliability	One of the key determinants in filing a regulatory submission within the established timeline.
GLP Compliance	Conducting qualification audit prior to making final decision should be done to insure current GLP status. Laboratory status changes over time and they may be experiencing some major GLP compliance issues.
Capacity	Overworked employees and over-loaded animal facilities will almost certainly lead to multiple mistakes or problems during the study conduct.
Reputation	Good laboratories will strive to maintain their reputation by meeting sponsor's demands. Time in the business is also a good indicator. Scientific meeting attendance is a good way to learn about the different laboratories.

right balance between the corporate needs and sound science while satisfying current regulatory agency expectations. This quest for the best compromise often leads to a series of unwise decisions, which eventually results in serious problems during the toxicology program. The serious problems may look to the untrained observer like a complete failure in planning due to severe strategic or scientific deficiencies. In reality, the problem is often the culmination of many small, apparently insignificant risks taken at different times during the development process for the wrong reasons rather than an inadequate plan to start with.

Nonclinical studies are performed at various stages of medicinal product development with the eventual goal of supporting the safety of the marketed product. Early in development, nonclinical studies for all pharmaceuticals are designed to allow determination of a reasonably safe starting dose and escalation scheme for use in humans by revealing the toxicity profile (i.e., the target organs, the dose-response and the reversibility of the observed toxicities) in appropriate animal models. In addition, nonclinical data identify the safety parameters that need to be monitored in the clinical trials. As clinical development proceeds, nonclinical studies are needed to continue to address the expanding risks and to eventually provide a complete safety profile that supports the marketing of the product. While there are many commonalities to the core battery of studies that are expected for most pharmaceuticals, there is no one approach that fits all. Formulating a nonclinical development plan specific for the pharmaceutical is thus a critical step. Although the purpose of nonclinical studies for biologic products is similar to drug products, the approach for obtaining relevant safety information may be much more challenging. Each biologic product has unique properties that should be considered when designing the safety program. The FDA encourages sponsors to discuss their product plans with the agency early in development in a pre-IND setting. Presentation and discussion of the nonclinical and clinical study plans with FDA scientists in a pre-IND meeting can facilitate the advancement of the product into clinical trials by identifying problematic areas prior to IND filing. Open communication with the FDA should continue throughout product development to assure that the proper strategy is being employed for achieving marketing approval.

Designing a toxicology program to support initial clinical trials is only the beginning of this critical component of overall development. Poor financial planning, inadequate design of studies, inappropriate species selection, non-optimized study scheduling, haphazard CRO selection, and inadequate monitoring activities can all introduce significant delays and risks of failure into the nonclinical safety development program. A cost-effective, time-efficient, scientifically sound, and information-rich nonclinical safety program should be the goal of all who endeavor to expedite the development of new pharmaceuticals.

Careful attention to the issues presented in this chapter should minimize the potential for major problems and allow for efficient integration of the nonclinical program into the overall development plan.

References

Cavagnaro, JA. Preclinical safety evaluation of biotechnology-derived pharmaceuticals. *Nat Rev Drug Discov.* 2002; 1:469-475.

Chirino AJ, Ary ML, Marshall SA. Minimizing the immunogenicity of protein therapeutics. *Drug Discov Today*, 2004; 9:82-90.

Darveau CA, Suarez RK, Andrews RD, Hochachka PW. Allometric cascade as a unifying principle of body mass effects on metabolism. *Nature*, 2002; 417:166-170.

Derelanko MJ, Hollinger MA. Handbook of Toxicology, Second Edition, New York: CRC Press, 2001.

Diehl KH, Hull R, Morton D, Pfister R, Rabemampianina Y, Smith D, Vidal J-M, Vorstenbosch CV. A good practice guide to the administration of substances and removal of blood, including routes and volumes, *J Appl Toxicol.*, 2001; 21:15-23.

Frederickson RM, Carter BJ, Pilaro AM. Nonclinical toxicology in support of licensure of gene therapies, *Mol Ther.*, 2003; 8:8-10.

Fredholm BB, Fleming WW, Vanhoutte PM, Godfraind T. The role of pharmacology in drug discovery, *Nat Rev Drug Discov.*, 2002; 1:237-238.

Gillooly JF, Brown JH, West GB, Savage VM, Charnov EL. Effects of size and temperature on metabolic rate, *Science*, 2001; 293:2248-2251.

Green JD, Black LE. Overview status of preclinical safety assessment for immunomodulatory biopharmaceuticals, *Hum Exp Toxicol.*, 2000; 19:208-212.

Haley, PJ. Species difference in the structure and function of the immune system, *Toxicology*, 2003; 188:49-71.

Hull RM. Guideline limit volumes for dosing animals in the preclinical stage of safety evaluation, *Human Exp Toxicol.*, 1995;14:305-307.

Imboden M, Shi F, Pugh TD, Freud AG, Thom NJ, Hank JA, Hao Z, Staelin ST, Sondel PM, Mahvi DM. Safety of interleukin-12 gene therapy against cancer: a murine biodistribution and toxicity study, *Hum Gene Ther.*, 2003; 14:1037-1048.

Koren E, Zuckerman LA, Mire-Sluis AR. Immune responses to therapeutic proteins in humans—clinical significance, assessment and prediction, *Curr Pharm Biotechnol.*, 2002; 3:349-360.

Leake, CD. The pharmacologic evaluation of new drugs, *JAMA*, 1929; 93:1632-1634.

Pilaro AM, Serabian MA. Preclinical development strategies for novel gene therapeutic products, *Toxicol Pathol.*, 1999; 27:4-7.

Roy D, Andrews PA. Nonclinical testing: from theory to practice, In: Anticancer Drug Development Guide: Preclinical Screening, Clinical trials, and Approval, 2nd Ed, BA Teicher and PA Andrews (eds), Totowa: Humana Press, 2004; pp 287-311.

Serabian M, Pilaro AM. Safety assessment of biotechnology-derived pharmaceuticals: ICH and beyond, *Toxicol Pathol.*, 1999; 27:27-31.

West GB, Brown JH, Enquist BJ. The fourth dimension of life: fractal geometry and allometric scaling of organisms, *Science*, 1999; 284:1677-1679.

Wierda D, Smith HW, Zwickl CM. Immunogenicity of biopharmaceuticals in laboratory animals, *Toxicology*, 2001;158:71-74.

United States Good Laboratory Practices Regulation. Title 21 of the *Code of Federal Regulations*, Part 58 (21 CFR part 58).

CHAPTER 5

Clinical Development Plans: Target Product Profile

By Janice M. Soreth, MD, and Steven E. Linberg, PhD

Proper planning is a critical component in the efficient and successful development of pharmaceuticals (drugs and biologics). Even the most modest home is planned well in advance of the start of construction. Blueprints list the location of everything from walls to light switches. Why should homes costing $80,000 have more planning than some drug development programs that will cost on average $800 million (averaging those that succeed, plus those that fail)? The answer is plain and simple: they probably should not.

There are two groups that possess expertise in drug development: the pharmaceutical industry and the FDA. The pharmaceutical industry is motivated to develop good products for the market that will meet a medical need and provide a return on investment that will support future development. Meanwhile, the FDA is charged with supporting better healthcare by fostering the development of safe and effective products, and protecting the public health by keeping other products off the market. The overlap is obvious: the FDA and the pharmaceutical industry have common goals in this process of developing beneficial future products.

The problem has been that communication between the two has not always been what it should be, and the quality and efficiency of pharmaceutical development has not always been what it could be. For that reason, the FDA and the pharmaceutical industry, represented by the Pharmaceutical Research and Manufacturers of America (PhRMA), collaborated in 1997 to develop a pilot program to address this need. That program was called the Targeted Product Information (TPI) pilot. The goal was to refine the "big picture" of development. This is similar to the analogy of taking a good look at the forest and not just the trees. Too many companies focus on building a development program study-by-study, without focusing on exactly where the development is going in the long term. Following the successful implementation of this Targeted Product Information pilot, the revised, full-scale Target Product Profile (TPP) program was expanded in January 2004, and is committed to address the common goal of the FDA and pharmaceutical companies to communicate on development more completely and clearly, with the end goal in mind.

Background and the FDA Perspective

Drug development has never been an easy task, and the FDA would like to do what it can to guide sponsors away from likely problems and toward efficient development. Obviously, the FDA can only address information brought to its attention. Communication is always a challenge, no matter what industry is involved. Part of the communication problem arises from the fact that FDA reviewers change. A sponsor cannot be guaranteed that the same FDA staff will be there through the entire development of a project. Likewise, members of the sponsor's drug development team change, so that the FDA also often has to deal with different players during a product's development. All of this may undermine communication between the sponsor and the FDA. To compound both of these problems, the direction of drug development often changes, so that unless there is a proper flow of information, one side or the other will suffer, often both. From the FDA point of view, poor communication helps no one, and no news is certainly NOT good news. A focused flow of critical information helps all parties involved. The TPI was to serve as the basis for an ongoing FDA-sponsor dialog.

As mentioned above, beginning in early 1997, a small group of FDA and industry representatives from PhRMA member companies embarked on a pilot program to improve the efficiency of pharmaceutical development. The result was a goal-oriented program that targeted the anticipated product description that the company wanted to achieve at product approval. What was known as the Targeted Product Information (TPI) pilot program supported the use of an evolving draft package insert that was to be used during all phases of development.

This concept was not completely new to many companies in the industry. The TPI was based on the idea of a "claims document," and was known by a variety of names, such as Target Product Profile, Target Package Insert, Draft Labeling,

Product Profile, and Concept Document, and in some companies the philosophy did not have a formal name because it was just the way of doing business. In reality, all of these approaches embodied the same principle: the combined interest of the FDA and industry was to formalize and expand this development philosophy into a more widely used practice by other pharmaceutical developers who had not yet been introduced to this concept.

What the TPP Is The sponsor should draft the TPP to guide the design, conduct and analysis of clinical trials. It should be used to summarize the specific studies supporting various indications and claims. At the end of the development program, the data should support the sponsor's desired outcome (i.e., the approval of the targeted labeling for the drug under development), assuming all goes according to plan. Generally, all does not always go according to plan. For that reason, the TPP evolves over time, incorporating new information and revised planning. The current TPP reflects the overall intent of the drug development program, given the totality of knowledge about the compound *at that time*. This serves as the basis for an ongoing dialogue between the FDA and the sponsor to facilitate a shared understanding of the goals of the drug development program, and the specific studies designed to achieve those goals.

The TPP is multidisciplinary, just as the final product label is multidisciplinary. It contains information about chemistry, pharmacology and toxicology, clinical efficacy and safety, and formulation information. As such, the TPP applies to all aspects of FDA oversight and can be used with all disciplines within the FDA. The TPP can also be used as a tool for facilitating early discussions and achieving a clear, shared understanding, with the review team at the FDA, of the evidence necessary to support the sponsor's desired labeling statements.

It should be obvious to many that the TPP would be a very useful document for the key FDA meetings during development. These meeting include the Pre-IND, End-of-Phase 1 (EOP 1), End-of-Phase 2 (EOP 2), and Pre-NDA meetings, as well as any discussions about efficacy supplements. The TPP can share both progress and planning as development progresses.

What the TPP Is Not The TPP is **not** required. As originally conceived, the TPI program was voluntary, and at this writing the TPP remains so. The TPP is not a required component of any regulatory submission. The FDA does not require that companies even follow this guidance, although it is strongly recommended.

The TPP should not be a long, burdensome document. The intent is to convey information. Clear and concise is best, particularly in the early stages. When the document becomes longer as more information becomes available, the FDA will also be more familiar with what it already contains.

Very importantly, the TPP should not be considered to represent an implicit or explicit obligation on the sponsor's part to pursue all stated claims. The FDA fully understands that initial hopes to market a product in certain markets are not always met. Internal company decisions that affect the range of indications sought do come into play, and the FDA respects that. Therefore, the TPP does not comprise a commitment on the part of the sponsor to develop any particular intended claim. Likewise, the TPP should not be construed to represent an agreement on the part of the FDA that the proposed development plan will be adequate to support each proposed indication or claim. That means the TPP cannot be considered to represent an implicit or explicit obligation on the FDA's part to accept for approval an indication that will eventually be supported (or not) by data from trials contained in the TPP. The FDA reserves that decision solely for the review process. What can be assured is that the sponsor will obtain the FDA's best-educated opinion, based on the general information provided to the agency at any time. The bottom line is that there are no commitments one way or the other. The TPP is strictly a tool for obtaining the best possible development options.

The TPP is also not subject to freedom of information access. The TPP represents confidential development information. When a product is finally approved for one or more indications, the final, approved label will be available through a variety of sources, including the freedom of information process, as is usually the case.

The TPP Template The FDA website currently contains a sample TPP template, and is available at www.fda.gov/cder/tpi. This website will soon be changed to reflect the transition to from the TPI to the TPP. A user-friendly template can be found at that site.

Implementation, and the Pharmaceutical Company Perspective

For the industry, the TPP serves many roles. First, the TPP is an internal document and represents "doing your homework." It is a planning tool. It helps identify the work to be done. It identifies the "target" of the development and tracks the progress. Additionally, the TPP is an extremely important project summary that every chief executive should demand. As you will see, the TPP embodies a high-level snapshot of the dynamic development of a prospective new drug. Everyone from development-team members to management can easily identify both the intended target and the current development status from one small, manageable document. From the project leader's perspective, this approach of being able to use one document simplifies life considerably, as will become more evident in the discussions below.

Second, and equally important, the TPP serves as a tool for communicating with the FDA exactly what the company hopes to do with a prospective new pharmaceutical. FDA reviewers see hundreds of products in development every year. They can better assess a drug development program if they understand the individual components or studies that comprise the "big picture." Without compromising any confidential data from other companies, the FDA can assist a company by helping to confirm the right path or redirecting a development program away from likely pitfalls. The FDA cannot provide this valuable advice unless it knows where a company is headed and how they hope to get there, however.

What Can a TPP Look Like? There is no one "flavor" of a TPP. There is a recommended approach from the FDA/PhRMA task force that has addressed this issue since 1997, but companies are free to design their own TPP to suit their own needs. The official TPP template is available for viewing, downloading and use at the TPP web site on the FDA's web site (go to http://www.fda.gov and enter TPP into the search box at the top of the page). If "TPP" does not work yet, try seaching for "TPI."

The "flavor" of TPP described here is one that was developed prior to the availability of the official TPP template. It is simpler and has a different look, but the end result is the same. It still represents "dong your homework," and meets senior management and FDA needs quite well.

As development progresses, the TPP evolves. Early in development, such as in preparation for the Pre-IND Meeting, the aspects of a label that are recommended for inclusion in a TPP include:

a) Description
b) Clinical Pharmacology
b)(2) Clinical Studies (proposed and/or completed)
c) Indications and Usage
f) Precautions (based on preclinical toxicology, if applicable)
j) Dosage and Administration
l) . Animal Pharmacology and/or Toxicology

The reader will note that the indexing above relates to the organization of a drug label in a current package insert (21 CFR 201). Later in development, such as in preparation for the End-of-Phase 2 Meeting, additional label topics can be added. Therefore, the TPP might include the following elements:

a) Description (updated based on formulation changes?)
b) Clinical Pharmacology
b)(2) Clinical Studies (proposed and/or completed)
b)(3) Patient-Reported Outcomes
c) Indications and Usage
d-i) (Depending on Toxicology, Phase 1-2 studies)
j) Dosage and Administration
l) Animal Pharmacology and/or Toxicology

The exhibits below present examples of how some of these might look. Begin by looking at the first exhibit below. This exhibit is designed to provide a look at some of the information that would appear under a) Description. What you should

Target	Annotations
[Trade name] (Sponsor) (Balderdash bromide inhalation solution) Bronchodilator Aerosol DESCRIPTION [Trade Name] in contained in a breath-actuated, pressurized metered-dose aerosol unit for oral inhalation. [Trade Name] contains a solution of balderdash in xyz propellant with [list excipients]. *Each actuation delivers 20pg of balderdash from the mouthpiece.* *Each canister provides 120 oral inhalations.*	**Proposed dosage strength** that is anticipated to emerge from Phase 2. **Number of actuations** per can has to be decided in conjunction with Marketing.

Comments: Italics represent text that is not yet supported by data. Bold is used for emphasis (internal and/or FDA).

note first is the use of *italics*. In this fictitious example of the TPP, *italics* denote any information that represents "wishful thinking," or is otherwise unknown or unsupported at present.

Italics indicate text that needs to be tested or confirmed at the time of that particular version of the document. In the example above, a dose of 20 pg is listed. Since Phase 2 has not yet been completed in this example, the stated dose simply means that a numerical value is needed for the dose at this point in the future label. 20 pg is merely a placeholder for the eventual number. By contrast, the number of actuations (or doses) per container is likely a specific target.

The right side of the TPP is used for annotations. For some sections, such as the Description above, this may be best used for simple notations. The use of bold lettering/colors can be added for further emphasis.

The two exhibits below illustrate the Indications and Usage, and the Dosage and Administration sections of this particular usage of the TPP.

Target	Annotations
INDICATIONS AND USAGE *Balderdash is indicated for* **long-term, once-daily administration** *in the maintenance treatment of asthma and in the prevention of bronchospasm in adults and children 3 years of age and older with reversible obstructive airways disease, including patients with symptoms of nocturnal asthma, who require regular treatment with inhaled, short-acting, beta 2 -agonists.* *Balderdash can be used to treat asthma concomitantly with short-acting beta 2-agonists, inhaled or systemic corticosteroids, and theophylline therapy.*	CT-11; CT-12; CT-13; CT-14 **Note: Dosing more frequently than once-daily will potentially compromise a successful marketing program. This is a major marketing need.** CT-13; CT-14; CT-15; CT-16

Target	Annotations
DOSAGE AND ADMINISTRATION *For Maintenance Treatment of Adult and Pediatric Asthma* *The usual dosage for adults and* **children 3 years of age** *and older is 2 inhalations repeated daily; in some patients, 1 inhalation daily may be sufficient. More frequent administration or the administration of a larger number of inhalations is not recommended. If symptoms arise between doses, an inhaled short-acting beta2-agonist should be taken for immediate relief.* *For Maintenance Treatment of Chronic Obstructive Pulmonary Disease (COPD).* *The usual dosage is two inhalations once daily using the inhaler. …*	CT-11; CT-12; **Dosing down to 3 years of age represents a significant advantage...** CT-19; CT-20

In these examples, the Annotations section on the right now takes on an added function. Here, the annotations are used to identify the clinical trials that are intended to provide support for and defend the text on the left. Studies (CT-11, CT-12, etc.) are identified as those studies that are intended to support the text on the left as it is stated. The use of wording such as "long-term" and "once-daily" will have to be supported by those particular trials. At least some of these trials will have to address the "long-term" issue by providing for stable treatment for some period of months or years, as the situation dictates. A "once-daily" claim will also have to be supported by one or more of these trials, possibly by testing against twice-daily dosing at lower doses, for instance. One or more of these studies must also include children as young as three years of age so that the intended target is supported. The specifics listed in these examples are not as important as the point that every word of the target information on the left needs to be addressed, and therefore defended or supported, by clinical data from trials listed on the right. Once the studies have been conducted and facts are known about aspects such as dosages, dosing frequency and long-term use, the text on the left can be corrected to make them factual (not wishful) and the font characteristics can be changed from italics to regular font to denote the change. Gradually, the entire left side of the TPP will be changed from italics to standard font as data are gathered and facts replace targets.

As is evident, the same studies can be used to target different parts of the TPP. In the examples above, studies CT-11 and CT-12 address both the Indications and Usage and the Dosage and Administration sections of the TPP. To avoid duplication of effort (and a major source of errors), the details of these trials are not listed each time they are used as a reference. Instead, one section of the label, the Clinical Studies section, is used as the "reference library." Trial details are kept in this one place, and the trial's abbreviated titles (e.g., CT-11) can be used in various places in the TPP to target or defend text, as indicated. The Clinical Studies section will list all of the intended trials on the right, and this section obviously can become longer (or shorter) and cover many pages as the number of trials increases (or decreases). The exhibit below provides an example of what the Clinical Studies section of the TPP might look like.

Target	Annotations
CLINICAL STUDIES *[Describe anticipated outcome of the trials, in italics]*	*CT-11: Adult Dose-Ranging Study* *Randomized, double-blind, placebo-controlled, single-dose 5-way crossover* *Balderdash pMDI: 20 pg, 40 pg* *Active control pMDI: 100 and 200 μg, QD* $N = 46$ *(Powered for* **equivalence** *hypothesis)* *Inclusion criteria:* 　　　*FEV1 =* **50***-80% of predicted* 　　　*Ages =* **18** *to 70 years* 　　　*Nocturnal asthma* 　　　*Regular use of inhaled short-term beta2 agonists* *Primary Endpoint:* 　　　*FEV1-AUC0-12 from same-day, pre-treatment baseline* *Secondary Endpoints:* 　　　*FVC, FEV1/FVC, PEFR, FEF25%, FEF25-75% …*

It is extremely important to keep in mind that, in the early stages, this all represents a company's best thinking. A particular clinical study may be divided into two studies, or vice versa, two studies may be combined into one. As thinking improves, and the plan changes, the TPP should be kept up-to-date. The TPP should always represent the best thinking at the time. It is a working document and, as such, is intended to be fluid and helpful.

This latter point cannot be overemphasized. As the data are obtained, what had been wishful thinking is either confirmed or discarded. It is likely that dosages, for instance, will change from the plans, and even entire target indications may change. A new therapy that is being developed to treat arrhythmias, for example, ultimately may turn out to be the significant therapeutic advance in an entirely different therapeutic area. If and when that happens, this should be reflected in the latest TPP.

Hopefully, one can picture how useful this document would be to anyone on the development team, including top management, *assuming* that the TPP is kept current. For the team leader, the TPP represents a true multifunctional planning and tracking document.

Taking this a step further, submitting this information to the appropriate FDA reviewing division on a regular basis will provide agency reviewers with the same information. Armed with specifics on what a company's plans are and how they are progressing, the FDA is in a position to review the overall development program at the appropriate milestone meetings as well as the details in individual protocols. Such communication between the FDA and sponsors is critical, and use of a tool like the TPP can help make it happen.

CHAPTER 6

Information Systems in Support of Pharmaceutical Development

By William Shipman

This chapter provides a broad understanding of the underlying information systems necessary to support the drug development process. It is written at a level that attempts to steer clear of information systems (IS) technical jargon and, for the purpose of readability, "geek speak" is kept to a minimum. The chapter was developed for clinical development personnel who need a better understanding of how IS is used in the drug development process, and IS personnel who are new to the clinical development process. [Note: IS and IT (information technology) can be used interchangeably in the real world.]

Computers have had a foothold in the research and development industry for a long time. Since there are so many uses for computers in this industry, it is difficult to imagine developing a drug without them. Unfortunately, there is one commonality that almost all pharmaceutical (biotech and traditional drug) companies seem to share with respect to computing—disparate information systems and applications. Companies generally have collections of systems and applications that are not integrated, but that are designed in a way to meet individual needs. Companies spend millions of dollars on computers, systems, applications, and other technology, but get so little "information." Many top executives have difficulty answering basic questions about their organization such as, "how many people do we currently employ?" much less a question such as, "how many patients in Europe are enrolled in the Crohn's trial?" This phenomenon is the same for companies of all sizes and levels of maturity. However, it seems like a more serious problem in larger companies, since the costs of managing large, disparate legacy applications are exorbitant. How does a company let its information systems get so far out of control that they cannot quickly answer basic questions about their business? Simple answer: there is often no information systems strategy as a part of the overall corporate strategy.

How can companies, large and small, learn something about designing information systems to meet the needs of pharmaceutical development? Further, how can companies avoid making costly mistakes, and information systems decision pitfalls that have plagued many other companies? In theory, small startups can learn a great deal studying the mistakes that older companies have made. But bridging the gap between theory and practice requires a company to focus some of its attention on information systems, and establish an information systems strategy. Unfortunately, monetary restraints and conflicting priorities often push a systems strategy to the back burner, or to be overlooked altogether.

Approach and Philosophy: Business and IS Partnership There is an obvious benefit when information system personnel have an increased understanding of the drug development process that they support. In addition, when clinical development personnel gain an appreciation and understanding of systems, they can work closer with the systems people when it comes time to prioritize projects or make difficult tradeoff decisions. Many companies struggle to answer the question, "who are the decision makers when it comes time to select information system applications?" This is an important question, especially in the early stages of a company's life. The decision making process should involve both IS and clinical staff. A solid partnership is the main ingredient in making worthwhile investments in information technology. A formal IS portfolio management process would probably be overkill at the early stages of a company. But, at the point that the company is deciding on making some big investments in IS, a formal process can be invaluable.

An IS Steering Committee and Portfolio Management To begin the formal process, an IS steering committee should be formed. This committee's main priority is governing the portfolio management process. A successful committee is made of director-level representatives from all of the functional areas. One important aspect of a portfolio management process is that it gets all of the business units involved in the decision-making process. For example, both the director of sales and marketing and the director of clinical operations should have a seat on the committee. This is helpful when making decisions on IS investments that overlap the two business units. A good example in this case is an application that stores extramural contact information, including research grants, university relationships, key opinion leaders, key investigators, and other key company contact information. Often, having a cross-functional perspective on IS investments can prove valuable for a long-term strategy. It is amazing to see the portfolio of IS investments at a large company and see how many overlapping and competing technologies are in place. With some careful planning, an efficient and cost-effective process can be implemented.

Process Before Technology The phrase "process before technology" has grown in popularity for many reasons. For one, during the technology bubble and hyper-growth period of technology companies in the late 1990s, companies were spending a lot of money on software and hardware. After this growth phase, companies looked back and were more critical of the investments that were made in information systems. Executives began asking questions such as, "what was the return on investment for that project." Unfortunately, the answer to that question was not what the executives had hoped. In fact, billions of dollars were spent on technology that was never implemented by companies because they did not have the capacity to absorb, adopt, and change their processes to fit the new technology.

Before discussing process and technology, there first has to be a strong business rational that drives the need for an initial analysis. Additionally, the business processes and work flow involved need to be examined closely before jumping into a technology solution. Many companies fail to see the significance of solving efficiency problems with practical changes in processes. While a number of factors contribute to this problem, the main issue is simple: some people do not like change. Of course, when translated into dollars and cents, the possibility of getting the executives' attention is great. For example, big pharmaceutical companies can spend upwards of $30 million on their sales force automation, and nearly all of them are unsuccessful implementations. The cause of this phenomenon is not the software or implementation; rather, it is the unwillingness of the company to change some of its legacy processes, and adopt a new way of doing business.

While conducting a detailed process analysis is not easy, it is a necessary step before making a technology decision. Information systems personnel are good at helping the business perform this task. A lot of IS people are engineers at heart, and are quick studies when it comes to process engineering. Also, IS has software tools that help capture various aspects of processes. Working in conjunction with business partners and modeling the process can have a good effect on the outcome of a software implementation.

Buy vs. Build A significant decision that companies face is whether or not to build a custom software solution as opposed to buying an off-the-shelf solution. This is a particular problem in the pharmaceutical industry, since not every aspect of the business has a readily available off-the-shelf package. The buy-versus-build decisions that companies face can be daunting. What adds to this dilemma is the fact that many off-the-shelf packages still require some degree of customization.

A colleague answers this "buy vs.build" question with the question, "what business are we in, the software business or the drug discovery business?" Further to that point, for every dollar you spend on software programming, it is one less you are spending on a pharm/tox study or a clinical trial. Not to pick on the sales and marketing people, but to spend $75 million on a sales force automation system for a new drug that a 'dog with a note in its mouth' could sell does not make a lot of business sense. The same can be said of a company that might spend two years and $10 million on a data warehouse for statistical analysis when its statisticians prefer to work on individual data sets locally.

Obviously, common sense is critical when deciding on spending money on software development projects. When reviewing large software project proposals, the IS steering committee should ask the one important question: will this software give the company a competitive advantage? If the answer is no, then buy available software and adopt processes to use it effectively.

Tactical vs. Long Term Strategic When determining the right mix of IS projects for the current 'in-plan' (the in-plan refers to the projects that are actively being resourced), the steering committee should identify what is needed tactically to solve the immediate needs of the company and what are considered longer-term projects that fit closer to the company's long-term strategy. For example, the company needs an email system, and access to the Internet—these are tactical projects. An example of a strategic project is a data warehouse for pharmacological vigilance.

How fast should companies invest in IS? A company needs to decide how aggressively it wants to pursue an IS strategy. If a company decides to bring more work in-house, and move away from an outsourcing model, the IS strategy accelerates accordingly. For example, if clinical work is slated to come in-house, suddenly there is the rush to implement a clinical trials database, a safety database and a document management system. If the company decides to bring manufacturing in-house, an Enterprise Resource Planning (ERP) system comes to the forefront. The corporate strategy and the surrounding decisions force IS to quickly morph their organizations. If a company approaches a hyper-growth stage, the IS department needs to have a good strategy as well as close relationships with the functional areas. It is this stage in the company's life cycle that the information systems need close attention, since many decisions are made as the different functional areas rush to get systems online quickly. Let me illustrate a possible scenario. The manufacturing division needs to quickly get a document management system in place, an ERP strategy, and other systems that deal with GMP compliance concerns. As a result, they hire consultants and contractors to help get these initiatives going. Unfortunately, at the same time, the clinical division is pursuing a document management system and a mechanism to file electronic submissions. The result is a company with two standards for electronic document management; this company has now entered the first phase of systems fragmentation, and the amount spent on document management just doubled.

As this last observation proves, this author is often accused of being the "master of the obvious." On the other hand, if this document management example is so obvious, then why do so few of the big pharma companies have one standard document management system? Sure, there might be a few companies that have standardized on a brand of document management software like Documentum, but they have not standardized the interface, the processes, and the use. System fragmentation is a virus, and its many causes are difficult to pinpoint. One huge cause is the perception that each different business unit has unique processes, along with a mindset that suggests, "we have special needs." If they are not careful, the only special need they will have is the need for more money to spend on separate IS solutions.

Another interesting factor in the decision over how fast a company should invest in IS is what is referred to as the "moving train" syndrome. The moving train syndrome describes a company that is in the middle of many research and development programs, and managing these programs through partnerships and contract research organizations (CROs). This stage in a company's lifecycle, added to the "hyper-growth" stage, complicates the company's ability to define its information systems strategy. What makes this stage interesting is that most of the company's data are held by its partners or contract research organizations. At this point, the smart strategy would be to identify the need to move the data in-house, regardless of who is collecting, analyzing, and reporting the information. Subsequently, the strategy should reflect the need to support the company transitioning from the outsourced model to the in-house model.

Information Systems: From Utility Through Strategic Advantage

The pyramid diagram below represents a hierarchy of approaches that companies can take with their information systems strategy. The utility layer represents the strategy of a company that wants to keep its investments to a minimum, while the competitive layer represents the strategy of a company that is a making a large commitment to using technology to gain a competitive advantage over competitors. Few companies have made it to the competitive layer, but the ones that did showed noticeable improvements over their competitors. Let's take a closer look at these layers as they are reflected in the biopharm industry.

The "technology implementation pyramid"

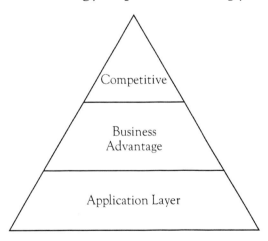

The Utility Layer The utility layer comprises the basic foundational systems, including networking capability, PCs, print services and other essential systems. Companies looking to stretch their IS budgets will look to get the basics in place to support minimum computing capability. For small biotech companies, this would include the phone system, the support for PCs, the local area network (LAN), printing services, and some level of system security. In addition, the utility layer includes such services as extending the LAN to support outsourced vendors by way of a virtual private network (VPN). This capability also gives the employees remote access to the network while at home or on the road. In addition to VPN, a company can also pursue a mechanism to provide secure email.

Expediting Drug and Biologics Development

The core applications supported in this layer would be the basic finance and accounting systems that include payroll, account payable/receivable, general ledger, and other functions required by the SEC.

The Application Layer The application layer comprises many of the core systems and applications on which the clinical development function relies in order to support the drug development process. The four core systems include the: clinical trials database (CTDB) system, clinical trials management system (CTMS), serious adverse events (SAE) system, and the document management/publishing system.

Clinical Trial Database System As a company begins to invest in the four core applications for clinical development, several factors must be considered. First, if the company only has money and resource to do one system at a time, it would be well advised to focus on the clinical trial database system first. Notable examples include Clintrial(tm), and Oracle(r) Clinical, among others. Getting this system in place provides plenty of flexibility for your outsource vendors, and provides the in-house repository for your clinical data. This is helpful even before you ramp up your clinical data management function, since it provides the means for the CRO to transfer data that it is collecting. In addition, you have the option of a contract with a CRO to perform the data management function, but stipulating that it should use your system remotely. This gives you real time access to data, and at the same time gives your clinical data management team time to learn the new CTDB system. Although there are only a few vendors that offer an off-the-shelf solution for a CTDB system, it is strongly recommended that a company does not attempt build its own system. The complexity and the regulatory compliance risk are too high. Ideally, the clinical data management department and the IS department can come to agreement on what off-the-shelf system will work best in the environment and be supportable. The following is a list of questions to ask in selecting the vendor and software for any big software purchase:

1. Vendor Viability. How long has the vendor been in business, what version of the software does it employ? What is the financial state of the company?
2. Does the vendor's software support the current environment? For example, a company may prefer to standardize all of its databases on Oracle.
3. What is the reoccurring maintenance cost for the software?
4. How much support will the vendor provide in the initial setup phase of the software? This would be an excellent line item in the contract with the vendor.
5. What kind of internal and external resources will be required to maintain and support this application?
6. A list of references from the vendor is helpful to uncover any stability and supportability issues.

Serious Adverse Events System The second significant decision regards the SAE system. Once again, there are few vendors that market an off-the-shelf solution for this function. But, as it is for the CTDB, the company is strongly advised to steer clear of developing its own in-house system. There are few companies that have successfully developed a custom solution, and the ones that did probably never recovered their investment.

There are several architecture considerations when deciding on an SAE system. For one, what is the initial requirement of integrating this system with the clinical trials database system? If, in the initial rollout of this system, you want to be able to reconcile SAEs that arrived separately (e.g., phone reports) with the adverse events entered in the clinical trials database (e.g., from case report forms), then that is something you might be able to negotiate with the vendor. Another architectural consideration relates to how the systems will be used. For example, will the system be accessed remotely by a CRO, or from other geographic locations within the company? If this is a requirement of the system, it should be accounted for within the official user requirements document, part of the system specification, and all the other documents that roll up into the official validation of the system.

When a company decides to implement a SAE system, there are important factors that must be considered. First, the project team should understand the resources it will take to validate the system, and subsequently add that cost to the overall implementation cost. Second, the safety department should have its processes determined and SOPs in place that train personnel. Third, the company should include, in the initial project, a plan to migrate any of the company's safety data from other sources.

Document Management and Publishing The third application on the horizon is the document management and publishing system. Actually, this is a suite of tools that enable the organization to author documents using version controls, to manage the documentation set, and to publish the final set of documents within the FDA guidelines. This includes both paper and electronic submissions. The main purpose of a well-designed document management and publishing solution is to provide a mechanism for a company to produce a submission to the FDA in the accepted format (e.g., the common technical document, CTD). In addition, the system should enable a company to provide an electronic version of the CTD, or an eCTD.

Chapter 6 - Information Systems in Support of Pharmaceutical Development

The eCTD is the electronic equivalent of the CTD (see chapter on eCTD). The eCTD provides a company with several advantages, including the ability to leverage many of the core elements of the marketing application by being able to submit them to regulatory agencies around the world. Another advantage of the eCTD is that, when companies amend an application, they can send a small electronic update. Reviewers can process the amendment faster, and track the history of changes more easily.

The electronic submission is a great opportunity for the applicant to leverage the "work style" of the FDA reviewer. It is one advantage for a company to understand the requirements and compliance issues with their submission; it is an even bigger advantage for the company to understand how the reviewer works. Understanding that, a company can begin to make the reviewer's job easier, and speed up the process. An important goal of the electronic submission is to make all the data and information contained in the application easily accessible by the FDA reviewer.

The eCTD specification has been developed by the ICH M2 Expert Working Group (EWG) under the ICH's international harmonization process. The technical specification for the eCTD is based upon the content defined within the CTD. The CTD describes the organizational content of information that makes up modules, sections and documents. This structure in the CTD has been used as the basis for defining the eCTD structure and content. The eCTD relies heavily on the use of open standards within the computer industry in the hopes of expanding the shelf life and usefulness of the eCTD specification. One open standard that the eCTD relies heavily upon is Extensible Markup Language (XML). Created by the MIT-founded group called the World Wide Web consortium (W3C), XML continues to gain support throughout the industry, and has fast become a de-facto standard as a data interchange framework. XML is the foundation of the eCTD, and is used to define the structure of the electronic submission. The structure is set up as a skeleton that includes the documentation-set hierarchy, underlying meta-data, a mechanism for navigating, and an overall usable table of contents.

The eCTD specification is designed to support the following high-level function for use by both the sponsor and the agency: viewing, exporting and printing documents; exporting data and information to databases; annotations; adaptability to change caused by amendments, supplements, or variations; copy and paste; searching information; and easy navigation throughout submission.

Implementing a document management system that integrates seamlessly with a publishing tool that has implemented the eCTD specifications is not easy. It might require a company to invest in several tools to fit the needs of the publishing department. Thanks to available off-the-shelf software, a company does not need to manually construct the eCTD, but can depend on the software to implement the specification.

The Clinical Trials Management Systems (CTMS) The CTMS is the sister application to the clinical trials database system. Unlike the CTDB, which is concerned with actual patient data (e.g., patient's blood pressure), the CTMS is designed to track the administrative information from the trial. Depending on the needs of the company, the CTMS can be designed to collect a variety of information. Typically, the information collected in a CTMS can be broken into three categories: financial; logistics; and administrative. The financial data managed throughout a trial includes investigator payment information, patient accruals, and other financial data. The logistics information that a company might want to track includes clinical drug supply levels, shipment information, and any other equipment that the site might need as part of the trial. The administrative information that is worth tracking includes all of the paperwork that a clinical research associate (CRA) needs to manage throughout the trial. Generally, the CTMS application is responsible for tracking everything from protocol amendments to the current enrollment status of the site.

Support for Statistical Analysis Setting up an environment for data analysis is fundamental to providing support for drug discovery and development. The technical infrastructure for analysis should include support for early discovery, data analysis in preclinical and later stage analysis in human trials, and the analysis needed for postmarketing research.

There are many analysis tools available, especially when considering all of the specialty tools designed for early discovery. Of course, further downstream in the clinical development world, SAS software for statistical analysis is recognized as a standard tool for the statistician. SAS is one of the few proprietary software programs that the FDA will ask for specifically (Adobe's Acrobat PDF format is another).

When designing the infrastructure for the environment supporting SAS, keep several things in mind that are specific to the type of analysis performed in the biopharmaceutical industry. First, a great deal of the analysis is performed on large amounts of data and extremely large data sets. For information systems, this translates into some important concepts. For one, the infrastructure should support ample disk space, and should be designed to be scalable. Nothing gives the IS department more of a black eye than running out of disk space, particularly during an important submission (is there any other type of submission?). All too often, for example, IS personnel are witnessed debating or questioning why the statisticians continue to make multiple copies of the same data sets, resulting in excessive disk space usage. This may be a legitimate concern, but it does not make sense to attempt to change the work habits of a company's statisticians when disk space is so inexpensive.

Another important design concept is determining the best performance option that fits the type of analysis being performed at your company. Although SAS has many capabilities and is often viewed as the "Swiss Army Knife" of software, it is not always the fastest software. The majority of SAS performance issues relate to I/O (input/output) issues associated with reading and writing the large data sets to disk (causing the disk drive to be the bottleneck). This suggests that the system should be designed with an architecture that takes advantage of multiple volumes of disk drives, and programs written to multi-thread SAS jobs that span across the different volumes. The latest versions of SAS provide support for this type of activity.

Occasionally, a need will arise that requires SAS to be used to write models and simulations that support an analysis plan. A red light should go on within the IS department when this request is made. I was visited on a Monday morning from an irate statistician claiming that his SAS job took all weekend to run and it still was not finished. Upon further research into this SAS job, the system administrators found that the job was running about 36 hours, and it had slowed the server down to the point that no other jobs were able to run. Even though SAS is probably not the best software to use for a simulation-type analysis such as this, often it is the only analysis tool that the statisticians know well enough to use. The question for the IS department is what can be done to provide this capability, without spending the entire IS budget. One approach that deserves serious consideration is designing the computing architecture using cheaper, more affordable Intel-based PCs. Much progress has been made in this arena, and many companies with restricted budgets and in search of high-level computing power are now turning to this option. The concept is simple, and with the arrival of more mature versions of the operating system Linux, what was once just a concept is now reality. The ability of IS departments to build a "bank" of Intel-based PCs, using the clustering technology concepts, is beginning to change the computing paradigm. No longer are companies forced to spend mega-millions on bigger mainframe computers and the accompanying application software. Linux clusters, at one time only popular in very specific applications and homegrown software developed in the early drug discovery world, are now being used in environments further downstream. For example, the latest version of Oracle's database products now can take advantage of Linux clusters. This opens up many avenues that can be explored by companies in search of high power at affordable prices. The economics of this architecture is extremely compelling.

Business Advantage Layer The business advantage layer is something a company's IS strategy should begin adressing after the core applications have been successfully implemented. The intent of this layer is to clearly define when IS investments begin improving the business model, either by providing the means to increase efficiencies or cut costs. IS investments that are classified as "business advantage" mean different things depending on what industry you were considering. For example, if you were discussing the customer goods service industry, a business advantage would be described as how efficient the IS systems were in support of the supply chain. IS might enable the company to more quickly handle the changing needs of its customers by using systems that better profile the different consumer groups. In the pharmaceutical industry, the concept of IS providing a business advantage takes on a different shape. A main consideration is the importance of moving important company data and information through the development and commercialization stream. A key factor at this stage is the systems' ability to share information and to integrate data. These systems and applications should support the data integration between organizational functions and better equip the company to make faster decisions. The underlying theme at this stage is building systems that add to the efficiencies of the company—making it faster, smarter, and more economical. Let's examine some examples that add to the efficiencies of a company and help reduce costs.

Integrating the Clinical Trials Database with the Safety Database Safety data from a clinical trial arrive by more than one mechanism (CRF entries, phone call from site), and often need to be reported by more than one mechanism (clinical study report, IND safety report). For a variety of reasons, data obtained for the same event by these different systems are often contradictory and need to be reconciled. By integrating these two systems, data entry can be saved, and the time personnel spend in verifying patient data is reduced. Often, a certain level of integration between these two systems requires customization. Several vendors offer a suite of products and tout the ability to do this out-of-the-box (Oracle Clinical/AERs, Clintrial/Clintrace). It needs to be confirmed whether or not a particular vendor's out-of-the-box integration will satisfy a particular company's exact needs. Fortunately, many advances have been made in the software toolsets to integrate applications, thus cutting down the programming time and level of expertise needed for a potential customization.

The integration of these two systems highlights an important requirement, namely the need for the clinical data management department and the safety department to agree on a clear process and ownership for this information being shared by the systems. Remember, the IS staff can make the software do almost anything, assuming sufficient time and programming resources. To make the investment cost effective, however, the solution has to match an established efficient process.

The Auto Encoding System An auto encoding system refers to the ability of an application, such as the adverse events tracking system, to automatically fill in the preferred term from the coding dictionary from a string of verbatim text. To understand how a basic auto-encoding system works, think of it in two simple steps:

1. The user inputs the verbatim text of the adverse event into the system. The system quickly checks an encoding history file for a match. If a match is found, the preferred term is entered into the database by the system, and the record is flagged as having been auto-encoded.

2. If the text string does not find a match in the encoding history file, the system runs some text string matching algorithms and makes some suggestions to the user who then verifies the right term. At this point, the system updates its coding history file.

Electronic Data Capture An electronic data capture (eDC) system is an application that provides the investigative site with a mechanism to enter patient data onto electronic CRFs (case report forms). The promise of this technology is that the sponsor obtains the data faster and cleaner by eliminating manual and duplicate processes. One obvious duplication that eDC eliminates is the data being entered manually at the clinical site, and then officially entered into the system electronically by the sponsor. A large part of the value proposition of eDC is its ability to cut down on incorrect data and the time it takes to resolve inconsistencies. A notable downside of eDC that has not been completely addressed is that vendors must build into their products the ability to link the electronically captured data (e.g., eDC) with an electronic regulatory submission capability (e.g., eCTD).

While the concept of eDC is simple and straightforward, and the value proposition seems possible, the rate of adoption by companies has been slow (see chapter on eDC concepts).

Clinical Drug Supply Tracking System Anyone who works in the pharmaceutical industry as an information systems person long enough is accustomed to hearing the familiar mantra, "our industry is special, we have special needs, and we are regulated." It is true that this industry is probably different in many ways from other industries. For one, the pharmaceutical industry seems to move at glacial speeds with regards to technology, and is extremely slow to adopt new technologies. Looking at the entire commercialization spectrum of a pharmaceutical company, the clinical development segment highlights this phenomenon perhaps best. As a vital aspect in the commercialization chain, clinical development constitutes the pivotal step in moving an experimental product into humans for the first time. Therefore, the needs of clinical development are highly specialized, particularly when considering the information technology used at this stage. One important system that a company relies on when it begins clinical trials in humans is logistics. This system is used to track the clinical drug and supplies that are shipped to the clinical sites participating in the program. Besides being a highly regulated system, it plays an important part in ensuring that the sites have enough clinical supplies to keep pace with the patients being enrolled into the trial.

When discussing the clinical drug supply system, it is common for personnel to ask "why can't we leverage the use of our ERP system that we already have in place." At an early but appropriate stage of a company's growth, one might suggest that the logistical needs of clinical development be considered when planning the ERP system that is being established for the manufacturing division. This makes a great deal of sense, but unfortunately, this type of planning is rarely done at small, growing companies. Because of the special needs of the clinical development processes, the ERP project team is usually afraid that the extra requirements will cost too much and risk delaying the implementation of the ERP system. Some of the special needs of clinical development include support for IVRS (interactive voice response system), and protocols that rely on randomization and drug blinding studies. As simple as these requirements seem to be, none of the major ERP systems provide this functionality out of the box. Besides the obvious extra expense of building a separate system to track clinical drugs and supplies, the main downfall of having more than one logistics system at a company is the unnecessary complexity that is added to forecasting manufacturing's needs. While it is hard to blame inadequate systems on a company's inability to forecast manufacturing, it makes a good argument for planning better systems.

When planning a clinical supply tracking system, what are the important components? The following is a list of must haves when planning for this type of system:

- Randomization: the system has to accommodate the randomization needs that the statisticians build into the protocol design of the study.
- Telephony: the system has to accommodate the use of telephony applications such as IVRS. Whether the remote clinical sites use a web-based system or the phone to order more supplies or

drugs, the system should be designed to allow for both. Many of the IVRS vendors have designed their products to use either the web or the telephone.

- Blinding: the system has to allow the company to ship product to clinical sites to service protocols designed for single or double blinding.
- Lot tracking: specifics on which drug lots were shipped to which sites represent information that is always necessary and sometimes critical for short-term recall.
- Bar coding: the system must be ready to handle bar coding, an excellent way to improve productivity and efficiency for everything from clinical supplies to paper documentation.

There can also be elements of the system that can provide extra value in addition to core functionality, including integration with the CTMS, lot-number tracking between the drug safety system and the system used in manufacturing, and inventory-level triggers.

Competitive Advantage Layer One might think that the "lofty" competitive advantage layer at the top of the pyramid is a place reserved for top companies, those that have excess revenue to spend on technologies in the hopes of separating themselves from their competitors. Actually, this layer is reserved for smart companies, regardless of size and revenue stream, that want to apply an IS strategy that will yield long-term benefits. These benefits come from slowly building a technology infrastructure that, together with good process discipline, returns efficiencies to the company. One reason why this layer is so difficult for a company to achieve is that too many companies spend time and resources "chasing" the latest technologies and techniques dictated by consultants rather than by internal planning. In fact, these "reactive" techniques usually yield only one thing—more revenue for the consultant companies.

The Importance of a Clear Data Architecture Leaders at a company have to realize that there is no silver bullet, magic system, or efficiency methodology that is going to suddenly make a difference to a company's P&L. For a company to get itself to a point where the information systems strategy is considered a competitive advantage will take painstaking time, careful planning, and resources to evaluate its corporate processes. In addition, a data architecture and vision will need to be determined, agreed upon, and implemented.

What type of IS strategy and data architecture separates a company from its competitors? This is the million-dollar question, and the answer depends on the many variables associated with a company's internal processes, existing systems, culture, and the complexity of its current operation. For larger, mature companies like the bigger pharmaceutical companies, the most significant variable is its ability to adapt to change. A corporate culture that can support a high rate of change can adapt to a new IS strategy and develop a systems architecture that enables it to function more efficiently. Of course, that is easier said then done. First, evaluate the size and complexity of the organization. If, for example, the company is large (over 10,000 employees) and has many disparate legacy systems, then the strategy must take on a "divide and conquer" mentality. In this scenario, there are no quick fixes, and it will require quite a bit of discipline on the part of the organization to begin to structure its strategy around centralizing many of its data sources.

A Central Source of Data Core to an IS strategy that builds on the concept of providing a company with a competitive advantage is the notion of one source of data. Larry Ellison, CEO of Oracle Corporation, has been known to preach this architectural concept. Oracle is a software company that specializes in applications designed for corporations to help manage and support all of their processes along the entire commercialization spectrum. Imagine Ellison's shock and horror long ago upon finding out that his company was not using a central-system architecture similar to what Oracle was attempting to sell to its clients. As it turns out, Oracle was in as bad a shape as the majority of other companies. Ellison realized the company had to change when he asked an executive working for him a simple question about the company's operation and could not get an answer. Apparently, Oracle had dozens of systems handling the basic operational functions of the company and was plagued with duplicate systems and data. Ellison began to quickly change the way the company ran its operation, and began to centralize all the databases into one database. What he wanted to accomplish was one data repository and one information source. That way, when he asked for the monthly sales figures from Europe, he would receive a timely and accurate answer. This last point—one information source—represents the foundation for any IS strategy that will enable a company to derive a competitive advantage from its information systems. Since a company with one source of information can make better and faster decisions, it will be able to react more rapidly to market variables and thus beat the competition.

Single Source Architecture: Big or Small Companies Whether your company is a big, established pharmaceutical company or a small startup, the need for one information source should be the underlying principle in your systems strategy. For the small startup company, it should be a part of your planning, and a part of every systems decision you make. Keep in mind that the decisions at this stage can have a significant effect on the future architecture of the company's systems, and can either help or hinder the future architectural foundation of its systems. Remember, when deciding on applications for specific functions in a company, those decisions affect all functions within the company. This last point is important and reverts back to the beginning of the chapter when the importance of setting up the corporate information steering committee was mentioned. To repeat that important theme, this committee's primary role is to make decisions on systems that make sense for the whole company, not just for one specific functional area. To illustrate this point, let's take a look at some of the decisions that a small company is faced with when building systems and applications to support the growth of the company.

Key Decision-Making by a Growing Company. As a company goes through a rapid growth period, information-system decisions are made quickly, and many times these quick decisions only give the company short-term results. We will take a look at a few examples to illustrate this point.

Scenario: Logistics and Manufacturing Company A is at a point in its corporate strategy that requires it to outsource all of its clinical manufacturing, while clinical logistics are handled by a small in-house department working closely with the clinical operations department that is managing the program. The problem the logistics team faces is that the clinical programs are getting larger and more complex at a faster pace. At some point, the logistics group will require a better system that allows it to work more efficiently.

Systems Decision I: One decision the company can make is what is commonly referred to as the "band aid" decision. In this circumstance, any hope or thought of a systems strategy is abandoned, and a quick fix is rapidly purchased to alleviate the immediate demands on the logistics team. Unfortunately, this is the system decision that the vast majority of all companies will make when faced with this problem. The system will cure the immediate needs of the tracking issues with which the department is faced, but will have few hopes of ever integrating effectively into an overall system architecture that supports the entire process. Unless there are serious regulatory risks at stake in this scenario, a good course of action is to take the simple approach of getting a better handle on the current processes and patch any tracking needs with a simple database or even excel spreadsheets.

Systems Decision II: A company that has an IS steering committee in place will be more likely to adopt another approach and reach a different decision. In this instance, a committee would have the opportunity to evaluate the overall business impact of selecting a point solution to solve the needs of the logistics team. Often, it is too convenient for the committee to approve the purchasing of a small-point solution, since the justification from the team can sometimes be quite compelling. Actually, this is a situation in which a red light should go off, and the committee should spend the needed time to analyze the decision. In some cases, even the IS steering committee may/should delegate a smaller working group to do further analysis of the situation. Two possible solutions can result from a working group's deliberation. For one, the team may find that the logistics department is in a legitimate crisis and needs to go forward with the purchase of a small system that will get them in compliance and get the process back on track. A second decision could include a strategy that advises the team to continue to use a "workaround" system while a team that includes other functional areas gets formed so that a broader understanding of the needs of the company are addressed. The second decision is one that a mature company, with patient leadership, will make, particularly if it is attempting to build an information architecture that will allow the company to scale-up appropriately.

Business Intelligence The theory of business intelligence builds on the concepts of one source of data for the company. Business intelligence is the ability of a company to understand enough about its own operations to make good, fast decisions. This section is included in the competitive intelligence pyramid because so few companies have this ability, and when present, it clearly differentiates that company from its competitors. Here are some examples of systems and the underlying architecture that support the concept of business intelligence within a company.

Example 1: A Project Management Methodology. The first example is a corporate, standard project management process and methodology that provides executives with access to quick information about important programs at the company. A small startup company does not necessarily need a project management system or a sophisticated methodology to be effective. In fact, at the very beginning phase of a company's formation, flexibility often is more effective. But if there is one area of a pharmaceutical company that can quickly spin out of control, it is project management. It is never the technical ability of the project managers; it is usually the fact that there are more projects starting up, each with greater complexity. A concise, standard methodology, coupled with a central project management system, can quickly deliver answers to questions that arise from the company's executive team.

Example 2: HR Employee Provisioning. One area of the company that is often overlooked and oversimplified is the human resource (HR) systems for tracking employees. Why would something so basic be included in the competitive advantage portion of the chapter? Because it is rarely done properly, and many operational man-hours are wasted in tracking employees. These wasted man-hours can be shifted to other activities that yield greater benefits to the company. In addition, once an efficient employee provisioning system and architecture is in place, many other systems and processes can take advantage and leverage its capability.

An employee provisioning system is extremely important in the pharmaceutical industry due to the dynamic nature of the discovery and development process of drugs. The importance of understanding to what teams employees are assigned is crucial, especially when programs need to shift resources quickly. While the true competitive advantage gets its roots from this system, it is used in an overall corporate strategy to best address the art of capacity management. Capacity management is the ability of a company to understand its workforce, understand the future demands of the company's priorities, and use systems to help track, anticipate and best utilize its employee base.

Competitive Intelligence It would not make much sense to have a section of the chapter that is dedicated to the highest part of the pyramid (i.e., designated Competitive Advantage) without having a discussion of "competitive intelligence," or CI. CI is a collection of data and information that increases a company's ability to make achievements faster than its competitors. It is the activity of monitoring the environment external to the firm for information that is relevant for the decision-making process of the company. It has the ability to separate a company from others by having a control of information that the others do not have.

Interest in CI has gained momentum in recent years, a phenomenon that is fueled by the increasing awareness of the abundant availability of information. True, the information age has fully enveloped the business world, and the availability of information through the Internet is extraordinary. This phenomenon, however, is a double-edged sword. The overwhelming amounts of data and the various techniques used to search and collect the data often hinder a company's ability to interpret the data and transform it into usable information. It is important to distinguish the idea that CI is not just a massive collection of data from the competitive marketplace, but an analytical process that transforms this disaggregated data into an accurate and strategic understanding of one's competitors. It is important also to point out that CI is not the art of espionage or stealing another company's secrets. Rather, it is an approach a company takes to better understand its competitors and their products. This could include a competitor's organizational structure, culture, strengths, weaknesses, and ability to execute in the market place.

Similar to the underlying theme of this chapter, CI can gain some traction in an organization if it is coordinated and if the organization adopts a standard approach. The first step, of course, is for the company to determine which business unit should adopt the function of CI and manage the resource, budget and direction of the program. This function (e.g., marketing research) can then engage representatives from the rest of the company to begin deciding on the company's approach. While it is important that the discussion on the approach include the type of technology that is going to be used, the primary goal of this newly formed team is to set the same goals for the use of CI at the company and, in doing so, avoid the temptation to "do it all." The team should select specific goals (e.g., identifying and understanding possible competitive threats, exploring new opportunities) and focus on these goals.

Chapter 7

Title 21 CFR Part 11

By Beverley Smith

The pharmaceutical industry is always looking for ways to make its business more effective and efficient. With the advent of computer systems, there was promise for improvement in the speed and accuracy of collecting, reporting, and sharing of information. As a result, many business processes have been re-engineered to reduce the use of paper and keep everything electronic. This transition from paper to electronic information has caused some concern among the world's regulators because the attributes of acceptable data applied to paper-based systems now need to be applied to the more complex world of computers. Traditionally, the FDA has defined the attributes of reliable data to be as follows:

- Attributable - who performed the observations and tests and subsequently recorded them
- Original - data are kept from the first point of recording the observation or test result
- Accurate - the data are reviewed before being considered final to ensure that no errors in recording have occurred
- Contemporaneous - the data are recorded "real-time" with the act of observation or testing
- Legible - the data can be easily read and reviewed, and changes to the data clearly allow the reader to see what was originally recorded, who recorded it, and why the data were changed.[bullet]

These principles must always be met for the regulators to accept the data submitted to them. To assist the pharmaceutical industry in understanding how the FDA expects the industry to demonstrate reliability of data submitted to them, they published a regulation entitled, "Electronic Records; Electronic Signatures Rule," which is also known as 21 CFR Part 11.

The challenge for the pharmaceutical industry is the maintenance of these principles when creating new processes that use one or more computer systems to support the creation, modification, maintenance, archiving, retrieval and transmission of data that support regulated activities.

Background The pharmaceutical industry lobbied the FDA to allow technical innovations in document management to begin to replace the paper-based processes. In 1991, the FDA began the regulatory process to meet pharmaceutical industry requests to move to the "paperless office." The industry was specifically interested in obtaining the agency's acceptance of electronic signatures. The requests to implement electronic signatures were strongest in the industry's manufacturing faction.

A task force was established with membership from the pharmaceutical industry and the regulators to explore the challenges of using electronic signatures. The outcome in July 1992 was that FDA published an advance notice of proposed rulemaking on the use of electronic signatures to gather further information from interested parties. Just over two years later, in August 1994, a proposed rule covering electronic signatures and electronic records was published. The justification for the expansion in scope from the original objective was that an electronic signature by definition can only be considered to be reliable and trustworthy if the associated electronic record also has the same attributes. The industry and other interested parties submitted their comments to the agency (FDA) and the responses the points raised can be read in 62 Federal Register 13429.

On March 20, 1997, the FDA published the final rule under Title 21, CFR Part 11, entitled, "Electronic Signatures; Electronic Records" with an effective date of August 20, 1997. The pharmaceutical industry was taken by surprise by the changes that had been made to the draft rule released in 1994 and the responses to the submitted questions and comments. A comparison of the draft and final regulation can be found at the following URL: http://www.fda.gov/ora/compliance_ref/part11/Frs/background/pt11pxf.htm

The key changes were as follows:

- The scope of the regulation was expanded to include records in electronic form that were retrieved

or archived as well as created, modified, maintained or transmitted. No grandfather clauses were included for existing legacy systems.
- The scope of the types of records that must comply with this rule was expanded to include those defined as records submitted to the agency under the requirements of the Federal Food, Drug, and Cosmetic Act and the Public Services Act, even if such records are not specifically identified in agency regulations.

Unusually, the final rule was not written as a stand-alone regulation, and cross-references predicate rules. This created concern within the industry as there is considerable variance within the regulations that cover pharmaceutical manufacturing, non-clinical research, clinical research and medical devices as to what is defined as a record, what constitutes acceptable change control practices, and what records require signatures. For computer systems that support more than one regulated area, the industry found itself having to apply the more stringent requirement for records to ensure compliance.

The agency also took a new approach in the final rule in defining electronic solutions for achieving reliability and trustworthiness of electronic records and signatures. In the past, the agency has defined principles and expectations rather than giving specific solutions. This allowed the industry some flexibility in choosing the best solution for its situation and then defending their choices during inspections (see discussions below).

What does 21 CFR Part 11 cover? The regulation, at first glance, appears to be brief and simple to follow. The agency provides the following definitions for key terms used in the regulation:
- Biometrics means a method of verifying an individual's identity based on measurement of the individual's physical feature(s) or repeatable action(s) where those features and/or actions are both unique to that individual and measurable;
- Closed system means an environment in which system access is controlled by persons who are responsible for the content of electronic records that are on the system;
- Digital signature means an electronic signature based upon cryptographic methods of originator authentication, computed using a set of rules and a set of parameters such that the identity of the signer and the integrity of the data can be verified.
- Electronic record means any combination of text, graphics, data, audio, pictorial or other information representation in digital form, that is created, modified, maintained, archived, retrieved or distributed by a computer system;
  - Note: there was much debate that this definition encompassed business tools, such as e-mail and voicemail when regulated topics were discussed in "conversations" rather than formal documents. Company policies must be written to define communication etiquette and what constitutes official records that must be maintained to demonstrate record compliance with the predicate rules.
- Electronic signature means a computer data compilation of any symbol or series of symbols, executed, adopted or authorized by an individual to be the legally binding equivalent of the individual's handwritten signature;
- Handwritten signature means the scripted name or legal mark of an individual, handwritten by that individual and executed or adopted with the present intention to authenticate a writing in permanent form. The act of signing with a writing or marking instrument such as a pen or stylus is preserved. The scripted name or legal mark, while conventionally applied to paper, may also be applied to other devices that capture the name or mark;
- Open system means an environment in which system access is not controlled by persons who are responsible for the content of electronic records that are on the system.

The regulation then goes on to define the FDA's expectations of open and closed computer systems. To demonstrate that an electronic record is authentic, has integrity and that the confidentiality has not been compromised, the closed computer system must: (1) be validated; (2) produce accurate and complete copies (paper or electronic) upon request; (3) use access controls and employ audit trails that are applied to the user and system administration interfaces that control key functionality, such as audit trails; (4) use system checks to ensure that only authorized users use the system in a predetermined way (for example, access level controls determine the user's ability to make changes to data and apply electronic signatures to records); and (5) be set up so that entered instructions and the data sources are checked for validity before execution.

The personnel responsible for the development and maintenance of the computer system as well as the users of the system must be able to demonstrate that they have the appropriate education, training and experience to perform their assigned roles. A mechanism must be in place to ensure that training is provided before users access the new system. Computer system that are used for recording staff training in topics covering regulated areas must therefore be compliant with 21 CFR Part 11.

If a computer system is considered open, the regulation adds the expectation that additional access controls must be employed to preserve the record's authenticity, integrity and confidentiality. Examples of these additional controls are the use of encryption, VPN (virtual private network) lines, or requiring digital signatures at key stages in the information processing life-cycle.

The largest part of the regulation covers the attributes of an electronic signature to ensure that it is equivalent to a handwritten signature. This part of the regulation was the only part that was initially expected by the industry. The stated requirements are expected to support the existing regulations where signatures are required.

The regulation defines that, when an electronic signature instead of a handwritten signature is used, the following information must be provided: the printed name of the signer; the date and time when the signature was executed; and the meaning of signature (acknowledgement, approval, acceptance, etc.) These attributes must never be separated from the signature or the electronic record to which they are associated, and must always appear on copies of the record (paper or electronic). In other words, the ability to copy and paste the signature to other records must be prohibited.

As with access controls, an individual's electronic signature must be unique and must employ two distinct identification components (i.e., identification code and password). Unlike handwritten signatures, the first signature employed during a session must use all electronic signature components, but subsequent signings in the same session may use only one component. This would be akin to writing your signature the first time it is used and then using initials thereafter in one signing session.

When companies use computer systems that span multiple time zones, date and time synchronization becomes extremely important to demonstrate that information was collected, modified, or had electronic signatures applied in the correct sequence. Therefore, workstations and servers must be regularly checked to ensure that the time and date synchronization has not been lost.

Security measures must be employed to ensure that electronic signature components remain unique and are changed periodically to prevent unauthorized use. The system administrators should also periodically verify that the access to, and application of signatures are appropriate and suspicious entries are promptly investigated.

What must a pharmaceutical company do to assess compliance of current systems with the requirements in 21 CFR Part 11? The following steps are recommended:

- Identify the predicate rules that govern the activities of the organization being assessed. A predicate rule, although not defined in 21 CFR Part 11, is a regulation published by the FDA that defines the acceptable standards for performance and the information that must be submitted to the FDA for a particular activity that the FDA regulates. The exhibit below provides a list of potentially relevant regulations for the pharmaceutical industry.

21 CFR	Subject
Part 50	Protection of Human Subjects
Part 54	Financial Disclosure
Part 56	Institutional Review Boards
Part 58	Good Laboratory Practice for Non-clinical Laboratory Studies
Part 210	Current Good Manufacturing Practice in Manufacturing, Processing, Packing, or Holding of Drugs, General
Part 211	Current Good Manufacturing Practice for Finished Pharmaceutical Products
Part 312	Investigational New Drug Application
Part 314	Applications for FDA Approval to Market a New Drug
Part 320	Bioavailability and Bioequivalence Requirements
Part 600	Biological Products: General
Part 601	Licensing

Note: The FDA also publishes supporting guidance documentation that provides more detail on how to comply with certain regulations, and these should also be referenced in preparing an analysis of the predicate rules. The guidance documents can be found at the following URL: http://www.fda.gov/cder/guidance.

- Perform a thorough analysis of the predicate rules to define what records are required to be maintained and where signatures are required. If internal business requirements expect a signature, these should be evaluated to ensure that they are really needed in an electronic system.
  Note: Since most companies do not operate only in the United States, and other regulatory authorities around the world have their own requirements on the use of electronic systems and electronic signatures, it would be wise to expand the scope of "predicate rule" to all regulatory authorities with whom the company interacts.
- Establish and maintain a complete inventory of all software and hardware used in all parts of the company, and highlight those used within a regulated environment. The process for maintaining the inventory should ensure that all upgrades or changes to the hardware or software that frequently occur are captured, including those that happen during routine maintenance.
- For each system in use, create and maintain a system description, at a high level, that describes what the system is used for and that can be shown to regulatory authority inspectors. Where necessary, also have a system interface diagram that shows how information moves between different systems from point of initial capture to archiving.
- Establish a company position for what predicate rule requirements will be applied to electronic systems that are used in multiple regulatory settings, such as non-clinical and manufacturing (e.g., the information that must be recorded when making a change to a record). Only the non-clinical research regulations (Good Laboratory Practices) require that the reason for a change be noted. Therefore, to achieve 21 CFR Part 11 compliance, the audit trail must capture not only who made the change, when the change was made, and the new and previous entry, but also the reason for why the change was made. When there is no such regulatory requirement, the decision to capture the reason for change will be driven by company preferences, cost, system performance and use, and storage space requirements.
- Define a risk model that will identify those electronic systems that are at most risk if the system fails in some way. Usually, the highest risk systems generate records that have no other source and are critical to the operation of a particular process or decision-making. These are the systems whose failure to comply with comply with the predicate rules will also fail to comply with the requirements of 21 CFR Part 11. Therefore, they should be the company's highest priority for remediation or replacement. GAMP has some useful definitions for risk that the reader should explore. See the following URL: http://www.ispe.org/gamp/.
- Rate all systems in the inventory using the risk model, and identify systems that are due for retirement, replacement, or remediation. All new systems added to the company should also be rated using the risk model. New systems should not be installed until the compliance gaps are resolved and the system is considered compliant.
- Establish and document a software development lifecycle that can provide the users of a system and external regulatory authorities with confidence that the system is designed, validated, implemented and maintained in a controlled state and that it performs the intended functions consistently. Develop templates for staff to use to ensure that each part of the software development lifecycle is performed and documented in accordance with company standards.
- Ensure that all documentation created for the system assessments and remediation activities are archived.
- Train the staff within the information technology and user departments on the processes and documentation expectations. Conduct periodic reviews to ensure that the established processes are followed.
- Installation qualification, operational qualification and performance qualification standards and documentation must be established for all systems. It is not adequate to rely on the manufacturer's engineering installation checks, and the users of the system must confirm appropriate intended performance before the system goes "live."
- The users are the key to success in the implementation of any compliant system. They drive the requirements the system must meet, how the system will be used and who will use it, and maintain oversight of the records created. It is very important that these individuals are cognizant of the predicate rules that govern their work and are appropriately trained in the proper use and maintenance of the system. Standard operating procedures play a key role in assisting staff in understanding their job performance expectations;

- One key aspect of 21 CFR Part 11 compliance is that the user must ensure that data integrity has been maintained from the point of capture to the submission of the data to the agency. To achieve this goal, the company's 21 CFR Part 11 plan must include assessments of all the systems, and data transfer protocols must be assessed to confirm that the integrity of the data is maintained;

- When data or documents are received from sources external to the company and the applications were created specifically for the company, it is advisable to have oversight of the system development and, where appropriate, conduct user acceptance tests before the system goes live.

- When systems are retired, the company must ensure that the archived information can be retrieved. Retrieval must include all the meta data that support the information, including the full audit trail and data capture settings. The FDA has stated that it does not expect companies to retain obsolete computer systems, although it does expect to be able to inspect the submitted information in the same way as if the system was still available.

Points to consider When outsourcing regulated activities, the contracted company must be assessed for 21 CFR Part 11 and predicate rule compliance. Any gaps should be addressed in the contract, and quality expectations should be defined.

Quality expectations should include the following: recruitment of appropriately qualified personnel who will receive adequate training before executing the contracted work; requirement for the presence of quality systems (standard operating procedures; quality control and quality assurance processes); prospective notification of any change in personnel, systems, or company situation; predicate rule requirements; established software development life-cycle; change control; logical and physical security; archiving procedures; disaster recovery; and business continuity.

Some outsourcing partners will be beyond the jurisdiction of the FDA. For example, in a clinical trial setting, an electronic medical records system and a central laboratory's laboratory information management system (LIMS) are regulated by government bodies other than the FDA. In these circumstances, the FDA can only take regulatory action against the sponsor of the clinical trial or the contract research organization that was delegated sponsor's obligations, or the investigator who performed the clinical trial. The responsibility for ensuring that the data used in submissions to the agency rests with the sponsor. It is, therefore, important to ensure that the electronic systems used to capture, generate, and transfer the data are assessed before the clinical trial commences. In some cases, the solution for a lack of compliance will be to recommend that procedural controls be implemented or that a paper-based data capture system be used instead.

Electronic data capture systems have their own unique challenges to meet predicate rule requirements. In the clinical research setting, for example, the investigator is responsible for all data generated for the research subjects under his or her care. Therefore, data integrity oversight must include the investigator's review and confirmation of the data before they are transmitted to the sponsoring company or contract research organization. In addition, after the clinical trial is completed, the investigator must have, in his or her care, the original data collected and all post-submission changes made by the sponsor or CRO. The challenge in this example is that the electronic data may physically reside at the location where the electronic system is hosted, and this may also be outsourced.

Record retention is probably the most challenging aspect of complying with the regulation. It has always been routine for companies to perform regular back-ups of electronic systems, but this usually involves the recycling of back-up tapes or disks at a predefined interval of time. Also, the back up generally is not organized in the same way, as a library might establish an inventory of the information to facilitate rapid retrieval. A company should, therefore, work with its professional archivists to establish the record retention process. For systems that reside at contracted companies, the company must establish if the archived information will reside at the point of generation or be transferred to the company at the conclusion of the work. Where predicate rules require that the contracted location keep the data, the method of record retention must ensure that all the data that define the original capture are kept. This means that audit trails, and "settings" used to capture the data are included.

The Future The FDA planned on holding an open meeting to review the current status of 21 CFR Part 11 in June 2004. With the unfortunate death of former president Ronald Reagan, however, that meeting was cancelled. There are no plans to re-organize the meeting, and any changes to 21 CFR Part 11 will be implemented only through the submission of written comments.

The general position of industry is that, while it supports the concepts of 21 CFR Part 11, it does not agree with the regulation being so specific in terms of technological solutions (such as the use of identification codes and passwords). In addition, the US government passed the Federal Electronic Signatures In Global and National Commerce Act (S.761) in June 2000, which would seem to overrule the requirements listed in 21 CFR Part 11.

Expediting Drug and Biologics Development

Industry will need to continue its remediation efforts and be able to demonstrate that all electronic information submitted to any regulatory authority is reliable. Good software design, testing, maintenance, and retirement practices will always be required. It is in the industry's best interests to ensure that new technologies are applied judiciously and are implemented only when proven to be satisfactory in meeting the requirements of the applicable predicate rules.

CHAPTER 8

Format and Content of the Common Technical Document (CTD)

By Diana Fordyce, Ph.D., and Leo Pavliv, R.Ph., M.B.A.

WHAT IS A CTD? The ultimate goal in the clinical development of a new medicinal product is to obtain regulatory agency authorization to sell and market the product. In the United States (U.S.), the Food and Drug Administration (FDA) must approve the marketing application. The marketing application is delineated in Form FDA 356h and defined in Title 21 of the United States (U.S.) Code of Federal Regulations (hereinafter referred to as 21 CFR) Part 312.3 as an application for a new drug (i.e., New Drug Application [NDA]) submitted under section 505(b) of the Act or a product license application for a biological product (Biologics License Application [BLA]) under the Public Health Service Act. The content of an NDA/BLA is described in 21 CFR Parts 314 and 601, associated FDA technical guidances, and International Conference on Harmonisation (ICH) technical guidances on safety (S), quality (Q) and efficacy (E).

The FDA has used format and content guidances to describe how companies should organize and submit all the information (specified on Form FDA 356h) required in an NDA/BLA or electronic NDA/BLA (eNDAs and eBLAs). Before the ICH's efforts to develop a harmonized marketing application format, each ICH region (e.g., European Union, Japan and U.S.) had different formats, thereby making it complex, costly and time-consuming for applicants to submit marketing applications in all the regions (e.g., reformatting large volumes of information into the various regional formats).

The Common Technical Document (CTD) is the ICH's term for a global dossier that provides a common format acceptable to all regions. Since July 2003, ICH initiatives for the CTD (mutltidisciplinary [M]4) have been in effect, with the CTD format being mandatory for marketing applications submitted in the EU and Japan and "highly recommended" in the United States. It is important to note that the CTD format does not substantially change the primary submission requirements for marketing applications, but comprises a submission format that is acceptable to regulatory authorities in the ICH regions.

The CTD comprises 5 modules:
- Module 1 is region-specific, and includes administrative information (e.g., in the U.S., it would include the Form-FDA 356 marketing application form) and labeling (e.g., in the U.S., it would include the proposed package insert).
- Module 2 (summary and overview information for each technical discipline)
- Module 3 (chemistry/pharmaceutical development, referred to as quality information)
- Module 4 (nonclinical reports, referred to as safety information)
- Module 5 (clinical reports, referred to as efficacy information)

The CTD's Pyramid Structure The pyramid concept for the construction of the NDA/BLA (shown below in the CTD format) can aid in developing a sense for the building blocks and organization of a marketing application. As shown below, the proposed labeling is developed at the IND stage (i.e., the Investigator's Brochure progresses to the proposed labeling). The data from each technical discipline (chemistry, nonclinical, and clinical) are collected according to the appropriate regulatory requirements as appropriate (GMP, GLP, GCP, respectively) and are then compiled into individual reports in each technical module (Module 3: Quality; Module 4: Nonclinical; and Module 5: Efficacy, respectively). Tabular and written summaries and overviews are then provided for each technical discipline in the summary module (i.e., in Module 2). This information is then provided as cross-references (annotation) to support the statements in the proposed labeling.

Expediting Drug and Biologics Development

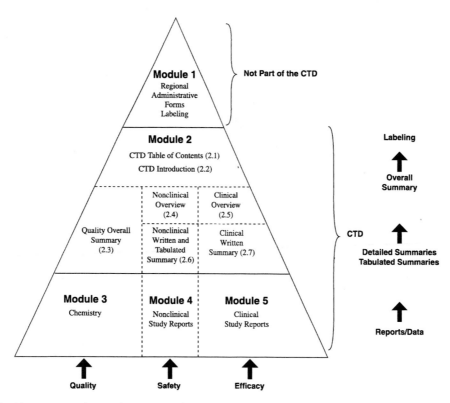

Reference Tools The ICH guidance documents that comprise the essential reference tools for constructing the CTD are listed below. The guidances were developed to parallel the CTD's "organization" (M4) and technical disciplines (M4Q Quality [chemistry], M4S Safety [nonclinical], and M4E Efficacy [clinical]). The organization guidance document (M4) indicates which components of the CTD are to be individual documents ("granularity"; important for the electronic structure), and the eCTD specifications indicate exact electronic naming. Each discipline has a related "questions and answers" document that tracks the questions received in each area along with the corresponding answers.

> Link: http://www.ich.org/
> - ICH - M4 - CTD - Organization
> - ICH - Questions and Answers - General
> - ICH - M2 - eCTD Specifications
> - ICH - M4Q - CTD - Quality
> - ICH - Questions and Answers - Quality
> - ICH - M4S - CTD - Safety
> - ICH - Questions and Answers - Safety
> - ICH - M4E - CTD - Efficacy
> - ICH - Questions and Answers - Efficacy

In addition to publishing the above guidance documents, the FDA has released a number of other agency-specific guidances on the submission of CTD-formatted marketing applications in the United States and on the submission of electronic applications in the CTD format (eCTD):

> Link: http://www.fda.gov/cder/guidance/index.htm......ICH
> - "Submitting Marketing Applications According to the ICH CTD Format - General Considerations"
> Link: http://www.fda.gov/cder/regulatory/ersr/ectd.htm.....Electronic Submission
> - "Providing Regulatory Submissions in Electronic Format-Human Pharmaceutical Product Applications and Related Submissions." This guidance refers to a series of specifications documents that include the M2 through M5 eCTD backbones and a U.S. regional Module 1 eCTD backbone. In moving toward the eCTD era, the FDA has accepted a hybrid eNDA (utilizing previous eNDA guidances) and CTD (utilizing the ICH eCTD specifications and FDA "General Considerations" Guidances).

Applicants should also reference product-specific reference tools (when available) when developing an NDA/BLA (e.g., specific guidances are available for inhalation products).

Chapter 8 - Format and Content of the Common Technical Document (CTD)

The NDA/BLA in CTD Format: Module 1 The fundamental theme of this book—plan with the endgoal in mind—is just as applicable to the marketing application development process as it is in earlier phases. Four documents should be used as "roadmaps" for the marketing application development plan. The documents will be used as or in components of Module 1 of the CTD: (1) marketing application form; (2) tracking of regulatory interactions and fulfillment of regulatory requirements/requests; (3) proposed product labeling; and (4) comprehensive table of contents for the CTD, including Module 1. These documents are described in more detail below.

Marketing Application Form (Form-FDA 356h) The Form FDA 356h (Application to Market a New Drug, Biologic, or an Antibiotic Drug for Human Use) is used for the NDAs, BLAs, and abbreviated new drug applications (ANDAs) in the United States. The form identifies the sections that can comprise an NDA/BLA to be submitted to the FDA (note: not all sections will be relevant to specific products or applications).

Product Description To avoid possible confusion and costly documentation changes later in development, product description information should be addressed and determined early in the development process. Doing so also forces the sponsor to consider key regulatory and marketing strategy issues that may arise following the decision on the proposed indication and classification.

PRODUCT DESCRIPTION		
NEW DRUG OR ANTIBIOTIC APPLICATION NUMBER, OR BIOLOGICS LICENSE APPLICATION NUMBER (If previously issued)		
ESTABLISHED NAME (e.g., Proper name, USP/USAN name)	PROPRIETARY NAME (trade name) IF ANY	
CHEMICAL/BIOCHEMICAL/BLOOD PRODUCT NAME (If any)	CODE NAME (If any)	
DOSAGE FORM:	STRENGTHS:	ROUTE OF ADMINISTRATION:
(PROPOSED) INDICATION(S) FOR USE:		

Abbreviations:
USP/USAN, United States Pharmacopeia/United States Adopted Names

replicated and extracted from Form FDA 356h

Establishing product name conventions may require early consultation with United States Pharmacopeia or United States Adopted Names (USP/USAN) and the FDA Nomenclature Standards Committee (Washington Drug Letter [1997] and ongoing FDA initiatives on product naming to avoid medication errors). Because the trade name may change at the time of FDA approval, the trade name should be used only in the proposed labeling, and the established or generic name should be used on all other NDA/BLA documentation.

The application number for drugs can be obtained prior to submission, but not for biologics. For drugs, application numbers in the range of 00001 to 49999 indicate original NDAs, 50000 to 59999 indicate original antibiotic NDAs, 60000 to 69999 indicate antibiotic ANDAs, and 70000 and up indicate ANDAs. The application number is then part of the FDA's Orange Book or "Approved Drug Products with Therapeutic Equivalence Evaluations" (the List) guide to obtaining information regarding the application. The Orange Book (http://www.fda.gov/cder/orange/default.htm; http://www.accessdata.fda.gov/scripts/cder/drugsatfda/index.cfm) includes the marketing status ([1] approved prescription drug products; [2] approved over-the-counter (OTC) drug products for those drugs not marketed without NDAs/ANDAs because they are not covered under existing monographs; [3] drug products with approval under Section 505 of the Act administered by CBER; [4] discontinued drug products). The Orange Book also includes the application number, the generic and trade names, the strengths, the applicant (holder of the application), patent number and expiration date, exclusivity code (including orphan drug) and expiration date, and equivalence evaluation information.

The indication is the part of the proposed product labeling that is used to guide expedient product development. The determination of the proposed indication(s) early in development will ensure adherence to appropriate treatment-related regulations and guidelines as well as provide a way of determining if the product has any existing comparator treatments. The existence and review of comparator treatments can be used early in the development program to determine the regulatory and marketing strategies involved. For example, clinical trials may involve comparator controls, and the proposed labeling claims may indicate no difference, equivalence, or superiority. In addition, the product and the proposed indication may have been the subject of a recent marketing application that was submitted or a marketing approval action (and/or have an active patent) and may, therefore, have terms of exclusivity that should be considered in the regulatory and marketing strategy considerations (exclusivity considerations are discussed in the next section of this chapter).

Expediting Drug and Biologics Development

The "uniform" terms provided in the Orange Book are helpful indicators of appropriate listing of dosage forms and routes of administration. The dosage form, strengths, and route of administration may affect the classification of the product which, in turn, may affect regulatory and/or marketing strategy considerations such as the application type, the associated development program, and exclusivity considerations. As an example, if XY is a fixed combination drug product being assessed for clinical product development, consider the scenarios described below:

- If X and Y are currently sold separately for the same indication
  - in the same formulation, then combination XY may be considered a new combination and must follow the regulations (21 CFR 300.50) for these types of products, which stipulate specific types of clinical trials. The application may be considered a 505(b)(1)-type or 505(b)(2)-type NDA or efficacy supplement application depending on the amount of, and right to reference, information from the original application(s).
  - in a different formulation, then combination XY may be considered both a new combination and a new formulation, which may require clinical trials for the new combination (21 CFR 300.50) as well as the new formulation. The application may be considered a 505(b)(1)-type or 505(b)(2)-type NDA or efficacy supplement application depending on the amount of, and right to reference, information from the original application(s).
- If X and Y are already sold as a fixed combination XY for the same indication
  - In the same formulation, then combination XY may be considered suitable for an ANDA (i.e., a generic product), which would require bioequivalence trials (21 CFR Part 320).
  - in a different formulation, then combination XY may be considered a new formulation, which may require clinical trials to demonstrate a comparison with the existing formulation. The application may be considered a 505(b)(1)-type or 505(b)(2)-type NDA or efficacy supplement application depending on the amount of, and right to reference, information from the original application(s).

Clearly, in this example, careful consideration of the product's classification, and appropriate consultation with the FDA, and the applicant's patent and exclusivity situation and/or ability to conduct a full development program are critical early in the development program.

Application Types (505(b)(1) NDA, 505(b)(2) NDA, ANDA and BLA) The application types (NDA, BLA, or ANDA) are provided on the Form 356h with the appropriate regulatory reference.

APPLICATION DESCRIPTION

APPLICATION TYPE

(check one) ☐ NEW DRUG APPLICATION (21 CFR 314.50)   ☐ ABBREVIATED APPLICATION (ANDA, 21 CFR 314.94)
☐ BIOLOGICS LICENSE APPLICATION (BLA, 21 CFR part 601)

IF AN NDA, IDENTIFY THE APPROPRIATE TYPE   ☐ 505 (b) (1)   ☐ 505 (b) (2)

IF AN ANDA, OR 505(b)(2), IDENTIFY THE REFERENCE LISTED DRUG PRODUCT THAT IS THE BASIS FOR THE SUBMISSION

Name of Drug   Holder of Approved Application

TYPE OF SUBMISSION

(check one)   ☐ ORIGINAL APPLICATION   ☐ AMENDMENT TO A PENDING APPLICATION   ☐ RESUBMISSION
☐ PRESUBMISSION   ☐ ANNUAL REPORT   ☐ ESTABLISHMENT DESCRIPTION SUPPLEMENT
☐ EFFICACY SUPPLEMENT ☐ LABELING SUPPLEMENT ☐ CHEMISTRY MANUFACTURING AND CONTROLS SUPPLEMENT ☐ OTHER

Abbreviations: *replicated and extracted from Form FDA 356h*
ANDA, Abbreviated New Drug Application

The type of NDA is specified according to the section of the Federal Food, Drug, and Cosmetic Act in which it is described (i.e., 505(b)(1), 505(b)(2)). The types of NDAs differ in terms of content (codified in 21 CFR Part 314 Subparts B and C) and possible terms of exclusivity (codified in 21 CFR 314.108). Exclusivity prevents the submission or effective approval of ANDAs or 505(b)(2) applications for similar conditions of approval; it does not prevent the submission or approval of a full NDA. Exclusivity provisions begin on the effective date of approval, which refers to the date of final approval and not to the date of tentative approval. Exclusivity considerations should be considered in concert with patent term information.

Briefly, the types of NDAs are described as follows:

505(b)(1) NDA

- The 505(b)(1) is characterized as a "full NDA."
- The required content is codified in 21 CFR 314.50; all information is required.
- Up to 5 years exclusivity (as codified in 21 CFR 314.108) may be received for a new chemical entity.

505(b)(2) NDA

- The 505(b)(2) is characterized as an NDA in which investigations other than bioavailability or bioequivalence trials are required for approval of a new indication or other change from a listed drug and an NDA in which some of the original investigations that are relied on for approval were not conducted by or for the applicant and the applicant has not obtained a right of reference or use from the original applicant. This type of application includes and has also been referred to as a "literature-based NDA" and is considered a modification of the former "paper NDA."
- The required content is codified in 21 CFR 314.3(b) and 314.54; all information is required as detailed in 21 CFR 314.50 (including appropriate patent information and certification) with the exception that nonclinical and clinical data are required as needed to support the safety and effectiveness. A 505(b)(2) cannot be filed for a product that could qualify as an ANDA (21 CFR 314.101(9)) or for inability to qualify as an ANDA due to differences from RLD (reference listed drug) that represent a poorly bioavailable product (less rate/extent of absorption compared with that of the RLD)(21 CFR 314.54).
- Up to 3 years exclusivity (as codified in 21 CFR 314.50(j)(4) and 314.108) may be received if the clinical investigations (other than bioavailability or bioequivalence) are:
  - New (i.e., the results of the clinical investigation(s) have not been relied on by the FDA to demonstrate substantial evidence of effectiveness of a previously approved drug product for any indication or of safety for a new patient population); and
  - essential to approval (i.e., certification that the applicant has thoroughly searched the scientific literature and, to the best of the applicant's knowledge, the list of published studies and publicly available reports of clinical investigations is complete and accurate and does not provide sufficient basis for the approval of the conditions for which the applicant is seeking without reference to the new clinical investigation(s). It should be noted that the FDA decides whether a study is essential to approval at the time of approval of the application and, therefore, scientific literature available after the time of submission and during the review process of the application is considered [Abbreviated New Drug Application Regulations: Patent and Exclusivity Provisions, Federal Register, Vol. 59, No. 190, October 3, 1994]); and
  - conducted or sponsored by the applicant (i.e., the applicant was named in the Form FDA 1571 for the Investigational New Drug Application [IND] under which the new clinical investigation(s) that is essential to approval of the application was conducted) and supported by the applicant (e.g., certification that the applicant provided 50% or more of the cost of conducting the study).

Interestingly, the 505(b)(2) is often described as a regulatory bridge between an ANDA and a full NDA because the 505(b)(2) provides a mechanism through which an applicant that is not the original listed drug applicant (innovator) of a product can gain approval for certain changes to that product. The 505(b)(2) is similar to a 505(b)(1) efficacy supplement except that the 505(b)(2) is sponsored by an applicant other than the original listed drug applicant and the investigations that are relied upon from the original listed drug application were not conducted by or for the applicant and there is not a right to reference or use. If the drug product is an active ingredient that has been previously approved (e.g., in a different formulation that allows a lower dose to achieve the same bioavailability as a higher dose of the RLD, or an extended release formulation) under another applicant and no longer under patent or exclusivity provisions, it may be helpful to consider referencing (and not repeating) some nonclinical and clinical work and filing a 505(b)(2)-type application that would allow reference to information in the previously approved application. This strategy would shorten development time, but would result in up to 3 years of exclusivity possible for investigations of safety and efficacy that may be required (compared with 5 years of exclusivity possible for a 505(b)(1)-type application). This type of application is described further in review articles such as U.S. Regulatory Reporter, Guide to 505(b)(2) Submissions (1995) and the Guidance for Industry: Applications Covered by Section 505(b)(2) and should be discussed with the FDA early in development of the product.

ANDA

Abbreviated applications (ANDAs) are categorized and the content codified in 21 CFR 314.94. Bioequivalence is defined as similar rate and extent of absorption at equimolar dose.

A suitability petition abbreviated applications (suitability petition ANDAs) is categorized and the content codified in 21 CFR 314.93 and FR 57 No 82 Apr 28 1992. Bioequivalence is defined as similar rate and extent of absorption at equimolar dose. This type of application would apply to products that are a new strength, new route, or new dose form of the RLD, and (for combination drug product) a change in a combination product of one of the active ingredients to a different one in the same class. A suitability petition ANDA can not be filed for only a difference in inactive ingredients/excipients from RLD (i.e., the differences in inactive ingredients/excipients have to be in accordance with 21 CFR 314.94(a)(9) for ANDAs or submitted as a 505(b)(2) NDA). A suitability petition ANDA will not be approved if safety and effectiveness investigations (information derived from animal or clinical studies or literature beyond BA/BE or limited confirmatory testing) are required (it should be submitted as a 505(b)(2) NDA).

Supplements

Supplemental applications are categorized and the content is codified in 21 CFR 314.70 for new drug applications (often referred to as sNDAs) and in 21 CFR 314.97 for abbreviated applications. Supplements to the original new drug application such as "efficacy supplements" may receive up to 3 years exclusivity (as codified in 21 CFR 314.50(j)(4) and 314.108) if the clinical investigations (other than bioavailability or bioequivalence) are new, essential to approval, and conducted or sponsored by the applicant as described above for 505(b)(2) applications. Efficacy supplements can be submitted for the following:

(1) A new indication or significant modification to the existing indication, including removal of a major limitation to use, such as second line status;

(2) A new dosing regimen, including an increase or decrease in daily dosage, or a change in frequency of administration;

(3) A new route of administration;

(4) A comparative efficacy or pharmacokinetic claim naming another drug;

(5) A change in sections other than the INDICATIONS AND USAGE section that would significantly alter the patient population to be treated, such as addition of pediatric use and/or dosing information or geriatric use and/or dosing information; or

(6) A proposed prescription-to-OTC switch.

Cross References

Cross references to related applications (License Applications, INDs, NDAs, and device applications) and drug or biologic master files (DMF or BMF) should be listed. The document type, number, holder, product, and other relevant information should be provided

Cross References (list related License Applications, INDs, NDAs, PMAs, 510(k)s, IDEs, BMFs, and DMFs referenced in the current application)

Abbreviations: replicated and extracted from Form FDA 356h

        IND, Investigational New Drug Application

        NDA, New Drug Application

        PMA, Pre-market Authorization

        IDE, Investigational Device Exemption

        BMF, Biologics Master File

        DMF, Drug Master File

Master files may be useful to cross reference as they may provide information about the substance, substance intermediate, and materials used in their preparation, and product (Type II), packaging materials (Type III), excipient, colorant, flavor, essence, and materials used in their preparation (Type IV), and FDA Accepted Reference Information (Type V), such that the information is updated in only one document rather than several applications. The holder of a master file can authorize an applicant to reference master file information (note: Type I DMFs [Manufacturing Site, Facilities, Operating Procedures, and Personnel] are no longer applicable per Final Rule published January 12, 2000 (65 FR 1776)).

Chapter 8 - Format and Content of the Common Technical Document (CTD)

It should be noted, however, that the master file information is not approved or disapproved by the FDA and will be reviewed only in conjunction with the marketing application. Important information regarding master files is located in the Guideline for Drug Master Files and in 21 CFR 314.420 (a DMF list is provided at website http://www.fda.gov/cder/dmf/).

It is also important to note that 7 years of exclusivity is possible, effective the date of FDA approval of a marketing application, for a product and indication that are the subject of orphan designation (codified in 21 CFR 316.31).

Rx, OTC

The applicant is required to state the proposed marketing status is prescription (Rx) or over-the-counter (OTC) status. Labeling requirements are codified, in 21 CFR 201 Subpart B and C respectively. A marketing application would be required for a product that deviates from the applicable OTC monograph (21 CFR 330.11). OTC monographs specific for some types of products are provided in 21 CFR Parts 331-358 and discussed in MAPP 6020.5.

Regulatory Information Consistent with the ICH guidance documents, the sponsor must acknowledge in the application those cases in which it received direct regulatory guidance from an agency, how it implemented such guidance. If the applicant did not implement an agency's recommendations, it must discuss and justify such deviations (M4S - 2.4; M4E - 2.5.1 and M4Q - QOS; FDA guidance on Clinical and Statistical Sections of New Drug Applications (1988)). For example, Module 5 (Section 2.5.1) indicates that, "Regulatory guidance and advice [at least from the region or regions where the Clinical Overview is being submitted] should be identified, with discussion of how that advice was implemented. Formal advice documents (e.g., official meeting minutes, official guidance, and letters from regulatory authorities) should be referenced, with copies included in the references section of Module 5." While the guidance does not specifically call for a tabular summary, a table can be used to list relevant regulatory guidances and any related regulatory interactions. The exhibit below provides an example of a tabular template to indicate regulatory interactions; this can be easily separated by technical discipline.

Summary Table of Regulatory Interactions (Meetings, Correspondence, Submissions)

Document Submitted	Submission Date ·	Details of Submission and Related Regulatory Agency Correspondence (noting deviations or fulfillment of Guidances/Requests)	Technical Discipline (/associated disciplines)		
			Chemistry	Nonclinical	Clinical/ Statistical

This type of tabular summary for regulatory interactions or regulatory data base output may be used in each CTD overview section by technical discipline. It can also be used as an attachment to the application's cover letter to document significant FDA instructions/decisions that affect the information contained in the NDA/BLA.

Targeted Product Profile - Annotated Labeling The marketing application is designed to provide evidence that the product is both safe and effective when used under specified conditions and when manufactured appropriately. Therefore, the application provides all the information that supports each statement in the proposed labeling for the product. Whether it is a paper-based or electronic submission and regardless of the ICH region in which it is submitted, the marketing application comprises many pages of documentation that support one to two pages of product labeling (e.g., the U.S. package insert or the European Summary of Product Characteristics, and labels on the containers) that physicians and the general public read and use.

The exhibit below provides a proposed template for final annotation of the U.S. package insert. FDA regulations require that the package insert provide annotations to the summary and technical sections (21 CFR 314.50(c) and (d)). Information supporting each statement in the package insert is annotated to the location of the information in a paper submission by volume and page number in a paper submission (FDA "Guideline for the Format and Content of the Summary for the New Drug and Antibiotic Applications" [1987]). In an electronic application, this information is hypertext linked (FDA Guidance "Providing Regulatory Submissions in Electronic Format - NDAs) to the supporting information in the electronic filing. In either case, each marketing application must provide the so-called "content of labeling" section in electronic format (FDA Guidance "SPL Standard for Content of Labeling," 2006). Preliminary annotation can be tracked throughout the development process by providing the study report number or comments in the annotation section that supports the proposed labeling statements. The exhibit below provides an example of a preliminary annotation.

This concept of utilizing the proposed product labeling as a means through which to track information and update the proposed labeling throughout product development is the subject of an FDA pilot program undertaken by CDER's Office of Drug Evaluation IV (i.e., the Targeted Product Information or Profile (TPI or TPP)). The Targeted Product Profile doc-

	Annotation	
	Item 3(Summary Section)	Technical Section

INDICATION AND USAGE (21 CFR 201.57(c))
PRODUCT is indicated [for the treatment of, OR prevention of, OR diagnosis of, OR as an adjunct to a specific mode of therapy] in patients with INDICATION, who are: list characteristics of patients if needed, to: relate to clinical endpoints.

preliminary annotation
   adequate and well-controlled studies:

prd1-cl-001-im; prd1-cl-003-im

ument is described on the FDA website as an evolving version of the proposed labeling that can be used by the sponsor to: (1) guide the design, conduct, and analysis of clinical trials; (2) facilitate communication with the FDA; and (3) promote a shared understanding of the sponsor's drug development program. The TPP is essentially a proposed package insert with the supporting study number information (i.e., preliminary annotation). The FDA expects the TPI to provide a greater amount of information than the General Investigational Plan submitted with the IND, and can: (1) be updated with the IND's annual report to the IND (the annual report regulations require a general investigational plan for the coming year); (2) be utilized at milestone meetings; and (3) enable communication about such critical subjects as the number of adequate and well-controlled studies required to support an indication and patient population.

A summary of the product and comparator products for treating the proposed indication(s) can be developed early in the development program and updated throughout development. This table should be presented in the form of a side-by-side comparison of the package inserts for the products for ANDAs (21 CFR 314.94(a)(8)) and 505(b)(2)s. The information can correspond to the preliminary annotation of the package insert to support components of the clinical development plan that are ongoing. This type of table can be used as a multipurpose tool for: (1) ensuring appropriate considerations and marketing strategy for the proposed labeling; and (2) inserting into the evaluation of the benefits/risk section of the clinical overview (CTD M4E Section 2.5.6).

Product Characteristic	Product X	Competitor Product Y	Competitor Product Z
Reference Information		Trade Name Application #/date/country Company	Trade Name Application #/date/country Company
Indication and Usage			
Dosage and Administration			
Route/Form/Delivery Active/Inactive Ingredients			
Effectiveness Profile			
Pharmacokinetic Profile			
Safety Profile			

Index (Comprehensive Table of Contents) and Compilation The following table provides a comparison of the formats that have been used previously for the organization of the NDA/BLA compared to the CTD. In the interim period (i.e., prior to the availability of final eCTD guidance), the FDA has accepted a hybrid eNDA/CTD in which the eNDA folder structure and a CTD/eCTD organization/file naming format are used. Knowledge of all the NDA/BLA requirements as listed in the Form-FDA 356h and the corresponding CTD components can guide the compilation of the NDA/BLA.

Index of NDA/BLA as per 21 CFR (Item #s as per Form FDA 356h)	eNDA Format	Location in CTD Format	eCTD Format Folder Name/File name
1. Index	main folder	Module 1	m1/
2. Labeling (check one) -Draft Labeling -Final Printed Labeling	labeling	Module 1	m1/
3. Summary (21 CFR 314.50 (c))	summary	Module 2	m2/
4. Chemistry section	cmc	Module 3 Module 2.3	m3/ m2/23-qos/

–continued–

Index of NDA/BLA as per 21 CFR (Item #s as per Form FDA 356h)	eNDA Format	Location in CTD Format	eCTD Format Folder Name/File name
A. Chemistry, manufacturing, and controls information (e.g. 21 CFR 314.50 (d) (1), 21 CFR 601.2)			
B. Samples (21 CFR 314.50 (e) (1), 21 CFR 601.2 (a)) (Submit only upon FDA's request)			
C. Methods validation package (e.g. 21 CFR 314.50 (e) (2) (i), 21 CFR 601.2)			
5. Nonclinical pharmacology and toxicology section (e.g. 21 CFR 314.50 (d) (2), 21 CFR 601.2)	pharmtox	Module 4 Module 2.4, 2.6	m4/ m2/24-nonclin-over/ m2/26-nonclin-sum/
6. Human pharmacokinetics and bioavailability (e.g. 21 CFR 314.50 (d) (3), 21 CFR 601.2)	cpbio	Module 5.3.1 - 4 Module 2.5, 2.7.1, 2.7.2, 2.7.5, 2.7.6	m5-clin-stud-rep/531-534... m2/25-clin-over/ m2/27-clin-sum/summary-biopharm.pdf, -clin-pharm.pdf
7. Clinical Microbiology (e.g. 21 CFR 314.50 (d) (4))	micro	Module 5 Module 2.5, 2.7	
8. Clinical data section (e.g. 21 CFR 314.50 (d) (5), 21 CFR 601.2)	clinstat	Module 5.3.5- Module 2.5, 2.7.3, 2.7.4, 2.7.5, 2.7.6	m5-clin-stud-rep /535... m2/25-clin-over/ m2/27-clin-sum/summary-clin-efficacy.pdf, summary-clin-safety.pdf, synopses-indiv-studies.pdf
9. Safety update report e.g. 21 CFR 314.50 (d) (5) (vi) (b), 21 CFR 601.2)	update	Module 5	
10. Statistical section (e.g. 21 CFR 314.50 (d) (6), 21 CFR 601.2)	clinstat	Module 5	
11. Case report tabulations (e.g. 21 CFR 314.50 (f) (1), 21 CFR 601.2)	crt	Module 5.3.7	m5-clin-stud-rep /537...
12. Case reports forms (e.g. 21 CFR 314.50 (f) (2), 21 CFR 601.2)	crf	Module 5.3.7	m5-clin-stud-rep /535...
13. Patent information-any which claims the drug (21 U.S.C. 355 (b) or (c)) (Form FDA 3542)	other	Module 1	m1/
14. Patent certification-any which claims the drug (21 U.S.C. 355 (b) (2) or (j) (2) (A)) (Form FDA 3542)	other	Module 1	m1/
15. Establishment description (21 CFR Part 600, if applicable)	other	Module 1	m1/
16. Debarment certification (FD&C Act 306 (k) (1))	other	Module 1	m1/
17. Field copy certification (21 CFR 314.50 (l) (3))	other	Module 1	m1/
18. User Fee Cover Sheet (Form FDA 3397)	other	Module 1	m1/
19. Financial Information (21 CFR Part 54) (Form FDA 3454, 3455)	other	Module 1	m1/
20. OTHER (specify)		Dependent on information	

Consistent with the ICH guidance, Module 1 should have a completed table of contents in the CTD including Module 1. A draft or "working" comprehensive table of contents should be developed at the start of a project and should be developed specifically for the medicinal product to be submitted. The table of contents should be based on a template of the CTD, including all required tables and the region-specific requirements for organization of the table of contents for Module 1. The table of contents should then be modified for the specific product (e.g., all reports planned and completed should be specified in the table of contents, all literature should be listed, etc). An extraction from an example draft or "working" comprehensive table of contents is provided in the exhibit below.

2.7.6	Synopses of Individual Studies
Table 2.7.6-1	Listing of Clinical Studies (Copy of Table 5.1)
2.7.6.1	GOOD COMPANY - BE Study Comparing Good Drug to RLD Study No. GD- CL-001]
2.7.6.2	*GOOD COMPANY - BE Study Comparing Good Drug 300 to 3x100 [Study No. GD- CL-002]*

Italics indicate that the study is not yet completed.
List studies in the same order as in Module 5. Table 5.1 should categorize and list in same order as in Module 5.
Studies not in italics indicates the study is completed and in the eCTD backbone Module 5.

FORMAT AND CONTENT OF THE CTD: MODULES 2-5 In many cases, documentation obtained during the development process is assembled on an as-needed basis, with the format and content dependent on the sponsor's preference at that time. Subsequently, the NDA/BLA is then compiled at the end of Phase 3, with considerable effort necessary to restructure the information in a similar format. For example, sponsors have been known to conduct five or more studies with five or more data collection and reporting standards (due to differences in contract research organizations and/or internal differences), something that requires the sponsor to embark on the time-consuming and costly effort of reworking key study information into a consistent format to logically display safety, pharmacokinetic, and efficacy information. Some information elements that often are compiled in the final months of development (but that should be compiled continuously throughout development) include the package insert, data set integration, report synopses and primary quantitative tabular summaries of results.

While each application presents unique issues, experience indicates that the submission of a marketing application would be delayed by approximately one to two months for every clinical study report that was not incorporated immediately after completion into a report, summary tables, and the proposed labeling. Similar delays transpire if specific development reports are not developed before writing the chemistry section. For an average marketing application, this translates into approximately a one-year delay.

The NDA/BLA project team assigned to the product should be very familiar with the components of the CTD. Typically, the team includes representatives from regulatory, project management, clinical, biopharmaceutics, biostatistics, pharmacology/toxicology, and chemistry. The team should discuss content issues, data presentation, and target dates. In addition, the team members should be aware that the NDA is a document that supports each statement of the labeling. Experience indicates that the team can ensure efficient project execution and change control with the use of status reports and meetings that review and track target completion dates of the modules of the CTD draft or "working" table of contents and related tasks (i.e., Gantt charts).

To expedite the completion of clinical information in the marketing application, the CTD modules should be started early in development and updated continually. It may be possible to submit the modules as portions of the investigational application (e.g., electronic IND) or marketing application (fast track/continuous marketing application). The following sections in this chapter provide a comprehensive table of contents (including required or suggested tables) for each of the CTD modules based on the CTD guidances (see section on "Reference Tools" above). In addition, the sections provide some experience-based tips for efficiency in compiling each module of the CTD.

CHEMISTRY (QUALITY) Module

Module 2: Quality Elements

2.3 QUALITY OVERALL SUMMARY (QOS)	
Introduction	
The introduction should include proprietary name, nonproprietary name or common name of the drug substance, company name, dosage forms, strengths, route of administration, and proposed indications.	Reference proposed labeling
2.3.S DRUG SUBSTANCE	
2.3.S.1 General information (name, manufacturer)	
2.3.S.2 Manufacture (name, manufacturer)	
Figure 2.3.S.2.1 Detailed flow diagram of manufacturing process	Copy Figure 3.2.S.2.2
Table 2.3.S.2.1 Raw materials used to manufacture API	Copy Table 3.2.S.2.3

–continued–

Table 2.3.S.2.2 Critical steps, acceptance criteria and tests	Copy Table 3.2.S.2.4
Table 2.3.S.2.3 Lot, use, scale, site, process, reason for change (if applicable) and impact	Copy Table 3.2.S.2.6
2.3.S.3 Characterization (name, manufacturer)	
Table 2.3.S.3.1 Studies performed to elucidate the structure of the API	Copy Table 3.2.S.3.1
2.3.S.4 Control of drug substance (name, manufacturer)	
Table 2.3.S4.15 API specification table including name of test, reference (if compendial or in-house) and specification limits	Copy Table 3.2.S.4.1
Table 2.3.S.4.2 Lot, use, scale and results	Copy Table 3.2.S.4.4
2.3.S.5 Reference standards or materials (name, manufacturer)	
Table 2.3.S.5.1 Specifications and characterization results for the reference standards	Copy Table 3.2.S.5
2.3.S.6 Container closure system (name, manufacturer)	
2.3.S.7 Stability (name, manufacturer)	
Table 2.3.S.7.1 Stability protocol time-points, conditions, and test to be conducted	Copy Table 3.2.S.7.2
Table 2.3.S.7.2 Stability results from registrational lots and supporting lots	Copy Table 3.2.S.7.3
2.3.P DRUG PRODUCT	
2.3.P.1 Description and composition of the drug product (name, dosage form)	
Table 2.3.P.1.1 Qualitative and quantitative composition of each strength (including quality (compendial or other) and function in the formulation)	Copy Table 3.2.P.1
2.3.P.2 Pharmaceutical development (name, dosage form)	
Table 2.3.P.2.1 Lot, dosage form (if changed), use, scale, site, process used, reason for change (if applicable) and impact	Copy Table 3.2.P.2.2.1
2.3.P.3 Manufacture (name, dosage form)	
Figure 2.3.P.3.1 Detailed flow diagram of manufacturing process	Copy Figure 3.2.P.3.3
Table 2.3.P.3.2 Critical steps, acceptance criteria and tests	Copy Table 3.2.P.3.4
2.3.P.4 Control of excipients (name, dosage form)	
Table 2.3.P.4.1 Specifications (For each excipient that is not USP with test, and reference (compendial or in-house). Where acceptance criteria are above compendial, provide list of those tests and specifications.)	Copy Tables 3.2.P.4.1
2.3.P.5 Control of drug product (name, dosage form)	
Table 2.3.P.5.1 Specifications (including name of test, reference (if compendial or in-house) and specification limits)	Copy Table 3.2.P.5.1
Table 2.3.P.5.2 Lot, use, scale and results	Copy Table 3.2.P.5.4
2.3.P.6 Reference standards or materials (name, dosage form)	
Table 2.3.P.6.1 Specifications and characterization results for the reference standards	Copy Table 3.2.P.6
2.3.P.7 Container closure system (name, dosage form)	
2.3.P.8 Stability (name, dosage form)	
Table 2.3.P.8.1 Stability protocol table with time-points, conditions, and tests to be conducted	Copy Table 3.2.P.8.2
Table 2.3.P.8.2 Stability results from the registrational lots as well as supporting lots	Copy Tables 3.2.P.8.3
2.3.A APPENDICES 2.3.A.1 Facilities and Equipment 2.3.A.2 Adventitious Agents safety Evaluation 2.3.A.3 Excipients	
2.3.R REGIONAL INFORMATION (EU)	
2.3.R REGIONAL INFORMATION (US)	

Module 3: Quality

3.1 MODULE 3 TABLE OF CONTENTS
3.2 BODY OF DATA
3.2.S DRUG SUBSTANCE (name of drug substance, manufacturer of drug substance)
3.2.S.1 General information (name, manufacturer)
3.2.S.1.1 Nomenclature (name, manufacturer)
3.2.S.1.2 Structure (name, manufacturer)
3.2.S.1.3 General Properties (name, manufacturer)
3.2.S.2 Manufacture (name, manufacturer)

–continued–

3.2.S.2.1 Manufacturers (name, manufacturer)
3.2.S.2.2 Description of manufacturing process and process controls (name, manufacturer) Figure 3.2.S.2.2 Detailed flow diagram of the manufacturing process
3.2.S.2.3 Control of materials (name, manufacturer) Table 3.2.S.2.3 Raw materials used to manufacture the API (including where used in the process and grade of material)
3.2.S.2.4 Controls of critical steps and intermediates (name, manufacturer) Table 3.2.S.2.4 Critical steps, acceptance criteria and tests
3.2.S.2.5 Process validation and/or evaluation (name, manufacturer)
3.2.S.2.6 Manufacturing process development (name, manufacturer) Table 3.2.S.2.6 Lot, use, scale, site, process, reason for change (if applicable) and impact
3.2.S.3 Characterization (name, manufacturer)
3.2.S.3.1 Elucidation of structure and other characteristics (name, manufacturer) Table 3.2.S.3.1 Studies performed to elucidate the structure of the API
3.2.S.3.2 Impurities (name, manufacturer)
3.2.S.4 Control of drug substance (name, manufacturer)
3.2.S.4.1 Specification (name, manufacturer) Table 3.2.S.4.1 API specification table including name of test, reference (if compendial or in-house) and specification limits
3.2.S.4.2 Analytical procedures (name, manufacturer)
3.2.S.4.3 Validation of analytical procedures (name, manufacturer)
3.2.S.4.4 Batch analyses (name, manufacturer) Table 3.2.S.4.4 Lot, use, scale and results
3.2.S.4.5 Justification of specification (name, manufacturer)
3.2.S.5 Reference standards or materials (name, manufacturer) Table 3.2.S.5 Specifications and characterization results for reference standards
3.2.S.6 Container closure system (name, manufacturer)
3.2.S.7 Stability (name, manufacturer)
3.2.S.7.1 Stability summary and conclusions (name, manufacturer)
3.2.S.7.2 Post-approval stability protocol and stability commitment (name, manufacturer) Table 3.2.S.7.2 Stability protocol table with time-points, conditions, and test to be conducted
3.2.S.7.3 Stability data (name, manufacturer) Table 3.2.S.7.3 Stability results from the registrational lots as well as supporting lots
3.2.P DRUG PRODUCT (name, dosage form) - Name (Product 1)
3.2.P.1 Description and composition of the drug product (name, dosage form) Table 3.2.P.1 Qualitative and quantitative composition of each strength (including quality (compendial or other) and function in the formulation)
3.2.P.2 Pharmaceutical development (name, dosage form) 3.2.P.2.1 Components of the drug product (name, dosage form) 3.2.P.2.1.1 Drug substance (name, dosage form) 3.2.P.2.1.2 Excipients (name, dosage form) 3.2.P.2.2 Drug product (name, dosage form) 3.2.P.2.2.1 Formulation development (name, dosage form) Table 3.2.P.2.2.1 Lot, dosage form (if changed), use, scale, site, process used, reason for change (if applicable) and impact 3.2.P.2.2.2 Overages (name, dosage form) 3.2.P.2.2.3 Physicochemical and biological properties (name, dosage form) 3.2.P.2.3 Manufacturing Process Development (name, dosage form) Table 3.2.P.2.3.1 Lot , use, scale, site, process used, reason for change (if applicable) and impact 3.2.P.2.4 Container closure system (name, dosage form) 3.2.P.2.5 Microbiological attributes (name, dosage form) 3.2.P.2.6 Compatibility (name, dosage form)
3.2.P.3 Manufacture (name, dosage form)
3.2.P.3.1 Manufacturers (name, dosage form)
3.2.P.3.2 Batch formula (name, dosage form)
3.2.P.3.3 Description of manufacturing process and process controls (name, dosage form) Figure 3.2.P.3.3 Detailed flow diagram of manufacturing process
3.2.P.3.4 Controls of critical steps and intermediates (name, dosage form) Table 3.2.P.3.4 Critical steps, acceptance criteria and tests
3.2.P.3.5 Process validation and/or evaluation (name, dosage form)

–continued–

3.2.P.4 Control of excipients (name, dosage form)
3.2.P.4.1 Specifications (name, dosage form)
Table 3.2.P.4.1 Specifications (For each excipient that is not USP with test, and reference (compendial or in-house). Where acceptance criteria are above compendial, provide list of those tests and specifications.)
3.2.P.4.2 Analytical procedures (name, dosage form)
3.2.P.4.3 Validation of analytical procedures (name, dosage form)
3.2.P.4.4 Justification of specifications (name, dosage form)
3.2.P.4.5 Excipients of Human or Animal Origin (name, dosage form)
3.2.P.4.6 Novel Excipients (name, dosage form)
3.2.P.5 Control of drug product (name, dosage form)
3.2.P.5.1 Specifications (name, dosage form)
Table 3.2.P.5.1 Specifications (including name of test, reference (if compendial or in-house) and specification limits)
3.2.P.5.2 Analytical procedures (name, dosage form)
3.2.P.5.3 Validation of analytical procedures (name, dosage form)
3.2.P.5.4 Batch analyses (name, dosage form)
Table 3.2.P.5.4 Lot, use, scale and results
3.2.P.5.5 Characterization of impurities (name, dosage form)
3.2.P.5.6 Justification of specifications (name, dosage form)
3.2.P.6 Reference standards or materials (name, dosage form)
Table 3.2.P.6 Specifications and characterization results for reference standards
3.2.P.7 Container closure system (name, dosage form)
3.2 P.8 Stability (name, dosage form)
3.2.P.8.1 Stability summary and conclusion (name, dosage form)
3.2.P.8.2 Post-approval stability protocol and stability commitment (name, dosage form)
Table 3.2.P.8.2 Stability protocol table with time-points, conditions, and test to be conducted
3.2.P.8.3 Stability data (name, dosage form)
Table 3.2.P.8.3 Stability results from the registrational lots as well as supporting lots
3.2.A APPENDICES
3.2.A.1 Facilities and equipment (name, manufacturer)
3.2.A.2 Adventitious Agents Safety Evaluation (name, dosage form, manufacturer)
3.2.A.3 Novel Excipients - Name
3.2.R REGIONAL INFORMATION (EU)
3.2.R.1 Process validation scheme for the drug Product
3.2.R REGIONAL INFORMATION (US)
3.2.R.1 Executed batch records
3.2.R.2 Method validation package
3.2.R.3 Comparability protocols
3.3. LITERATURE REFERENCES

Tips for Efficiency

CTD Table of Contents Maintain a detailed CTD draft or "working" table of contents for the project. The chemistry/quality scientist/leader of the project team should provide an update of the CTD table of contents periodically. Some techniques that may assist in updating this information and utilizing the CTD table of contents as a tracking tool including the following:

- Consistent with the CTD M4 guidances, no elements of the CTD table of contents should be deleted or reordered; however, it may be that some categories of information are "not applicable" or were "not conducted" for the product and should be listed as such in the table of contents.
- Ensure that all team members are aware of the differences in scope between the NDA and CTD and that more focus is provided for the CTD

Labeling Ensure that the statements in the labeling associated with the chemistry information (e.g., description, ingredients and excipients, how supplied, etc.) are supported by and consistent with the tabular data and summaries. This must be completed for each strength, size, and package. This information should be provided in a quality overview summary (QOS) in CTD Section 2.3.

Regulatory Interactions and Guidances Ensure that the chemistry program is consistent with the regulatory guidances used. As stated above, regulatory interactions can be categorized and shown by technical discipline (2.4.1 for nonclinical and 2.5.1 for clinical); it is often beneficial to show this information and indicate that previous regulatory advice has been obtained and followed.

Expediting Drug and Biologics Development

Pharmaceutical Development Studies throughout the development process should be undertaken with this section in mind to ensure timely completion. Individual reports should be completed as the studies are done.

Novel Excipients Ensure that all known names for planned excipients are searched and stated (e.g., using CHEM ID or other chemistry database). Search inactive FDA Ingredient List, GRAS list, ingredients in approved products and other sources to determine if the planned excipients are listed and/or in approved products and in a similar quantity and form. If excipients are novel (including new routes of administration for existing excipients), ensure that all supporting data are available and that correspondence with regulatory authorities is initiated early to avoid potentially significant delays.

Abbreviations Acronyms and abbreviations should be defined the first time that they are used in each module. Ensure that acronyms and abbreviations that are used across chemistry, nonclinical, and clinical sections are consistent (e.g., the abbreviation for sponsor name, product name, etc.).

Hypertext linking rules Hypertext linking strategies should be developed in advance to assist authors and those coordinating the publishing and submission of the eCTD.

Tabular Summaries Some time-saving approaches include the following:
- Create all tabular summaries prior to written text.
- All key data should be tabulated and the tables should be updated continuously throughout product development (i.e., the table should be constructed for the IND/CTA and be updated throughout the process to the CTD submission).
- Batch history tables should be comprehensive, and should include lot number, date of manufacture, use, size, process used, site, and key results. Specific detailed analysis should be performed regarding impurities for each batch and justification of their limits. In addition, ensure that data are available for all other drug substance and drug product critical characteristics.
- If significant changes to analytical methods have been employed, ensure that all data can be compared. This may entail duplicate testing using old and new methods.
- Consistent with the guidance:
  - Unit conversions and relationships to human dosing should be clear.
  - Studies conducted to assess formulation, impurities, degradants, or novel excipients should be cross-referenced as appropriate in the nonclinical/quality sections.
  - Formulations and batch numbers should be tracked according to their use in nonclinical and clinical studies (and cross-referenced to these studies); manufacturing changes should be clearly described.

NONCLINICAL (SAFETY) Module

Module 2: Safety Elements

2.4 NONCLINICAL OVERVIEW

2.4.1 Overview of the nonclinical testing strategy*
- GLP status
- Association with clinical results
- Impurity and excipient information and cross-reference to supporting quality and safety
- Concordance or lack of concordance with current research regarding design of studies or analysis
  - Literature search and results (references provided in Module 5)
  - Regulatory guidance and advice (list, references provided in Module 5)*

2.4.2 Pharmacology

2.4.3 Pharmacokinetics

2.4.4 Toxicology

2.4.5 Integrated overview and conclusions

    Implications of the nonclinical findings for the safe human use of the pharmaceutical (i.e., as applicable to   Reference proposed labeling labeling).

2.4.6 Literature references

---

* While a table is not specified in the guidances; a table can be used to effectively summarize the required information.

2.6 NONCLINICAL WRITTEN AND TABULATED SUMMARY

2.6.1 INTRODUCTION
- Brief information concerning the pharmaceutical's structure and pharmacologic properties   Reference proposed labeling
- Information concerning the pharmaceutical's proposed clinical indication, dose, and duration of use

2.6.2 PHARMACOLOGY WRITTEN SUMMARY

    2.6.2.1 Brief Summary

    2.6.2.2 Primary Pharmacodynamics

    2.6.2.3 Secondary Pharmacodynamics

    2.6.2.4 Safety Pharmacology

    2.6.2.5 Pharmacodynamic Drug Interactions

    2.6.2.6 Discussion and Conclusions

    2.6.2.7 Tables and Figures (embedded in the text, or at the end of the section)

2.6.3 PHARMACOLOGY TABULATED SUMMARY

    Table 2.6.3.1 Pharmacology: Overview

    Table 2.6.3.2 Primary Pharmacodynamics*

    Table 2.6.3.3 Secondary Pharmacodynamics*

    Table 2.6.3.4 Safety Pharmacology

    Table 2.6.3.5 Pharmacodynamic Drug Interactions*

2.6.4 PHARMACOKINETICS WRITTEN SUMMARY

    2.6.4.1 Brief Summary

    2.6.4.2 Methods of Analysis

    2.6.4.3 Absorption

    2.6.4.4 Distribution

    2.6.4.5 Metabolism

    2.6.4.6 Excretion

    2.6.4.7 Pharmacokinetic Drug Interactions

    2.6.4.8 Other Pharmacokinetic Studies

    2.6.4.9 Discussion and Conclusions

    2.6.4.10 Tables and Figures (embedded in the text, or at the end of the section)

2.6.5 PHARMACOKINETICS TABULATED SUMMARY

    Table 2.6.5.1 Pharmacokinetics: Overview

    Table 2.6.5.2 Analytical Methods and Validation Reports*

    Table 2.6.5.3 Pharmacokinetics: Absorption after a Single Dose

    Table 2.6.5.4 Pharmacokinetics: Absorption after Repeated Doses

    Table 2.6.5.5 Pharmacokinetics: Organ Distribution

    Table 2.6.5.6 Pharmacokinetics: Plasma Protein Binding

    Table 2.6.5.7 Pharmacokinetics: Study in Pregnant or Nursing Animals

    Table 2.6.5.8 Pharmacokinetics: Other Distribution Study

    Table 2.6.5.9 Pharmacokinetics: Metabolism In Vivo

    Table 2.6.5.10 Pharmacokinetics: Metabolism In Vitro

    Table 2.6.5.11 Pharmacokinetics: Possible Metabolic Pathways

    Table 2.6.5.12 Pharmacokinetics: Induction/Inhibition of Drug-Metabolizing Enzymes

    Table 2.6.5.13 Pharmacokinetics: Excretion

    Table 2.6.5.14 Pharmacokinetics: Excretion into Bile

    Table 2.6.5.15 Pharmacokinetics: Drug-Drug Interactions

    Table 2.6.5.16 Pharmacokinetics: Other

2.6.6 TOXICOLOGY WRITTEN SUMMARY

    2.6.6.1 Brief Summary

        Tabular Listing of Toxicology Program

    2.6.6.2 Single-Dose Toxicity

    2.6.6.3 Repeat-Dose Toxicity (including supportive toxicokinetic evaluation)

    2.6.6.4 Genotoxicity

    2.6.6.5 Carcinogenicity (including supportive toxicokinetics evaluations)

    2.6.6.6 Reproductive and Developmental Toxicity (including range-finding supportive toxicokinetics evaluations)

    2.6.6.7 Local Tolerance

    2.6.6.8 Other Toxicity Studies

    2.6.6.9 Discussion and Conclusions

    2.6.6.10 Tables and Figures (embedded in the text, or at the end of the section)

–continued–

2.6.7 TOXICOLOGY TABULATED SUMMARY
Table 2.6.7.1 Toxicology: Overview
Table 2.6.7.2 Toxicokinetics: Overview of Toxicokinetics Studies
Table 2.6.7.3 Toxicokinetics: Overview of Toxicokinetics Data
Table 2.6.7.4 Toxicology: Drug Substance
Table 2.6.7.5 Single-Dose Toxicity
Table 2.6.7.6 Repeat-Dose Toxicity: Non-Pivotal Studies
Table 2.6.7.7 Repeat-Dose Toxicity: Pivotal Studies
Table 2.6.7.8 Genotoxicity: In Vitro
Table 2.6.7.9 Genotoxicity: In Vivo
Table 2.6.7.10 Carcinogenicity
Table 2.6.7.11 Reproductive and Developmental Toxicity: Non-Pivotal Studies
Table 2.6.7.12 Reproductive and Developmental Toxicity - Fertility and Early Embryonic Development to Implantation
Table 2.6.7.13 Reproductive and Developmental Toxicity - Effects on Embryo-Fetal Development
Table 2.6.7.14 Reproductive and Developmental Toxicity - Effects on Pre- and Postnatal Development, Including Maternal Function
Table 2.6.7.15 Studies in Juvenile Animals
Table 2.6.7.16 Local Tolerance
Table 2.6.7.17 Other Toxicity Studies

2.6.8 LITERATURE REFERENCES**

*In accordance with M4S, a tabulated summary is optional. It is preferable to include text tables and figures with the Written Summary.
**Section for Reference List can be added if needed

Module 4: Safety

4.1 MODULE 4 TABLE OF CONTENTS
4.2 STUDY REPORTS
(Note: Each Study report needs to be part of TOC so should be #ed accordingly in TOC)
4.2.1 PHARMACOLOGY
    4.2.1.1 Primary Pharmacodynamics
        Study ID   Title
    4.2.1.2 Secondary Pharmacodynamics
        Study ID   Title
    4.2.1.3 Safety Pharmacology
        Study ID   Title
    4.2.1.4 Pharmacodynamic Drug Interactions
        Study ID   Title
4.2.2 PHARMACOKINETICS
    4.2.2.1 Analytical Methods and Validation Reports (if separate reports are available)
        Study ID   Title
    4.2.2.2 Absorption
        Study ID   Title
    4.2.2.3 Distribution
        Study ID   Title
    4.2.2.4 Metabolism
        Study ID   Title
    4.2.2.5 Excretion
        Study ID   Title
    4.2.2.6 Pharmacokinetic Drug Interactions (nonclinical)
        Study ID   Title
        4.2.2.7 Other Pharmacokinetic Studies
        Study ID   Title
4.2.3 TOXICOLOGY
    4.2.3.1 Single-Dose Toxicity (in order by species, by route)
        Study ID   Title
    4.2.3.2 Repeat-Dose Toxicity in order by species, by route, by duration, including supportive toxicokinetics evaluations)
        Study ID   Title
    4.2.3.3 Genotoxicity
        4.2.3.3.1 In vitro

–continued–

Study ID   Title

4.2.3.3.2 In vivo (including supportive toxicokinetics evaluations)

Study ID   Title

4.2.3.4 Carcinogenicity

4.2.3.4.1 Long-term Studies

(in order by species; including range-finding studies that cannot appropriately be included under repeat-dose toxicity or pk)

Study ID   Title

4.2.3.4.2 Short- or Medium-term Studies

(including range-finding studies that cannot appropriately be included under repeat-dose toxicity or pk)

Study ID   Title

4.2.3.4.3 Other Studies

4.2.3.5 Reproductive and Developmental Toxicity

(including range-finding studies and supportive toxicokinetics evaluations)

(If modified study designs are used, the following sub-headings should be modified accordingly.)

4.2.3.5.1 Fertility and Early Embryonic Development

Study ID   Title

4.2.3.5.2 Embryofetal Development

Study ID   Title

4.2.3.5.3 Prenatal and Postnatal Development, including Maternal Function

Study ID   Title

4.2.3.5.4 Studies in which the Offspring (Juvenile Animals) are Dosed and/or Further Evaluated

4.2.3.6 Local Tolerance

Study ID   Title

4.2.3.7 Other Toxicity Studies (if available)

4.2.3.7.1 Antigenicity

4.2.3.7.2 Immunotoxicity

4.2.3.7.3 Mechanistic Studies (if not included elsewhere)

4.2.3.7.4 Dependence

4.2.3.7.5 Metabolites

4.2.3.7.6 Impurities

4.2.3.7.7 Other

4.3 LITERATURE REFERENCES

AUTHOR et al (YEAR) TITLE. JOURNAL ABBREV. VOL: Page-Page

Tips for Efficiency

CTD Table of Contents Maintain a detailed CTD draft or "working" table of contents for the project. The nonclinical scientist/leader of the project team should provide an update of the CTD table of contents periodically. Some techniques that may assist in updating this information and utilizing the CTD table of contents as a tracking tool include the following:

- Consistent with the CTD M4 guidance, no parts of the CTD table of contents should be deleted or reordered; however, it may be that some categories of studies are "not applicable" or were "not conducted" for the product and should be listed as such in the table of contents.
- Show completed studies in the table of contents. Show planned/ongoing studies in the table of contents but in *italics* to indicate to the team that the study reports are not yet available. Use a uniform study identifier structure to refer to all reports in-text (e.g., Study ID number) and ensure that it is clear if there is a distinction (if necessary) between applicant-sponsored reports, right-of-reference reports, and literature reports (e.g., Literature Study Author Year). Use a uniform structure to refer to all reports in Module 4 (i.e., Study ID and Title). The CTD guidance indicates that literature citations should be consistent with the Uniform Requirements for Manuscripts Submitted to Biomedical Journals, International Committee of Medical Journal Editors (ICMJE)

Labeling Ensure that the statements in the labeling associated with the nonclinical information (e.g., pregnancy nonclinical study information, carcinogenicity, etc) are supported by and are consistent with the nonclinical study tabular data and summaries. This information should be provided in overview in CTD Section 2.4 and in summarized in CTD Section 2.6.1.

Regulatory Interactions and Guidances Ensure that the nonclinical program is consistent with the regulatory guidances used and the regulatory advice received. As stated above, regulatory interactions can be categorized and shown by technical discipline (2.4.1 for nonclinical and 2.5.1 for clinical); it is often beneficial to show this information and indicate that previous regulatory advice has been obtained and followed.

Expediting Drug and Biologics Development

Abbreviations Acronyms and abbreviations should be defined the first time they are used in each module. Ensure that acronyms and abbreviations that are used across chemistry, nonclinical, and clinical sections are consistent (e.g., the abbreviation for sponsor name, product name, etc).

Hypertext linking rules Hypertext linking strategies should be developed in advance to assist authors and those coordinating the publishing and submission of the eCTD. Some time-saving approaches include the following:
- For literature not used as reports:
  1. The reference in-text links to the citation on the literature (bibliography) list.
  2. The citation links directly to the reprint of the publication.
- For reports:
  1. The in-text reference to the report links to the tabular summary where the report is listed (in accordance with the CTD guidance M4S; Table X.X, Study/Report Number).
  2. The study identifier in the table links to the actual report

Tabular Summaries Some time-saving approaches include the following:
- Create all tabular summaries prior to written text.
- The overview table of studies should be updated continuously
throughout the product's development (i.e., the table should be constructed for the IND/CTA and be updated throughout to the CTD).
- The nonclinical guidance currently does not specifically state that an overall table is required, but a listing can be placed in Section 2.6 (similar to that suggested for toxicology in Section 2.6.6.1).
- Consistent with the guidance:
  - The categorization of the studies and the order in which they are presented should be the same as the categorization and order of reports in Module 4.
  - Studies should be listed only once in Module 4 and cross-referenced as needed to other categories.
  - Consistent with the guidance, the CTD Table 2.6.7.1 can be used to extract the table needed for 2.6.6.1 and for subsequent tables in 2.6.7.
  - Unit conversions and relationships to human dosing should be clear.
  - Studies conducted to assess formulation, impurities, degradants, or novel excipients should be cross-referenced to the appropriate Quality section.
  - The GLP status of the studies should be clear.
  - Species order should be as follows: Mouse, Rat, Hamster, Other rodent, Rabbit, Dog, Nonhuman primate, Other nonrodent mammal, Nonmammals.
  - Routes of administration order should be as follows: Intended route for human use, Oral, Intravenous, Intramuscular, Intraperitoneal, Subcutaneous, Inhalation, Topical, Other

Report summaries/synopses Ensure that report summaries are written such that they can be directly related to the CTD summary sections (2.6.2, 2.6.4, 2.6.6)

Literature reports In some cases, such as 505(b)(2) NDAs, literature may be used to support some aspect of the nonclinical or clinical information in addition to, or in lieu of, sponsor-conducted studies. If the literature can qualify as supportive or in place of an investigation conducted by the sponsor (reference the CTD M4S - 2.4 Nonclinical Overview, FDA Guidance on Clinical Effectiveness), then it should be placed as a study report, but should be clearly identified as literature in the written and tabular summaries in Module 2 and in Module 4.

CLINICAL (EFFICACY) Module

Module 2: Efficacy Elements

2.5 CLINICAL OVERVIEW	
2.5.1 Product Development Rationale	Reference proposed
• Pharmacological class	labeling
• Targeted indication	
• Scientific background/support for investigations	
• Clinical Development Program	
• Concordance or lack of concordance with current research regarding design of studies or analysis	
• Literature search and results (references provided in Module 5)	
• Regulatory guidance and advice (list, references provided in Module 5)*	

–continued–

2.5.2 Overview of Biopharmaceutics
- Critical analysis of important issues related to BA (e.g., dose, strength proportionality, food-effect) of formulations used in clinical trials and to-be-marketed formulation

2.5.3 Overview of Clinical Pharmacology
- Critical analysis of important issues related to PK/PD

2.5.4 Overview of Efficacy
- Critical analysis of important issues related to Efficacy

2.5.5 Overview of Safety
- Critical analysis of important issues related to Safety

2.5.6 Benefits and Risks Conclusions*

2.5.7 References

* While a table is not specified in the guidances; a table can be used to effectively summarize the required information.

2.7 CLINICAL SUMMARY

2.7.1 SUMMARY OF BIOPHARMACEUTIC STUDIES AND ASSOCIATED ANALYTICAL METHODS

2.7.1.1 Background and Overview

2.7.1.2 Summary of Results of Individual Studies

(The narrative descriptions should be similar to an abstract for a journal article and should describe critical design features and critical results; they may be abstracted from the ICH E3 synopsis. Provide links to the full report.)

Table 2.7.1.1 Summary of Bioavailability Studies

Table 2.7.1.2 Summary of In Vitro Dissolution Studies

2.7.1.3 Comparison and Analyses of Results Across Studies

- effects of formulation and manufacturing changes on in vitro dissolution and BA and conclusions regarding BE.
- food effects on BA and conclusions regarding BE with respect to meal type or timing of the meal (where appropriate).
- correlations between in vitro dissolution and BA, including the effects of pH, and conclusions on specifications
- comparative bioavailability, including BE conclusions, for different dosage form strengths.
- comparative BA of the clinical study formulations (for clinical studies providing substantial evidence of efficacy) and the formulations to be marketed.
- source and magnitude of observed inter- and intra-subject variability for each formulation in a comparative BA study.

2.7.1.4 Appendix (embedded in the text, or at the end of the section)

2.7.2 SUMMARY OF CLINICAL PHARMACOLOGY STUDIES

2.7.2.1 Background and Overview

2.7.2.2 Summary of Results of Individual Studies

(The narrative descriptions should be similar to an abstract for a journal article and should describe critical design features and critical results; they may be abstracted from the ICH E3 synopsis. Provide links to the full report.)

Table 2.7.2.1 Summary of Drug Interaction PK Studies

2.7.2.3 Comparison and Analyses of Results Across Studies
- in vitro drug metabolism and in vitro drug-drug interaction studies and their clinical implications
- human PK studies, including the best estimates of standard parameters and sources of variability. The focus should be on evidence supporting dose and dose individualization in the target patient population and in special populations (e.g., pediatric or geriatric patients, patients with renal or hepatic impairment).
- comparison between single and repeat-dose PK
- population PK analyses, such as results based on sparse sampling across studies that address interindividual variations in the PK or PD of the active drug substances that may be due to extrinsic or intrinsic factors
- dose-response or concentration-response relationships. This discussion should highlight evidence to support the selection of dosages and dose intervals studied in the important clinical trials. In addition, information that supports the dosage instructions in the proposed labeling should be discussed in Section 2.7.3.4.
- major inconsistencies in the human biomaterial, PK, or PD database
- PK studies that were performed to determine whether foreign clinical data could be extrapolated to the new region (see ICH E5). The result of the studies and analysis of the similarity of the PK data between regions or races should be summarized in this section. Studies that use PD biomarkers (but do not evaluate clinical efficacy) can also be summarized here. An independent subsection can be created to summarize these kinds of data.

2.7.2.4 Special Studies

2.7.2.5 Appendix (embedded in the text, or at the end of the section)

–continued–

2.7.3 SUMMARY OF CLINICAL EFFICACY (INDICATION)

2.7.3.1 Background and Overview of Clinical Efficacy

2.7.3.2   Summary of Results of Individual Studies

(The narrative descriptions should be similar to an abstract for a journal article and should describe critical design features and critical results; they may be abstracted from the ICH E3 synopsis. Provide links to the full report.)

Table 2.7.3.1 Description of Clinical Efficacy and Safety Studies

Table 2.7.3.2 Results of Efficacy Studies

2.7.3.3   Comparison and Analyses of Results Across Studies

2.7.3.3.1 Study Populations

2.7.3.3.2 Comparison of Efficacy Results of All Studies

2.7.3.3.3 Comparison of Results in Subpopulations

2.7.3.4 Analysis of Clinical Information Relevant to Dosing Recommendations   Reference proposed labeling

2.6.3.5 Persistence of Efficacy and/or Tolerance Effects

2.7.3.6 Appendix (embedded in the text, or at the end of the section)

2.7.4 SUMMARY OF CLINICAL SAFETY

2.7.4.1 Exposure to the Drug

2.7.4.1.1 Overall Safety Evaluation Plan and Narratives of Safety Studies

Listing of Safety Studies (Note: or cross-reference to 2.7.3.2 and/or Table 5.1)

2.7.4.1.2 Overall Extent of Exposure

Table 2.7.4.1 Study Subject Drug Exposure by Mean Daily Dose and Duration of Exposure

2.7.4.1.3 Demographic and Other Characteristics of Study Population

Table 2.7.4.2 Demographic Profile of Patients in Controlled Trials

2.7.4.2 Adverse Events

2.7.4.2.1 Analysis of Adverse Events

2.7.4.2.1.1 Common Adverse Events

Table 2.7.4.3 Incidence of Adverse Events in Pooled Placebo and Active Controlled Trial Database

Table 2.7.4.4 Incidence of Adverse Events in Individual Studies

Table 2.7.4.5 Patient Withdrawals by Study: Controlled Trials

2.7.4.2.1.2 Deaths

Table 2.7.4.6 Listing of Deaths

2.7.4.2.1.3 Other Serious Adverse Events

2.7.4.2.1.4 Other Significant Adverse Events

2.7.4.2.1.5 Analysis of Adverse Events by Organ System or Syndrome

2.7.4.2.2 Narratives

2.7.4.3 Clinical Laboratory Evaluations

2.7.4.4 Vital Signs, Physical Findings, and Other Observations Related to Safety

2.7.4.5 Safety in Special Groups and Situations

2.7.4.5.1 Intrinsic Factors

2.7.4.5.2 Extrinsic Factors

2.7.4.5.3 Drug Interactions

2.7.4.5.4 Use in Pregnancy and Lactation

2.7.4.5.5 Overdose

2.7.4.5.6 Drug Abuse

2.7.4.5.7 Withdrawal and Rebound

2.7.4.5.8 Effects on Ability to Drive or Operate Machinery or Impairment of Mental Ability

2.7.4.6 Post-marketing Data

2.7.4.7 Appendix (embedded in the text, or at the end of the section)

2.7.5 REFERENCES

2.7.6 SYNOPSES OF INDIVIDUAL STUDIES

Table 2.7.6.1 (Copy of Table 5.1) Listing of Clinical Studies

2.7.6.X Individual Study Synopses (same order as in Module 5)

Chapter 8 - Format and Content of the Common Technical Document (CTD)

Module 5: Efficacy

5.1 TABLE OF CONTENTS OF CLINICAL STUDY REPORTS AND RELATED INFORMATION

5.2 TABULAR LISTING OF ALL CLINICAL STUDIES

Table 5.1 Listing of Clinical Studies

5.3 CLINICAL STUDY REPORTS AND RELATED INFORMATION

(Note: Each Study report needs to be part of TOC so should be #ed accordingly in TOC)

5.3.1 Reports of Biopharmaceutic Studies

    5.3.1.1 Bioavailability (BA) Study Reports

Study ID	Title

    5.3.1.2 Comparative BA and Bioequivalence (BE) Study Reports

Study ID	Title

    5.3.1.3 In Vitro-In Vivo Correlation Study Reports

Study ID	Title

    5.3.1.4 Reports of Bioanalytical and Analytical Methods for Human Studies

Study ID	Title

5.3.2 Reports of Studies Pertinent to Pharmacokinetics Using Human Biomaterials

    5.3.2.1 Plasma Protein Binding Study Reports

Study ID	Title

    5.3.2.2 Reports of Hepatic Metabolism and Interaction Studies

Study ID	Title

    5.3.2.3 Reports of Studies Using Other Human Biomaterials

5.3.3 Reports of Human Pharmacokinetic (PK) Studies

    5.3.3.1 Healthy Subject PK and Initial Tolerability Study Reports

Study ID	Title

    5.3.3.2 Patient PK and Initial Tolerability Study Reports

    5.3.3.3 Intrinsic Factor PK Study Reports

Study ID	Title Mild, Moderate and Severe Hepatic Dysfunction

Study ID	Title Renally Impaired Subjects

    5.3.3.4 Extrinsic Factor PK Study Reports

    5.3.3.5 Population PK Study Reports

5.3.4 Reports of Human Pharmacodynamic (PD) Studies

    5.3.4.1 Healthy Subject PD and PK/PD Study Reports

Study ID	Title

    5.3.4.2 Patient PD and PK/PD Study Reports

5.3.5 INDICATION A - Reports of Efficacy and Safety Reports

    5.3.5.1 Study Reports of Controlled Clinical Studies Pertinent to the Claimed Indication

Study ID	Title

    5.3.5.2 Study Reports of Uncontrolled Clinical Studies

Study ID	Title

    5.3.5.3 Reports of Analyses of Data from More than One Study

Study ID	Title

    5.3.5.4 Other Study Reports

Study ID	Title

5.3.6 Reports of Post-marketing Experience

5.3.7 Case Report Forms and Individual Patient Listings

(Case report forms and individual patient data listings that are described as appendices 16.3 and 16.4 in the ICH clinical study report guideline, should be placed in this section when submitted, in the same order as the clinical study reports and indexed by study.)

5.4 LITERATURE REFERENCES

Include copies of referenced articles in the Module 2 Clinical Overview/Summary, include copies of referenced guidances, include copies of official meeting minutes

AUTHOR et al (YEAR) TITLE. JOURNAL ABBREV. VOL: Page-Page

Tips for Efficiency

CTD Table of Contents Maintain a detailed CTD draft or "working" table of contents for the project. The clinical scientist/leader of the project team should provide an update of the CTD table of contents periodically. Some techniques that may assist in updating this information and utilizing the CTD table of contents as a tracking tool include the following:

- Consistent with the CTD M4 guidance, no parts of the CTD table of contents should be deleted or reordered; however, it may be that some categories of studies are "not applicable" or were "not conducted" for the product and should be listed as such in the table of contents.
- Show completed studies in the table of contents. Show planned/ongoing studies in the table of contents, but do so in italics to indicate to the team that the study reports are not yet available. Use a uniform study identifier structure to refer to all reports in-text (e.g., Study ID number) and ensure that it is clear if there is a distinction (if necessary) between applicant-sponsored reports, right-of-reference reports, and literature reports (e.g., Literature Study Author Year). Use a uniform structure to refer to all reports in Module 5 (i.e., Study ID and Title). The CTD guidance states that literature citations should appear in the Uniform Requirements for Manuscripts Submitted to Biomedical Journals, International Committee of Medical Journal Editors (ICMJE))

Labeling Ensure that the statements in the labeling associated with the clinical information (e.g., indication, dosing, etc) are supported by and consistent with the clinical study tabular data and summaries. This information should be provided in overview in CTD Section 2.5 and in summary in CTD Section 2.7.3.

Regulatory Interactions and Guidances Ensure that the clinical program is consistent with the regulatory guidances used and the regulatory advice received. As stated above, regulatory interactions can be categorized and shown by technical discipline (2.4.1 for nonclinical and 2.5.1 for clinical); it is often beneficial to show this information and to indicate that previous regulatory advice has been followed.

Abbreviations Acronyms and abbreviations should be defined the first time they are used in each module. Ensure that acronyms and abbreviations that are used across chemistry, nonclinical, and clinical sections are consistent (e.g., the abbreviation for sponsor name, product name, etc).

Hypertext linking rules Hypertext linking strategies should be developed in advance to assist authors and those coordinating the publishing and submission of the eCTD. Some time-saving approaches include the following:

- For literature not used as reports:
  1. The reference in-text links to the citation on the literature (bibliography) list.
  2. The citation links directly to the reprint of the publication.
- For reports:
  1. The in-text reference to the report links to the tabular summary where the report is listed/summarized (Table 5.1).
  2. The study identifier in the table links to the actual report (synopsis).

Tabular Summaries Some time-saving approaches are listed below.

- Create all tabular summaries prior to written text.
- The overview table of studies should be updated continually throughout development of the product (i.e., the table should be constructed for the IND/CTA and be updated throughout to the CTD).
- Table 5.1 can be modified (see example below) to include results and then can be used to extract sub-tables that summarize information by category of study (e.g., for Tables 2.7.1.1, 2.7.1.2, 2.7.2.1, 2.7.3.1).
- Consistent with the guidance:
  - The guidance specifies that the overall table (Table 5.1 Listing of Clinical Studies) is to be reproduced in the synopsis section (Section 2.7.6).
  - The categorization of the studies and order in which they are presented in module 2.7.6 (Synopses) and Table 5.1 (Listing of Clinical Studies) should be the same as the categorization and order of reports in Module 5.
  - Studies should be listed only once in Module 5 and cross-referenced as needed to other categories.
  - Unit conversions and relationship to human dosing should be clear.

Table 5.1 (example as provided in CTD Guidance)

Type Study	Study Identifier	Location of Study Report	Objective(s) of the Study	Study Design and Type of Control	Test Product(s); of Dosage Regimen; Route of Administration	Number of Subjects	Healthy Subjects or Diagnosis of Patients	Duration of Treatment	Study Status; Type of Report

Modified Table 5.1 (modified example to enable extraction for Tables 2.7.1.1, 2.7.1.2, 2.7.2.1, 2.7.3.1)

Type of Study	Study Identifier Study Title No. Site(s) Investigator(s) Country IND/CTA No.	Status/Date cut-off date GCP status Report type	Subject Population Total No. Age range (yr) mean Gender M/F (%) Race B/W/O (%)	Design/ Control Objectives/Endpoint(s)	Dose, Form, Route, Regimen [Product ID/ Formulation Batch/Lot No.]	Clinical Outcome Pharmacology						Cross-Reference Location of Report

Sub-table within "Clinical Outcome":

Cmax (mg/L)	Tmax (hr)	AUC* (mg/L x hr)	Cmin** (mg/L)	T1/2 (hr)	Other

Efficacy
Safety
AEs
Discontinued due to AEs
SAEs

- GCP status of the studies should be clear.

Report summaries/synopses Ensure report synopses are written such that they can be directly copied into the synopsis section (Section 2.7.6) and related to the CTD summary sections (2.7.1.2, 2.7.2.2, 2.7.3.2, and 2.7.4.1.1).

- The CTD guidance M4E specifies that all synopses should be consistent with the ICH E3 standard and include study summary tables and figures as appropriate.
- While not specifically discussed in the CTD M4E guidance, some reports may have been written prior to ICH E3; if this is the case, it may be necessary to rewrite the synopsis in ICH E3 format and then specify on the synopsis, in bold print, that the synopsis has been rewritten for the purposes of the CTD and to provide the original synopsis/report in Module 5.
- It should be noted that the previous U.S. requirement for an integrated analysis of safety and efficacy (referred to as and ISS, ISE or more recently the IAS, IAE) is now likely satisfied by 2.7.3.3, 2.7.3.4, and 2.7.4,or may require a separate report described in 5.3.5.3. If the integrated analysis requires a separate report, it does not require a separate synopsis (i.e., Section 2.7.6 is for 'Synopses of Individual Studies'). The following FDA guidance should also be consulted: "Conducting a Clinical Safety Review of a New Product Application and Preparing a Report on the Review" (2005).

Literature reports In some cases, such as 505(b)(2) NDAs, literature may be used to support some aspect of the nonclinical or clinical information in addition to or in lieu of sponsor-conducted studies. If the literature can qualify as supportive (CTD M4S; CTD M4E and FDA Guidance on "Providing Clinical Evidence of Effectiveness for Human Drug and Biological Products"), then it should be placed as a study report, but clearly identified as literature in the written and tabular summaries in Module 2 and in Module 5.

The guideline for Item 8 of the NDA/BLA ("Guideline for the Clinical and Statistical Sections of New Drug Applications" [1988]) indicates that literature should be summarized as part of the controlled, uncontrolled, and other studies with a description of the search strategy used to assess the world literature. In addition, regulatory requirements to demonstrate that clinical investigations are "essential" for claims of exclusivity indicate that the applicant provide a "list of all published studies or publicly available reports of clinical investigations known to the applicant through a literature search that are relevant to the conditions for which the applicant is seeking approval" and a "certification that the applicant has thoroughly searched the scientific literature" (21 CFR 314.50(j)(4)(ii)). It is also important to note what date was used as a cut-off date for the incorporation of literature search information into the marketing application. A tabular template to show literature search strategies is provided below; this type of table can be organized into clinical, nonclinical, and chemistry sections and can be provided with the associated items of the marketing application to facilitate review of the information.

Topic	Key Words/Strategy	Databases Search cut-off date(s)	Technical Discipline (/associated disciplines)		
			Chemistry	Nonclinical	Clinical/ Statistical

PRE- AND POST-SUBMISSION PROCESSES

The marketing application requires maintenance not only before submission, but after submission, during the review process, and after approval as well. Some of the pre-submission and post-submission processes that affect the NDA/BLA content are outlined below.

Pre-NDA/BLA Meetings Pre-NDA/BLA meetings (i.e., End-of-Phase 2 and Pre-NDA/BLA meetings) are important meetings to exchange information with the FDA regarding the product's development and resulting data and to indicate the sponsor's intentions regarding the format and content of the NDA/BLA. The FDA guidance document entitled, "Formal Meetings with Sponsors and Applicants for PDUFA Products" identifies the procedures for requesting and holding meetings, and outlines recommended content for pre-meeting information packages.

Consistent with FDA guidance, a table of contents for the pre-NDA/BLA meeting information package may comprise the following:

- Form FDA 1571 (if being submitted to IND) or 356h (if being submitted to NDA/BLA)*
- Product Background/Overview, including:
    1. Product name and application number (if available)*
    2. Chemical name and structure*
    3. Proposed indication(s)*; dosage form, route, regimen (frequency and duration)
    4. Type of meeting to be requested (Type A, B, or C)*
    5. Statement of the purpose of the meeting (e.g., general nature of questions to be asked, how the meeting fits in with the development plan) *
    6. Specific objectives/outcomes expected from the meeting*
    7. Agenda* (note: Meetings conducted at FDA currently are focused on the specific questions)
    8. Specific questions, grouped by discipline*
    9. Attendees list from Sponsor*
    10. Attendees list requested from FDA*
- Proposed labeling** (including annotations to rationale, studies in development plan, and regulatory information (include references to previous regulatory interactions and resolution of action items)
- Proposed NDA/BLA table of contents (in CTD format)**
- Clinical data summary
- Nonclinical data summary
- Chemistry data summary

* This information will be included in the request for the meeting and should be updated in the pre-meeting information package.

** Although this information is not specifically cited in the aforementioned guidance document, it may be appropriate to include this information to obtain FDA feedback on critical elements of labeling and the plan for submission of the application (e.g., plans to submit abbreviated reports). Regulatory information should be organized by discipline and include previous agreements, requests for information and subsequent responses, and reference components of the submission that address any outstanding issues.

The pre-meeting information package should be as concise as possible. It should be fully paginated with a table of contents and appropriate tabs, cross-references, indices, and appendices. The FDA's guidance indicates that the specific questions should frame much of the meeting content and, therefore, the specific questions should be as precise and comprehensive as possible.

Safety Update In accordance with 21 CFR 314.50(d)(5)(vi)(b) and 21 CFR 601.2, safety updates are required four months (120 days) after the sponsor files the application, after the sponsor receives an approvable letter, and at other times as requested by the FDA (e.g., some FDA divisions request two safety updates within a standard review of an application. The safety updates must be submitted in the form of the integrated analysis of safety information. In addition, case report forms for all patients who died during a clinical study or who discontinued due to an adverse experience are required. According to the FDA's "Guideline for Format and Content of the Clinical and Statistical Sections of an Application," if the total exposure has changed substantially, generally increased by 25% or more, the overall analysis of both new and old data is required. Since a substantial increase in exposure could greatly affect the conclusions of the application, it is appropriate to consider data cut-off/lock dates (reference ICH E9) so that the information is inclusive up to several months before the submission.

AKNOWLEDGEMENTS

Diana Fordyce wishes to thank colleagues for assistance and support in learning the CTD process: David Driver, Catherine Maher, Ann Gooch, Holly Buchanan, Jason Horn, Stephen Truocchio, Karl Whitney and Ted Murphy.

REFERENCES

Approved Drug Products with Therapeutic Equivalence Evaluations. 18th edition. "Orange Book." U.S. Department of Health and Human Services, Public Health Service, FDA. 1998. http://www.fda.gov/cder/orange/default.htm or http://www.accessdata.fda.gov/scripts/cder/drugsatfda/index.cfm

Drug Applications: http://www.fda.gov/cder/regulatory/applications/default.htm

Electronic Drug Applications: http://www.fda.gov/cder/regulatory/ersr/default.htm, http://www.fda.gov/cder/regulatory/ersr/ectd.htm, http://www.fda.gov/cder/guidance/index.htm...Electronic Submissions

Federal Register. Abbreviated New Drug Application Regulations: Patent and Exclusivity Provisions, Vol. 59, No. 190, October 3, 1994 http://www.accessdata.fda.gov/scripts/oc/ohrms/index.cfm

Form FDA 356h, Application to Market a New Drug, Biologic, or Antibiotic Drug for Human Use. http://www.fda.gov/opacom/morechoices/fdaforms/cder.html

Guide to 505(b)(2) Submissions. U.S. Regulatory Reporter. Vol 11, No. 11, May 1995. http://www.fda.gov/cder/guidance/index.htm.....Procedural.

Washington Drug Letter. FDA to Issue (How-To) Guide for Naming Drugs. August, 1997. http://www.fda.gov/cder/mapp.htm....Risk Management

REGULATIONS:

http://www.access.gpo.gov/cgi-bin/cfrassemble.cgi?title=200421

http://www.accessdata.fda.gov/scripts/cdrh/cfdocs/cfCFR/CFRSearch.cfm

Title 21 Code of Federal Regulations 201. Labeling

Title 21 Code of Federal Regulations 314. Applications for FDA approval to market a new drug or an antibiotic drug

Title 21 Code of Federal Regulations 600 and 601. Biological products: general; Licensing

Title 21 Code of Federal Regulations 320. Bioavailability and bioequivalence requirements

Title 21 Code of Federal Regulations 330. Over-the-Counter (OTC) human drugs which are generally recognized as safe and effective and not misbranded

GUIDELINES:

SELECTED FDA GUIDELINES:

http://www.fda.gov/cder/guidance/index.htm, http://www.fda.gov/cber/guidelines.htm

Submitting Marketing Applications According to the ICH CTD Format - General Considerations http://www.fda.gov/cder/guidance/index.htm....ICH

Providing Regulatory Submissions in Electronic Format - Human Pharmaceutical Product Applications and Related Submissions. http://www.fda.gov/cder/regulatory/ersr/ectd.htm, http://www.fda.gov/cber/regulatory/esub/esub.htm

SPL Standard for Content of Labeling Technical Qs & As http://www.fda.gov/cder/guidance/index.htm....Electronic Submissions

Applications Covered by Section 505(b)(2) http://www.fda.gov/cder/guidance/index.htm....Procedural

Drug Master Files http://www.fda.gov/cder/guidance/index.htm....Chemistry

Fast Track Drug Development Programs (Designation, Development, and Application Review http://www.fda.gov/cder/guidance/index.htm....Procedural

Continuous Marketing Applications http://www.fda.gov/cder/guidance/index.htm....Procedural

Formal Meetings with Sponsors and Applicants for PDUFA Products http://www.fda.gov/cder/guidance/index.htm....Procedural

Expediting Drug and Biologics Development

Guideline - Format and Content of the Summary for New Drug and Antibiotic Applications: February 1, 1987 http://www.fda.gov/cder/guidance/index.htm....Clinical/Medical

Guideline - Format and Content of the Chemistry, Manufacturing and Controls Section of an Application: February 1, 1987 http://www.fda.gov/cder/guidance/index.htm....Chemistry

Guideline - Format and Content of the Nonclinical Pharmacology/Toxicology Section of an Application: February 1, 1987 http://www.fda.gov/cder/guidance/index.htm....Pharmacology/Toxicology

Guideline - Format and Content of the Human Pharmacokinetics and Bioavailability Section of an Application: February 1, 1987 http://www.fda.gov/cder/guidance/index.htm....Clinical Pharmacology, http://www.fda.gov/cder/guidance/index.htm....ClinicalBiopharmaceutics

Guideline - Format and Content of the Microbiology Section of an Application: February, 1987 http://www.fda.gov/cder/guidance/index.htm....Microbiology

Guideline - Format and Content of the Clinical and Statistical Sections of New Drug Applications: July 1, 1988 http://www.fda.gov/cder/guidance/index.htm....Clinical/Medical, http://www.fda.gov/cder/guidance/index.htm....Drug Safety

Providing Regulatory Submissions in Electronic Format NDAs http://www.fda.gov/cder/guidance/index.htm....Clinical/Medical

Providing Clinical Evidence of Effectiveness for Human Drug and Biological Products http://www.fda.gov/cder/guidance/index.htm....Clinical/Medical

SELECTED ICH GUIDELINES:

http://www.ich.org/ (http://www.fda.gov/cder/guidance/index.htm......ICH)

ICH - M4 - CTD - Organization

ICH - Questions and Answers - General

ICH - M2 - eCTD Specifications

ICH - M4Q - CTD - Quality

ICH - Questions and Answers - Quality

ICH - M4S - CTD - Safety

ICH - Questions and Answers - Safety

ICH - M4E - CTD - Efficacy

ICH - Questions and Answers - Efficacy

CHAPTER 9

Streamlining the Drug Development and Approval Process

By Michele Bronson, Ph.D.

Over the past 25 years, various medical crises and political pressures prompted the Food and Drug Administration (FDA) to develop and implement several programs to provide earlier access to drugs being developed for life-threatening conditions and to provide more expedient paths to approval. The major precipitating factor was the Acquired Immune Deficiency Syndrome (AIDS) crisis of the late 1980s and early 1990s. From 1987 through 1992, public and political pressure spurred the FDA to develop and implement four programs to expedite patients' access to emerging therapies: the treatment IND (Investigational New Drug Application), a mechanism that provides patients with access to promising, but as-yet unapproved, drugs for serious and life-threatening diseases; parallel track, a plan that provides patients suffering from AIDS or AIDS-related diseases with early access to experimental-stage therapies; an accelerated drug development program for drugs designed to treat life-threatening and seriously debilitating diseases; and an accelerated drug approval program for therapies designed to treat serious or life-threatening illnesses.

The FDA's Accelerated Drug Development Program (Subpart E) By mid-1988, the FDA had successfully implemented several initiatives designed to make drugs more accessible through both preapproval availability plans and speedier reviews. At that time, the treatment IND regulations were in effect, and seven experimental therapies had been available to patients with AIDS, cancer, Parkinson's disease, and other life-threatening conditions. In addition, the agency had established a new level of review priority for all AIDS products, and had created a new drug review division to focus on evaluating these therapies. The FDA credited such initiatives with the rapid availability and review of AZT, which the agency approved only 107 days after the submission of Burroughs Wellcome's NDA.

In August 1988, then-Vice President George Bush, in his capacity as the chairman of the Presidential Task Force on Regulatory Relief, asked the FDA to build on these "successes" by developing procedures for expediting the marketing of new therapies intended to treat AIDS and other life-threatening illnesses. In the two months that followed, FDA officials met with representatives from other government agencies, AIDS groups, and consumer, health, and academic organizations to obtain input on developing this program.

The FDA released such a plan on October 21, 1988: its *Interim Rules on Procedures for Drugs Intended to Treat Life-Threatening and Severely Debilitating Illnesses*, or Subpart E procedures. The interim rule, which the FDA claimed was based on its experience with AZT, was described by the agency as an attempt "to speed the availability of new therapies to desperately ill patients, while preserving appropriate guarantees for safety and effectiveness. These procedures are intended to facilitate the development, evaluation, and marketing of such products, especially where no satisfactory therapies exist. These procedures reflect the recognition that physicians and patients are generally willing to accept greater risks or side effects from products that treat life-threatening and severely debilitating illnesses than they would accept from products that treat less serious illnesses. These procedures also reflect the recognition that the benefits of the drug need to be evaluated in light of the severity of the disease being treated. The procedures apply to products intended to treat acquired immunodeficiency syndrome (AIDS), some cancers, and other life-threatening and severely debilitating illnesses."

Essentially, there are four key components to the FDA's "expedited drug development plan": (1) early and increased FDA and sponsor consultation aimed at formulating agreements on the design of preclinical and clinical studies needed for marketing approval; (2) the "compression" of Phase 3 clinical trials into Phase 2 testing; (3) the FDA's adoption of a modified medical risk-benefit analysis when assessing the safety and effectiveness of qualifying drugs; and (4) the use of Phase 4 postmarketing studies to obtain additional information about drug risks, benefits, and optimal use.

Expediting Drug and Biologics Development

The limited data that are available suggest that, over the last decade, the Subpart E program may have become less relevant given the availability of other options for industry. According to research by the Tufts Center for the Study of Drug Development, the FDA had approved 48 drugs under the Subpart E regulations from October 1988 through December 1999. The study also indicates, however, that only 2 of these 48 drugs were approved from 1997 through 1999. The program appeared to have reached its peak of approval activity in 1991, when the FDA approved 12 drugs under the Subpart E program.

Recent FDA data suggest that the Subpart E program has remained at least somewhat active for biological products. CDER, for example, recently listed those therapeutic biological products (inherited by CDER as part of CDER/CBER consolidation) that have been approved under the Subpart E program. These included Erbitux (approved in February 2004), Fabrazyme (April 2003), Zevalin (February 2002), and Campath (May 2001). From January 1998 through February 2004, the FDA had approved seven biological products under the Subpart E program.

By most accounts, however, the Subpart E program has become less relevant given the agency's successes under the prescription drug user fee program and given the availability of the fast track program and related provisions under FDAMA. In addition, the agency now routinely works with sponsors of all drugs so early in the development process that the accelerated development program's focus on early sponsor-FDA interaction likely is no longer viewed as a worthwhile incentive to participate.

The Accelerated Approval Rule (Subpart H) With its accelerated drug development program in place, the FDA wanted to take "additional steps...to facilitate the approval of significant new drugs...to treat serious or life-threatening diseases." The agency did so under final regulations (Subpart H) published in December 1992. Today, the accelerated approval program remains perhaps the most active and relevant of the accelerated development and early/expanded access programs that the FDA introduced in the late 1980s and early 1990s.

Unlike the FDA's accelerated development program, which focused largely on expediting the drug testing process, the Subpart H regulations focused on accelerating the agency's review and approval of drugs for serious or life-threatening illnesses, by modifying the criteria for both. The Subpart H regulations establish procedures "under which FDA will accelerate approval of certain new drugs and biological products for serious or life-threatening illnesses, with provision for required continued study of the drugs' clinical benefits after approval or for restrictions on distribution of use, where those are necessary for safe use of the drugs. These procedures are intended to provide expedited marketing of drugs for patients suffering from such illnesses when the drugs provide meaningful therapeutic advantage over existing treatment."

Specifically, the accelerated approval regulations allow the FDA to base marketing approval on a drug's effect on a surrogate endpoint or on an effect on a clinical endpoint other than survival or irreversible morbidity. According to the regulation, "FDA may grant marketing approval for a new drug product on the basis of adequate and well-controlled clinical trials establishing that the drug product has an effect on a surrogate endpoint that is reasonably likely, based on epidemiologic, therapeutic, pathophysiologic, or other evidence, to predict clinical benefit or on the basis of an effect on a clinical endpoint other than survival or irreversible morbidity. Approval under this section will be subject to the requirement that the applicant study the drug further, to verify and describe its clinical benefit, where there is uncertainty as to the relation of the surrogate endpoint to clinical benefit, or of the observed clinical benefit to ultimate outcome. Postmarketing studies would usually be studies already underway. When required to be conducted, such studies must also be adequate and well controlled."

In its April 1992 proposed procedures for accelerated approval, the FDA discussed the benefits of not requiring companies to study the effects of desperately needed new drugs on primary endpoints (i.e., mortality or morbidity). "Approval of a drug on the basis of a well-documented effect on a surrogate endpoint can allow a drug to be marketed earlier, sometimes much earlier, than it could if a demonstrated clinical benefit were required... Approval could be granted where there is some uncertainty as to the relation of that endpoint to clinical benefit, with the requirement that the sponsor conduct or complete studies after approval to establish and define the drug's clinical benefit."

Eligibility for Accelerated Approval Under the FDA's regulations, the accelerated approval program "applies to certain new drug and antibiotic products that have been studied for their safety and effectiveness in treating serious and life-threatening illnesses and that provide meaningful therapeutic benefit to patients over existing treatments (e.g., the ability to treat patients unresponsive to, or intolerant of, available therapy, or improved patient response over available therapy)."

Although the agency stated in its April 1992 proposal that it would apply the terms "serious" and "life-threatening" as it had in its treatment IND program and other programs, the FDA did discuss their application once again in the context of the accelerated approval plan. "The seriousness of a disease is a matter of judgement, but generally is based on its impact on such factors as survival, day-to-day functioning, or the likelihood that the disease, if left untreated, will progress from a less severe condition to a more serious one. Thus, acquired immunodeficiency syndrome (HIV) infection, Alzheimer's dementia, angina pectoris, heart failure, cancer, and many other diseases are clearly serious in their full manifestations. Further, many chronic illnesses that are generally well managed by available therapy can have serious outcomes. For example, inflammatory bowel disease, asthma, rheumatoid arthritis, diabetes mellitus, systemic lupus erythematosus, depression, psychoses, and many other diseases can be serious for certain populations or in some or all of their phases."

Approval Based on a Surrogate Endpoint The Subpart H regulations were important in that they codified the FDA's ability to approve a drug based on a surrogate endpoint that is reasonably likely, based on epidemiologic, therapeutic, pathophysiologic, or other evidence, to predict clinical benefit or on the basis of an effect on a clinical endpoint other than survival or irreversible morbidity. Prior to the accelerated approval regulations, the agency had, in a number of instances, approved drugs based on surrogate endpoints. The FDA did not define, within the regulations, what acceptable surrogate endpoints were and instead, according to the 1992 proposal, said the "sponsor must persuasively support the reasonableness of the proposed surrogate as a predictor and show how the benefits of treatment will outweigh the risks."

When an application is approved under Subpart H, postmarketing studies confirming the product's clinical benefit are required. In addition, to make clear that the approval was based on a surrogate endpoint, the agency requires clarifying statements in product labeling, such as: "The effectiveness of DRUG X is based on response rates (see CLINICAL STUDIES section). There are no controlled trials demonstrating a clinical benefit, such as an improvement in survival."

Subpart H and Postmarketing Commitments Following an accelerated approval, a sponsor must verify the approved product's clinical benefit. According to the regulations, "postmarketing studies would usually be studies already underway" at the time of approval. "When required to be conducted, such studies must also be adequate and well-controlled," and "the applicant shall carry out any such studies with due diligence." In fact, there are provisions allowing the FDA to withdraw a drug from the market if a postmarketing study fails to verify clinical benefit, if the studies are not conducted in a timely manner, or if other evidence shows the drug is not safe or effective. Although no drug has been removed from the market following an accelerated approval to date, there were discussions of a withdrawal after postmarketing studies for the oncology agent Iressa failed to confirm a survival benefit for the drug (see discussions below).

In addition to postmarketing studies, there are certain restrictions placed on the distribution of promotional materials for products approved via accelerated approval. Promotional materials for products cleared under the accelerated approval program require preapproval, and must be submitted to the FDA at least 30 days prior to the intended time of initial dissemination.

Experience to Date with the Subpart H Program The FDA's accelerated approval program has been the most active of the agency's expedited development and review initiatives in recent years. According to FDA data, the agency has approved at least 57 NDAs and 22 supplemental NDAs (additional indications) under the Subpart H program from its inception through July 2005. Not surprisingly, the majority of the accelerated approvals have been in HIV- and oncology-related indications.

AIDS Since pressure from AIDS patient advocacy groups was a major impetus for the FDA to propose the accelerated approval regulations, it is not surprising that the first drug approved under the principles and procedures was zalcitabine (commonly known as ddC, approved June 19, 1992). In addition, the majority of the accelerated approvals to date have been for AIDS and AIDS-related indications. Although a decrease in CD4 cell counts (a reflection of immune system strength) was used originally as a surrogate endpoint for the accelerated approval of anti-viral HIV drugs, this endpoint was supplanted by viral load level (plasma HIV RNA levels) more recently. Most of the early approvals were based on an interim analysis of a surrogate endpoint in a randomized, controlled trial, with conversion to standard approval coming after the trial was completed.

Oncology After HIV, the greatest number of accelerated approvals has been granted for cancer drugs. In contrast to AIDS drugs, the accelerated approvals of cancer drugs usually have relied on response rate (percentage of patients that document >50% decrease in tumor burden) as the surrogate endpoint in non-randomized trials (Phase 2 studies enrolling limited numbers of patients). Generally, the studies that supported accelerated approval were in "refractory" patient populations—patients who had not responded to prior therapies and who had no further treatment options. Subsequently, clinical benefit is demonstrated in separate randomized trials after drug approval, usually in a less refractory patient population.

Recently, the FDA has stated that time to progression (TTP) "may be a preferred endpoint for evaluating cytostatic agents because it does not require tumor size reduction. TTP, unlike survival, is documented before patients receive additional therapy." Therefore, TTP results are not "obscured by subsequent or cross-over therapies." In addition, "TTP is measured

NDAs Approved Under CDER's Accelerated Approval Program (Subpart H), 1992-June 2005

Drug	Indication	Approval Time (months)
Hivid	Combination w/ zidovudine in advanced HIV	7.6
Biaxin (suspension)	Disseminated mycobacterial infections	13.7
Zerit	Advanced HIV in adults	5.9
Zinecard	Reduce incidence/severity of cardiomyopathy assoc. w/ doxorubicin administration in certain breast cancer patients	9.7*
Casodex	Combination w/ LHRH analogue for treating advanced prostate cancer	12.7
Epivir	HIV infection	4.4
Doxil	AIDS-related Kaposi's sarcoma in unresponsive patients	14.3
Invirase	Advanced HIV in combination w/ nucleoside analogues	3.2
Norvir (2 NDAs)	HIV infection as monotherapy or in combination w/ nucleoside analogues	2.3
Crixivan	HIV infection in adults	1.4
Taxotere	Patients with locally advanced or metastatic breast cancer who have relapsed or progressed during anthracycline-based therapy	21.6
Camptosar	Refractory colorectal cancer	5.6
Viramune	Combination w/ nucleoside analogues for HIV-1-infected adults experiencing clinical or immunologic deterioration	3.9
Serostim	AIDS wasting assoc. w/ catabolism loss or cachexia	11.4
ProAmatine	Symptomatic orthostatic hypotension	11.4**
Viracept (2 NDAs)	HIV infection	2.6
Rescriptor	Treatment of HIV infection in combination w/ antiretroviral agents	8.7
Xeloda	Treatment of patients w/ metastatic breast cancer who are resistant to both paclitaxel and an anthracyline-containing chemotherapy regimen or resistant to paclitaxel and for whom further anthracycline therapy may be contraindicated	6
Sulfamylon	Adjunctive topical antimicrobial agent to control bacterial infection of excised burn wounds	14.2***
Priftin	Pulmonary tuberculosis	6
Thalidomide	Cutaneous manifestations of erythema nodosum leprosum	18.8
Sustiva	Use in combination w/ other antiretroviral agents for HIV-1	3.2
Actiq	Breakthrough cancer pain	23.7
Ziagen	Treatment of HIV-1 in combination w/ other antiretroviral agents	5.8
DepoCyt	Intrathecal treatment of lymphomatous meningitis	5.9
Temodar	Adults w/ refractory anaplastic astrocytoma	5.9
Synercid	Vancomycin resistant Enterococcus faecium	7.8****
Mylotarg	Treatment for patients 60 or older with CD33 positive acute myeloid leukemia in first relapse	6.6
Kaletra (2 NDAs)	Treatment of HIV in combination w/ other antiretroviral agents	3.5
Mifeprex	Termination of pregnancy through 49 days of pregnancy	18.0†
Trizivir	Alone or in combination w/ other antiretroviral agents in treating HIV	10.9
Gleevec	Treatment of chronic myeloid leukemia	2.4
Viread	In combination w/ other antiretrovirals to treat HIV	5.9
Tracleer	Primary pulmonary arterial hypertension	12.1
Remodulin	Primary pulmonary hypertension	19.1
Xyrem	Cataplexy associated w/ narcolepsy	21.5
Eloxatin	Metastatic carcinoma of colon or rectum	1.5
Fuzeon	HIV-1	5.9
Gleevec	Chronic myeloid leukemia	4.0
Iressa	Non-small cell lung cancer	9.0
Velcade	Multiple myeloma	3.7
Plenaxis	Palliative treatment of advanced symptomatic prostate cancer	35.4
Truvada	HIV-1	4.7
Aptivus	HIV-1	6.0
Clolar	Leukemia	8.9
Luveris	Stimulation of follicular development	41.3

* Review time based on date of submission of significant new clinical data. ** Review time based on date of submission of significant new clinical data. *** Review time based on date of submission of significant new clinical data supporting a new indication. **** Total approval time adjusted because of negative plant inspection. †Time adjusted due to manufacturing issues, submission of final study report late in review.

Source: CDER

in all patients (not just responders) and may be a better predictor of overall benefit than response rate." It has been further recommended that, "an alternative to the nonrandomized trial in refractory patients is to implement the paradigm used in AIDS. Accelerated approval is based on an interim analysis of a surrogate endpoint (e.g., response rate and TTP) in a randomized trial, with the ultimate clinical benefit (e.g., survival) demonstrated at the trial's completion."

Many of the sponsors for the oncology products approved via accelerated approval have not yet completed their post-approval commitments and, therefore, confirmed the clinical benefits of the drugs cleared under Subpart H. In one recent controversial case, however, two postmarketing studies failed to confirm the survival benefit of the oncologic therapy Iressa, which was cleared under the accelerated approval program. Rather than withdraw Iressa from the market, however, the agency approved more limited Iressa labeling, and agreed to a sponsor-proposed limited distribution program for the product. The FDA has not yet withdrawn any product approved under Subpart H.

Claiming that the Iressa case highlighted the importance of confirmatory studies conducted following approval, critics of the accelerated approval program once again expressed concern over the fact that so many companies marketing drugs approved under the accelerated approval program had failed to complete the mandatory postmarketing studies. Earlier, during a March 2003 meeting, members of CDER's Oncologic Drugs Advisory Committee indicated that they might be more reluctant to recommend that cancer drugs receive accelerated approval based on limited clinical evidence, given the fact that only four of the 15 oncology drugs approved under Subpart H at that time had been shown to have clinical benefits in confirmatory trials. The committee agreed that the FDA needs a mechanism to ensure that companies complete these trials. At a November 2005 meeting, the same advisory committee applauded both FDA and industry in proactively undertaking such trials, which the members noted seemed to reverse the so-called "foot dragging" noted in 2003. Given the challenges in testing treatments for rare cancers, including a dearth of patients, however, committee members recommended that FDA and sponsors consider establishing an "exceptional approval strategy" for therapies for which the completion of confirmatory trials is unlikely.

Given the importance of the accelerated approval program in oncology, CDER Division of Oncologic Drug Products Director Richard Pazdur, M.D., had been quite vocal about both challenges for oncology products and industry practices under the Subpart H program. In recent years, Pazdur has tried to encourage companies to initiate confirmatory studies earlier in the development process. "The reason why I want these trials initiated earlier is [because] the truly successful trials that we saw that completed their trials in a very expedited fashion were those trials that were ongoing when we approved the drug," Pazdur noted. At a November 2005 meeting, Pazdur noted his concerns about industry's use of what he called "creative indications," which he said is "a reflection of how people want to use or misuse accelerated approval." Rather than focusing on niche, highly refractory patient populations in accelerated approval efforts, companies should instead focus on broader populations in which the drug will be used in practice, said Pazdur.

Again given the importance of oncology product development to the accelerated approval program, it is not surprising that much of the program's recent evolution has responded to concerns related specifically to oncology product development. The FDA, for example, has attempted recently to revise or clarify its interpretation of the eligibility criteria for the accelerated approval and fast track programs to eliminate what it saw as a barrier to the development of products under these plans. Because an accelerated approval or fast track designation could be granted only for a drug that essentially meets an unmet medical need, the FDA held that the approval of a first drug for this unmet indication was, in effect, a grant of market exclusivity (i.e., because other drugs for the same indication could not then meet the unmet medical need criterion). At a May 2003 oncology meeting, then-FDA Commissioner Mark McClellan, M.D., Ph.D., noted that the agency had modified its accelerated drug approval policies to permit the agency to clear multiple cancer drugs for a single indication. McClellan noted that the agency took this step "so that for cancer drugs that have met accelerated approval, other products will also be able to get accelerated approval status for that indication until one of these therapies actually demonstrates in its Phase 4 study commitments a confirmatory clinical benefit in patients." [Editor's Note: In reality, the FDA's eligibility criteria for Subpart H do not use the term "unmet medical need," but instead refer to treatments that are for "treating serious and life-threatening illnesses and that provide meaningful therapeutic benefit over existing treatments."]

Other Indications In addition to HIV and cancer indications, the FDA has granted Subpart H approvals for other serious and life-threatening conditions, including infectious diseases, orthostatic hypotension and pulmonary arterial hypertension (PAH). Some of these additional indications were approved in accordance with 21 CFR 314.520, which allow the FDA to impose restrictions to assure safe use. Under these provisions, the FDA can limit distribution to facilities or physicians with special training or experience or make the distribution conditional on the performance of specified medical procedures to ensure the safe use of the drug product.

Expediting Drug and Biologics Development

Other Mechanisms to Streamline Drug Development Since 1992, when the FDA enacted the accelerated approval regulations, the agency has continued to create additional initiatives to streamline certain aspects of drug development.

The Oncology Initiative Unveiled in March 1996, CDER's Oncology Initiative was, at least in part, a response to public criticism and congressional inquiries regarding why there was such an imbalance of agency resources dedicated to the review of therapies for AIDS compared to the review of drugs for illnesses that kill far more Americans each year, including cancer and heart disease. Responding to such inquiries, then-FDA Commissioner David Kessler, M.D., agreed to evaluate the perceived inequalities in resource allocations and to evaluate methods of expediting cancer drug reviews.

Introduced as "a uniform policy" rather than as a regulation, CDER's Oncology Initiative (formally called "Reinventing the Regulation of Cancer Drugs") was designed to reduce cancer drug development times by at least a year and to cut FDA oncology drug review times from an average of 12.4 months to 6 months. The initiative itself comprised four separate elements, each of which the FDA claimed to have the authority to implement immediately:

- Accelerated Approval for Cancer Drugs. "To speed the availability of cancer drugs, FDA may now rely on partial response (such as measurable but incomplete shrinkage of a tumor) to a therapy, in addition to the current criteria such as a patient's survival and improved quality of life," the agency stated in the policy document. "While the predictive value of partial responses may still be a matter of discussion and study for all types of cancer patients, FDA has concluded that for patients with refractory malignant disease or for those who have no adequate alternative, clear evidence of anti-tumor activity is a reasonable basis for approving the drug. In these cases, studies confirming a clinical benefit may appropriately be completed after approval. By basing accelerated approval on surrogate markers such as tumor shrinkage for patients who have no satisfactory alternative therapy, and by allowing more definitive data on survival or other criteria to be developed after marketing approval, FDA believes that many cancer therapies will reach patients sooner." Under the policy, the agency can apply the accelerated approval provisions to certain products intended to remove a serious or life-threatening toxicity associated with a particular cancer treatment.

  In effect, this aspect of the Oncology Initiative simply extended the accelerated approval process (Subpart H) to cancer drugs. While the FDA pointed out that the accelerated approval regulations were applicable to drugs for cancer patients who did not benefit from or could not tolerate available therapy, the agency stressed that, in the past, "this approval mechanism has not been frequently utilized, largely because general agreement on reasonable surrogate endpoints has been lacking." Post-approval studies would be required for most drugs approved on the basis of tumor shrinkage and for all products that remove treatment-associated toxicities.

- Expanded Access for Drugs Approved in Other Countries. Under this aspect of the Oncology Initiative, the FDA was to contact the U.S. sponsor and encourage the company to pursue an expanded access protocol "whenever a cancer therapy for patients who are not curable, or well-treated by currently available therapies, is approved by a recognized foreign regulatory authority." To qualify, a drug must be in a controlled clinical trial in the United States and be approved by "an identified regulatory agency in a foreign country." Although the FDA did not specifically identify any "recognized" regulatory authorities, it did state that the authorities must have "review practices, review standards, and access to specialized expertise in the evaluation of agents for use in cancer treatment that are sufficient to allow FDA to conclude that a marketing approval action by that authority is likely to provide an adequate basis for proper consideration of an expanded access protocol for U.S. patients."

  In considering such expanded access protocols, the agency will accept an English-language version of the data submitted to the foreign regulatory authority. The expanded access protocols should be directed at the "same general type of patient condition and similar dosage and schedule" as approved by the foreign regulatory authority.

- Cancer Patient Representation at FDA Advisory Committee Meetings. The FDA agreed to expand the "consumer member" concept in the context of its advisory committees, each of which typically includes a consumer member. "Because cancer is not one disease but many, FDA will now include a person who has experienced the specific cancer on each cancer-therapy advisory committee... FDA will now ensure that an individual who has personal experience with the specific cancer being studied be included as an ad hoc member of each cancer therapy committee."

- Clarification of the FDA's Policy for Studies of Marketed Cancer Products. To reduce the number of unnecessary INDs submitted by clinical investigators, the agency clarified its policy on INDs for studies of marketed drugs and announced that it would now refuse to accept INDs for exempt studies of marketed drugs. The agency stated that it will not accept an IND for a study of a lawfully marketed drug if: (1) the study is not intended to support approval of a new indication or a significant change in product labeling or advertising; (2) the study does not involve a route of administration or dosage level or use in a patient population or other factor that significantly increases the risks (or decreases the acceptability of the risks) associated with the use of the product; and (3) the study meets the requirements for IRB approval and informed consent and does not commercialize the investigational product. The agency also clarified that it will not view a drug company's act of providing a marketed drug free of charge for an investigator-initiated study as constituting a promotional activity.

In recent years, the focus on the Oncology Initiative as a distinct program or initiative has faded to some degree, especially with the advent of FDAMA. During this time, however, the Division of Oncologic Drug Products has assimilated the Oncology Initiative's goals and provisions into standard divisional practices and policies.

The FDA Modernization Act and the "Fast Track" Program The most recent evolution in the FDA's various expanded access/accelerated development programs came through a new program authorized under the FDA Modernization Act of 1997 (FDAMA). Through this law, Congress added a new program designed to expedite the development and approval of new drugs that demonstrate the potential to address unmet medical needs in the treatment of serious or life-threatening conditions. The new program, called the "fast track" program, incorporates and, therefore, mirrors the accelerated approval program and similar programs in many respects.

Through its fast track provisions, FDAMA authorizes CDER to:

- Approve a new drug that qualifies for fast track status "upon a determination that the product has an effect on a clinical endpoint or on a surrogate endpoint that is reasonably likely to predict clinical benefit." The agency has pointed out that this element of FDAMA in effect codifies in law the Subpart H program, which permits the agency to approve a new drug product on the basis of the product's effect "on a surrogate endpoint that is reasonably likely, based on epidemiologic, therapeutic, pathophysiologic, or other evidence, to predict clinical benefit or on the basis of an effect on a clinical endpoint other than survival or irreversible morbidity." Similar to approvals under the Subpart H program, drugs approved under the fast track program may require appropriate postapproval studies to validate the surrogate endpoint or otherwise confirm the effect on the clinical endpoint.
- Accept for review portions of a marketing application prior to the receipt of the complete application. Sponsors of designated fast track products can request, by submitting clinical data indicating that the product may be effective, that the agency accept for formal review completed portions of an NDA before the other sections of the application are submitted. If the agency permits this submission—sometimes called a rolling submission—the sponsor is required to provide a schedule for submitting the information necessary to make the NDA submission complete.

Although industry encouraged Congress to include the fast track program in FDAMA, it was unclear to many what real advantages the program offered aside from those that were already available under other programs. The agency itself concedes that, with the exception of the "rolling NDA" provisions, other elements of the fast track program have been available under regulations authorizing the other accelerated development/approval programs. In many ways, FDA officials note, the fast track program is an amalgamation of the provisions of these various other programs.

Still, industry had sought over 500 fast track designations as of mid-2005, and companies appeared to be fairly aggressive in seeking such designations. In FY2005, for example, CDER received 83 requests from sponsors seeking fast track designations for their products.

While many industry officials did not see the benefits offered under the fast track program as intrinsically valuable, they had begun to view a fast track designation as a valuable "staging mechanism" for what they increasingly saw as the real gateway to rapid drug approval—priority review status. With priority NMEs being approved, on average, 9.6 months faster than their standard counterparts (i.e., for 2004-approved drugs), companies are attempting to get whatever edge they can in obtaining the prized priority status for their products. Although priority review status is not necessarily automatic once a firm obtains a fast track designation, industry officials note that such a designation does seem to help a company set the expectation at the agency that the drug will be a significant new therapy—an expectation that the company can use to its advantage. CDER's 1998 guidance entitled, "Fast Track Drug Development Programs-Designation, Development, and

Expediting Drug and Biologics Development

Application Review" (updated in July 2004) specifically notes that "a fast track product would ordinarily meet [the agency's] criteria for priority review." And, since a fast track designation can be sought and obtained so early in the development process (as early as the IND filing), a firm can leverage that designation throughout the process to obtain meetings and to set the stage for seeking priority review status for an NDA. The agency has noted in other guidance documents, however, that it will not automatically bestow priority review status on fast track products.

Qualifying for Fast Track Status To become eligible for the benefits offered under the fast track program, a drug sponsor must first apply for, and obtain, a fast track designation for its drug product. In its fast track guidance, the agency established the specific eligibility criteria that sponsors, drug, and product development programs must meet to qualify for designation.

In outlining the fast track eligibility criteria, which industry has applauded as being fairly liberal, the agency emphasized that a fast track classification applies not to a product alone, but to a combination of the product and specific indication for which it is being studied. "The indication, for the purposes of [the fast track guidance], includes both the condition for which the drug is intended (e.g., heart failure) and the anticipated or established benefits of use (e.g., improved exercise tolerance, decreased hospitalization, increased survival)," the agency states. "It is therefore the development program for a specific drug for a specific indication that will receive fast track designation. Such a program is referred to...as a fast track drug development program."

Although the fast track program applies to drugs that are designed to treat, diagnose, or prevent serious or life-threatening conditions and that demonstrate the potential to address unmet medical needs, the agency chooses not to distinguish between serious or life-threatening conditions in its guidance. Rather, the agency points out that all life-threatening conditions, as defined under the accelerated drug development (Subpart E) program, automatically qualify as serious conditions, which the guidance document focuses on defining.

To qualify for a fast track development program, a drug must "not only be used in patients with a serious condition, it must be intended to treat a serious aspect" (i.e., either a serious manifestation or serious symptom) of the condition, the agency emphasizes. Products intended to ameliorate or prevent a side effect of therapy of a condition would be considered to treat a serious condition if the side effect is serious (e.g., serious infections in patients receiving immunosuppressive therapy).

The agency notes that a preventive product will be considered to treat a serious condition if it is being evaluated for its ability to prevent a serious manifestation of the condition, or if it is being studied for its ability to prevent the condition and it is scientifically reasonable to assume that prevention of the condition would prevent its serious consequences. "A product intended and being studied for its ability, to treat a condition while avoiding the side effects of currently accepted treatments of the condition may be considered to treat a serious condition if such side effects were serious (e.g., a less myelosuppressive treatment for a tumor or an anti-inflammatory drug that does not cause gastrointestinal bleeding)," the guidance states. "The potential for a new drug to avoid the serious sequelae of existing drugs would qualify that drug development program for fast track designation only in limited circumstances. Many therapies, even those intended to treat non-serious conditions, are associated with rare, serious, adverse reactions, and new therapies, despite initial hopes, often are associated with their own set of serious reactions. Nonetheless, some adverse reactions are significant public health problems, and the development of therapies that do not cause such serious reactions would merit close attention."

In addition to being intended for a serious or life-threatening condition, a drug must also meet a second critical criterion—it must demonstrate the potential to address an unmet medical need—to qualify for fast track status. While an unmet medical need is obvious when no therapy exists for a qualifying condition, it is not as apparent when alternative therapies exist. In such cases, the agency's guidance indicates that programs for new agents would qualify if they evaluate any of the following:

- improved effect(s) on serious outcomes of the condition that are affected by alternate therapies;
- effect(s) on serious outcomes of the condition not known to be affected by the alternatives;
- the ability to provide benefit(s) in patients who are unable to tolerate or are unresponsive to alternative agents;
- the ability to provide benefits similar to those of alternatives while avoiding serious toxicity present in existing therapies, or avoiding less serious toxicity that is common and causes discontinuation of treatment of a serious disease; or
- the ability to provide benefit(s) similar to those of alternatives but with improvement in some factor, such as compliance or convenience, that is shown to lead to an improved effect on serious outcomes.

Seeking a Fast Track Designation As noted, a firm must apply for and obtain a formal fast track designation before its drug becomes eligible for the program's benefits. According to the FDA's fast track guidance, designation requests can be made as early as the IND submission stage, but generally should not be made later than the pre-NDA meeting. The request must be submitted either with the IND or as an IND amendment.

Regarding the content of the designation request, the agency states that the sponsor should "identify the serious condition and the unmet medical needs, provide a plausible basis for the assertion that the drug has the potential to address such unmet medical needs, and include in the development plan (at a level of detail appropriate to the stage of development) trials designed to evaluate this potential." Although the agency claims that the submission "should not be voluminous," it should contain the discussion and supporting documentation necessary to allow a reviewer to assess whether the criteria for fast track designation are met without having to refer to information located elsewhere.

The nature and quantity of data submitted in a designation request will depend on several factors, including whether the drug is designed to treat a fatal or non-fatal condition (i.e., less discussion/data if for a fatal condition), the availability of alternative therapies (i.e., less discussion/data if no alternatives available), and the stage of a drug's development (i.e., only animal and pharmacology data may be available). The evidentiary standard for obtaining a fast track designation was modest by design so that firms would be able to seek designation as early as the IND submission (i.e., because many of the benefits of designation are more valuable early in the development process).

The FDA will respond to a designation request within 60 calendar days of receiving the request. If the agency determines that the sponsor and drug/development program have met the criteria for fast track designation, it will forward a "designation letter" to inform the sponsor that designation has been granted and that the sponsor must design and perform studies that can show whether the product fulfills unmet medical needs, and to emphasize that the develement program must continue to meet the fast track designation criteria. Alternatively, the agency may issue a "non-designation letter" informing the sponsor that the request was incomplete or that the development program failed to meet the criteria for fast track designation. Sponsors can re-apply for designation after receiving non-designation letters.

FDA performance data released in 2005 showed that CDER had taken action on well over 80% of fast track designations within the 60-day goal. At the time, CDER had taken action on the requests in a median time of just over 50 days.

Fast Track and the Rolling NDA As noted above, the right to submit rolling NDAs is really the only new element of the fast track program that was not already available under previous accelerated drug development and approval regulations. The theory behind the rolling NDA, which some CDER review divisions have accepted in the past, is that the review process may be expedited if the agency can begin its review of parts of an NDA while the final elements of the application are being completed. Although the rolling NDA is addressed under FDAMA's fast track provisions, CDER officials have maintained that FDAMA permits the rolling NDA's use under existing programs, including the priority review and accelerated approval programs.

It is important to note that FDAMA establishes only that the FDA "may consider" a sponsor's request that the agency accept and begin the review of portions of a marketing application before the complete NDA is submitted. According to the fast track guidance, "after the sponsor submits to the IND a preliminary evaluation of data from the clinical trials, the Agency may consider accepting portions of the application if (i) the clinical trials that would form the basis for the Agency's determination of the safety and effectiveness of the product and that would support drug labeling are nearing completion or have been completed, (ii) the Agency agrees that the product continues to meet the criteria for fast track designation, and (iii) the Agency agrees that preliminary evaluation of the clinical data supports a determination that the product may be effective." Typically, the sponsor's request to submit a rolling NDA should be included in the company's information package submitted in advance of the pre-NDA meeting (i.e., so that the firm and review division can discuss relevant issues during the meeting).

Applicants seeking to submit a rolling NDA must first provide a schedule for the submission of portions of the NDA and obtain the agency's agreement to accept portions of the application as well as its agreement to the submission schedule. Regarding the standards that partial NDA submissions must meet, the agency states that, "it is expected that a section submitted for review will be in a form adequate to have been included in a complete...NDA submission. Drafts should not be included in a submission. Occasionally, the Agency may, at its discretion, accept less than a complete section (e.g., a CMC section lacking final consistency lot data and long-term stability data; an acute toxicology section lacking chronic toxicology data or final study reports for some or all of the principal controlled trials without integrated summaries) if it determines that such a subsection would constitute a reviewable unit and would be useful in making the review process more efficient overall." The agency also emphasizes that its acceptance of a rolling NDA does not necessarily guarantee that its review will begin prior to the complete dossier's submission, and that review assignments are based on several factors, including staffing and workload.

A sponsor must submit the full user fee associated with an NDA when it submits the initial portion of the application for review. In addition, the review clock applicable to the NDA (i.e., likely the six-month timeframe for priority products) will not begin until the complete application is submitted, the agency notes.

The agency established in its 2004 guidance that applicants with fast track drug programs can seek traditional approval based on data demonstrating an effect on clinically meaningful endpoints or well-established surrogate endpoints, or under the existing accelerated approval regulations based on evidence of a drug's effect on a less than well-established surrogate endpoint. Generally, approval based on clinical endpoints other than survival or irreversible morbidity would be granted under traditional procedures rather than under the accelerated approval process. Approval based on clinical endpoints other than survival or irreversible morbidity would "be considered under the accelerated approval regulations only when it is essential to determine effects on survival and irreversible morbidity in order to confirm the favorable risk/benefit judgement that led to approval," the agency noted in quoting the accelerated approval regulations.

Assessing the Activity of the Fast Track Program Although it seemed that industry was somewhat slow to embrace the fast track program, perhaps due to poorly defined benefits and the lack of a formal guidance document initially, there has been considerable effort to seek designations in the program's first four years. As noted, drug and biologic companies had submitted an estimated 500 fast track designation requests as of mid-2005 (150 for biologics). Based on the designation requests acted on as of 2005, industry is enjoying a roughly 73% success rate in obtaining fast track designations for their drugs.

Although a 2000 study found that just over half of all designation requests were submitted to either the Division of Antiviral Drug Products or the Division of Oncologic Drug Products, more recent studies are showing that other indications are accounting for a growing number of fast track designations. In a 2003 study, the Tufts Center for the Study of Drug Development found that fast track designations for products aimed at treating diseases other than cancer and HIV/AIDS grew from more than 30 in 2001 to more than 50 in 2003. Further, more than 10% of fast track designations in 2003 were for diabetes and obesity, 21% were for rare inherited conditions affecting children, and 21% were for infectious diseases, the study found.

With the growing number of approvals for drugs with fast track designations (CDER had approved 52 NDAs and BLAs under the program as of September 30, 2005), the first studies on the impact of the program on development and approval times are becoming available. According to the Tufts Center for the Study of Drug Development study, the clinical development times of fast track drugs approved between 1998 and 2003 were, on average, 2 to 2.5 years shorter than those for non-fast track drugs. Mean FDA approval times for fast track drugs were about a third of those of standard drugs (non-fast track) and about half of those of priority drugs (non-fast track).

References

1. Shulman, S.R. and Brown, J.S. (Tufts Center for the Study of Drug Development), The Food and Drug Administration's Early Access and Fast-Track Approval Initiatives: How Have They Worked? *Food and Drug Law Journal*, 1995, pp. 503-531.

2. Ibid.

3. Hewitt, P. (Tufts Center for the Study of Drug Development). Data from Tufts Center for the Study of Drug Development Marketed Drugs and Expedited/Accelerated Datasets, March 1997.

4. Johnson, JR; Williams G, Pazdur R. End Points and United States Food and Drug Administration Approval of Oncology Drugs. *Journal of Clinical Oncology*, 21(7):1404-1411, 2003.

CHAPTER 10

Meeting with the Food and Drug Administration (FDA)

by Steven Hirschfeld MD, PhD & Andrea Wright, BA

One of the most effective mechanisms available to the regulated industry and academic investigators for understanding regulatory requirements and expectations is to meet with the FDA. The intent of meetings is to clarify issues and improve understanding. Additionally, companies and individuals who participate in meetings have the potential to utilize the collective experience of other sponsors as filtered through the FDA staff. Meetings can occur in person, through a video-conference, or by telephone, and are offered as a courtesy to prospective and current IND sponsors. Meetings are not required, but are optional and are initiated at the request of the sponsor.

One exception is an advisory committee meeting, which is initiated at the request of the FDA. An advisory committee meeting is generally a public meeting through which the expert committee provides advice to the FDA. If the advice being requested pertains to a product approval, then a sponsor will be invited to the meeting to present data and answer questions regarding a licensing application that is under review. Advisory committees and meetings are regulated under the Federal Advisory Committee Act of 1972, and are sufficiently different from all other meetings that they will not be further discussed in this chapter (see chapter on advisory committee meetings elsewhere in this text).

Communications with the FDA, including meetings and teleconferences, are confidential, and the FDA will not acknowledge either publicly or to a third party that an interaction occurred or even that an IND exists.

The exhibit below provides a general overview of the product development process. The upper portion lists the sponsor's responsibilities along a hypothetical timeline, while the lower portion lists FDA roles and responsibilities. Noted in boxes are landmarks in the product development process at which meetings may occur. The description concludes with the initial filing of a biologic licensing application (BLA) or new drug application (NDA), although the paradigm also applies to supplemental filings. Not included are post-licensing interactions.

Overview of Therapeutic Development

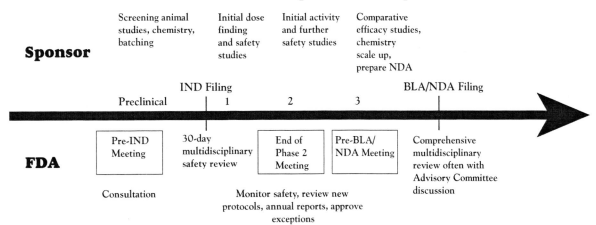

This chapter provides some general comments on participating in FDA meetings, and includes specific comments on selected types of meetings

General Comments on Meeting with the FDA The optimal time to solicit FDA input on product development is when a particular landmark is reached in the therapeutic development process. The typical landmarks are pre-IND, End of Phase 2, and pre-BLA/NDA.

Expediting Drug and Biologics Development

All meetings are sponsor initiated. Meeting requests are made in writing to the appropriate review division responsible for a product's IND. The FDA must respond to the meeting request within 14 days. Since the passage of the Prescription Drug User Fee Act (PDUFA), meetings have been grouped into three categories based on priority (see exhibit below).

Meeting Type	Description	Time Frame
A	Critical to proceed with a stalled development program	within 30 calendar days
B	Pre-IND, end of Phase 2 or end of Phase 1 for accelerated approval, pre licensing application submission	within 60 calendar days
C	Any other type of meeting	within 75 calendar days

A Type A meeting is considered urgent and critical to move an otherwise-stalled development program forward. Type B meetings are considered major landmark meetings. Typically, a sponsor is permitted only one Type B meeting for each landmark. Type C meetings comprise all other meetings.

A sponsor's meeting request should contain the following: (1) a brief statement of the purpose and type of meeting; (2) a requested range of meeting dates based on the type of meeting; (3) a listing of the specific objectives and outcomes the requester expects from the meeting; (4) a proposed agenda, including estimated times needed for each agenda item; (5) a listing of planned external attendees; (6) a listing of requested FDA participants by name or discipline type; and (7) the approximate time that supporting documentation for the meeting will be sent to the center.

The FDA generally agrees to honor meeting requests that it believes will serve a useful purpose. A request for a Type B meeting that is the first for a given landmark in a development plan is almost always honored. Generally, meeting requests would be denied if the proposed agenda has already been discussed at a prior meeting between the sponsor and the FDA, if there would be no new regulatory consequences from the discussion, and if the question would not warrant the commitment of resources that a meeting entails (i.e., could otherwise be addressed by submitting an amendment to the IND).

A sponsor should submit a background or briefing package, which should arrive at the agency at least four weeks in advance of the meeting. The exception to this is Type A meetings, for which the briefing package is expected two weeks in advance. The briefing package should contain: (1) the product name and application number (if applicable); (2) the product's chemical name and structure; (3) the proposed indication(s); (4) the dosage form, route of administration, and dosing regimen (frequency and duration); (5) a brief statement of the purpose of the meeting (this brief statement could include a discussion of the types of completed or planned studies or data that the sponsor or applicant intends to discuss at the meeting, the general nature of the critical questions to be asked, and where the meeting fits in overall development plans; (6) a list of the specific objectives/outcomes expected from the meeting; (7) a proposed agenda, including the estimated amounts of time needed for each agenda item and designated speaker(s); (8) a list of specific questions grouped by discipline; (9) a clinical data summary (as appropriate); (10) a preclinical data summary (as appropriate); (11) chemistry, manufacturing, and controls information (as appropriate); and (12) a list of sponsor attendees with names and affiliations.

While sponsors can request up to 90 minutes for a meeting (the maximum granted), the assumption is that a meeting will last an hour. Due to time constraints and the knowledge that the FDA will have studied and discussed the material prior to the meeting, formal sponsor presentations are discouraged because these presentations can take time that could be devoted to more useful discussions. If a sponsor believes that a presentation is absolutely necessary, the presentation should be restricted to a summary of the submitted material. No new material should be introduced, no new questions should be considered, and no discussions regarding updates to the submitted material should be anticipated. The presentation should be as brief as possible—generally five minutes or less—and should have as few presenters as possible (preferably only one).

The biggest challenge for sponsors is framing and then phrasing the specific questions. Questions should be discipline specific, meaning that if an issue has a clinical component, a statistical component, a pharmacokinetic component and a toxicology component, it should be separated into four separate questions. The value of FDA advice is contingent upon the focus and clarity of the questions. Broad questions are difficult to answer and may not yield the specific information necessary to satisfactorily complete product development. Forward-looking questions (e.g., the sufficiency of data for product approval?) are discouraged because the FDA cannot answer such questions until the review of a licensing submission (BLA or NDA) is completed. In addition, speculative questions cannot be answered (e.g., whether a particular series of possible future events would affect the product's approval).

Questions that can be answered in a productive discussion at a meeting include those regarding product specifications and processes, clinical trial designs, appropriate comparator arms, pharmacokinetic characterization, clarification on regulatory pathways, electronic data requirements, the need for independent review of data and the adequacy of safety monitoring. Additional examples are provided in the specific meeting sections below. While there is no specific limitation on the number of questions that can be answered in a meeting, the questions should be sufficient in number to elicit information that can be used to guide the development plan for the product's stage of development, yet not so many that there would not be adequate time to discuss them thoroughly during the meeting.

Although not required, it is common practice for sponsors to phrase questions in ways that elicit a yes or no answer, and to include qualifiers inquiring whether the FDA agrees to a particular statement or proposal. The challenge in constructing and answering questions with a yes or no answer is that the message is often complex and the answers may have several acceptable alternatives. Questions that have multiple components and modifying clauses are particularly difficult, and the phrasing may trigger "no" responses.

While briefing packages can vary in structure, it is typical that a single volume will contain the background information, rationale for proceeding, and specific questions for the FDA. Supplemental volumes, if necessary, may contain additional detailed data, such as line listings and copies of literature articles. For ease of organization and review, sections may be separated by tabs. Sponsors should not anticipate that materials sent or faxed less than 30 days prior to the meeting date will be reviewed or discussed.

General FDA Meeting Practices and Policies Each FDA-sponsor meeting is actually two meetings—an internal FDA meeting to reach consensus (pre-meeting) followed by the formal meeting with sponsor. Generally, the internal or pre-meeting, which is coordinated by the regulatory project manager, includes the primary reviewers and team leaders of each relevant discipline, the division or deputy division director, the office or deputy office director, and internal and external consultants, which might include patient representatives as needed (in person or by telephone). The FDA pre-meeting's agenda is determined by the sponsor's questions, and its goal is to determine the best response for each question and to reach a consensus on the language used to convey the response.

Some FDA divisions/offices inform the sponsor of the draft responses prior to the meeting, while other divisions/offices provide the draft responses during the meeting.

Sponsors should be prompt in arriving for or telephoning in for a meeting. FDA resources are limited and in demand, so it is often not possible to extend the meeting beyond the scheduled time. When arriving for a face-to-face meeting, sponsor representatives should allow sufficient time for the necessary security clearance process.

To initiate the meeting, the regulatory project manager usually will ask all participants to introduce themselves by name and affiliation. Generally, the FDA participants will be the same individual who participated in the pre-meeting, except the external consultants, whose participation generally is not anticipated.

The meeting agenda will consist of the sponsor-submitted questions and the FDA's responses, followed by a discussion of each response. It is best for sponsors to allow the agenda and discussion to be completed before addressing any new issues. New issues should be introduced for informational purposes, without any expectation for an FDA response, which will require review, discussion and consensus.

The purpose of any meeting is to exchange information and to provide advice. FDA advice is offered in good faith with the realization that circumstances may change. Meeting discussions do not constitute a binding agreement for a regulatory action. All regulatory actions are based upon the strength of the data submitted for review and compliance with the relevant regulations.

At the close of a meeting, the points of agreement and action items are summarized. Following the meeting, the FDA will convey formal minutes to the sponsor within 30 days, and these will comprise the minutes of record. While sponsors may take their own minutes, the FDA will not consider these to be the official meeting minutes.

Types of Meetings The most common types of FDA-sponsor meetings are: pre-IND meetings; end of Phase 2 meetings; chemical and manufacturing/product meetings; pre-BLA/NDA meetings; and advisory committee meetings. Each of these meeting types is discussed below.

Usually, IND sponsors do not seek advice or meet with the FDA for the initiation of Phase 2 studies. Once data are available from Phase 2 studies, sponsors may request a meeting to discuss approaches to formally establish efficacy for the registration of a use claim.

Pre-IND Meeting Before filing an IND to initiate clinical trials, sponsors may find it helpful to solicit FDA advice regarding the requirements for pre-clinical studies and to discuss clinical development scenarios. This may be particularly the case when a company is developing a new molecular entity or new biological product.

Expediting Drug and Biologics Development

The goal of a pre-IND meeting is to ascertain what types of pre-clinical and non-clinical studies would be helpful and would satisfy regulatory requirements, discuss the general framework for a clinical development plan, and specifically discuss the Phase I study design. Once it begins to contemplate human clinical studies, a company may request a pre-IND meeting to discuss with the FDA the possible approaches to product preparation, recommended animal and other pre-clinical studies, and approaches to determine human dosing and preliminary toxicity characteristics for initial clinical studies.

The briefing document may comprise proposed or preliminary animal and other preclinical studies as well as details on product characterization and preparation, planned Phase 1 studies in outline or draft form, and perhaps outlines of further clinical studies. Specific questions should seek FDA advice to ensure compliance with pertinent regulations, particularly with regard to product sterility, provide an adequate scientific basis for the initiation of the proposed clinical studies, and address any issues regarding the appropriate patient population, dose escalation schema, and safety monitoring.

Chemistry Manufacturing/Product Meeting Although the focus of a chemistry and manufacturing or product meeting can vary, its usually involves issues relating to production standards, stability, compliance, microbiology, sterility, purity, potency and scale up procedures. As product and clinical development proceeds, the FDA anticipates greater detail and specifications to be submitted for review.

The End of Phase 2 Meeting If, in the course of performing Phase 2 studies, the sponsor obtains preliminary data to support a potential claim for clinical benefit, it can request a formal meeting to discuss further clinical development, including clinical trial design and analysis plans for formal efficacy studies. It is quite possible that this discussion could be the most critical in product's development.

The goals of an end of phase 2 (EOP2) meeting are to discuss the overall development plan, study designs for formal efficacy studies (usually Phase 3), and the general requirements for a BLA/NDA filing with regard to the anticipated number and types of studies. This may include not only clinical studies, but pharmacokinetic and non-clinical studies as well. In addition, any outstanding product issues, including characterization, purity and potency, must be addressed.

The major focus of a development plan is to gather data to support a health claim. The ultimate goal of an end of phase 2 meeting is to design a plan that would produce the relevant data.

An end of Phase 2 meeting package would typically include: (1) summaries of Phase 1 and Phase 2 studies; (2) summaries of non-clinical experience, including animal studies; (3) summaries of relevant product data; (4) brief reviews of the current treatment options for the disease or condition for which a claim is being sought; and (5) draft proposals for the diseases or conditions to be studied

The questions that should be considered in formulating an EOP2 meeting package include the following:
- What is the nature of the anticipated benefit? Is it clinically meaningful?
- What are the key clinical endpoints?
- Is clinical benefit measured directly or through a surrogate endpoint? Is the surrogate endpoint validated in the relevant patient population?
- Is the comparator arm for a multi-arm study reasonable and appropriate?
- Is the proposed study population representative of individuals with the disease or condition (e.g., with regard to age, gender, race, disease severity, prior therapy)?
- What is the anticipated burden of visits and tests?
- Dose the proposed data analysis plan address the endpoints and potential benefits, study dropouts, missing data, and any planned interim analysis, and does it distinguish between primary and exploratory analyses?
- Is accelerated approval (using a likely surrogate) considered? If so, what is(are) the proposed follow up study(ies)?
- Are there any additional regulatory issues?

Ideally, the EOP2 meeting's outcome will include answers to all the questions posed by the sponsor as well as the framing of a plan for developing the necessary data for a marketing application. Often, the sponsor agrees to follow up with the submission of detailed clinical protocols. Product issues should be sufficiently resolved so that, when the clinical studies begin to enroll subjects, the studies employ the same product that is intended for marketing.

The FDA has a program called Special Protocol Assessment that allows sponsors to submit carcinogenicity protocols, stability protocols, and clinical protocols for trials whose data will form the primary basis of an efficacy claim for in depth review. The time frame for such a review is 45 days with the outcome that the FDA can enter into a binding agreement regarding the acceptability of the protocol design if both parties agree. An FDA Guidance document referenced at the end of this chapter describes the program in greater detail. Any subsequent protocol amendments would require FDA review and a new agreement.

Pre-BLA/NDA Meeting Before an NDA or BLA is submitted, the FDA will meet with a sponsor in a pre-BLA/NDA meeting to: review the portfolio of studies; discuss which components of a potential submission package are present and which still require development or completion; discuss the time frame for submission; discuss the filing strategy; and discuss formatting and data specifications.

While the pre-NDA/BLA briefing package contents will depend upon the nature and number of studies and the nature of the product's proposed indication, it should include information such as:

- What are the clinical questions being asked in each of the studies?
- Do the studies answer the questions?
- How were the studies designed to answer the question?
- What are the claimed benefits?
- What proportion of the enrolled patients demonstrated the benefit?
- How durable is the benefit?
- Are the results consistent from study to study?
- Is the manner in which the data are expressed consistent?
- What are the perceived risks of product exposure?
- Was the patient population representative of those patients for whom a claim is sought?
- Was the data analysis that was performed the one that was planned?
- Was a Special Protocol Assessment performed by the FDA?
- Were there any additional agreements?

The goal of a pre-NDA/BLA meeting will be to reach agreement on the formatting, timing, and content of a marketing application. It will not be possible for the FDA to comment on the outcome of the review process until the submission is formally submitted and reviewed.

Bibliography

Guidance for Industry: Formal Meetings With Sponsors and Applicants for PDUFA Products, http://www.fda.gov/cder/guidance/2125fnl.htm#Type%20C%20Meeting

Section 735(1) of the Federal Food, Drug, and Cosmetic Act (the Act) (21 U.S.C. 379g(1)) (PDUFA products).

March 1996 (MAPP 4512.1, Formal Meetings Between CDER and External Constituents) http://www.fda.gov/cder/mapp/4512-1.pdf

Guidance for Industry: Special Protocol Assessment, http://www.fda.gov/cder/guidance/3764fnl.htm

CHAPTER 11

The IND

by Paul R. Hartmann, R.Ph.

As specified in Section 312 of the U.S. Code of Federal Regulations, an investigational new drug application (IND) is required before clinical trials of a new drug or biologic may be initiated. Aside from a possible pre-IND package (see Chapter 6), the IND is the first formal document the FDA sees from many new companies, and thus represents a firm's first opportunity to create a favorable impression with FDA reviewers. Care in drafting and assembling a complete and professional document will enhance this first impression, will make the reviewer's job easier, and will help pave the way for a smooth, professional interaction with the FDA in the future. Established companies, which have filed numerous INDs, have learned the benefits of drafting INDs with consistent formats and contents.

This chapter provides a basic outline for an investigational new drug application. This outline can also be used to prepare an action item list and to budget, schedule, and plan the tasks that are critical in obtaining the required information. The chapter's main goal is to provide general guidance on the important issues confronting the individuals responsible for developing an IND, and to offer a blueprint for drafting the document. At the core of the chapter is the sample IND template (see below), which follows the guidance provided by the FDA in 21 CFR 312.23. The template is intended to serve as a general outline for both drug and biologic IND submissions, although sponsors may have to modify the proposed format and content to accommodate particular situations.

Like NDAs and BLAs, INDs are evolving due to many factors, including international harmonization efforts, electronic submission initiatives, scientific advances, and concerns over new drug safety. While marketing applications were the initial focus of the ICH/FDA's adoption of a common application format (common technical document, or CTD), the agency quickly moved to extend the CTD principles and format to other applications, including the IND. In their most recent calls for electronic INDs, for example, CDER officials are encouraging companies to provide electronic INDs (eIND) in the CTD format. While industry had limited interest in submitting electronic INDs as recently as early 2005, agency officials were hoping that such interest would rise with the development of new electronic tools. Meanwhile, the FDA continues to encourage industry to submit pharmacogenomics information in INDs and other applications to help FDA reviewers and scientists understand the relevant scientific issues in this emerging field. Further, as part of the FDA's focus on risk management under PDUFA III, some sponsors may choose to submit, as early as the IND submission, a draft version of a so-called "risk minimization action plan (RiskMAP)," which is defined as "a strategic safety program designed to meet specific goals and objectives in minimizing known risks of a product while preserving its benefits" upon marketing.

The "IQ" Curve When preparing the IND, the sponsoring company needs to consider the information vs. question (IQ) curve presented below. When inadequate information is submitted, the FDA obviously will have many comments and, more importantly, may place the IND on "clinical hold." When the company submits additional—and more adequate—information, the FDA will have fewer questions. Obviously, a company wants to be on the IQ curve at the point at which the questions are few. At least theoretically, however, one never reaches the point at which no questions are posed. The fact is that FDA reviewers are paid to ask them.

There is also a point of diminishing returns, where supplemental information will result in additional, not fewer, questions and comments. Consequently, it is a waste of effort and precious resources to prepare either inadequate or too much information. With experience, a company will learn what information answers the relevant questions sufficiently. Until sponsors develop a sense of how much information to provide, they should pay careful attention to the requirements presented in 21 CFR 312.23 regarding IND content and FDA guidance documents.

Undoubtedly, the one IND section that is most likely to suffer from too much or too little information is the chemistry section (Item 7 in the sample IND outline below). Developers should consider the information presented in Chapter 6, which discusses the extent of product and assay development needed for different clinical phases at the time of the IND filing. The IND's preclinical section represents another section in which the amount of information presented is critical (Item 8 in the sample outline below). The information provided in this section must be sufficient to support the initiation of testing in humans. It need not be exhaustive, but it must be sufficient. Chapter 4 of this book addresses the general and specific issues relevant for compiling the needed nonclinical information.

Writing for the Reviewer The goal of the IND is to allow FDA reviewers to quickly read their assigned sections during the 30-day review period for the initial submission. Doing so will allow the sponsor to initiate its clinical trial(s) as scheduled. Therefore, although this may sound simplistic, the sponsor should prepare the IND with the reviewer in mind by assembling a submission that is well-organized, has a consistent theme, and addresses the salient points clearly and efficiently.

Keep in mind that sponsor-employed project experts can represent a double-edged sword in the IND preparation process. In many cases, what is totally obvious to the "expert author" may be presented in a manner that is not understandable to an outside reviewer. Compounding the problem is the fact that various individuals and departments normally prepare different sections of the IND. Therefore, unless the IND sponsor takes particular care, considerable discontinuity between the various sections of the application can result. Assigning a regulatory affairs specialist to review the entire IND and edit it for consistency is the best means of addressing this potential problem.

Information vs. Questions

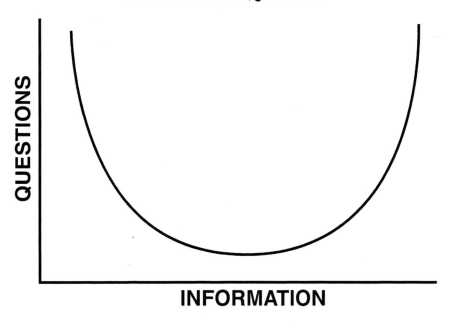

Important Clinical Issues
- From the project's outset, the sponsor should have a draft package insert to use as the guide for the clinical plan.
- The investigational plan must contain:
    - the scientific rationale for the product being developed;
    - the clinical indication(s) to be studied;
    - an approach for evaluating the product;
    - the clinical trials to be conducted;
    - the number of subjects/patients to be treated in the trials; and
    - an approach for addressing the risks based on animal data or prior human experience.
- The clinical trials must:
    - contain a hypothesis to be addressed;
    - list subject/patient exclusion and inclusion criteria;
    - list clearly defined clinical (and surrogate) endpoints;
    - address the need for (or lack of) active or placebo control groups;
    - contain a study outline/table that clearly describes what procedures will be conducted during each study visit;

- contain a means of safety monitoring;
- contain a detailed statistical analysis plan;
- build upon previously generated clinical data;
- be supported by preclinical safety data; and, most importantly,
- generate data that are needed for product approval.

Important Chemistry, Manufacturing and Controls (CMC) Issues Information pertaining to the drug substance should contain the following:

- Manufacturing information (flowcharts and narratives) that is easy to follow and that clearly demonstrates that the key manufacturing steps have appropriate in-process controls. This information should be for the lot of material(s) that will be evaluated in clinical trials. If manufacturing steps do not have appropriate in-process controls, prior agreement with the FDA must be obtained;
- Physical and chemical data demonstrating that the product is properly characterized;
- Acceptance specifications for key intermediates and final bulk product (see the next section);
- Lot comparison data (physical/chemical data) and changes in the manufacturing process among the lots if multiple lots have been manufactured;
- Data regarding impurities and degradation products (include a discussion of theoretical degradation pathways);
- Stability data;
- Descriptions of the assay methods; and
- Bulk product lot release data.

Information for the Drug Product (Final Dosage Form) should include:

- Manufacturing information of the same detail as that presented for the drug substance;
- A product development summary (i.e., excipient evaluation and compatibility testing) to demonstrate that the formulation is acceptable;
- A description of the primary container and closure system (that part of the packaging that directly contacts the drug product);
- Acceptance specifications (see next section);
- Lot comparison data (physical/chemical data) and changes in the manufacturing process among the lots if multiple lots have been manufactured;
- Stability data that demonstrate that the drug product will be stable during its use in the clinical trials;
- Descriptions of the assay methods (the assays must be able to quantify the amount of drug substance that is in the final product); and
- Lot release data (either certificates of analysis or release protocols).

Developing all of these data and ideas into an informative and easily reviewable IND is essential for the initiation of a successful development program. The use of a format such as the one in the following template (and the accompanying suggested content) should help both the sponsor in preparing the IND and the FDA in reviewing the submission.

Sample IND Template After each IND item is completed, all pages for that item can be numbered. In this example, pages are numbered in the lower right using an electric page stamper. The suggested format for page numbering is a two-part number. The first two digits (e.g., "01") represent the IND item number and the last set of numbers (e.g., "001") represents the page number within the item. This allows each IND item to be independently page numbered as it is completed without having to wait for the previous items to be completed. This number is used in the IND table of contents (IND Item 2) and in the table of contents for each IND item. This is also the page number that is used when referencing an IND page number in the text of the IND.

A table of contents for each IND item should be prepared first. Each item's tables of contents can then be electronically copied and consolidated into IND item 2.

A format for IND tables of contents follows below.

Expediting Drug and Biologics Development

Company Name
Product Code and Name
IND Serial No. 000, IND Item 2, Table of Contents

TABLE OF CONTENTS

> The page number in the lower right-hand corner of each page is a two part number. The first number is the IND Item number and the second number is the page number within the IND Item. For example, 07 035 is for IND Item 7, page 35.

Description	IND Volume	Page
IND Item 1		
Form FDA 1571 01		01 001
IND Item 2		
IND Table of Contents 01		02 001
IND Item 3		
3.0 Introductory Statement 01		03 001
3.1 Overview		
3.1.1 Name of the Drug Substance, Structure and Chemical Properties.................		
3.1.2 Dosage Formulation		
3.1.3 Route of Administration		
3.1.4 Broad Objectives and Planned Duration of the Proposed Investigations		
3.2 Summary of Previous Human Experience		
IND Item 4		
4.0 General Investigational Plan 01		04 001
4.1 Scientific Rationale for the Product and the Research Study		
4.2 Indications(s) to be Studied		
4.3 General Approach to Evaluate the Product		

Company Name
Product Code and Name
IND Serial No. 000, IND Item 2, Table of Contents

4.4 Clinical Trials to be Conducted in the First Year Following the IND Submission		
4.5 Estimated Number of Subjects/Patients to be Treated		
4.6 Anticipated Special Risks Based on Animal Data or Prior Human Experience.................		
IND Item 5		
5.0 Investigator's Brochure 01		05 001
IND Item 6		
6.0 Protocol 01		06 001
6.1 Investigational Site Documentation...............		
6.1.1 Investigator's Curriculum Vitae		
6.1.2 Form FDA 1572		
6.1.3 IRB Approval Documents		
6.1.4 Informed Consent Forms		
IND Item 7		
7.1 Introduction...........................02		07 001
7.1.1 Drug Substance		
7.1.2 Names and Addresses of the Manufacturers and Facilities Description		
7.1.3 Summary Manufacturing/Synthetic Flow Chart		
7.2 Drug Substance		
7.2.1 Description................		
7.2.1.1 Names		
7.2.1.2 Formula		
7.2.1.3 Appearance		
7.2.1.4 Physical and Chemical Properties................		
7.2.2 Name and Address of Manufacturer/Testing Facility............		
7.2.3 Method of Preparation		
7.2.3.1 Raw Materials Used in Manufacture................		
7.2.3.2 Major Pieces of Manufacturing Equipment................		

Company Name
Product Code and Name
IND Serial No. 000, IND Item 2, Table of Contents

7.2.3.3 Manufacturing Flow Diagram	
7.2.3.4 Description of Manufacturing Process................	
7.2.4 Reference Standard - Characterization of the Drug Substance	
7.2.5 Specifications................	
7.2.6 Release/Analytical Data	
7.2.7 Container/Closure System	
7.2.8 Stability Data	
7.2.8.1 Protocol	
7.2.8.2 Summary of Results	
7.3 Drug Product	
7.3.1 Qualitative and Quantitative Composition	
7.3.2 Component Specifications	
7.3.3 Name and Address of Manufacturer/Testing Facility and Packaging Facility	
7.3.4 Method of Manufacture and Packaging	
7.2.4.1 Description of the Manufacturing Process - Flow Diagram................	
7.3.4.1 Description of the Manufacturing Process - Narrative	
7.3.5 Specifications................	
7.3.6 Release/Analytical Results - Lot/Batch Comparison Data.......	
7.3.7 Container and Closure................	
7.3.7.1 Intermediate Packaging	
7.3.7.2 Final Primary Packaging Material................	
7.3.8 Stability	
7.3.8.1 Protocol	
7.3.8.2 Summary of Results	
7.3.9 Labeling	
7.4 Diluent................	
7.5 Placebo................	
7.6 Test Procedures................	
7.6.1 Drug Product Test Procedure Descriptions	
List titles here	

Company Name
Product Code and Name
IND Serial No. 000, IND Item 2, Table of Contents

7.6.2 Final Product Test Procedure Documents		
List titles here		
7.7 Environmental Assessment................		
IND Item 8		
8.0 Pharmacology and Toxicology Data 02		08 001
8.1 Nonclinical Pharmacology Summary		
8.2 Toxicology Summary		
8.3 Good Laboratory Practice Statement of Compliance		
8.4 Bibliography................		
IND Item 9		
9.0 Previous Human Experience 02		09 001
9.1 Overall Clinical Summary		
9.2 Clinical Investigations		
9.3 Marketing Experience		
9.4 Bibliography................		
IND Item 10		
10.0 Additional Information 02		10 001
10.1 Drug Dependence and Abuse Potential		
10.2 Radioactive Drugs		
10.3 Other Information		

Company Name
Product Code and Name
IND Serial No. 000 IND Item 3, Introductory Statement

TABLE OF CONTENTS

Description	IND Volume	Page
3.0 Introductory Statement 01		03 001
3.1 Overview		
3.1.1 Name of the Drug Substance, Structure and Chemical Properties		
3.1.2 Dosage Formulation		
3.1.3 Route of Administration		
3.1.4 Broad Objectives and Planned Duration of the Proposed Investigations		
3.2 Summary of Previous Human Experience		
3.3 Withdrawal From Investigational Trials or Marketing		

This Item is an executive summary of information extracted from other IND Items (4, 5, 7, and 9). It should be no more than eight to ten pages.

Company Name
Product Code and Name
IND Serial No. 000 IND Item 3, Introductory Statement

3.0 Introductory Statement — 21 CFR 312(a)(3)

3.1 Overview — 21 CFR 312.23(a)(3)(i)

3.1.1 **Name of the Drug Substance, Structure and Chemical Properties**

This information is extracted from IND Item 7.

List the name and product code of the drug substance (drug or biologic).

State the class of drug or biologic.

If known, provide the structural formula.

3.1.2 **Dosage Formulation**

This information is extracted from IND Item 7.

• **Final Product Composition and Container/Closure**

List the qualitative and quantitative composition. List the grades (e.g., USP, NF, EurP) of the excipients and the quantitative composition of the final product (e.g., tablet, capsule, vial, ampule, tube, etc.) and a typical lot size (see IND Item 7).

Example:

Composition

	Batch	Dosage Unit
Active Substance	X g	X mg (or mg/mL)
Excipient A (Name and Grade)	X kg	X g (or mg/mL)
Excipient B (Name and Grade)	X kg	X g (or mg/mL)
Excipient C (Name and Grade)	X kg	X g (or mg/mL)

Company Name
Product Code and Name
IND Serial No. 000 IND Item 3, Introductory Statement

Container and Closure System

Example:

Material/Grade	Manufacturer
Tubing vial, Type I glass	
Rubber stopper, grey butyl	
Aluminum seal	

Diluent Composition and Container/Closure

List the qualitative and quantitative composition if it is not commercially available (using the format described above). If it is commercially available, only list the diluent name (e.g., 0.9% Sodium Chloride Injection, USP).

3.1.3 **Route of Administration**

This information is extracted from IND Item 5.

List the route of administration (e.g., oral, intramuscular, intravenous, etc.).

3.1.4 **Broad Objectives and Planned Duration of the Proposed Investigations**

This is a summary (no more than one page) of the objectives and planned trials presented in IND Item 4.

3.2 **Summary of Previous Human Experience — 21 CFR 312.23(a)(3)(ii)**

This is a summary (no more than one page) of the information presented in IND Item 9.

3.3 **Withdrawal from Investigational Trials or Marketing — 21 CFR 312.23(a)(3)(iii)**

State either:

"This product has not been withdrawn from investigation or marketing in any country for any reason related to safety or efficacy."

OR -

"This product has been withdrawn from investigation or marketing in *list countries* due to *list the safety or efficacy reasons.*"

Company Name
Product Code and Name
IND Serial No. 000 IND Item 4, General Investigational Plan

TABLE OF CONTENTS

Description	IND Volume	Page
4.0 General Investigational Plan 01		04 001
4.1 Scientific Rationale for the Product and the Research Study		
4.2 Indications(s) to be Studied		
4.3 General Approach to Evaluate the Product		
4.4 Clinical Trials to be Conducted in the First Year Following the IND Submission		
4.5 Estimated Number of Subjects/Patients to be Treated		
4.6 Anticipated Special Risks Based on Animal Data or Prior Human Experience		

This is an executive summary that gives the FDA an overview of the following year's clinical plan and the types of clinical trials to be initiated.

Expediting Drug and Biologics Development

4.0 General Investigational Plan — 21 CFR 312.23(a)(3)

4.1 Scientific Rationale for the Product and the Research Study — 21 CFR 312.23(a)(3)(iv)(a)

Discuss why the product is being developed and provide the following:

- a brief history of the condition(s) to be treated by the product;
- why current therapies are not adequate or non-existent; and
- how this product is a potential improvement over current treatment.

4.2 Indication(s) to be Studied — 21 CFR 312.23(a)(3)(iv)(b)

List of the indications to be studied.

4.3 General Approach to Evaluate the Product — 21 CFR 312.23(a)(3)(iv)(c)

Discuss how the product is to be evaluated.

4.4 Clinical Trials to be Conducted in the First Year Following the IND Submission — 21 CFR 312.23(a)(3)(iv)(d)

List and describe the types of clinical trials that will be conducted. Copies of the clinical protocols and their supporting documents are submitted in IND Item 6. If the plans are not developed for the entire year, this needs to be stated.

4.5 Estimated Number of Subjects/Patients to be Treated — 21 CFR 312.23(a)(3)(iv)(e)

List the number and types of subjects and patients that will be enrolled in the trials that were discussed previously in Section 4.4.

4.6 Anticipated Special Risks Based on Animal Data or Prior Human Experience — 21 CFR 312.23(a)(3)(iv)(f)

List the anticipated risks of particular severity or seriousness that are based on animal toxicological data or prior human experience with the product or related products (i.e., products of the same chemical class).

TABLE OF CONTENTS

Description	IND Volume	Page
5.0 Investigator's Brochure	01	05 001

The table of contents for this item varies according to the investigator's brochure being submitted. It lists the IND page number for the major sections in the brochure. For additional information on the investigator's brochure, see Chapter 14.

Investigator's Brochure — 21 CFR 312.23(a)(5)

Since the investigator's brochure is given to investigators as a "free-standing" document without a copy of the rest of the IND, it may not reference any other IND Items.

Introduction

Provide an overview of:

- the disease that is to be treated by the product;
- the results from previously conducted clinical trials; and
- the plans for the clinical trials to be conducted under the IND.

Description of the Product and its Formulation — 21 CFR 312.23(a)(5)(i)

Provide:

- a brief description and structural formula of the drug substance; and
- a description of the final product formulation.

OPTIONAL INFORMATION:

- a description of the container/closure system (i.e., vial size and type, closure type);
- a description of the diluent;
- storage condition requirements; and
- instructions to prepare and administer a dose to the subject.

Summary of Pharmacology and Toxicology — 21 CFR 312.23(a)(5)(ii)

Provide a summary of the pharmacological and toxicological effects of the product in animals and humans (if known).

Summary of the Pharmacokinetics and Biological Disposition — 21 CFR 312.23(a)(5)(iii)

Provide a summary of the pharmacokinetics and biological disposition of the product in animals and humans (if known).

Summary of Previous Human Experience, Safety and Effectiveness — 21 CFR 312.23(a)(5)(iv)

Provide a summary of human safety and effectiveness information obtained from clinical trials.

Possible Risks and Side Effects — 21 CFR 312.23(a)(5)(v)

Provide a description of possible risks and side effects based on experience with the product or related products in animals and humans. Discuss precautions or special monitoring that may be needed.

References

Provide a list of all published and unpublished reports cited in the body of the brochure. Copies of all published articles are located in IND Item 10.

Company Name
Product Code and Name
IND Serial No. 000, IND Item 6, Protocol

TABLE OF CONTENTS

Description	IND Volume	Page
6.0 Protocol 01		06 001
6.1 Investigational Site Documentation		
6.1.1 Investigator's Curriculum Vitae		
6.1.2 Form FDA 1572		
6.1.3 IRB Approval Documents		
6.1.4 Informed Consent Forms		

Company Name
Product Code and Name
IND Serial No. 000, IND Item 6, Protocol

The following information must be provided in the IND:

- final approved protocol [21 CFR 312.23(a)(6)(i) through (iii) for protocol requirements];
- investigator's name and qualifications (curriculum vitae) [21 CFR 312.23(a)(6)(iii)(b)];
- subinvestigator's name(s) [21 CFR 312.23(a)(6)(iii)(b)];
- research facility's name and address [21 CFR 312.23(a)(6)(iii)(b)]; and
- IRB's name and address [21 CFR 312.23(a)(6)(iii)(b)].

21 CFR Part 312 does not require the following information to be submitted to the FDA. However, you may be asked to provide the following documents:

- case report forms;
- a completed FDA Form 1572 that is signed by the investigator;
- the IRB approved informed consent; and
- the record of IRB approval to initiate the trial.

6.0 Protocol

Provide a *brief* overview of the protocol (one or two paragraphs discussing the purpose, patient population, end-points, etc.). Phase 1 study protocols may be less detailed and more flexible than protocols for Phase 2 and 3 studies. Provide a copy of the protocol.

6.1 Investigational Site Documentation

6.1.1 Investigator's Curriculum Vitae

The sponsor is required to submit only the CV for the investigator(s). There is no requirement to submit CVs for subinvestigators, but it is advised that the sponsor obtain copies of these CVs for its file. 21 CFR 312.3 states that an *investigator* is "an individual who actually conducts a clinical investigation (i.e., under whose immediate direction the drug is administered or dispensed to a subject)." In the event an investigation is conducted by a team of individuals, the investigator is the responsible leader of the team. *Subinvestigator* includes any other individual member of that team.

The documents listed below do not need to be submitted to the FDA, but must be maintained in the sponsor's files. If these are not filed, the sponsor should state, "The investigator has signed Form FDA 1572 and the IRB has approved initiation of the protocol and the informed consent form. The sponsor has a copy of the Form FDA 1572 and IRB approval and the IRB approved informed consent in our files."

Company Name
Product Code and Name
IND Serial No. 000, IND Item 6, Protocol

6.1.2 Form FDA 1572

This form provides the information required by 21 CFR 312.23(a)(6)(iii)(b).

6.1.3 IRB Approval Documents

If it is not available at the time that the IND is to be submitted, submit it later in an IND amendment.

6.1.4 Informed Consent Forms

This is a copy of the IRB approved informed consent form. However, this may not be available when the IND is ready for submission. In that case, submit a model informed consent that the sponsor has written for use by the investigator(s).

Company Name
Product Code and Name
IND Serial No. 000, IND Item 7, Chemistry, Manufacturing, and Control Data

This is a general guideline/boilerplate for assembling an IND Item 7. This section is to be modified in accordance with the type of product being developed.

DRUG MASTER FILES

Sponsors must obtain letters from Drug Master File (DMF) holders authorizing the FDA to reference documents in their DMFs in support of the IND. These letters are addressed to the FDA. Copies of these letters are submitted behind the FDA Form 1571.

INSTRUCTIONS FOR ITEM 7

The intention of this item is to demonstrate that the manufacturing processes are fully documented and adequately controlled. This section must present a well-organized description of all of the critical manufacturing steps, in-process controls, specifications, release tests, and stability data.

Expediting Drug and Biologics Development

Company Name
Product Code and Name
IND Serial No. 000, IND Item 7, Chemistry, Manufacturing, and Control Data

TABLE OF CONTENTS

Description	IND Volume	Page
7.0 Chemistry, Manufacturing and Control Data 02		07 001
7.1 Introduction		
7.2 Drug Substance		
7.3 Final Product/Dosage Form.		
7.4 Diluent.		
7.5 Placebo.		
7.6 Test Procedures.		
7.7 Environmental Assessment.		

Company Name
Product Code and Name
IND Serial No. 000, IND Item 7, Chemistry, Manufacturing, and Control Data

7.1 INTRODUCTION

TABLE OF CONTENTS

Description	IND Volume	Page
7.1 Introduction 02		07 XXX
7.1.1 Drug Substance/Product		
7.1.2 Names and Addresses of the Manufacturers and Facilities Description		
7.1.3 Summary Manufacturing/Synthetic Flow Chart		

Company Name
Product Code and Name
IND Serial No. 000, IND Item 7, Chemistry, Manufacturing, and Control Data

7.1   Introduction — 21 CFR 312.23(a)(7)

7.1.1   Drug Substance/Product

This is a brief description (no more than a few paragraphs) of the product providing:

- descriptive name (e.g., generic name);
- chemical names (e.g., Chemical Abstract Service name and registry number);
- chemical structure, molecular formula, molecular weight/size;
- physical description;
- name(s) of the manufacturer(s) of the drug substance and final product (if not the sponsor);
- the names and amounts of the drug substance in the final product;
- how the final product is manufactured;
- the names and amounts of the inactive ingredients (including preservatives);
- a description of the container and closure; and
- if used, a description of diluent that will be used to reconstitute the product prior to administration.

7.1.2   Names and Addresses of the Manufacturers and Facilities Description

This section provides the names and addresses for all manufacturing sites along with the number of the IND or DMF describing the facility or manufacturing process. If an IND or DMF is not available, this description contains:

- facilities' names and addresses;
- facilities description to include floor plans and HVAC (e.g., air pressure gradients, temperature and particulate control);
- major pieces of equipment (by department); and
- storage and flow of materials through the facilities.

7.1.3   Summary Manufacturing/Synthetic Flow Chart

This is a one to two page flow chart that provides an overview of the manufacturing process showing starting materials, reactants, and key intermediates.

Company Name
Product Code and Name
IND Serial No. 000, IND Item 7, Chemistry, Manufacturing, and Control Data

7.2 DRUG SUBSTANCE

TABLE OF CONTENTS

Description	IND Volume	Page
7.2 Drug Substance. 02		07 XXX
7.2.1 Description.		
7.2.1.1 Names		
7.2.1.2 Formula		
7.2.1.3 Appearance		
7.2.1.4 Physical and Chemical Properties.		
7.2.2 Name and Address of Manufacturer/Testing Facility.		
7.2.3 Method of Preparation		
7.2.3.1 Raw Materials Used in Manufacture.		
7.2.3.2 Major Pieces of Manufacturing Equipment		
7.2.3.3 Manufacturing Flow Diagram		
7.2.3.4 Description of Manufacturing Procedures		
7.2.4 Reference Standard - Characterization of the Drug Substance . . .		
7.2.5 Specifications		
7.2.6 Release/Analytical Data		
7.2.7 Container Closure System		
7.2.8 Stability Data.		
7.2.8.1 Protocol		
7.2.8.2 Summary of Results		

Company Name
Product Code and Name
IND Serial No. 000, IND Item 7, Chemistry, Manufacturing, and Control Data

7.2 Drug Substance — 21 CFR 312.23(a)(7)(a)

References to published literature may be used and copies of the articles provided in IND Item 10.

7.2.1 Description

7.2.1.1 Names

List accepted names for the drug substance (e.g., IUPAC, CAS, etc.).

7.2.1.2 Formula

Provide the structural formula, molecular formula, and molecular weight/size.

7.2.1.3 Appearance

List the physical appearance (e.g., white crystalline powder).

7.2.1.4 Physical and Chemical Properties

List the physical and chemical properties, such as solvability in various solvents and melting point.

7.2.2 Name and Address of Manufacturer/Testing Facility

List the physical location of the sites.

7.2.3 Method of Preparation

7.2.3.1 Raw Materials Used in Manufacture

This is a list of all the raw materials showing their grades (e.g., ACS, reagent grade, compendial, etc.) and strength (e.g., molarity, normality, etc.). This list is in the same order that the materials are used in the manufacturing process. The following is an example:

Step 1	Grade
Sodium Chloride	
Glycerin	
Acetone	
Sodium Hydroxide	
Phenol	
Dehydrated Alcohol	
Magnesium Sulfate	

Company Name
Product Code and Name
IND Serial No. 000, IND Item 7, Chemistry, Manufacturing, and Control Data

7.2.3.2 Major Pieces of Manufacturing Equipment

This is a list of the major pieces of equipment showing their size/capacity and manufacturer. The following is an example list:

In order to allow flexibility in the equipment that can be used, state that equivalent equipment from other suppliers may be used.

Step 1	Supplier
Glass-Lined Multipurpose Reaction Tank (800 L) with cooling jacket	
Centrifuge	
Filter Press	

Company Name
Product Code and Name
IND Serial No. 000, IND Item 7, Chemistry, Manufacturing, and Control Data

7.2.3.3 Manufacturing Flow Diagram

The following is an example of a manufacturing description.

Manufacturing Steps	In-Process Controls
1.0 FERMENTATION	
1.1 Growth Medium Preparation	
1.2 Working Seed Inoculation	Strain Identity (API No.)
1.3 Fermentation	pH, Growth Monitoring, CO2/O2 content and Culture Purity
1.4 Cell Harvest	
2.0 EXTRACTION OF LIPOPOLYSACCHARIDE (LPS)	
2.1 Phenol Extraction No.1	
2.2 Dialyze Pellet	
2.3 LPS Harvest and Lyophilization	Endotoxin and SDS PAGE

7.2.3.4 Description of Manufacturing Procedures

This report contains a "cookbook" description of each manufacturing step. It must have ranges in manufacturing conditions that are acceptable to the FDA and provide sufficient flexibility for the IND sponsor.

Information in this report includes, but is not limited to:

- major pieces of manufacturing equipment (not testing equipment and materials);
- reasonable variations;

Company Name
Product Code and Name
IND Serial No. 000, IND Item 7, Chemistry, Manufacturing, and Control Data

- intermediates' storage conditions, container/closure, and holding time limits;
- reprocessing steps;
- yields/acceptance limits; and
- in-process control procedures (IPCs).

The primary objective is to demonstrate that all of the manufacturing processes are under control and the sponsor (or contract manufacturer) can reproducibly manufacture product lots/batches that consistently meet specifications.

The following is an example of a manufacturing description.

STEP X: TITLE

Raw Materials   **Grades**

List

Major Manufacturing Equipment (equivalent equipment from other manufacturers may be used)

List

Methods

Warm the material from the previous step to 30 to 40°C and incubate for 10 to 12 hours with the addition of 100 mg per liter each of XXX and XXY. Add 500 mg per liter of XXZ and allow the mixture to incubate for 5 to 7 hours. Diafilter the material against eight volumes of 0.05 M XYZ, pH 6.0, using an ultrafiltration system equipped with 16,000 nominal molecular weight cut-off filters.

In-Process Controls

IPC:	Endotoxin Test (SOP No. XX-XXXX)
Method:	LAL
Requirement:	Endotoxin level is noted for informational purposes.
IPC:	UF Integrity Test (SOP No. XX-XXXX)
Method:	Capillary Precipitation
Requirement:	A lack of precipitation demonstrates integrity of the ultrafiltration system.

7.2.4 Reference Standard - Characterization of the Drug Substance

This section presents data supporting the structure of key intermediates. Some examples of the type of data to be generated are:

- nuclear magnetic resonance spectroscopy;
- infrared spectroscopy;
- mass spectrometry;
- thin layer chromatography; and
- high-pressure liquid chromatography.

7.2.5 Specifications

Provide a copy of the product specifications. As stated on Table 1, product specifications will evolve during the development process. Initially broad, but scientifically defendable, specifications are set. As additional lots/batches of product are manufactured and the assay results are assessed, these specifications are tightened.

7.2.6 Release/Analytical Data

Provide a copy of the certificate of analysis for the drug substance. If several lots/batches have been manufactured, even if different lot/batch sizes were produced, it is appropriate to present lot/batch comparison data.

7.2.7 Container and Closure

Provide a description of the container and closure.

7.2.8 Stability Data

This section is a summary of the stability data that has been completed prior to the submission of the IND. When available, accelerated stability data from stressed conditions are presented. Additionally, forced degradation data (e.g., reflux in concentrated acid or base) are presented to demonstrate that there is a stability-indicating assay.

This section also states, "As additional stability data are generated, these data will be submitted in amendments to this IND."

7.2.8.1 Protocol

This section is a tabular listing of the validated stability- indicating assays that will be conducted, the storage conditions, and the sampling times. Insert the document into this section.

7.2.8.2 Summary of Results

This section is a tabular listing of the available stability data, along with a review of the data and a conclusion concerning the proposed shelf life.

7.3 DRUG PRODUCT

TABLE OF CONTENTS

Description	IND Volume	Page
7.3 Drug Product 02		07 XXX
7.3.1 Qualitative and Quantitative Composition		
7.3.2 Component Specifications		
7.3.3 Name and Address of Manufacturer/Testing Facility and Packaging Facility.		
7.3.4 Method of Manufacture and Packaging		
7.3.4.1 Description of the Manufacturing Process - Flow Diagram		
7.3.4.1 Description of the Manufacturing Process - Narrative		
7.3.5 Specifications.		
7.3.6 Release/Analytical Results - Lot/Batch Comparison Data.		
7.3.7 Container and Closure		
7.3.7.1 Intermediate Packaging		
7.3.7.2 Final Primary Packaging Material.		
7.3.8 Stability		
7.3.8.1 Protocol		
7.3.8.2 Summary of Results		
7.3.9 Labeling		

Company Name
Product Code and Name
IND Serial No. 000, IND Item 7, Chemistry, Manufacturing, and Control Data

7.3 **Drug Product — 21 CFR 312.23(a)(7)(b)**

7.3.1 **Qualitative and Quantitative Composition**

This section is a tabular listing of the qualitative and quantitative composition of the final product. This listing is for an individual dosage form and for the lot. For example:

Components	Vial	500 Vials (or Liters)
Drug Substance	50 mg	XX mg
Excipient 1, NF	X mg	XX mg
Excipient 2, USP	X mg	XX mg
Water for Injection	2 mL	q.s. to XX Liters

7.3.2 **Component Specifications**

Component	Grade
Drug Substance	
Excipient 1	e.g. USP/NF, Ph Eur, etc.
Excipient 2	e.g. USP/NF, Ph Eur, etc.
etc.	

7.3.3 **Name and Address of Manufacturer/Testing Facility and Packaging Facility**

List the physical location of the sites.

7.3.4 **Method of Manufacture and Packaging**

7.3.4.1 **Description of the Manufacturing Process - Flow Diagram**

The following is an example of a manufacturing description.

Manufacturing Steps	In-Process Controls
1.0 Materials and Equipment	
1.1 Vial Preparation	
1.2 Stopper Preparation	
1.3 Vial Filling Equipment Preparation	
1.4 Other Equipment Preparation	

Company Name
Product Code and Name
IND Serial No. 000, IND Item 7, Chemistry, Manufacturing, and Control Data

2.0 Preparation of the Phosphate
Buffer Solution (pH 7.0 ± 0.2)   Monitor pH and Filter Integrity Test

3.0 Preparation/Formulation of Bulk Solution

Etc.

7.3.4.2 **Description of the Manufacturing Process - Narrative**

This section presents a well-organized description of all:

- manufacturing processes;
- in-process controls;
- reasonable variations;
- reprocessing steps;
- yields;
- acceptable limits; and
- example container labels.

It is essential to present all relevant manufacturing and control information in order to demonstrate that the manufacturing process is fully documented, well-controlled and capable of producing lots of consistent quality. See the "FDA Guidelines of the Preparation of Investigational New Drug Products (Human and Animal)". The following is an example for a manufacturing step.

STEP X: PREPARATION OF pH 6.0 BUFFER SOLUTION

Materials	Grade
Salt 1	USP
Salt 2	USP
Water for Injection (WFI)	USP

Company Name
Product Code and Name
IND Serial No. 000, IND Item 7, Chemistry, Manufacturing, and Control Data

Equipment

List

Methods

1. Determine the total amount of buffer solution to prepare.

2. Add WFI to the container to approximately 80% of the total volume needed from Step 1.

3. Add an amount of Salt 1 to provide a concentration of 0.25 gm/L. Add an amount of Salt 2 to provide a concentration of 1.25 gm/L. Mix thoroughly until dissolved.

4. q.s. with WFI to the final volume.

5. IPC: pH Measurement. Requirement: 5.5 to 6.3.

6. Filter the solution through a 0.2 m filter into a tared, sterile receiving vessel.

7. IPC: Conduct filter integrity testing (bubble point) — See below.

In-Process Controls

IPC: Filter Integrity testing

Method: Bubble Point

Requirement: > 45 PSIG.

7.3.5 **Specifications**

This section provides the "regulatory or shelf-life" specifications (there must be tighter in-house specifications for potency). This section provides product specifications and test methods to evaluate:

- potency (immunogenicity/antigenic activity (21 CFR 610.10);
- general safety (21 CFR 610.11);
- sterility (21 CFR 610.12);
- purity (21 CFR 610.13);
- moisture content (21 CFR 610.13(a)(1));
- pyrogenicity (21 CFR 610.13(b)) for rabbit testing and the "FDA Guideline on Validation of the Limulus Amebocyte Lysate Test as an End-Product Endotoxin Test for Human and Animal Parenteral Drugs, Biological Products, and Medical Devices," for LAL);

Company Name
Product Code and Name
IND Serial No. 000, IND Item 7, Chemistry, Manufacturing, and Control Data

- identity (21 CFR 610.14); and
- any other relevant testing criteria.

7.3.6 **Release/Analytical Results - Lot/Batch Comparison Data**

Insert these documents into this section. If several lots/batches have been manufactured, this section should include lot/batch comparison data in a tabular format.

7.3.7 **Container and Closure**

7.3.7.1 **Intermediate Packaging**

Normally the bulk dosage form (or bulk formulated liquid) is stored in bulk waiting for release testing prior to packaging in the final container and closure. Provide a description of this bulk container. In addition to the final container and closure (listed below) stability of the product in this bulk intermediate container should be generated.

7.3.7.2 **Final Primary Packaging Material**

Provide a description of the final container and closures, the following is an example.

Material/Grade	Manufacturer (Manufacturers of equivalent materials may be used)
Tubing vial, Type I glass (1 mL)	Company Name
Rubber stopper, grey butyl	Company Name
Aluminum seal	Company Name

7.3.8 **Stability**

This section is a summary of the stability data that have been completed prior to the submission of the IND. When available, accelerated stability data from stressed conditions are presented. The intention is to demonstrate that the material is stable while it is being evaluated in clinical trials. Additionally, forced degradation (e.g., reflux in concentrated acid or base) data are presented to demonstrate that there is a stability-indicating assay.

This section also states, "As additional stability data are generated, these data will be submitted in amendments to this IND."

7.3.8.1 **Protocol**

This section is a tabular listing of the validated stability-indicating assays that will be conducted, the storage conditions, and the sampling times.

Company Name
Product Code and Name
IND Serial No. 000, IND Item 7, Chemistry, Manufacturing, and Control Data

7.3.8.1 Protocol

This section is a tabular listing of the validated stability-indicating assays that will be conducted, the storage conditions, and the sampling times.

7.3.8.2 Summary of Results

This section is a tabular listing of the available stability data along with a review of the data and a conclusion concerning the proposed shelf life.

7.3.9 Labeling 21 CFR 312.23(a)(7)(d)

The following information is required on the label:

- product generic/chemical name;
- quantity and strength of the drug substance and dosage unit (vial);
- lot number;
- storage conditions;
- adequate directions for use and route of administration (this can be provided in the Investigator's Brochure);
- names of all inactive ingredients (if it is for other than oral use) with the exception of flavorings, perfumes and color additives except for additives prescribed in 21 CFR 201.20 and Title 21 Chapter I, Subchapter A (21 CFR 201.100(a)(5)(iii) which states, "Trace amounts of harmless substances added solely for individual product identification need not be named. If it is intended for administration by parenteral injection, the quantity or proportion of all inactive ingredients, except that ingredients added to adjust the pH or to make the drug isotonic may be declared by name and a statement of their effect; and if the vehicle is water for injection it need not be named.";
- manufacturer, packer or distributor's name and address; and
- The IND caution statement, "Caution: New Drug Limited by Federal Law to Investigational Use."

Company Name
Product Code and Name
IND Serial No. 000, IND Item 7, Chemistry, Manufacturing, and Control Data

7.4 DILUENT

TABLE OF CONTENTS

Description	IND Volume	Page
7.4 Diluent.. 02		07 XXX

Company Name
Product Code and Name
IND Serial No. 000, IND Item 7, Chemistry, Manufacturing, and Control Data

7.4 Diluent — 21 CFR 312.23(a)(7)(b)

The use of commercially available diluents is strongly recommended. If the diluent is not a commercially available product, this section presents:

- the qualitative and quantitative composition;
- a description of the container/closure system;
- manufacturing instructions;
- specifications;
- release data;
- stability protocol and stability data; and
- example container label.

When a non-commercial diluent is used, the same detailed manufacturing and control information that is presented for the active product must be presented for the diluent. See Section 7.3 for the format.

Company Name
Product Code and Name
IND Serial No. 000, IND Item 7, Chemistry, Manufacturing, and Control Data

7.5 Placebo

TABLE OF CONTENTS

Description	IND Volume	Page
7.5 Placebo... 02		07 XXX

Company Name
Product Code and Name
IND Serial No. 000, IND Item 7, Chemistry, Manufacturing, and Control Data

7.5   Placebo — 21 CFR 312.23(a)(7)(b)

If a placebo is used that is not commercially available, this section presents:

- a brief description of the adjuvant;
- the qualitative and quantitative composition;
- a description of the container/closure system;
- manufacturing instructions;
- specifications;
- release data;
- stability protocol and stability data; and
- example container label.

The same detailed formulation and control information that is presented for the active product must be presented for the placebo. See Section 7.3 for the format.

Company Name
Product Code and Name
IND Serial No. 000, IND Item 7, Chemistry, Manufacturing, and Control Data

7.6 TEST PROCEDURES

TABLE OF CONTENTS

Description	IND Volume	Page
7.6 Test Procedures.................................02		07 XXX
7.6.1 Drug Substance Test Procedure Descriptions		
List titles here		
7.6.2 Drug Product Test Procedure Descriptions		
List titles here		

Company Name
Product Code and Name
IND Serial No. 000, IND Item 7, Chemistry, Manufacturing, and Control Data

7.6   Test Procedures

7.6.1   Drug Substance Test Procedure Descriptions

Provide a summary description of each test procedure. These should be detailed enough (no more than one page) to demonstrate that the test procedure will provide the desired data, but provide the ability to modify procedures as required.

If the sponsor so desires, copies of the test procedures can be submitted. However, this would require the sponsor to submit new versions of the test procedures every time they are updated.

7.6.2   Drug Product Test Procedure Descriptions

Provide a summary description for each test procedure. The same comments from the previous section apply to this section.

Company Name
Product Code and Name
IND Serial No. 000, IND Item 8, Pharmacology and Toxicology Data

7.7 ENVIRONMENTAL ASSESSMENT

This section requests a categorical exclusion for the preparation of an environmental assessment in accordance with 21 CFR 25.24(c)(4). The following paragraph is used:

"The sponsor is claiming an exemption from the requirement for preparing an environmental assessment. This is based upon 21 CFR 25.24(c)(4) which allows a categorical exclusion for an action on an Investigational New Drug Application provided that the drug or biologic is intended to be used for clinical studies or research in which waste will be controlled or the amount of waste expected to enter the environment may reasonably be expected to be nontoxic."

Expediting Drug and Biologics Development

Company Name
Product Code and Name
IND Serial No. 000, IND Item 8, Pharmacology and Toxicology Data

TABLE OF CONTENTS

Description	IND Volume	Page
8.0 Pharmacology and Toxicology Data		08 001
8.1 Nonclinical Pharmacology Summary		
8.2 Toxicology Summary		
8.3 Good Laboratory Practice Statement of Compliance		
8.4 Bibliography		

Refer to Chapter 2 for definitive information that must be included in this section.

Company Name
Product Code and Name
IND Serial No. 000, IND Item 9, Previous Human Experience

8.0 Pharmacology and Toxicology Data — 21 CFR 312.23(a)(8)

8.1 Nonclinical Pharmacology Summary — 21 CFR 312.23(a)(8)(i)

This is a review of the nonclinical pharmacology studies. The purpose of this section is to present initial pharmacology data obtained from nonclinical studies. The information that should be included must be tailored for the product. For more detailed information the reader is referred to Chapter 2.

All published and unpublished literature cited in this review is given a citation number (e.g., 1,2,3,etc.).

8.2 Toxicology Summary — 21 CFR 312.23(a)(8)(ii)

This is an integrated summary of the toxicological effects of the product in animals. Depending on the nature of the product and the phase of the clinical trials, this discussion should contain the results from acute, sub-acute and chronic toxicity tests; carcinogenicity; effects on reproduction and fetal development; any special toxicity tests related to the mode of administration or conditions of use; and in vitro studies. Discuss additional information such as general safety, pyrogenicity and immunogenicity testing.

All published and unpublished literature cited in this review is given a citation number (e.g., 1, 2, 3, etc.). A bibliography is located at the end of Item 8 (see Section 8.4). Each toxicology study that is intended to support the safety of the proposed clinical trial must have a full tabulation of data suitable for a detailed review [21 CFR 312.23(a)(8)(ii)(b)].

8.3 Good Laboratory Practice Statement of Compliance — 21 CFR 312.23(a)(8)(iii)

All nonclinical laboratory studies subject to good laboratory practice (GLP) regulations must contain a statement that the study was conducted in compliance with the GLP regulations. If the study was not conducted under GLP, provide a brief statement explaining what is not in compliance and the reason(s).

Provide a list giving the location (IND page number) of the GLP compliance statements.

8.4 Bibliography

List in this section all supporting published and unpublished literature that was cited in the integrated review (see Section 8.2) in the same order as it is cited. The references are in the same order as the citations in the integrated review.

Provide copies of the nonclinical literature in IND Item 10. Each toxicology report that is intended to support the safety of the clinical investigations must contain a full tabulation of data suitable for detailed review.

Company Name
Product Code and Name
IND Serial No. 000, IND Item 9, Previous Human Experience

TABLE OF CONTENTS

Description	IND Volume	Page
9.0 Previous Human Experience	02	09 001
9.1 Overall Clinical Summary		
9.2 Clinical Investigations		
9.3 Marketing Experience		
9.4 Bibliography		

Company Name
Product Code and Name
IND Serial No. 000, IND Item 10, Additional Information

9.0 Previous Human Experience — 21 CFR 312.23(a)(9)

9.1 Overall Clinical Summary — 21 CFR 312.23(a)(9)(i) and (ii)

This is a review of the clinical studies and experience with the product (this is particularly relevant if the product was studied or being marketed outside of the United States). It may be useful to present clinical data for compounds that are of the same class as the one being evaluated under the IND.

All published and unpublished literature cited in this review is given a citation number (e.g., 1, 2, 3, etc.). A bibliography is located at the end of Item 9 (see Section 9.4).

9.2 Clinical Investigations — 21 CFR 312.23(a)(9)(i) and (ii)

If the product has been previously investigated or marketed, this is a detailed summary providing information relevant to the rationale and safety of the investigation. If controlled clinical trials have been conducted, provide detailed safety and efficacy information in order to assess the product's proposed investigational use.

All published and unpublished literature cited in this summary is given a citation number (e.g., 1, 2, 3, etc.). A bibliography is located at the end of Item 9 (see Section 9.4). Submit full copies of all published literature that are relevant to the safety of the proposed trials or an assessment of the product's effectiveness in Item 10. Although optional, submit all published literature that is indirectly relevant to the product's safety and effectiveness, but provides useful supporting information.

9.3 Marketing Experience — 21 CFR 312.23(a)(9)(iii)

This is a list of all countries where the product has been marketed and a list of the countries in which the product has been withdrawn from the market for reasons potentially related to safety or effectiveness.

9.4 Bibliography

All supporting published and unpublished literature cited in the integrated review (see Section 9.2) is listed in this section in the same order as it is cited there.

The bibliography for literature that was not cited in the summary, but is relevant to the product's safety and effectiveness, is arranged in alphabetical order by first author's last name.

Provide copies of the clinical literature in IND Item 10.

Company Name
Product Code and Name
IND Serial No. 000, IND Item 10, Additional Information

TABLE OF CONTENTS

	Description	IND Volume	Page
10.0	Additional Information		10 001
10.1	Drug Dependence and Abuse Potential		
10.2	Radioactive Drugs		
10.3	Other Information		
10.4	Bibliography and Reprints		

10.0 Additional Information — 21 CFR 312.23(a)(10)

10.1 Drug Dependence and Abuse Potential — 21 CFR 312.23(a)(10)(i)

If the product has psychotropic properties or abuse potential, this section presents relevant clinical and nonclinical studies and experience.

10.2 Radioactive Drugs — 21 CFR 312.23(a)(10)(ii)

If the product is radioactive, this section presents sufficient information from animal or human studies to allow a reasonable calculation of radiation-absorbed dose to the whole body and to critical organs.

10.3 Pediatric Studies — 21 CFR 312.23(a)(10)(iii)

Plans for assessing pediatric safety and effectiveness.

10.4 Other Information — 21 CFR 312.23(a)(10)(iv)

This section briefly provides any other information that would aid evaluation of the safety or design of the proposed clinical investigations and their potential as controlled clinical trials supporting a product marketing application.

10.5 Bibliography and Reprints

This section contains copies of all published articles and unpublished reports that were cited in the previous IND Items. They are divided into the following sections:

- Clinical — Published Articles;
- Clinical — Unpublished Reports;
- Preclinical — Published Articles;
- Preclinical — Unpublished Reports; and
- Other.

The list for published literature is arranged in alphabetical order by the first author's last name. The list for unpublished reports is also arranged alphabetically by originating organization's name.

CHAPTER 12

The Investigator's Brochure

By Deborah I. Scott, MIM, MIB, RAC

An investigator's brochure (IB) provides a summary of available information for an investigational product (drug or biologic), and is initially prepared concurrently with the other sections of the investigational new drug application (IND). The information presented in the IB must be factual, concise, scientifically sound and balanced. In essence, the IB serves multiple purposes. Most importantly, it is intended to provide the investigator, the investigator's staff and the institutional review board (IRB) with all of the available information regarding an investigational product, including the intended use and the rationale for clinical development. Included within the rationale should be an overview of where the product fits within the medical armamentarium. Ultimately, the IB serves as a prototype for the package insert.

The IB's focus evolves during an investigational product's development. During the early clinical phases, there is a greater emphasis on nonclinical pharmacology and toxicology data in the absence of clinical data. As additional clinical experience is gained, there is a shift to emphasize the clinical data, particularly with respect to the observed safety profile. Although nonclinical data remain an important component in the IB, the level of detail provided for each study can be reduced. As a result, the IB is a document that requires continual updating and maintenance to ensure that the various clinical investigators, IRBs and research subjects are provided with the most current information available to ensure the product's safe use in clinical trials.

Title 21 of the Code of Federal Regulations (21 CFR 312.23) requires that sponsors include the following information within an IB:

- A brief description of the drug substance and formulation;
- A summary of the pharmacological and toxicological effects in animals and humans;
- A summary of the pharmacokinetics and biological disposition in animals and humans;
- A summary of the safety and effectiveness in humans; and
- A description of possible risks and anticipated side effects based upon prior experience with the drug or similar drugs as well as any precautions or special monitoring to be performed.

International harmonization efforts have attempted to refine the IB's format and content to provide consistency among drug sponsors within the United States and internationally. An outline, as described in the ICH's "Good Clinical Practice: Consolidated Guideline" (E6) appears in the exhibit below.

The drafting of an IB for the IND addresses information from all areas of R&D, including pharmaceutical operations, toxicology and pharmacology, clinical research and drug safety. Utilizing report synopses for both the nonclinical and the clinical sections is an efficient means of compiling the data and presenting each study in a systematic and consistent manner. However, the sponsor must integrate, interpret, and discuss the limitations of the available data. This is particularly critical during the early phases of the clinical development.

Potential toxicity and side effects should be presented within both the Safety and Efficacy sections, as well as in the Guidance to the Investigator sections in the IB. In instances in which limited or no clinical data are available, the Guidance to the Investigator section should describe potential events associated with similar products, if there are any. It is often useful to include references on similar products. The intent is not to imply or make any promotional claims, but rather to provide a broad basis of working knowledge for the product. Practical information concerning possible safety risks, including the clinical management of these events, should also be described. Likewise, this section should address any special monitoring requirements (e.g., laboratory tests) or precautions imperative to maintaining patient safety.

A well-written Guidance to the Investigator section within the IB can save the sponsor time and effort in the safety reporting area, since both telephone/fax and written safety reports to the FDA are based directly on whether the event is "unexpected"—that is, whether or not it is identified in the IB (21 CFR 312.32). An unexpected adverse experience means any adverse experience with a severity or specificity that is not consistent with the current IB. The intent is to identify events that have not been previously observed and to remove the idea of defining "expectedness" based on the pharmacological properties of the product. Care in identifying potential adverse experiences may reduce the number of events that must be considered as unexpected, minimizing the need to submit safety reports under the IND. A conservatively drafted IB can also assist the investigator in preparing well-written informed consent forms.

Given the numerous contributors involved in the creation of the IB, any review and sign-off procedures should reflect this multidisciplinary process. Drafts of the IB should have a fairly broad circulation within the sponsoring company. Any requested changes should be rapidly incorporated into the document and approved by management so that the IB can be included in the IND submission and distributed to the project team and investigators.

Since the IB is such an important document that is central to the efficient development of an investigational program, it is a good idea to place the responsibility for overseeing the IB's development and continual updating in the hands of the senior clinical scientist responsible for the overall project—the project leader (PL). Working in collaboration with all areas of R&D, the PL should identify the nonclinical and clinical data to be included and integrate this information into the IB. To assist the PL in this endeavor, a system for tracking all nonclinical and clinical reports must be in place to aid in the updating process. This system must include a medical/scientific review of all new reports, a decision on whether or not each report contains new information that should be incorporated into the next revision of the IB, and a mechanism for storing this information for the next update. A tracking system maintained by either clinical research or regulatory affairs can accomplish this goal.

Sponsors should adopt policies that permit a two-tier approach to updating IBs. The first tier addresses the immediate need to notify all participating investigators when a reportable adverse event or other reportable safety issue has been identified (as outlined in 21 CFR 312.32). This new safety information is generally conveyed by the sponsor to the investigator by letter and, as explained below, must be incorporated into the current IB when it arises. This satisfies the condition that a particular adverse event be, from that point forward, identified within the IB as "expected" (i.e., not "unexpected") so that it will no longer qualify as "unexpected" and possibly trigger the need for another IND safety report, as described below.

As required by the regulations, all currently participating investigators need to be informed of all serious adverse events associated with the use of the drug that are serious, related and "unexpected" (i.e., not in the IB). As mentioned above, sponsors generally notify participating investigators of previously unexpected and serious adverse events in what are termed "Dear Investigator" letters. In addition to alerting the investigators regarding a previously unexpected and serious adverse event in a clinical trial, these letters should instruct the investigators to append a copy of the letter to the IB. From that point on, the IB can be considered as containing information regarding that adverse event. A tab can be included with the first adverse event report letter identifying a new section of the IB as "Adverse Event Updates." Each subsequent letter should also include an updated serious adverse event table of contents. An explanatory paragraph should precede the table of contents and contain a standard statement noting that, "The following adverse events have not been previously described in the current IB. The sponsor is providing this information to ensure that investigators and consultants are aware of these events." The table of contents should include a unique serial number identifying each event, the date of the "Dear Investigator" letter, the adverse event reported and the location of the letter within the update section of the IB. Each time a letter is sent to all participating investigators, a new table of contents should be generated and distributed concurrently with the new "Dear Investigator" letter. New investigators will receive an IB containing the "Adverse Event Update" tab, the explanatory paragraph page, a complete adverse event update table of contents, and all "Dear Investigator" letters distributed to date. By appending the adverse event reports ("Dear Investigator" letters) to the IB in this manner, similar future events will not be considered "unexpected," and will not require the written notification of all participating investigators. All the "Dear Investigator" letters appended to the IB should be summarized and incorporated into the main body of the IB at the time it is revised.

The second tier addresses the routine review and incorporation of new information acquired since the last update of the IB was released. This requires updated literature listings as well as identifying nonclinical and clinical reports that have been completed and finalized during the updating interval. Consequently, by adhering to a two-tier approach, sponsors should be able to meet the information needs of the medical community with respect to providing available knowledge on the product in a timely and efficient manner.

Ideally, routine revisions to the IB should coincide with the IND annual report (21 CFR 312.33). This process could be initiated as follows: Sixty days before the anniversary date of the original filing, the project's regulatory affairs representative should send a notification to the project leader to request a determination as to whether the IB should be updated.

The project leader should, in turn, obtain a listing of all reports and publications for the product since the last version of the IB was released, according to the earlier determination that the report's findings should be included in the next IB (second tier, see above). Once a determination has been made that the IB requires updating, the project leader should revise the IB as appropriate, incorporating available results for both effectiveness and safety. For IB revisions, review and sign-off procedures should be the same as they were for the document's initial creation. Once the revised IB has been approved, the document can be submitted to the FDA as part of the IND's annual report. All current and future investigators should receive the latest version of the IB. Investigators whose research on the product spanned more than one version of the IB should keep all applicable IBs in their files for a possible FDA site audit.

Administrative Issues During the investigational phase of a product's development, the IB will most likely require revision several times. An archival record of each IB and the distribution records of each revision should be maintained within the sponsor's files. This will aid the preparation process for clinical site audits. Including the date of the original edition as well as all revision dates on the title page of the IB will help the clinical monitor reviewing the files at the clinical site ensure that the site has the most appropriate version(s) of the IB.

An investigator's signature page can be inserted immediately after the title pages. This provides a mechanism to record and document the investigator's receipt of a specific edition of the IB. The sponsor can then maintain copies of the signed pages to ensure that sites have the appropriate editions throughout the duration of the study.

Citing all relevant references within the IB not only provides the reader with information concerning the source of the data, it also can serve as a useful tool when preparing the annotated package insert. The sponsor should consider the following general approaches concerning the use of citations within the IB:

- As a rule, if specific information about the product has been presented in both an unpublished report and a published article, the citation for the published article should be used. The unpublished report may also be cited if it contains additional information apart from the article.
- If the same study is the subject of more than one unpublished report and/or publication, the citation that reflects the most comprehensive information or the latest document should be cited. The other documents may also be cited if they provide additional relevant information.
- Data that have been neither quality assured nor incorporated into a report or publication should be noted as preliminary data if they are used. Text and any associated tables should indicate that the data are considered to be preliminary.

Conclusions The underlying objective for creating and maintaining a well-written IB for a product is to ensure that investigators have the necessary product knowledge to perform rational clinical research. Given the cost of this research and the importance of subject welfare, extra effort and diligence invested at this stage will provide benefits for all parties involved.

Outline of an Investigator's Brochure

Title Page

Confidentiality Statement (optional)

Signature Page (optional)

1. Table of Contents

2. Brief Summary (no more than 2 pages)

3. Introduction

4. Pharmaceutical Data
   Description of product substance
   Chemical and/or structural formula
   Pharmaceutical properties
   Formulation
   Storage and Handling Instructions

–continued–

Outline of an Investigator's Brochure continued–

5. Nonclinical Studies
   Pharmacology
   Pharmacokinetic and Product Metabolism in Animals
   Toxicology

6. Effects in Humans
   Pharmacokinetics and Product Metabolism in Humans
   Clinical Trials (Phase I-IV) Safety and Efficacy
   Marketing Experience (including regulatory history of approvals, withdrawals and registrations)

7. Summary of Data and Guidance for the Investigator

8. Appendices (if required, including Serious Adverse Event updates)

   Adapted from the ICH's "Good Clinical Practice: Consolidated Guideline" (E6), May 1997

CHAPTER 13

The Phases of Clinical Development

by Mark Mathieu

The Structure of Clinical Trials

The design of a clinical trial will differ significantly from one drug and disease state to another. The nature of a drug, the product's proposed use, the results of the preclinical testing, principles of medical practice, patient preferences, biostatistical considerations, and the availability and quality of existing standard treatments are among the factors considered in designing a clinical trial or a global drug development program.

Although clinical trials for different drugs can vary greatly in design, they are often similar in structure. Since researchers may know little about a new compound prior to its use in humans, testing the drug through serially conducted investigations permits each phase of clinical development to be carefully designed to use and build upon the information obtained from the research stage preceding it. In its October 1988 *Plan for Accelerated Approval of Drugs to Treat Life-Threatening and Severely Debilitating Illnesses*, the FDA discussed the structure of clinical trials and the basis for this structure:

"[The clinical] drug development process is generally thought of, in simplified terms, as consisting of three phases of human testing to determine if a drug is safe and effective: Phase 1 with 10 to 50 patients to study how the drug is tolerated, metabolized, and excreted; Phase 2 with 50 to 200 patients in which the safety and efficacy of the drug are first evaluated in controlled trials; and Phase 3 with 200 to 1,000 or more patients to confirm and expand upon the safety and efficacy data obtained from the first two phases... The three phases describe the usual process of drug development, but they are not statutory requirements. The basis for marketing approval is the adequacy of the data available; progression through the particular phases is simply the usual means the sponsor uses to collect the data needed for approval. The statute itself focuses on the standard of evidence needed for approval, as derived from adequate and well-controlled clinical investigations, with no mention of phases 1, 2, and 3."

While acknowledging that clinical testing is often classified into these primary "temporal phases," the ICH's final E8 *Guidance on General Considerations for Clinical Trials* (December 1997) also points out that the phases are descriptive rather than prescriptive. For some drugs, this "typical sequence" may be inappropriate or unnecessary, the guidance states (see exhibit below).

Phase 1 Clinical Trials

The earliest Phase 1 clinical trials, sometimes called "first-in-man studies," represent the first introduction of a new drug into human subjects. While the focus at this stage is the assessment of clinical safety, researchers usually obtain pharmacokinetic data as well and frequently assess a drug's effect on a well-established biomarker (e.g., ACE inhibition, blood pressure). Except for extrapolations based on the safety profile obtained from animal studies, investigators may know little about the drug's possible clinical effects prior to these studies.

Phase 1 testing of a new drug is considered highly exploratory because there are often no human safety data available. For this reason, these studies are entered into very cautiously, with the drug being used in an escalating fashion and at fractions of the predicted therapeutic doses in small numbers of subjects, each of whom must submit to close clinical observation for drug effects. While healthy adults whose schedules permit short-term confinement are ideal subjects, stable patients with the target disease or condition can also be studied in Phase 1 trials. Although male volunteers have dominated Phase 1 study populations traditionally, the FDA continues to push for as much as an equal number of females in early-stage trials, unless there is a specific reason to exclude females (see discussion above).

Phase 1 clinical trials provide an initial clinical indication of whether a drug is sufficiently well tolerated to be used in further human testing. According to FDA regulations, "Phase 1 includes the initial introduction of an investigational new drug into humans... These studies are designed to determine the metabolism and pharmacologic actions of the drug in humans, the side effects associated with increasing doses, and, if possible, to gain early evidence on effectiveness. During

Phases of Clinical Investigation

(from the ICH's December 1997 Final Guideline on General Considerations for Clinical Trials)

Phase 1 (Most typical type of study: Human Pharmacology). Studies in Phase 1 typically involve one or a combination of the following assessments:

- *Estimation of initial safety and tolerability.* The initial and subsequent administration of an investigational new drug into humans is usually intended to determine the tolerability of the dose range expected to be needed for later clinical studies and to determine the nature of adverse reactions that can be expected. These studies typically include both single and multiple-dose administration.
- *Determination of pharmacokinetics* (PK). Preliminary characterization of a drug's absorption, distribution, metabolism, and excretion is almost always an important goal of Phase 1. PK studies are undertaken to assess the clearance of the drug and to anticipate the possible accumulation of parent drug or metabolites and potential drug-drug interactions.
- *Assessment of pharmacodynamics* (PD). Depending on the investigational drug and the endpoint under study, PD studies and studies relating drug blood levels to response (PK/PD studies) may be conducted in healthy volunteer subjects or in patients with the target disease. In some studies involving patients, PD data can provide early estimates of drug activity and potential effectiveness and can guide the dosage and dose regimen in later studies.
- *Early measurement of activity.* Preliminary studies of activity or potential therapeutic benefit may be conducted in Phase 1 as a secondary objective. Such studies may be appropriate when effectiveness is readily measurable with a short duration of drug exposure.

Phase 2 (Most typical kind of study: Therapeutic exploratory). Generally, Phase 2 is considered to comprise studies in which the primary objective is to explore therapeutic effectiveness in patients. Initial therapeutic exploratory studies may use a variety of study designs, such as concurrent controls and comparisons with baseline status. Subsequent trials are usually randomized and concurrently controlled to evaluate the efficacy of the drug and its safety for a particular therapeutic indication. The goals of Phase 2 studies include determining the dose(s) and regimen for Phase 3 studies and the evaluation of potential study endpoints, therapeutic regimens (including concomitant medications), and target populations (e.g., mild versus severe disease) for further study in Phase 2 or Phase 3 trials.

Phase 3 (Most typical kind of study: Therapeutic confirmatory). Usually, Phase 3 is considered to begin with the initiation of studies in which the primary objective is to demonstrate, or confirm, therapeutic benefit. Phase 3 studies are designed to support marketing approval by confirming the preliminary evidence collected in Phase 2 that shows the drug to be safe and effective for use in the intended indication and population. Studies in Phase 3 may also further explore the dose-response relationship, or explore the drug's use in a broader population, in different disease stages, or in combination with another drug.

Phase 4 (Variety of studies: Therapeutic Use). Phase 4 includes all postapproval studies (other than routine surveillance) related to the approved indication. These studies, which are not considered necessary for approval but are often important for optimizing the drug's use, include additional drug-drug interaction, dose-response, or safety studies and studies designed to support use under the approved indication (e.g., mortality/morbidity studies).

Phase 1, sufficient information about the drug's pharmacokinetics and pharmacological effects should be obtained to permit the design of well-controlled, scientifically valid Phase 2 studies. The total number of subjects and patients included in Phase 1 studies varies with the drug, but is generally in the range of 20 to 80. Phase 1 studies also include studies of drug metabolism, structure-activity relationships, and mechanism of action in humans, as well as studies in which investigational drugs are used as research tools to explore biological phenomena or disease processes." These studies can also provide basic pharmacokinetic information, which allows for the comparison of human drug disposition to that of animals so that nonclinical findings can be correlated and verified.

It is worth noting that the term Phase 1 can refer not only to a stage of development (i.e., earliest human exposure), but also to a type of study (i.e., generally any clinical pharmacology study). This type of study may occur at various times throughout a drug's clinical development, and sometimes after the drug has been introduced into the market.

Testing certain drugs in healthy adults is not considered ethical. Because of the known toxicity of certain classes of drugs, such as those used in treating AIDS and cancer, some Phase 1 studies are conducted with patients who have, or are at risk of having, the condition for which the drug is being studied. Because healthy volunteers have no opportunity to benefit from a treatment, the administration of highly toxic compounds to such individuals is considered an unacceptable risk. Even if the subjects are patients, Phase 1 trials are not efficacy studies, but focus on safety/tolerability and effects on preclinical biomarkers.

The FDA advises that investigators performing Phase 1 tests involving "normal" volunteers should be skilled in the "initial evaluation of a variety of compounds for safety and pharmacological effect." In those cases in which diseased patients are studied under a Phase 1 protocol, investigators should be, or should work with co-investigators who are, experts in either the particular disease categories to be treated or in the evaluation of drug effects on the disease process. It is also important that such investigators carefully consider the influence of any active disease state on the pharmacokinetic and pharmacodynamic findings.

PK/PD and Phase 1 Trials Based on the FDA's review experience in the early 1990s, the selection of the starting dose for clinical trials was recognized as a weakness of many clinical programs. Traditional dose-based comparisons between animals and humans are considered inadequate largely because of major differences between species in the disposition and metabolism of drugs. Thus, calculations based on animal half-lives and dosing intervals and their relationship to toxicity often led to errors in selecting the starting dose for Phase 1 trials. For these reasons, the "first-in-man" dose is usually a fraction (often as small as one-tenth) of the highest no-effect dose in pertinent animal toxicity studies.

In a July 2005 guidance, however, the agency outlines a process, or algorithm, for deriving the maximum recommended starting dose (MRSD) for "first in human" clinical trials of new molecular entities in adult healthy volunteers, and recommends a standardized process through which researchers can select the MRSD. The MRSD selection process advocated under the guidance, entitled *Estimating the Maximum Safe Starting Dose in Clinical Trials for Therapeutics in Adult Health Volunteers*, employs observed toxicities, administered doses, and an algorithmic approach, and involves five key steps.

> An FDA focus on early-stage pharmacokinetic/pharmacodynamic studies, which was championed under former CDER Director Carl Peck, M.D., has continued many years after Peck's departure from CDER. In the 1994 final guideline entitled, E4 Dose-Response Information To Support Drug Registration, the ICH parties stated that dose-response data "are desirable for almost all new chemical entities," and that "assessment of dose-response should be an integral component of drug development with studies designed to assess dose-response as an inherent part of establishing the safety and effectiveness of the drug."

The FDA's efforts to develop additional guidelines provide further evidence of the agency's continuing interest in promoting the importance of dose-response studies during Phase 1 and Phase 2 clinical trials. In April 2003, for example, the agency supplemented the ICH's E4 guidance with its own guidance entitled, *Exposure-Response Relationships—Study Design, Data Analysis, and Regulatory Applications* to provide recommendations to IND and NDA sponsors on the use of exposure-response information in the development of new drugs.

In a pair of guidances—*In Vivo Drug Metabolism/Drug Interaction Studies-Study Design, Data Analysis, and Recommendations for Dosing and Labeling* (November 1999) and *Drug Metabolism/Drug Interaction Studies in the Drug Development Process: Studies In Vitro* (April 1997)—the agency encourages sponsors to develop information on a drug's metabolic profile early in clinical trials. A May 1998 CDER guidance entitled, *Pharmacokinetics and Pharmacovigilance in Patients with Impaired Renal Function: Study Design, Data Analysis, and Impact on Dosing and Labeling* specifies when PK studies of patients with impaired renal function should be performed, and discusses the design and conduct of PK/PD studies in such individuals. In a May 2003 guidance entitled, *Pharmacokinetics in Patients with Impaired Hepatic Function: Study Design, Data Analysis, and Impact on Dosing and Labeling*, CDER provides recommendations to companies planning to conduct studies to assess the influence of hepatic impairment on the pharmacokinetics and, where appropriate, the pharmacodynamics of experimental drugs. In a February 1999 guidance entitled, *Population Pharmacokinetics*, the agency offers recommendations on the use of population pharmacokinetics to identify differences in safety and effectiveness among population subgroups in drug development programs.

Sponsor Information/Data Submissions During Clinical Trials Although the clinical program becomes the primary focus of a drug's development once Phase 1 trials begin, other activities continue to support these trials. As clinical trials progress, FDA reviewers continually reassess the safety of these studies. Because the FDA wants these assessments to be based on the latest available data and information, the agency requires that sponsors submit periodic reports on completed and upcoming research. During clinical trials, at least four important types of data and information flow regularly from the sponsor to the FDA:

- New Animal Data. As mentioned previously, animal testing continues during clinical development. Submitted in the form of information amendments to the IND, additional toxicology and pharmacokinetic data may be needed from animal studies to support the safety of new and/or modified clinical studies. For example, longer-term toxicology studies are required as the duration of treatment in humans is extended.

- Protocols and Protocol Amendments. Because protocols for Phase 2 and Phase 3 trials are not normally included in the original IND, protocols for these studies must be forwarded to the FDA subsequently. Also, whenever sponsors want to make changes to previously submitted protocols, they must submit protocol amendments.
- Annual Reports. Current regulations require sponsors to submit brief annual reports on the progress of the investigations. These reports must include information on individual studies, provide a summary of the clinical experience with the drug, and provide information on the general investigational plan for the upcoming year, changes in the investigator's brochure, and foreign regulatory and marketing developments.
- IND Safety Reports. The drug sponsor must notify the FDA and all participating investigators about information that the company receives from any source indicating or suggesting significant hazards, contraindications, side effects, or precautions that are associated with the use of the drug. All significant safety findings must be reported.

Ideally, trial sponsors will establish a collegial relationship with the FDA reviewing team, participate in frequent, informal communications to keep the reviewers apprised of developing data, and engage in a progressive exchange of ideas to facilitate the execution of the clinical development program.

Phase 2 Clinical Trials

Phase 2 clinical trials represent a shift away from testing focused on safety to testing designed to provide a preliminary indication of a drug's effectiveness. In Phase 2 studies, a drug is used, often for the first time, in patients who suffer from the disease or condition that the drug is intended to prevent, diagnose, or treat.

FDA regulations state that "Phase 2 includes the controlled clinical studies conducted to evaluate the effectiveness of the drug for a particular indication or indications in patients with the disease or condition under study and to determine the common or short-term side effects and risks associated with the drug. Phase 2 studies are typically well-controlled, closely monitored, and conducted in a relatively small number of patients, usually involving no more than several hundred subjects."

Typical Phase 2 studies are well-controlled and randomized trials that compare the experimental drug, often at several different doses, to placebo or, in some cases, to an active drug. The studies can provide evidence of effectiveness, a preliminary look at dose-response for effectiveness and the more common adverse drug reactions, and a firm basis for selecting the dose or, ideally, the dose-range to be studied in Phase 3.

In many ways, Phase 2 studies provide the foundation for several key aspects of the study design for the all-important Phase 3 trials. The observed magnitude of the treatment effect in Phase 2 trials is a critical factor in Phase 3 sample size calculations, for example.

Given the costs associated with Phase 3 studies and the perception that Phase 3 success rates have declined for new drugs, some firms have announced that they are focusing more intently on Phase 2 studies—for example, to characterize or fine-tune the dose for the pivotal studies. In fact, agency officials such as CDER's Associate Director for Medical Policy Robert Temple, M.D., have criticized industry for not taking full advantage of Phase 2 trials in designing pivotal Phase 3 studies. Too frequently, says Temple, sponsors fail to conduct comprehensive Phase 2 studies that explore a complete dose range and a drug's effects on biomarkers and then confirm the Phase 2 impressions in well-designed Phase 3 studies that examine the dose range of interest. Instead, he notes, companies tend to "do a little bit" of Phase 2 work and then simultaneously conduct multiple Phase 3 studies, sometimes at a single selected dose and sometimes at a number of doses, but rarely using several doses in a trial to obtain a good picture of dose-response for favorable and unfavorable effects. Temple argues that companies, by obtaining more complete data from Phase 2 trials in advance, could focus on the appropriate dose range in Phase 3 and, therefore, increase the likelihood of success.

While FDA officials concede that they are not absolutely certain of the reasons for declining Phase 3 success rates, many suspect that it can be traced directly to insufficient exposure-response work in Phase 2 studies. Because of this, agency reviewers are now making themselves available to consult with sponsors following the conclusion of so-called "Phase 2A studies," which examine a drug's absorption, metabolism, and pharmacodynamics in patients. Under the new pilot program (see discussion of end-of-Phase 2A meetings below), the agency will provide input on drug-dosing issues before a sponsor initiates Phase 2B studies, which will study a drug's safety and effectiveness in a somewhat larger patient population.

As noted above, Phase 2 trials that are well-controlled studies may provide the basis on which certain drugs are approved for marketing either under the traditional full approval or the accelerated approval model. When a new drug is the first effective treatment for, or is a significant advance in the treatment of, a serious or life-threatening disease, the sponsor may file an NDA at the completion of Phase 2. In such cases, however, the data must be statistically sound, and a post-marketing surveillance requirement may be a condition of approval. In recent years, this model has been used several times for antiviral treatments directed against the human immune deficiency virus (HIV) as well as for some cancer drugs, whose accelerated approvals have been based on reasonable surrogate endpoints (e.g., tumor response, 24-week viral load).

Since Phase 2 trials also involve the first meaningful assessment of a drug's effects on key clinical endpoints (i.e., clinical events or measurements used to assess drug effectiveness), these studies can provide valuable information on the utility of a variety of clinical endpoints and markers. Sponsors and investigators then can use this information to select the most appropriate endpoints—those most reflective of the disease and responsive to therapy, for example—for Phase 3 trials (see discussion of clinical endpoints below).

Generally, Phase 2 study objectives should also include developing a description of the dose-response for favorable and unfavorable effects. This information is critical to dose selection (e.g., a very well-tolerated drug may be dosed on the plateau of the dose-response curve, while a drug with toxicity might be given at a lower dose or started at a lower dose). Well-conducted Phase 2 studies of pharmacokinetic and pharmacodynamic parameters may provide useful insights as to whether different subpopulations (e.g., defined by gender, age, or concomitant illness) require different dosing regimens. It is critical to note that the relatively small numbers of patients in Phase 2 studies will usually not allow definitive conclusions about dose-response. Phase 3 studies are necessary to confirm Phase 2 findings and to detect less-common dose-related events.

Because a drug's short-term side effects remain primary concerns during Phase 2 investigations, the compound is administered to a limited number of patients who are closely monitored by the investigators. The use of the drug in larger numbers of subjects (i.e., compared to Phase 1) may reveal less-frequent side effects and provide for better estimates of the dose-toxicity relationships for the more frequently observed adverse effects. Dose-ranging may reveal type 1 target-organ toxicity at the higher doses. Such findings are used to refine the safety surveillance monitoring plans for Phase 3.

Generally speaking, given the comparatively small numbers of patients enrolled in Phase 2 trials, these studies usually are unable to provide the definitive evidence of efficacy and safety necessary to support approval. Under the FDA's expedited development (Subpart E) program, however, Phase 2 trials for products designed to treat life-threatening and severely debilitating diseases may be prospectively designed to support marketing approval.

End-of-Phase 2 Meetings and Other FDA-Sponsor Communication During Clinical Trials Under FDAMA and FDA/industry agreements associated with the user-fee program, the FDA has committed to several goals relevant to both end-of-Phase 2 meetings and other important meetings and communications (e.g., protocol reviews). In addition, the agency is actively participating in two pilot programs regarding agency/sponsor interactions during the clinical development process—an end-of-Phase 2A pilot program and a frequent scientific interaction pilot program (see discussions below).

End-of Phase 2 Meetings Although the agency had emphasized in the past that end-of-Phase 2 meetings were designed primarily for sponsors of NMEs and important new uses of marketed products, the FDA has since made the conferences available to all new drug sponsors, regardless of the classification of their products. Federal regulations state that the purposes of end-of-Phase 2 meetings are to determine the safety of proceeding to Phase 3, to evaluate the Phase 3 plan and protocols and the adequacy of current studies and plans to assess pediatric safety and effectiveness, and to identify any additional information necessary to support a marketing application for the uses under investigation. The ultimate goal of such a meeting is for the sponsor and the FDA to reach agreement on plans for the conduct and design of Phase 3 trials.

Under PDUFA III, the FDA has agreed to respond to meeting requests and hold requested meetings, including end-of-Phase 2 meetings, within specified timeframes. Within 14 calendar days of receiving a formal meeting request (i.e., a scheduled face-to-face meeting, teleconference, or videoconference), CDER should notify the sponsor by letter or fax of the date, time, and place for the meeting, as well as the expected CDER participants. The center will attempt to meet this goal for at least 90% of such requests during the PDUFA III years (FY2003-FY2007).

The agency's new meetings management system requires CDER to meet with sponsors within specific timeframes based on the type of meeting requested:

Type A Meeting: "A meeting which is necessary for an otherwise stalled drug development program to proceed (a 'critical path' meeting)." These meetings should take place within 30 days of CDER's receipt of a sponsor's request.

Type B Meeting: An end-of-Phase 2, pre-IND, end-of-Phase 1 (i.e., for Subpart E or Subpart H or similar products), or pre-NDA meeting. Type B meetings should occur within 60 calendar days of the agency's receipt of a meeting request.

Expediting Drug and Biologics Development

Type C Meeting: Any other type of meeting. Type C meetings should be held within 75 calendar days of the agency's receipt of a meeting request.

For a meeting request to qualify under these performance goals, it must be made in writing and fulfill certain informational standards (e.g., statement of purpose, approximate schedule for submission of supporting documentation). In addition, CDER must agree that the meeting "will serve a useful purpose (i.e., it is not premature or clearly unnecessary)." The agency notes, however, that Type B meetings will be honored "except in the most unusual circumstances."

As its name implies, the end-of-Phase 2 meeting takes place after the completion of Phase 2 clinical trials and before the initiation of Phase 3 studies. Since agency recommendations may bring about significant revisions to a sponsor's Phase 3 trial plans, the agency suggests that these meetings be held before "major commitments of effort and resources to specific Phase 3 tests are made." The FDA adds, however, that such meetings are not intended to delay the transition from Phase 2 to Phase 3 studies.

As they should in all such communications with the FDA, sponsors should attempt to obtain from agency reviewers and officials specific recommendations during the meeting. Agency staffers advise that sponsors develop highly specific questions or well-formulated proposals, and that they focus questions not only on safety issues regarding Phase 3 protocols, but on what studies and data will be necessary for the ultimate approval of the drug as well. Under PDUFA III commitments, the FDA has agreed to prepare the meeting minutes and make them available to the sponsor within 30 days after the meeting (i.e., for at least 90% of meetings). The minutes should "clearly outline the important agreements, disagreements, issues for further discussion, and action items from the meeting in bulleted form and need not be in great detail," the agency states.

End-of-Phase 2A Meetings. Under a new voluntary pilot program, CDER is participating in so-called end-of-Phase 2A meetings in an effort to address drug-dosing issues earlier in a product's development process. Specifically, such meetings are designed "to improve the design and use of dose-response and pharmacokinetics-pharmacodynamics studies and data, and to discuss the overall biopharmaceutics and clinical pharmacology development strategy needed to support drug dosing and NDA approval."

In a November 2003 concept paper, the agency said that such meetings would take place after the completion of Phase 1 and the first set of exposure-response studies in patients, but before the initiation of Phase 2B and Phase 3 clinical studies. An outgrowth of the FDA's strategic action plan, the pilot program is designed to provide for FDA/sponsor discussions at a critical juncture—before a company has initiated definitive dose-ranging studies and before it has started planning for the all-important Phase 3 trials.

Continuous Marketing Application Pilot 2—Frequent Scientific Feedback/Interaction. Under PDUFA III's so-called Pilot 2 program, the FDA and applicants of eligible fast track products can enter into an agreement to engage in "frequent scientific feedback and interactions during the IND (or clinical development) phase of a product's development." To qualify for frequent scientific feedback and interactions with FDA under PDUFA III's Pilot 2, companies must submit a Pilot 2 application describing how their fast track products could significantly benefit the public health and how their proposed clinical development program could benefit from frequent FDA communication.

Given the resources and level of commitment anticipated in Pilot 2 programs, the FDA established that each product review division could participate in only a single Pilot 2 project over the course of PDUFA III. As of mid-2004, only 7 of CDER's 17 new drug and biologics review divisions had received an "acceptable" application and enrolled a Pilot 2 project, however.

After a division accepts a Pilot 2 project, the division and the applicant will finalize an agreement on the nature of and timelines for feedback and interactions. The FDA outlines Pilot 2 further in an October 2003 guidance entitled, *Continuous Marketing Applications: Pilot 2—Scientific Feedback and Interactions During Development of Fast Track Products Under PDUFA*.

Special Protocol Assessment and Agreement Process. As part of its "special protocol question assessment and agreement" process introduced under PDUFA II and continued under PDUFA III, the agency also agreed to evaluate Phase 3 clinical trial protocols (as well as carcinogenicity and stability protocols) to determine whether a trial's design and size are adequate to meet scientific and regulatory requirements identified by the sponsor. Within 45 days of receiving such a protocol and specific sponsor questions, the agency will provide a written response that includes "a succinct assessment of the protocol and answers to the sponsor's questions." Under PDUFA III, the agency has committed to responding to at least 90% of such requests within the 45-day timeframe.

According to text that accompanied the agency's original commitments, "the fundamental agreement here is that having agreed to the design, execution, and analyses proposed in protocols reviewed under this process, the Agency will not later alter its perspective on the issues...unless public health concerns unrecognized at the time of protocol assessment under this process are evident." Related language in the FDA Modernization Act of 1997 seemed to be even stronger: "Any agreement regarding the parameters of the design and size of clinical trials of a new drug...that is reached between the [FDA] and a sponsor or applicant shall be reduced to writing and made part of the administrative record...[and] shall not be changed after the testing begins, except-(i) with the written agreement of the sponsor or applicant; or (ii) pursuant to a decision...by the director of the reviewing division, that a substantial scientific issue essential to determining the safety or effectiveness of the drug has been identified...."

In a May 2002 final guidance entitled, *Special Protocol Assessment*, the FDA attempts to establish the process through which special protocol assessments will be conducted and agreements will be reached. CDER generally recommends that a sponsor submit a protocol intended for a special protocol assessment to the agency at least 90 days prior to the study's anticipated start date. A separate request in the form of an IND amendment should be forwarded for each protocol that the sponsor wants to have reviewed under this process.

To ensure that the CDER review division "is aware of both the developmental context in which the protocol is being reviewed and the questions that are to be answered," the sponsor should seek a meeting with the agency. In the request for protocol assessment, the sponsor should pose focused questions concerning specific issues regarding the protocol, protocol design (including proposed size), study conduct, study goals, and/or data analysis for the proposed investigation. The request should also discuss, in reasonable detail, all data, assumptions, and information needed for an adequate evaluation of the protocol.

Within 45 calendar days of receiving an applicant's request for a special protocol assessment, the review team responsible for the drug product should forward its comments to the applicant. If the applicant wants to discuss any remaining issues (e.g., disagreements) or issues regarding the protocol following the special assessment, it can request a meeting (i.e., a Type A meeting). All agency/sponsor agreements and disagreements should be documented clearly in the special protocol assessment letter and/or the minutes of the Type A meeting.

According to the May 2002 guidance, "documented special protocol assessments should be considered binding on the review division and should not be changed at any time, except as follows:"

- Failure of a sponsor to follow a protocol that was agreed upon with the agency will be interpreted as the sponsor's understanding that the protocol assessment is no longer binding on the agency.
- If the relevant data, assumptions, or information provided by the sponsor in a request for special protocol assessment change are found to be false statements or misstatements or are found to omit relevant facts, the agency will not be bound by any assessment that relied on such data, assumptions, or information.
- A documented special protocol assessment can be modified if (1) the FDA and the sponsor agree in writing to modify the protocol (section 505(b)(4)(C) of the Act) and (2) such modification is intended to improve the study. A special protocol assessment modified in this manner will be considered binding on the review division, except under the circumstances described in the bullet below.
- A clinical protocol assessment will no longer be considered binding if the director of the review division determines that a substantial scientific issue essential to determining the safety or efficacy of the drug has been identified after the testing has begun (section 505(b)(4)(C) of the Act). If the director of the review division makes such a determination, (1) the determination should be documented in writing for the administrative record and should be provided to the sponsor, and (2) the sponsor should be given an opportunity for a meeting at which the review division director will discuss the scientific issue involved (section 505(b)(4)(D) of the Act).

Phase 3 Clinical Trials

In Phase 3 investigations, a drug is tested under conditions more closely resembling those under which it would be used if approved for marketing. During this phase, an investigational compound is administered to a significantly larger patient population (i.e., from several hundred to several thousand subjects) to, in the FDA's words, "gather additional information about effectiveness and safety that is needed to evaluate the overall benefit-risk relationship of the drug and to provide an adequate basis for physician labeling."

Expediting Drug and Biologics Development

The larger patient pool and the genetic, lifestyle, environmental, and physiological diversity that it brings allow the investigators to identify potential adverse drug reactions and to determine the appropriate dosage of the drug for the more diverse general population. Patient population criteria for Phase 3 trials may also be expanded to include those with concomitant therapies and conditions.

Even with the expanded eligibility criteria, the patient population studied in Phase 3 trials will always be a subset of the overall population with a particular disease or condition. The study population in Phase 3 must be sufficiently homogeneous so that variability in response(s) is minimized and so that the study has adequate power to demonstrate an effect. At the same time, the study population must be adequately representative to enable the generalization of the results to the patient population at large.

For certain drugs, principally those for serious and life-threatening illnesses, Phase 3 also marks the point at which clinical trial sponsors must make another important decision: The sponsor often must consider whether to make the study drug available to patients who desperately need therapeutic alternatives and who are unable to enroll in the formal clinical trials. Such availability, sometimes called "expanded access" or "compassionate use," can be provided under several mechanisms that the agency has established, including treatment INDs and emergency use INDs. Reached in consultation with the FDA, the decision to make a drug available in this manner is a function, first and foremost, of what is known about a drug's safety and, secondly, what is known about its efficacy. This decision is also based upon the availability of satisfactory therapeutic alternatives in the marketplace and the severity of the disease and its potential for causing disability or death.

Pivotal Clinical Studies Phase 3 testing may produce data from controlled and uncontrolled trials conducted at several hospitals, clinics, or other sites outlined in the protocol. But the clinical data that the FDA will review most closely and upon which the agency will base its approval/disapproval decision are those derived from tests specified in federal regulations as "adequate and well-controlled studies."

The focus on adequate and well-controlled studies as the criterion for assessing the effectiveness of new drugs flows directly from the Federal Food, Drug and Cosmetic Act, which states that "the term 'substantial evidence' means evidence consisting of adequate and well-controlled investigations...on the basis of which it could fairly and responsibly be concluded by...experts that the drug will have the effect it purports or is represented to have under the conditions of use prescribed, recommended, or suggested in the labeling or proposed labeling thereof."

The concept of substantial evidence has a second important component. With rare exceptions, at least two adequate and well-controlled studies are necessary to obtain FDA approval for a new drug. According to the FDA's *Guideline for the Content and Format of the Clinical and Statistical Sections of an Application*, "the requirement for well-controlled clinical investigations has been interpreted to mean that the effectiveness of a drug should be supported by more than one well-controlled trial and carried out by independent investigators. This interpretation is consistent with the general scientific demand for replicability. Ordinarily, therefore, the clinical trials submitted in an application will not be regarded as adequate support of a claim unless they include studies by more than one independent investigator who maintains adequate case histories of an adequate number of subjects."

It is important to note, however, that the adequate and well-controlled studies submitted in support of a drug need not be identical. In some cases, for example, they might be carried out in patient populations with different expressions of the same target illness to be treated by the investigational drug.

In late 1997 and early 1998, an FDA guidance document and the FDA Modernization Act clarified the concept of the "substantial evidence" of effectiveness necessary for approval. In the November 1997 reform legislation, Congress established that data from a single adequate and well-controlled study, together with confirmatory evidence, may, at the FDA's discretion, comprise substantial evidence of effectiveness.

Then, with its release of a May 1998 *Guidance for Industry - Providing Clinical Evidence of Effectiveness for Human Drug and Biological Products*, the FDA took another important step in clarifying—some might say evolving—this standard. The agency stated that it was appropriate to re-articulate its current thinking concerning the "quantitative and qualitative standards for demonstrating effectiveness of drugs" because "the science and practice of drug development and clinical evaluation have evolved significantly since the effectiveness requirement for drugs was established, and this evolution has implications for the amount and type of data needed to support effectiveness in certain cases... At the same time, progress in clinical evaluation and clinical pharmacology has resulted in more rigorously designed and conducted clinical efficacy trials, which are ordinarily conducted at more than one clinical site. This added rigor and scope has implications for a study's reliability, generalizability, and capacity to substantiate effectiveness.

"The usual requirement for more than one adequate and well-controlled investigation reflects the need for independent substantiation of experimental results..., [which is] often referred to as the need for 'replication' of the finding. Replication may not be the best term, however, as it may imply that precise repetition of the same experiment in other patients by other investigators is the only means to substantiate a conclusion. Precise replication of a trial is only one of a number of possible means of obtaining independent substantiation of a clinical finding and, at times, can be less than optimal as it could leave the conclusions vulnerable to any systematic biases inherent to the particular study design. Results that are obtained from studies that are of different design and independent in execution, perhaps evaluating different populations, endpoints, or dosage forms, may provide support for a conclusion of effectiveness that is as convincing as, or more convincing than, a repeat of the same study."

This important guidance also identifies situations in which the agency will consider approving new drugs, or new uses of approved medicines, without data from two adequate and well-controlled studies. To the pharmaceutical industry, the guidance's most intriguing aspect was a discussion of the situations in which a single pivotal study could provide the basis for marketing approval. Although the agency had issued a 1995 statement specifying when a single, multicenter study could support approval, the FDA points out that it had not "comprehensively described the situations" in which a single study might be used or the characteristics of a single study that would make it adequate to support approval.

While the FDA contends that none of the characteristics "is necessarily determinative," the presence of one or more of five characteristics can contribute to a conclusion that a single pivotal study would be adequate to support approval: certain large multicenter studies; consistency across study subsets; multiple "studies" in a single study; multiple endpoints involving different events; and statistically very powerful findings.

The guidance also offers several caveats regarding the use of a single pivotal trial for approval. Reliance on a single study, the agency points out, generally will be limited to situations in which a trial has demonstrated a clinically meaningful effect on mortality, irreversible morbidity, or prevention of a disease with a potentially serious outcome, such that confirmation of the result in a second trial would be ethically difficult or impossible.

Although they concede that the use of a single clinical trial is more common or even typical in certain cases (e.g., oncology drugs, outcome studies), senior FDA officials note that the approach is employed only in a "tiny minority" of all cases today.

A 2001 Tufts Center for the Study of Drug Development (CSDD) found that over 80 percent of major pharmaceutical companies surveyed had used or planned to employ regulatory provisions allowing the use of a single controlled trial to gain product approval. The study found that 8 of the 15 top worldwide pharmaceutical companies surveyed used the single controlled trial (SCT) approach for product applications submitted in 1998 and 1999. The Tufts CSDD identified ten approved drug applications employing the SCT approach—six NDAs, four of which were NDAs for new molecular entities, and four supplemental NDAs. Two of the NME-NDAs were submitted to and approved by the Division of Oncologic Drug Products, while the Division of Gastrointestinal and Coagulation Drug Products received four applications using the SCT approach—three supplemental NDAs and one original NDA. Many, but not all, of the drugs employing the SCT approach were products for indications for which SCTs "were expected to be acceptable to FDA," including orphan drugs, pediatric indications, and drugs reviewed under the accelerated approval process.

The Tufts CSDD study also noted that nine of the 12 identified applications (i.e., ten NDAs and two biologics applications) supplemented the SCT data with confirmatory evidence from related adequate and well-controlled studies. Five of these nine applications included data from studies on different doses, regimens, or dosage forms. A third of the applications used just one type of related study, 55 percent used two or three types of related studies, and 11 percent used as many as five types of related studies to support the SCT. Interestingly, all three of the applications that included data from an SCT alone (i.e., without confirmatory evidence) had been approved. Tufts CSDD noted that the sponsors of these three applications all self-rated their SCTs as being very strong in regard to two of the five study characteristics that the FDA claims are of particular importance when an SCT is used: (1) no single site was disproportionately responsible for the positive effect; and (2) there was consistency of important covariates across study subsets.

Standards for Pivotal Trials Because of their central importance to the FDA's approval decision, pivotal studies must meet particularly high scientific standards: "The purpose of conducting clinical investigations of a drug is to distinguish the effect of a drug from other influences, such as spontaneous change in the course of the disease, improvements in supportive care, placebo effect, or biased observation," the agency states. Therefore, adequate and well-controlled trials are designed to isolate the drug's effects from extraneous factors that might otherwise undermine the validity of the trials' results.

Expediting Drug and Biologics Development

Generally, a study must meet four criteria to be considered pivotal:

1. A pivotal study must be a controlled trial. As previously discussed, a controlled trial, in many cases, compares a group of patients treated with a placebo or standard therapy against a group of patients treated with the investigational drug. The FDA specifies in federal regulations, and the ICH parties recognize in a July 2000 guidance (*E10 Choice of Control Group and Related Issues in Clinical Trials*), five types of controls: placebo concurrent controls; dose-comparison concurrent controls; no treatment concurrent controls; active (positive) treatment concurrent controls; and historical (external) controls. The E10 guidance notes that, "the choice of control group is always a critical decision in designing a clinical trial. That choice affects the inferences that can be drawn from the trial, the ethical acceptability of the trial, the degree to which bias in conducting and analyzing the study can be minimized, the types of subjects that can be recruited and the pace of recruitment, the kind of endpoints that can be studied, the public and scientific credibility of the results, the acceptability of the results by regulatory authorities, and many other features of the study, its conduct, and its interpretation" (see exhibit below). The guidance also notes that it is increasingly common for more than one type of control group to be used in a development program. The 2000 guidance was criticized by industry, principally because it failed to harmonize the various control group preferences of the ICH regions (e.g., the FDA's preference for placebo controls and European regulators' preference for active comparators). The FDA has acknowledged that the guidance, although it discusses the appropriateness of the various controls in specific situations, does not address the requirements in any of the three regions.

2. A pivotal study must have a blinded design when such a design is practical and ethical. According to the ICH's September 1999 final guideline entitled, *Statistical Principles for Clinical Trials*, "blinding, or masking, is intended to limit the occurrence of conscious and unconscious bias in the conduct and interpretation of a clinical trial arising from the influence that the knowledge of treatment may have on the recruitment and allocation of subjects, their subsequent care, the attitudes of subjects to the treatments, the assessment of end points, the handling of withdrawals, the exclusion of data from analysis, and so on. The essential aim is to prevent identification of the treatments until all such opportunities for bias have passed." Double-blind trials are those in which the subjects and the investigator and sponsor staff involved in treating and evaluating patients are kept from knowing which subjects are receiving the experimental drug and which are receiving the placebo/standard therapy. When double-blind trials are not feasible (e.g., because the pattern of administration differs), studies may employ single blinds, in which only the subjects are kept from knowing which treatment is administered. In some cases, however, only an open-label study is possible because of ethical or practical factors. In certain instances, studies employ a mechanism of blinding often referred to as a "double dummy" design that is intended to eliminate the biases that might otherwise result from the comparison of different formulations or routes of administration. In such a design, each study subject receives two formulations, only one of which contains the active moiety. This might be used, for example, when an intravenous antibiotic is being compared to an oral antibiotic. Half the subjects might receive the active oral formulation and a placebo intravenous formulation, while the remaining subjects would receive the oral placebo and the active intravenous formulation.

3. A pivotal study must be randomized. This means that clinical subjects are assigned randomly to the treatment and control groups. Therefore, each subject has an equal chance of being assigned to the various treatment and control groups to be studied in a particular trial. In combination with blinding, randomization helps prevent potential bias in the selection and assignment of trial subjects.

4. A pivotal study must be of adequate size (see discussion below). The study must involve enough patients to provide statistically significant evidence of a new drug's safety and effectiveness. According to the FDA's *General Considerations for the Clinical Evaluation of Drugs*, the size of a pivotal study is dependent upon factors such as: (1) the degree of response one wishes to detect; (2) the desired assurance against a false positive finding; and (3) the acceptable risk of failure to demonstrate the response when it is present in the population. Sample size calculations require many assumptions about the results to be obtained with the treatment and the population being studied. Because considerable clinical judgment is employed in making these assumptions, FDA officials warn that faulty presumptions frequently result in studies of inadequate statistical power. Most recently, the FDA and ICH have discussed the difficulties and factors involved in study sample

sizes, largely from the safety perspective, in guidance documents such as the ICH's E1A *The Extent of Population Exposure to Assess Clinical Safety: For Drugs Intended for Long-term Treatment of Non-Life-Threatening Conditions* (March 1995) and the FDA's March 2005 *Premarketing Risk Assessment* (see discussion below).

These criteria also are included in FDA regulations, which add that the "characteristics" of adequate and well-controlled studies include the following:

- a clear statement of the objectives of the study;
- a design that permits a valid comparison with a control to provide a quantitative assessment of the drug effect;
- a method of subject selection that provides adequate assurance that subjects have the disease or condition being studied, or that they show evidence of susceptibility and exposure to the condition against which prophylaxis is directed;
- a method of assigning patients to treatment and control groups that minimizes bias and that is intended to assure comparability of the groups with respect to pertinent variables such as age, sex, severity of disease, duration of disease, and the use of drugs or therapy other than test drugs (*Author's note*: It is important to note that significant improvements in concomitant therapies or mortality rates may drastically alter the conditions of a long-term treatment study involving a chronic disease. The population characteristics of those enrolled near the end of a study may be entirely different from those found in patients enrolled at the beginning of the study);
- adequate measures to minimize bias by the subjects, observers, and analysts of the data;
- well-defined and reliable methods for objectively assessing subjects' responses; and
- an adequate analysis of the study results to assess the effects of the drug (this should not involve so called "data-dredging" to find a positive effect).

The FDA wrote in 1987 that it "has long considered [these] characteristics as the essentials of an adequate and well-controlled study... In general, the regulation on adequate and well-controlled studies has two overall objectives: (1) To allow the agency to assess methods for minimizing bias; and (2) to assure a sufficiently detailed description of the study to allow scientific assessment and interpretation of it."

It is worth noting that federal regulations do not provide a comprehensive discussion of the testing conditions necessary for pivotal trials. Mentions of other standards that the FDA sees as necessary for pivotal studies are scattered throughout a variety of agency guidelines. Although it does not address pivotal trials directly, the ICH's September 1998 guideline entitled, *E9 Statistical Principles for Clinical Trials* offers a useful discussion regarding important aspects of later-phase study design issues, including study configuration (e.g., cross-over and parallel group), trial comparisons (e.g., superiority, equivalence), and sample size.

Determining Adequate Study Sizes

Against the backdrop of high clinical study costs and difficulties in recruiting study subjects, determining adequate trial sizes remains a complex and problematic process that continues to bedevil many product development programs. In mid-2003, for example, Division of Oncologic Drug Products Director Richard Pazdur, M.D., warned that undersized, or statistically "underpowered," clinical trials for oncology drugs were rapidly becoming a larger problem. "Many times, patient populations and number of patients are calculated more or less from a practical perspective of how many patients one can realistically accrue [within a specific time period], rather than putting a true estimation of what is the treatment effect or what is the proposed effect," Pazdur said at the time.

Over the last several years, a handful of international and FDA guidance documents have addressed the trial-size issue. Under a March 1995 ICH guidance entitled, *E1A The Extent of Population Exposure to Assess Clinical Safety: For Drugs Intended for Long-Term Treatment of Non-Life-Threatening Conditions*, the FDA and ICH generally recommended that 1,500 subjects be exposed to an investigational product (with 300 to 600 exposed for six months, and 100 exposed for one year) intended for the long-term treatment (e.g., chronic or recurrent intermittent) of non-life-threatening conditions. For those products that the E1A guidance characterized as chronic use products, the FDA recommends that the 1,500 subjects include only those who have been exposed to the product in multiple doses, since many adverse events of concern (e.g., hepatotoxicity, hematologic events) do not appear with single doses or very short-term exposure. Also, the 300 to 600 subjects exposed for six months and 100 patients exposed for one year should be exposed to "relevant doses," with a reasonable representation of subjects exposed at the highest proposed dose.

Expediting Drug and Biologics Development

The E1A guidance, however, specifies a number of circumstances in which a safety database larger than 1,500 may be appropriate, including:

1. When there is concern that the drug would cause late-developing adverse events, or cause adverse events that increase in severity or frequency over time. Such concern could be triggered by data from animal studies, clinical information on other agents with related chemical structures or from a related pharmacologic class, or pharmacokinetic or pharmacodymamic properties known to be associated with such adverse events.

2. When there is a need to quantitate the occurrence rate of an expected specific low-frequency adverse event. Examples would include situations in which a specific serious adverse event has been identified in similar products or when a serious event that could represent an alert event is observed in early clinical trials.

3. When a large database would help make risk-benefit decisions in situations in which the benefit from the product is small (e.g., symptomatic improvement in less-serious medical conditions), will be experienced by only a fraction of the treated patients (e.g., certain preventive therapies administered to healthy populations), or is of uncertain magnitude (e.g., efficacy determination on a surrogate endpoint).

4. When there this concern that a product may add to an already significant background rate of morbidity or mortality, and clinical trials should be designed with a sufficient number of patients to provide adequate statistical power to detect prespecified increases over the baseline morbidity or mortality.

More recently, the agency provided its perspectives on the appropriate size of premarketing safety databases in a March 2005 guidance entitled, *Premarketing Risk Assessment*, which it developed as part of its push in the risk management area under PDUFA III. In this guidance, the agency acknowledges the complexities of determining an adequate size for safety databases and the practical limitations of clinical development programs.

"Providing detailed guidance on what constitutes an adequate safety database for all products is impossible," the agency notes. "The nature and extent of safety data that would provide sufficient information about risk for purposes of approving a product are individualized decisions based on a number of factors...."

The Choice of Clinical Trial Controls

(from the ICH's July 2000 guidance entitled, *The Choice of Control Group and Related Issues in Clinical Trials*)

Placebo Concurrent Control "In a placebo-controlled study, subjects are randomly assigned to a test treatment or to an identical-appearing treatment that does not contain the test drug. The treatments may be titrated to effect or tolerance, or may be given at one or more fixed doses. Such trials are almost always double-blind. The name of the control suggests that its purpose is to control for "placebo" effect (improvement in a subject resulting from thinking that he or she is taking a drug), but that is not its only or major benefit. Rather, the placebo control design, by allowing blinding and randomization and including a group that receives an inert treatment, controls for all potential influences on the actual or apparent course of the disease other than those arising from the pharmacologic action of the test drug. These influences include spontaneous change (natural history of the disease and regression to the mean), subject or investigator expectations, the effect of being in a trial, use of other therapy, and subjective elements of diagnosis and assessment. Placebo-controlled trials seek to show a difference between treatments when they are studying effectiveness, but may also seek to show lack of difference (of specified size) in evaluating a safety measurement."

No-Treatment Concurrent Control "In a no-treatment controlled study, subjects are randomly assigned to test treatment or to no (i.e., absence of) study treatment. The principal difference between this design and a placebo-controlled trial is that subjects and investigators are not blind to treatment assignment. Because of the advantages of double-blind designs, this design is likely to be needed and suitable only when it is difficult or impossible to double-blind (e.g., treatments with easily recognized toxicity) and only when there is reasonable confidence that study endpoints are objective and that the results of the study are unlikely to be influenced by [any of the problems associated with knowledge of treatment assignment (e.g., unblinded subjects on active drug might report more favorable outcomes because they expect a benefit or might be more likely to stay in the trial)]. Note that it is often possible to have a blinded evaluator carry out endpoint assessment, even if the overall trial is not double-blind. This is a valuable approach and should always be considered in studies that cannot be blinded, but it does not solve the other problems associated with knowing the treatment assignment...."

Dose-Response Concurrent Control "In a randomized, fixed-dose, dose-response trial, subjects are randomized to one of several fixed-dose groups. Subjects may either be placed on their fixed dose initially or be raised to that dose gradually, but the intend-

—continued—

ed comparison is between the groups on their final dose. Dose-response studies are usually double-blind. They may include a placebo (zero dose) and/or active control. In a concentration-controlled trial, treatment groups are titrated to several fixed-concentration windows; this type of trial is conceptually similar to a fixed-dose, dose-response trial."

Active (Positive) Concurrent Control "In an active control (or positive control) trial, subjects are randomly assigned to the test treatment or to an active control treatment. Such trials are usually double-blind, but this is not always possible; many oncology trials, for example, are considered difficult or impossible to blind because of different regimens, different routes of administration, and different toxicities. Active control trials can have two distinct objectives with respect to showing efficacy: (1) To show efficacy of the test treatment by showing it is as good as a known effective treatment or (2) to show efficacy by showing superiority of the test treatment to the active control. They may also be used with the primary objective of comparing the efficacy and/or safety of the two treatments. Whether the purpose of the trial is to show efficacy of the new treatment or to compare two treatments, the question of whether the trial would be capable of distinguishing effective from less effective or ineffective treatments is critical."

External Control (Including Historical Control) "An externally controlled study compares a group of subjects receiving the test treatment with a group of patients external to the study, rather than to an internal control group consisting of patients from the same population assigned to a different treatment... External (historical) control groups, regardless of the comparator treatment, are considered together as the fifth type [of control group] because of serious concerns about the ability of such trials to ensure comparability of test and control groups and their ability to minimize important biases, making this design usable only in exceptional circumstances. The external control can be a group of patients treated at an earlier time (historical control) or a group treated during the same time period but in another setting. The external control may be defined (a specific group of patients) or nondefined (a comparator group based on general medical knowledge of outcome). Use of this latter comparator is particularly trecherous (such trials are usually considered uncontrolled) because general impressions are so often inaccurate. So-called baseline-controlled studies, in which subjects' status on therapy is compared with status before therapy (e.g., blood pressure, tumor size), have no internal control and are thus uncontrolled or externally controlled."

The ICH guidance also notes that it is often possible and "advantageous" to employ more than one type of control in a single study (e.g., using both an active control and a placebo). Some trials might use several doses of a test drug and several doses of an active control with or without placebo. Such a design, says the guidance, may be useful for active drug comparisons when the relative potency of the two drugs is not well established, or when the trial's purpose is to establish relative potency.

The appropriate size of a safety database supporting a new product, the agency notes, will depend on a number of product-specific factors, including:

- The product's novelty (i.e., whether it represents a new treatment or is similar to available treatment)
- The availability of alternative therapies and the relative safey of these alternatives as compared to the new product
- The intended population and condition being treated
- The product's intended duration of use.

Safety databases for products intended to treat life-threatening disease are "usually" smaller than those for products supporting symptomatic treatment of a nonserious disease, the agency emphasizes. A larger safety database may be appropriate if a product's preclinical assessment or human clinical pharmacology studies identify signals of risk that warrant clinical data to properly define the risk.

In its *Premarketing Risk Assessment* guidance, the FDA notes that it is "difficult" to offer general guidance on the appropriate target size of clinical safety databases for products intended for short-term or acute use. "This is because of the wide range of indications and diseases (e.g., acute strokes to mild headaches) that may be targeted by such therapies," says the agency.

Although the FDA uses the *Premarketing Risk Assessment* guidance to emphasize E1A's provisions regarding clinical database sizes for products intended for the long-term treatment of non-life-threatening conditions (see discussion above), it specifies additional circumstances in which a larger database may be appropriate:

"1. The proposed treatment is for a healthy population (e.g., the product under development is for chemoprevention or is a preventive vaccine).

2. An effective alternative to the investigational product is already available and has been shown to be safe."

"The FDA is not suggesting that development of a database larger than that described in E1A is required or should be the norm," the agency points out. "Rather, the appropriate database size would depend on the circumstances affecting a particular product... Therefore, FDA recommends that sponsors communicate with the review division responsible for their product early in the development program on the appropriate size of the safety database. FDA also recommends that sponsors revisit the issue at appropriate regulatory milestones (e.g., end-of-phase 2 and pre-NDA meetings)."

The agency also uses the March 2005 guidance to emphasize that premarketing safety databases should include, to the extent possible, "a diverse population" in Phase 3 studies. "We recommend that, to the extent feasible, only patients with obvious contraindications be excluded from study entry in phase 3 trials," says the agency. "Inclusion of a diverse population allows for the development of safety data in a broader population that includes patients previously excluded from clinical trials, such as the elderly (particularly the very old), patients with concomitant diseases, and patients taking usual concomitant medications. Broadening inclusion criteria in phase 3 studies enhances the generalizability of study findings and may, therefore, allow the product to be labeled for broader use. Although some phase 3 efficacy studies may target certain demographic or disease characteristics (and have narrower inclusion and exclusion criteria), overall, the phase 3 studies should include a substantial amount of data from less restricted populations."

Phase 4 Clinical Studies

In a very real sense, the clinical development process continues long after a product's approval. The further collection and analysis of adverse experience information and other data provide the sponsor and the FDA with a continuing flow of information so that a drug's safety and effectiveness can be reassessed periodically in light of the latest data.

PDUFA III and several agency initiatives have brought a renewed regulatory focus on the postapproval phase of a product's life cycle. Although the two earlier iterations of the FDA's user-fee program focused largely on the clinical testing and FDA review stages of product development, a primary focus of PDUFA III was on the postapproval phase and drug safety. Among other concepts, PDUFA III introduced the concept of the "risk minimization action plan" (RiskMAP), a strategic safety program designed to minimize a product's "known risks," and the so-called "peri-approval period," a two-year period (following a product's approval) during which the FDA can monitor an applicant's implementation of a RiskMAP. Meanwhile, both the ICH and the FDA have released separate guidances on pharmacovigilance practices and planning.

Today, Phase 4 clinical studies have become almost a standard element of the development programs for new drugs, as companies and the FDA seek to further characterize a drug's effects following approval. A Tufts Center for the Study of Drug Development analysis showed that the FDA formally requested postmarketing studies for 73% of the new molecular entities (NME) approved from 1998 through 2003, for example. Further, a *U.S. Regulatory Reporter* study of the approval letters for the 50 NMEs approved from 2001 through 2003 showed that the prevalence of Phase 4 postmarketing commitments has risen from 75% to almost 90% over this three-year period.

Phase 4 clinical trials, which are studies initiated after a drug's marketing approval, have become an increasingly important and common method through which sponsors obtain new information about their marketed drugs. A drug manufacturer may undertake postmarketing clinical studies for any one of several reasons, including the following:

- To satisfy an FDA request made prior to an NDA's approval that Phase 4 trials be conducted following approval. For example, the FDA may want the sponsor to better characterize the drug's safety and/or effectiveness in patient groups that may not have been widely represented in pivotal trials (e.g., children, pregnant women, persons using concomitant medications). Sponsor commitments made at the time of a drug's approval may also become, in effect, postmarketing requirements. Often called "Phase 4 commitments," these commitments—and sponsors' progress in fulfilling them—are actively tracked by the FDA following approval.
- To develop pharmacoeconomic, or cost-effectiveness, data that can be used to support marketing claims highlighting the advantages of a drug over competing therapies. Given the emergence of managed care and the increased focus on health care costs, however, growing numbers of companies are incorporating the study of pharmacoeconomic parameters into their premarketing studies.
- Other post-marketing studies are carried out to support the publication of articles in different medical specialty journals and presentations at medical specialty meetings. The goal of these studies, which are often conducted by opinion leaders in various specialties, is to provide information to less-experienced practitioners. These studies are sometimes called "Phase 5" studies.
- Finally, there are Phase 4 studies that characterize new formulations, dose regimens and routes of administration for already proven therapeutic indications.

Aside from the fact that they are conducted after approval, Phase 4 studies may differ in a number of important respects from Phase 1, 2, and 3 trials. Phase 4 studies are often of a larger scale than are pre-marketing studies. Also, they may be less rigorously controlled than key, pre-approval studies, although the FDA is monitoring the scientific integrity of these studies, particularly those to be used in support of comparative efficacy and pharmacoeconomic claims and those that become the basis for articles that company sales forces use to promote drug products.

In August 2004, both the Pharmaceutical Research and Manufacturers of America (PhRMA) and the Biotechnology Industry Organization (BIO) asked the FDA to reassess the necessity of Phase 4 postmarketing testing requirements in many cases. With the increase in Phase 4 studies required by the FDA as part of new drug approvals, the organizations claim that firms will initiate fewer development projects. PhRMA asked the agency to consider establishing "a process for ongoing review by therapeutic area to distinguish necessary Phase IV studies from those that are informative but not required for the safe use of a drug... Absent this process, sponsors can be faced with escalating Phase IV programs with little or no offsetting reduction in the Phase III testing program."

CHAPTER 14

Clinical Trials Enrolling Children

By Steven Hirschfeld, MD PhD

The very basis for performing clinical trials in children is that children are not small adults. Observations and conclusions from adult studies may not apply to children due to differences in physiology, anatomy, pharmacokinetics, and response to therapy. In addition, some diseases or conditions primarily or exclusively occur in specific age groups.

Children are a biological work in progress beginning *in utero*, continuing through birth and into adolescence. Some age-dependent variables that affect physiology, metabolism and, therefore, drug disposition are listed in the exhibit below.

Selected Age-Dependent Physiologic Variables

- Body size
- Surface to volume ratio
- Penetrability of the CNS
- Maturation of neuro-humoral-immune axis
- Body composition
- Growth rate
- Cognitive/motor function
- Integrity of skin and mucosal barriers
- Protein binding and displacement
- Developmental changes in metabolism (including the Phase I and II enzyme activities
- Receptor expression and function
- Organ functional capacity

The physiologic factors are among the reasons for studying drugs in children of various ages, due to the increased risk of adverse reactions or decreased effectiveness related to inappropriate dose. Other reasons for studying drugs in children are the potential reluctance of practitioners to prescribe potentially useful products without adequate information and ensuring that drug use in children is medically appropriate.

During the 20th century, the principles for the protection of clinical research participants were established and became international policy. The exhibit below compares some of the factors involved in research that enrolls adults to research enrolling children. Children participate in research only if a parent or guardian— normally the person or party who would authorize medical care—grants permission. In the United States and some other countries, researchers directly address school-age children by requesting their assent (in addition to obtaining parental or guardian permission). Assent is generally considered a voluntary process. The process of obtaining permission is always imperfect, and can be especially complex in research studies in which patients may be randomized to different treatments because all possibilities should be discussed, even if neither the subject nor the researcher knows which therapy is being consented or what the possible risks may be. The process of being "informed" should not be considered complete following a signature on a form. The need to educate parents and patients about clinical trials in general, and the study protocol in particular, should be an ongoing component of the process.

Adult vs. Pediatric Research

Adults	Pediatric
Consent-patient	Permission-parent
	Assent (optional)-child
Risk-patient	Risk-child/parent (indirectly through any potential harm to child)
Benefit-patient, future patients	Benefit-child, parent, future patients
All components potentially in same individual plus professional risk and benefit to investigator	All in separate individuals plus professional risk and benefit to investigator

Expediting Drug and Biologics Development

In December 2000, the International Conference on Harmonization (ICH) issued a guidance entitled, "Clinical Investigations of Medicinal Products in the Pediatric Population" (E11), which has been adopted in the three ICH regions (U.S., EU, and Japan). The general principles within E11 are that pediatric patients should be given medicines that have been properly evaluated for their use in the intended population; that product development programs should include pediatric studies when pediatric use is anticipated; that pediatric development should not delay adult studies nor adult availability; and that pediatric development is a shared responsibility among companies, regulatory authorities, health professionals, and society as a whole.

Protecting Children Participating in Clinical Research In the United States, all clinical research must be approved by an institutional review board (IRB); in many other regions, a local ethics committee performs the same function. The institutional approval of pediatric studies is a challenge, and requires pediatric expertise on IRBs and ethics committees to provide appropriate protection. At the same time, that process must also be balanced to permit children to participate in studies and not deny pediatric populations the opportunity to gain access to medical advances. Studies using investigational agents or approved products in a setting in which the risks are unknown also require permission from the Food and Drug Administration, and must be performed under an investigational new drug (IND) application.

In 1999, an FDA advisory panel discussed the issue of appropriate pediatric populations for clinical studies. The consensus was:

(1) In general, pediatric studies should be conducted in subjects who may benefit from participation in the trial. This is interpreted as the study participant having or being susceptible to the disease under study. A flexible definition of eligibility may apply in some circumstances. For example, almost any child has the potential to benefit from a treatment for otitis media, and could potentially participate in a clinical study directed at otitis media. The implication of the recommendation requiring that there be the potential for benefit means that study participants in pediatric clinical research are *patients*, and should be referred to as such rather than under the more general term of study subjects.

(2) In general, children who can give assent should be enrolled in a study in preference to, or prior to, children who cannot give assent. Careful consideration must be given to the importance of the study's potential benefit. In certain circumstances, the potential benefit that may be derived from studying children who cannot give assent may override the preference for first enrolling assenting children.

(3) The final recommendation was that the regulations that protect children enrolled in research studies that receive federal funding be adapted and extended to pediatric studies that do not receive federal funding (e.g., industry-sponsored research).

Federal regulations covering research enrolling human subjects were published in the early 1980s. They addressed research that was funded by the federal government, including educational research, and are published in the Code of Federal Regulations (CFR) in Title 45 Part 46 (45 CFR 46). These regulations include a section—Subpart D—that specifically applies to protections for children. The salient feature of the regulations is the categorization of research according to risk and potential benefit. Research that has minimal risk, defined as those risks routinely encountered in daily life, does not require the prospect of benefit for participation. If the risks are considered to be greater-than-minimal risks, then the study should offer the prospect of direct benefit to the participant or, if the risk is a minor increase over minimal risk, the study should offer the likelihood that it will yield generalizable knowledge about the disease or condition. In all cases, IRB approval, and FDA permission if applicable, is required prior to study initiation. If a proposed study does not fit any of the three categories (minimal risk, greater than minimal risk with prospect of direct benefit, or minor increase over minimal risk with generalizable knowledge), it may be possible to proceed if a federal panel is convened and recommends that the study be initiated.

Central to the determination of whether a study can proceed is the assessment of risk. For pediatric studies, the major sources of risk assessment are experience in human adults, non-clinical animal studies, and prediction based on known biological mechanisms. A recommended definition of minimal risk for children is considered absolute, and is described as the risks in daily activities or routine medical examinations that a prudent parent would allow for an average, normal, and healthy child. In contrast, the definition of a minor increase over minimal risk is considered relative to the condition of the patient and available treatments. Nonetheless, there are some risks that are considered unacceptable, including but not limited to increased pain, decreased interpersonal interaction, or shortened lifespan.

In 2001, the FDA published an interim final rule/adaptation of Subpart D to apply to all FDA-regulated research, independent of funding source. Some critical aspects of the interim adaptation are outlined in the following sections.

Definitions

Children are persons who have not attained the legal age for consent to treatments or procedures involved in clinical investigations, as determined under the applicable law of the state in which the research will be conducted. This provision means that the applicable state law for the research site will determine the participant's legal age of consent.

Parent is defined as a child's biological or adoptive parent.

Ward is a child who is placed in the legal custody of the State or other agency, institution, or entity, consistent with applicable federal, state, or local law.

Guardian is an individual who is authorized under applicable state or local law to consent on behalf of a child to general medical care.

Permission is the agreement of a parent(s) or guardian to their child's or ward's participation in a clinical investigation. Permission must be obtained in compliance with FDA regulations, and must include the elements of informed consent established.

Assent is a child's affirmative agreement to participate in research. FDA's definition also states that the mere failure to object to participation in clinical investigations should not, absent affirmative agreement, be considered assent.

Minimal Risk is defined as in 45 CFR 46, and includes the types of procedures that might be used in a clinical investigation, such as clean-catch urinalysis, obtaining stool samples, administering electroencephalograms, requiring minimal changes in diet or daily routine, a taste test of an excipient or tests of devices involving temperature readings orally or in the ear or the use of standard psychological tests.

IRB Approval Process for Pediatric Research

- The FDA-adopted version of Subpart D differs from 45 CFR 46 because it does not allow an IRB to waive the parental permission requirement for participation in research.
- The general criteria for IRB approval based on FDA regulations are the same for initial review and continuing review, and include a determination by the IRB that: (1) risks to subjects are minimized; (2) risks to subjects are reasonable in relation to anticipated benefits; (3) selection of subjects is equitable; (4) informed consent is adequate and appropriately documented; (5) where appropriate, the research plan makes adequate provisions for monitoring the data collected to ensure the safety of subjects; (6) where appropriate, there are adequate provisions to protect the privacy of subjects and to maintain the confidentiality of data; and (7) appropriate safeguards have been included to protect vulnerable subjects.
- For a clinical investigation in which no greater than minimal risk is presented, approval can occur only if an IRB finds and documents that adequate provisions are made for soliciting the assent of the children involved and the permission of their parents or guardians.
- For clinical investigations in which an IRB finds that there is greater than minimal risk to children, but that presents the prospect of direct benefit to individual subjects, approval can occur only if the IRB finds and documents that: (1) the risk is justified by the anticipated benefit to the subjects; (2) the relation of the anticipated benefit to the risk is at least as favorable to the subjects as that presented by available alternative approaches; and (3) adequate provisions are made for soliciting the assent of the children and the permission of their parents or guardians. These clinical investigations generally are performed in children with the disease or condition for which the product is intended.
- For a clinical investigation in which the IRB finds that greater than minimal risk to children is presented (1) by an intervention or procedure that does not hold out the prospect of direct benefit for the individual subject or (2) by a monitoring procedure that is not likely to contribute to the well-being of the subject, the clinical investigation may be approved only if the IRB finds and documents that: (a) the risk represents a minor increase over minimal risk; (b) the intervention or procedure presents experiences to subjects that are reasonably commensurate with those inherent in their actual or expected medical, dental, psychological, social, or educational situations; (c) the intervention or procedure is likely to yield generalizable knowledge about the subjects' disorder or condition that is of vital importance for the understanding or amelioration of the subjects' disorder

or condition; and (d) adequate provisions are made for soliciting the assent of the children and the permission of their parents or guardians.

While the level of risk in a clinical investigation may change during the course of a study, appropriate strategies may be included in the study design to mitigate risks. These might include individual patient exit strategies in the case of particular adverse events or a lack of efficacy, or the use of a data monitoring committee (DMC) to review ongoing data collection and recommend study changes, including stopping a trial on the basis of safety information.

Evaluation of Efficacy in Pediatric Research Efficacy is generally considered the capacity to produce a desired effect or benefit in a controlled clinical trial. Effectiveness applies to the general use of a product in medical practice. To establish efficacy, a trial must assess a clinical endpoint that is disease- and aged-specific, and that changes in both a positive and negative direction with clinical outcome. While objective measures are preferred over subjective measures, patient-reported outcomes or clinical observations can be used if properly controlled and validated.

Validation can have two meanings in clinical medicine. One is that a particular test provides reproducible results within acceptable specifications, and can be performed and interpreted independent of location and personnel. The other meaning of validation is that the results of a test are predictive of a clinical outcome. Examples of objective measures that can function as clinical endpoints in pediatric research are infection rates, microbial culture results, serum chemistries, hematology counts, blood pressure, urine output, and medical imaging. Almost all objective measures have age-dependent parameters to provide context for interpretation.

Patient-reported outcomes should be disease-related and specifically validated for disease and population, including the improvement and worsening of clinically meaningful changes. The assessments should be in real time—that is, not based on recall, and ideally confirmed by other assessments, such as physical signs like respiratory rate, retractions, or other objective measures. Patient-reported outcomes can be direct or indirect (observed), particularly in younger children.

Several variables have been reported to affect the interpretation of patient-reported outcomes, including age, gender, geographic location, and the type of instrument used. Variables that affect outcome must be accounted for in the design and analysis of studies that measure patient-reported outcomes. The validation of patient-reported outcomes is context- and treatment-specific. Standard statistical analyses may not apply.

In some circumstances, borrowed data can either confirm and/or provide a basis for determining efficacy. Under a 1994 regulation and 1996 guidance document, the FDA permits the extrapolation of adult efficacy data to a pediatric population if the course of the disease and the beneficial and adverse effects of the drug are "sufficiently similar" in the pediatric and adult population. The principles were subsequently codified in the Food and Drug Administration Modernization Act and the Best Pharmaceuticals for Children Act (BPCA). The determination of "sufficiently similar" depends on numerous factors, including pathophysiology, natural history, drug action and metabolism, and is considered to be easier to conclude for brief or acute disorders than for chronic disorders or those with a lengthy and variable history.

Some factors that may provide supporting evidence for extrapolation include non-clinical evidence, pathophysiology, natural history, and response to therapy. Although no consistent framework for extrapolation currently exists, if one is effectively developed it could contribute to the sharing of data among study populations and would diminish the resource burden for conducting clinical trials.

Evaluation of Safety in Pediatric Research Due to the various physiologic factors noted above, the pediatric adverse event profile of a product may differ from the adult profile in types of events, magnitude of severity, or duration. Careful monitoring and scheduled clinical assessments in the relevant population are, therefore, necessary for safety evaluation. Unintended exposure, such as accidental ingestion, may provide additional opportunity for dose and safety information. Long-term or surveillance studies should be considered, particularly for chronic therapies, to observe effects on growth and development. Factors that should be considered include skeletal growth, cognitive function, emotional state, immunologic function and sexual maturation.

Considerations of Trial Design As in other domains of clinical research, the guiding principles in pediatric study design are to minimize bias and uncertainty. In addition to meeting the requirements for good clinical practice as outlined in ICH E6 and ICH E11, consideration must be given to population-specific medical and ethical issues.

In 1995, the American Academy of Pediatrics issued guidelines on placebo-controlled studies. These guidelines state that placebo or untreated observational control groups can be used in pediatric studies if their use does not place children at increased risk. Placebo controls are acceptable in pediatric studies, according to the guidelines, when there is no commonly accepted therapy for the condition, when the commonly used therapy is of questionable efficacy, or when the commonly used therapy has a high frequency of undesirable side effects and the risk may be greater than the benefits. A placebo is also considered acceptable in a comparative add-on study design where a new treatment or placebo is added to an established regimen.

In 2000, an FDA panel discussed placebo controlled studies in children as well. The major points of discussion were that comparison with a placebo may be acceptable if there are no approved or adequately studied therapies for children with the condition under study. For studies involving serious or life-threatening illnesses, a data monitoring committee and planned interim analyses and study stopping rules should be used. In all studies, each patient should have escape criteria to minimize exposure to ineffective treatment. If an adult and pediatric condition are similar in history, response to therapy, and outcome, a placebo should be considered primarily for symptomatic or pharmacodynamic endpoints. Add-on trials that do not deny any elements of the standard of care are appropriate if individual patient discontinuation rules are outlined. For minor illnesses or illnesses with uncomfortable symptoms, a randomized withdrawal study may minimize exposure to placebo. Individual patient escape rules should be defined. A data monitoring committee would generally not be needed, unless there were specific safety concerns.

Except for studies enrolling children with cancer, general criteria for enrolling children in Phase 1 or initial exposure studies do not exist. The oncology framework was discussed by an FDA advisory panel in 2002, and pertains to children who have cancer and who have relapsed or who are refractory to available anti-cancer therapy, and would be candidates for investigational drugs. The consensus was that the evidence burden for initiating clinical studies in children with cancer should include the biological plausibility of the product having activity against a pediatric tumor (which could be obtained from preclinical data), some expectation of potential benefit, a reasonable expectation of safety, and sufficient information to choose an appropriate starting dose. If a scientific rationale and a population of pediatric cancer patients with no available anti-cancer therapeutic alternative exists, then pediatric oncology clinical studies should be initiated, in most cases, immediately following adult Phase 1 studies.

General requirements for pediatric Phase 1 studies can be inferred from the oncology example, but must be discussed and evaluated on a case-by-case basis. First and foremost, do no harm. As in all clinical research, benefit and risk must be estimated prior to patient enrollment. The challenges and complexities of Phase 1 studies in children include the reality that relevant data can be quite limited, although typically human adult Phase 1 data and perhaps other adult data are available. For diseases that are only found in pediatric populations, the pertinent data may only be non-clinical. The minimum requirement for considering benefit is biological plausibility in treating the underlying disease. In addition, there is a need to identify appropriate doses and preliminary safety information, define dose-limiting or unacceptable toxicities, and develop exit strategies for individual patients and stopping rules for the entire study. Depending on the level of risk, the need for a data monitoring committee should be evaluated.

Although the ideal circumstances for using a data monitoring committee in pediatric research vary, some general recommendations based on the oncology model include:
- when the risks are greater than minimal risk or are unknown;
- when a study is multi-institutional, and particularly when international in scope;
- when the study is in the later stages of clinic development for a product, particularly registration or Phase 3 studies; and
- when the disease is life threatening.

The purpose of a data monitoring committee is to provide independent, scheduled assessments and analysis of adverse events, and recommendations regarding study modification, including changes in monitoring and accrual.

Obtaining parental or guardian permission for a child to enroll in a Phase 1 study can be difficult unless there is a clear understanding by all parties of the goals and expectations. Parents may anticipate direct benefits that are quite unlikely, and investigators may assume a level of safety that is not supported by the available evidence. Parents should be counseled that, in early-phase clinical studies, it is not known whether there will be a direct benefit with respect to the underlying disease, but that there is the advantage of participating in a study and receiving careful observation and attentive care.

Timing of Initiation of Pediatric Studies in a Product Development Program The ICH's E11 guideline states that the most important factor is the presence of a serious or life-threatening disease for which the medicinal product represents a potentially important advance in therapy, something that should trigger an urgent and early introduction of pediatric studies in the development program. Other circumstances would normally warrant waiting until initial exploratory studies are completed in adults to avoid exposing children to ineffective or unacceptably toxic products.

Expediting Drug and Biologics Development

Development of Pediatric Formulations If a product is intended for the highly variable pediatric population, it should be available in age-and physiologically appropriate dosage forms. This is particularly necessary for oral medications. The practical issues that must be addressed include the ability to swallow pills or capsules, providing the correct dose (concentration) in the relevant ranges, and anticipating the need to change doses for children of different sizes, which is especially important for chronic medications, such as antihypertensives or anticonvulsants. Other factors include the development of a dosage form that ensures compliance and that is stable when stored.

Multiple technical factors must be addressed and solved in preparing a pediatric formulation, including the age-appropriate volume and vehicle. Differences in metabolism and permeability to body compartments, such as the central nervous system, limit options. Nonetheless, a successful pediatric formulation can have broad applicability to many other populations, including handicapped and geriatric patients.

Federal Initiatives to Promote Pediatric Development Although the major principles of federal regulation of biologics, foods and drugs were developed in the 20th century in response to health crises involving children, children have not been the beneficiaries of incentives designed to spur commercial development, as the table below indicates. Children were termed "therapeutic orphans," and for the better part of the last 100 years, only about 20% of the licensed products had pediatric-specific information in the approved package insert.

Development of Major Regulatory Principles

Principle	Year	Legislation	Contributing Factor
Labeling of biologics	1902	Biologics Control Act	Tetanus antitoxin
Labeling of drugs	1906	Pure Food and Drug Act	Opium
Safety	1938	Food, Drug and Cosmetic Act	Sulfanilamide
Efficacy	1962	Amendment to FD&C Act	Thalidomide
Incentives	1983	Orphan Drug Act	Tourette's syndrome

It was not until 1979 that a pediatric use section was added to the approved package insert, also known as the product label, and not until 1994 that a regulation was written to explicitly encourage pediatric information in the product label. Since the effort was voluntary and the response to the regulation was less than anticipated, during the 1990s an incentive program and a requirement that pediatric studies be performed were instituted in certain cases. These programs have evolved into the current Best Pharmaceuticals for Children Act and the Pediatric Research Equity Act.

The Best Pharmaceuticals for Children Act The core goal of the Best Pharmaceuticals for Children Act (BPCA) is the public dissemination of pediatric information. The BPCA contains several sections to implement the overall aim, and provides for two programs to generate new pediatric data. These programs—one for on-patent drugs and the other for off-patent drugs—will be discussed in some detail below.

The general mechanism is that the FDA sends a written request to the sponsor or manufacturer of a product asking for pediatric data that addresses a public health need. Therefore, the program is voluntary. Qualifying products are mostly small molecule drugs, but not particular antibiotics or biologics. In many, but not all, cases, the written request will ask for new studies. Almost always, the FDA requests dosing and safety information for various age groups and, in some cases, a new formulation. The disease or condition to be studied need not have any relationship to the approved adult uses of the product, and may be for a pediatric-specific condition. While some written requests are FDA-initiated, the majority are issued in response to proposals from the product sponsor or, occasionally, other interested parties acting with permission of the pharmaceutical sponsor. The process is summarized in the exhibit below.

If the product is on patent or still has marketing exclusivity, the sponsor has 180 days to make a commitment to provide the requested information—that is, while the pediatric data are not due in 180 days, a written commitment to provide the data is expected. If no letter is received by the FDA when the 180-day deadline passes or if the sponsor formally declines, the FDA can publicly disclose that the sponsor is not willing to provide requested pediatric information. The written request can then be referred to the Foundation for the National Institutes of Health, a non-profit foundation that receives private donations from non-governmental sources, including the pharmaceutical industry. The Foundation can then provide study grants for the conduct of the FDA-requested studies.

If, however, the sponsor of a product that is still on patent or has remaining marketing exclusivity agrees to provide the FDA with the requested pediatric information by the due date in the written request, the sponsor can qualify for a six-month extension of marketing exclusivity for all dosage forms of the product with the same active ingredient. This is the incentive in the program, and translates into a substantial amount of additional revenue for some products.

General Process for FDA to obtain pediatric information under the Best Pharmaceuticals for Children Act

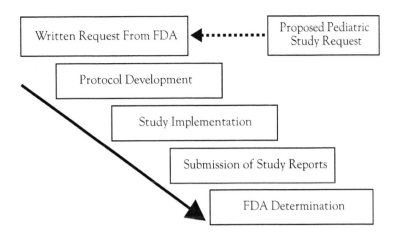

If the product is not on patent, the process is more complex and does not involve an incentive because there is no patent or marketing exclusivity to extend. Products for the off-patent program are selected by a consensus following an annual consultation between the FDA and the NIH's National Institute for Child Health and Human Development (NICHD) and that involves a panel of experts in the areas within which products are being considered. After a list of priority products is made public, the FDA prepares its written requests from the list. The FDA-generated written requests are sent to all current manufacturers, which are given 30 days to reply. Because there is no incentive and because all costs would accrue to the manufacturer, the expectation is that each written request will be declined. The absence of an affirmative response or a formal refusal results in the written request being forwarded to the NICHD. The NICHD will then issue a request for proposals and, based on the responses, select an applicant that, under a contract, will perform the requested studies and submit the data, initially to the NICHD. Subsequently, an NICHD-funded data coordinating center will prepare the data for submission to the public docket.

All FDA written requests are prepared initially by disease experts in the FDA's Center for Drug Evaluation and Research (CDER). The draft written requests are then forwarded to a multidisciplinary review committee that can provide scientific and regulatory advice and that can ensure consistency. The written requests are then sent to the sponsor by the appropriate CDER office director. Listings of approved products for which written requests have been issued, as well as sample templates for written requests, are provided on the FDA's web site under "Pediatrics."

Pediatric written requests should neither impact nor delay a product's development for adults. All written requests have a due date that is based upon the scope of the information requested. If new studies are required and the disease or condition is relatively rare, the due date can be several years after the written request's issue date. For an on-patent product that would qualify for an incentive, the sponsor may submit the data anytime until the due date. Written Request due dates are based on estimates of the time required to address the scientific issue. Patent and existing marketing exclusivity expirations are not taken into consideration in this process.

A study report comprises the formal response to a written request. Initially, the study report is assessed by the relevant review division. The lone goal of the assessment is to determine if the required components of the Written Request have been submitted; given the brief timeframe, an assessment of safety and/or efficacy cannot be undertaken. The review division then forwards a recommendation to an FDA review board that will determine whether the conditions of the written request were fairly addressed. The review board is an internal FDA multidisciplinary body comprised of scientific and legal experts. If the review board determines that the information sought in the written request was provided, then the sponsor is notified, and a formal notification is posted on the FDA web site. If the study report is considered inadequate, the sponsor is notified that pediatric exclusivity has been denied and no Internet posting is made.

To qualify for the incentive, all of the requested information must be provided, although the results from clinical studies do *not* require a demonstration of efficacy. Negative study results are also considered informative, provided that the data are of sufficient quality and quantity to yield a conclusion. A summary of the clinical and biopharmaceutic FDA reviews is posted on the FDA web site. Study results that cannot be interpreted are not considered adequate to address the public health need, and indeed the studies that produced them can be considered unethical because children will have been placed at risk without any meaningful result.

Expediting Drug and Biologics Development

If the written request sought a new formulation and the sponsor found that it was not possible to produce one, the sponsor should provide detailed documentation of its good-faith effort to preserve its eligibility for the incentive.

In exchange for receiving the incentive, the sponsor must anticipate that the results of the written request will be made public. This is done through several mechanisms, including the results' inclusion in the product label (even if the data are negative), publication of the FDA's reviews, and public discussion. If the sponsor resists including the information in the product label, an available dispute resolution mechanism involves public discussion before an FDA advisory panel. Since the proceedings of such discussions are published on the Internet, the information will enter the public domain.

The Pediatric Research Equity Act (PREA) Basically, PREA requires that each new drug or biological product application for a new active ingredient, new indication, new dosage form, new dosing regimen, or new route of administration contain data adequate to assess the safety and effectiveness of the drug or biological product for its claimed indications, and to support dosing and administration for each pediatric subpopulation (i.e., age group) for which the product is safe and effective, using appropriate formulations for each age group. If a product sponsor can submit evidence that the drug or biological product is likely to be ineffective or unsafe in children, or does not confer a significant benefit for pediatric patients, then a sponsor can request a waiver or partial waiver (typically for certain pediatric age groups, such as infants and neonates).

If a disease or condition exists in both adult and pediatric patients, then one of two additional conditions must be met before the FDA can invoke the requirement: Either the prevalence of the disease must be greater than 50,000 children, or the product must be considered a therapeutic advance. Since, for most childhood diseases that are rare, the prevalence condition will not apply, the therapeutic advance provision is pertinent. The FDA can issue waivers for some or all pediatric populations, and in no case should pediatric development delay development for adults.

It is possible for a sponsor to receive a mandate under the Pediatric Research Equity Act and also receive a written request under the Best Pharmaceuticals for Children Act. A comparison of the two programs appears below.

Comparison of FDA Pediatric Initiatives

Pediatric Mandate (Pediatric Research Equity Act)	Pediatric Incentive Program (Best Pharmaceuticals for Children Act)
• Applies to all drugs and biologics, except orphan designation	• Biologics and some drugs excluded, but includes orphan designation
• Only applies to the drug product and indication under review	• Applies to all products with same active moiety
• Only applies if an approved or pending indication occurs in adults and children	• Eligible indications for study must occur in pediatric populations
• Only applies if there is a therapeutic advance or widespread use	• Only applies when there is underlying patent or exclusivity protection
• May be used more than once if a public health need is identified	• Limited use in a product lifetime
• Mandatory—compliance expected	• Voluntary - no compliance required
• No expiration stated in legislation	• Program expires in 2007

Acknowledgements

Drs. Sarah Goldkind and Dianne Murphy are gratefully acknowledged for careful reading of the manuscript and helpful suggestions and comments.

Bibliography

International Conference on Harmonization, "Clinical investigation of medicinal products in the pediatric population" (E11), December 2000. (http://www.fda.gov/cder/guidance/4099FNL.pdf)

Best Pharmaceuticals for Children Act. Public Law No. 107-109. (http://www.fda.gov/cder/pediatric/PL107-109.pdf)

Pediatric Research Equity Act. Public Law No. 108-155. (http://www.fda.gov/cder/pediatric/S-650-PREA.pdf)

Federal Regulations for the Protection of Human Subjects participating in federally funded research. (http://www.hhs.gov/ohrp/humansubjects/guidance/45cfr46.htm)

FDA Regulations for the Protection of Human Subjects participating in FDA regulated research. (http://www.accessdata.fda.gov/scripts/cdrh/cfdocs/cfcfr/CFRSearch.cfm?CFRPart=50)

The Ethical Conduct of Clinical Research Involving Children—Board on Health Sciences Policy, Institute of Medicine. (http://www.nap.edu/books/0309091810/html/)

CHAPTER 15

Clinical Study Reports

By Christine Kochi, Pharm.D.

A clinical study report (CSR) describes the objective(s), design, rationale, methodology, statistical considerations, organization, results, discussion, and conclusions of a clinical study. Ideally, the CSR's development will begin as early as the protocol development phase. Initiating the process early facilitates and expedites the overall CSR development process and results in a higher quality document.

This chapter discusses two aspects of the CSR: (1) establishing the CSR format and content to set the target for the study's clinical documentation; and (2) the process of completing a CSR once the trial is finished.

Establishing the Format and Content: The ICH's "Structure and Content of Clinical Study Reports" (E3)
The ICH's E3 guideline makes recommendations for the CSR's structure, format, and content, and this chapter will be based on those recommendations. It provides a table of contents, template forms for some sections of the CSR, and instructions for the content of each section within a CSR. The proposed model can be organized differently, as long as all topics are presented and apply to the objectives of the study. As will be discussed later, however, generally it is best not to deviate from the template.

The ICH E3 guidance is recommended and has been adopted by regulatory agencies within the United States, European Union (EU), and Japan. Today, the CSR format/content recommended within the guidance is also used by most pharmaceutical and biotechnology companies.

Technical issues arise in developing the CSR for any study. These issues should be addressed before the formal development begins. The table of contents presented in the E3 guidance applies to CSRs for Phase 3 studies (e.g., there are sections that do not apply to earlier phases of drug development). These sections can be either removed from the CSR or left in the CSR with appropriately added "not applicable" notations. (It is recommended that sections not be removed, and that the numbering of sections remain as it appears in the template. This will aid the eventual reviewer, who will know immediately where to look for various elements of information.)

For earlier-phase studies, additional subsections can be added, as necessary, without altering the existing template numbering system. For example, in template Section 9.5.3 Primary Efficacy Variables, multiple primary variables can be added to the template as Sections 9.5.3.1 for the first of the primary variables, 9.5.3.2 for the second, and so on. As another example, a pharmacokinetic study may have pharmacokinetic variables substitute for efficacy variables, and Section 9.5.3 might be labeled Primary Pharmacokinetic Variables instead of Primary Efficacy Variables.

Further, the E3 guideline includes the serious adverse listings and narratives in two different sections of the CSR (Sections 12.3.1 and 14.3.2), yet one location suffices. The location can either be standardized in all CSRs written within the company (or institution) or be adapted to each CSR. If few serious adverse events (SAE) were reported during the study, listings and narratives can be included within the text in the safety results section (Section 12). If numerous SAEs were reported, listings and narratives may be better presented in the CSR section that includes the summary tables, figures, and graphs (see E3).

FDA guidance documents propose additional CSR formats (e.g., abbreviated CSR) that can be used to support a marketing application under certain circumstances (see http://www.fda.gov/cber/gdlns/abbrev.pdf).

The Overall Development of a Clinical Study Report: The Clinical Study Report Template A CSR template should be in place before the writing of a CSR begins, and should specifically reflect the needs of a company or institution. The CSR template should be developed in coordination with a study protocol template to ensure that most of the study information and methodology required in a CSR have already been included in the study protocol and can be easily transferred to the CSR. A well-formatted CSR template is indispensable when CSRs are part of an electronic submission.

Expediting Drug and Biologics Development

A quality CSR template includes the format and content discussed in this chapter, facilitates the CSR development, standardizes the CSR format within a company, and may improve the review process at regulatory agencies.

Clinical Study Development Phase As early as possible during the protocol development, data to be included in the CSR should be described in the protocol. During the study development phase, an understanding of CSR requirements facilitates the CSR development later on and ensures that all appropriate information and documents have been collected. For example, study documents such as investigator curriculum vitae (CV) should be limited to a maximum of two pages when included in the CSR; study information, such as protocol deviations and lot numbers of study drug used in the study, should be collected during the study and be presented in the CSR.

Statistical Analysis Plan The study's statistical analysis plan (SAP) should be available at the time the study begins to ensure that study data are collected appropriately to meet the study objectives. Furthermore, the statistical analysis plan can be incorporated into the CSR early during the CSR development.

Overall Timelines The CSR's development very much involves a team effort. To ensure that this team is successful, timelines should be established. Timelines for the CSR development can be outlined at the beginning of a clinical study. Prior to a study's database lock, detailed timelines should be established and the responsibilities of each member of the CSR development team should be defined.

The following principal steps of the CSR development process should be included in a timeline:
- Prepare the CSR *Shell*
- Run the statistical analysis and produce tables, figures, and listings
- Write the results and incorporate all tables, figures, and listings
- Complete all CSR appendices
- Finalize Discussion, Conclusion, and CSR synopsis
- Complete internal reviews, audits, and approval of the CSR.

Format and Content of a Clinical Study Report: The Outline A CSR can be divided into five principal elements, each of which is discussed below. The section numbers, as they appear in the table of contents of the ICH's E3 guideline, are presented in *italics* for reference:
- "CSR Shell" (*Sections 1, 3-9, 15*)
- Results (*Sections 10-13*)
- Summary Source Tables, Figures, Graphs, and Narratives (*Section 14*)
- Source Documents (*Section 16*)
- Synopsis (*Section 2*)

Although it is located in the beginning of a CSR, the Synopsis is described last because it summarizes the entire document and should be completed after all other sections in the CSR are finalized.

The CSR Shell The CSR Shell includes information on the study's conduct. It can be written long before the study results are available (it is recommended that it start as soon as the study starts). It includes Sections 1, 3 through 9, and 15 of the ICH CSR Template:

Section 1: CSR title page

Here, it is important to note the relevance of generating, during the protocol development process, a study title that provides an adequate description of the study design. A good title can be used for both the Protocol and the CSR. Otherwise, the CSR title page should include a brief description of the study design. The statement regarding compliance, another element of the title page, should refer to the ICH's Good Clinical Practices guidance (E6) and the related sections of Title 21 of the U.S. Code of Federal Regulations, Part 312 (21 CFR 312). For international studies, the compliance statement can also refer to other applicable standards for the protection of human subjects and the integrity of clinical data.

Sections 3 through 5: These sections include the table of contents, a list of abbreviations, and a statement of ethical considerations.

Section 6: Investigators and study administrative structure

All investigators and any other key participants (e.g., coordinating investigator, advisory committee members) should be listed. The rationale for designating the coordinating (principal) investigator for the study should be presented.

Any laboratories, other than the sponsor's, that were used to perform testing for the study, and any contract research organization involved, should be mentioned here. Any external personnel (e.g., statistician, medical writer) who authored the

CSR or participated in the CSR process (e.g., programming of tables) should also be listed.

The information required in this section should be available in the study protocol.

Section 7: Introduction

This section can be adapted directly from the protocol. It should present a brief statement concerning the study's position in the drug's development, the rationale for choosing the indication, the patient population, the study design, and treatment.

Section 8: Study objective

This section can be taken directly from the protocol, and should match the protocol exactly. There should be no reason to change the protocol wording, except the tense of the verbs.

Section 9: Methodology used in the study (Investigational Plan Information) in this section corresponds to the study protocol and SAP. It explains what data were collected (as well as their frequency and the methodology), monitored, entered, validated, and analyzed. It also presents how the eligibility of the study subjects was determined, how subjects were randomized (where applicable), how the blind was maintained, and how subjects' treatment compliance was evaluated. The determination of the sample size and how the study was powered (e.g., determination of sample size) should be described. For blinded studies, the degree of blinding should be clearly explained.

This section of the CSR is critical in evaluating the efficacy and safety results. It provides information on the quality of the data and of their analyses, and supports the validity of the results presented in the CSR. This information, with the exception of the SAP, should have been clearly stated in the protocol to ensure the proper conduct of the study. Any changes to the conduct of the study or planned analyses after the start of the study should be described.

Section 15: References

This section provides a list of any references included in the text of the report, including any publications based on the study.

Results The results sections of the ICH CSR Template include text and primary tables, figures and graphs. These sections are:

Section 10: Disposition of patients and protocol deviations

This section should present a clear account of all subjects who entered the study, how they were randomized and dosed, and whether they completed or discontinued the study. For a blinded study, this section should mention whether or not the blind was broken and if so, under what circumstances. It should also account for subjects who were screened but failed enrollment, and should indicate the reasons for failing enrollment.

Important protocol deviations should be summarized in this section, and details of any deviations should be provided in listings by subject in the CSR appendices (in *Section 16.2*). It is critical that the study monitors collect and report any and all protocol deviations during the course of the study. All protocol deviations should be presented in the CSR to support the validity of the study data.

Note that demographic data, baseline characteristics, and treatment compliance may easily be included in *Section 10* instead of *Section 11*, as proposed in the ICH CSR guidance model.

Section 11: Demographics and efficacy results

This section may also include the results from studies evaluating pharmacokinetics and/or pharmacodynamics.

Section 12: Safety results

Narratives for SAEs, deaths, and other significant events must be included in the CSR. Some other significant events can be defined as standards for all CSRs within the company (or institution), such as adverse events (AE) leading to study drug discontinuation. Some events may be product specific, such as events that are likely inherent to the drug's mechanism of action. Finally, some events may be selected on a case-by-case basis (e.g., unusual nature of the event and/or its severity).

Section 13: Overall discussion and conclusions

In this section, the results of the study should be discussed in the context of the overall drug development program.

Summary Source Tables and Serious Adverse Event Narratives *Section 14* of the ICH CSR template includes tables, figures, and graphs referred to, but not included in, the text of the CSR. These are the non-primary summary tables, figures, and graphs. Listings and narratives of SAEs and other significant adverse events may be presented in this section or in *Section 12*.

Expediting Drug and Biologics Development

Source Documents In the ICH CSR template, the source documents are divided into four parts:

Section 16.1: Study information

Section 16.2: Patient data listings

Section 16.3: Patient case report forms

Section 16.4: Individual patient data listings

The source documents (referred to as appendices in the ICH CSR guidance) are voluminous and may be prepared early in the CSR development process. It is essential that these documents be collected appropriately during the study. They should be available as early as possible during the CSR development.

Study Information

Section 16.1.1: Protocol and amendment(s).

The version of the protocol under which the first subject was enrolled, and all subsequent amendments, should be included in this section.

Section 16.1.2: Sample case report form (CRF).

The sample CRF presented should include all unique and any revised forms.

Section 16.1.3: List of Institutional Review Boards (IRBs) or Institutional Ethics Committees (IECs) and sample (or model) informed consent form(s) (ICF(s)).

For each investigational site, the IRB or IEC involved in reviewing the protocol and ICF should be identified. If several versions of the model ICF(s) exist, the latest version submitted may be chosen for inclusion in the CSR (the rest are kept in the study files at the site). If a separate model ICF and written information for patients were created for a region other than North America (e.g., EU), they should be included in the CSR as well. If no model ICF(s) is(are) available, a sample ICF from an investigational site (e.g., in the US and in Europe for an international study) should be presented.

Section 16.1.4: List and description of investigators and other important participants, and the curriculum vitae.

During the investigational site initiation process, the study monitors should request a single-page *Curriculum Vitae* (CV) from the investigators and sub-investigators (maximum of two pages). Brief CVs will facilitate their inclusion in the CSR.

Section 16.1.5: Signature of sponsor's responsible medical officer and/or coordinating investigator(s).

The signatures can be located in this section or at the beginning of the CSR. For European submissions, the signature of the coordinating investigator should accompany the signature of the sponsor's responsible medical officer.

Section 16.1.6: Listing of patients receiving drug and lot numbers.

When several lots were used during the study, the lot number should be specified for each subject who received the test article (study drug).

Section 16.1.7: Randomization scheme and code.

Section 16.1.8: Audit certificates.

The certificate of investigational site audit(s) should be included in this section. Audit reports should not be included, however.

Section 16.1.9: Documentation of statistical methods.

Any additional documentation not presented in Section 9.7 should be included here.

Section 16.1.10: Documentation of inter-laboratory standardization methods and quality assurance procedures.

Any specific laboratory testing (other than routine laboratory tests) or medical procedures should be presented in this section.

Section 16.1.11: Publications based on the study.

Publications based on the study should be included in this section. If a publication has not been published when the final CSR is completed, the section can indicate that the publication is "in press."

Section 16.1.12: Important Publications Referenced in the CSR.

Scanned copies of publications referenced in the CSR should be included in this section. A company (or institution) should decide whether all publications should be included in the CSR or only selected ones.

Patient Data Listings

Section 16.2: The ICH Guidance suggests that the patient data listings be included in this section. Additional listings can be included as deemed appropriate.

Patient Case Report Forms

Section 16.3: Case report forms can be particularly voluminous. For that reason, they may be included in this section or be provided under a separate cover. Selected subjects' CRFs (e.g., subjects who experienced an SAE or withdrew due to an AE) may be presented. The selection of CRFs for inclusion in the CSR should be consistent within the company (or institution) for a study drug and indication.

Individual Patient Data Listings

Section 16.4: Individual patient data listings should be provided for U.S. submissions.

Synopsis The synopsis of a CSR (*Section 2*) summarizes and reflects the content of the CSR, and includes sections on the methodology (from the CSR *shell*), results, and conclusion. During the CSR development, the content of the synopsis should be checked systematically for consistency with other CSR sections. When the CSR is nearing completion, it is critical that any changes in the body of the document be added to the synopsis, when appropriate. The synopsis should remain concise and be meticulously prepared.

Clinical Study Report Writing

This section addresses the "realization" of the CSR, or "making it happen." As stated above, the CSR's development should begin long before the study's completion. The development of a quality CSR can be challenging in a deadline-driven environment like the pharmaceutical industry. The reporting of a study is part of the overall study management, which starts with the protocol development and ends with the final CSR. As with any project, the development of a CSR requires careful planning and the implementation of well-established processes to be successful.

Project Planning: Establishing Roles and Responsibilities The roles and responsibilities of each member of the CSR team should be clearly established.

The main players in the CSR's development usually are the medical writer, biostatistician, study medical officer, and study project manager and/or lead clinical research associate. Additional participants may include representatives from regulatory affairs, drug safety, statistical programming, data management, pharmacokinetics (if any pharmacokinetic data were to be collected during the study), and laboratory personnel for specific laboratory assays performed during the study. The quality assurance (QA) group should also be involved in the CSR development so that it can check data output (tables, figures, and listings) and review the completed CSR document.

When an electronic document management system is used, multiple authors may contribute simultaneously to the writing of the CSR. Such a system significantly expedites the writing process, provided that there is effective coordination and communication between authors.

For each review cycle, the personnel responsible for reviewing the CSR should be identified. Their availability for the CSR review period should be confirmed in advance, and the date of the reviews should be communicated to the reviewers. This becomes essential when filing for a new drug application (NDA) or market authorization application (MAA), since several CSRs and other documents usually must be reviewed within a brief period of time.

Developing Timelines Detailed timelines for the CSR's development should be established long before the database lock is implemented for a study. The CSR timelines should include, at a minimum, the critical tasks to be performed to complete the CSR, and the personnel responsible for each task. Critical tasks may be outlined as follows:

- completion of the CSR *shell*
- completion of programming the data tables and analyses
- completion of data necessary for the finalization of all CSR sections (e.g., tables, figures, listings, narratives for serious adverse events, and narratives for other significant events)
- completion of writing and inclusion of study source documentation in all CSR sections
- CSR review cycles and audit
- CSR team meetings to discuss reviewers' comments
- revisions of the CSR to incorporate reviewers' comments

- technical steps necessary for compiling the CSR or publishing the CSR when submitted electronically
- approval and sign-off.

After the CSR if finalized, additional activities are necessary to prepare the document for an electronic submission. These activities should be addressed in establishing a timeline for the CSR's availability for submission to a regulatory agency.

The CSR timelines should be updated and distributed to the team on an ongoing basis. Regular team meetings should be held to discuss the status of the CSR development and any issues that must be resolved. The CSR review cycles should be clearly established so that the CSR team reviews a complete draft CSR before the document is forwarded for senior management review.

Clinical Study Report Development Process To expedite CSR development, any information or documents that can be included in the CSR or prepared before the database lock for the study should be completed. After database lock, the CSR team may focus on processing the data, and the authors may focus on presenting the results in the CSR. A CSR's message should be clearly defined and communicated to the authors before they begin writing the results sections.

Prior to Study Completion The CSR *shell*, which is written from the protocol and the statistical analysis plan (SAP), can be prepared during the course of the study. Some CSR source documents (e.g., protocol, amendment(s), informed consent forms (ICF), list of ethic committees (IEC)/institutional review boards (IRB), curriculum vitae (CV) for investigators and other significant participants, inter-laboratory standardization methods, publications) may be available at the initiation of the study and may, therefore, be included in the CSR early on. The CSR *shell* may also include some bullet-point text in the results sections before the study results are available, and this may later facilitate the completion of these sections.

At Study Completion A study is completed when either: (1) the last subject enrolled in the study has completed his/her last visit (or last treatment); or (2) the study ends prematurely. Further information may be incorporated into the CSR *shell* at study completion, including protocol deviations and some source documents (e.g., study drug lot number(s), audit certificates). A review of the CSR *shell* should be performed early in the CSR development process, before study results are available. This initial review reduces the number of comments generated during subsequent reviews of the completed CSR and permits faster review cycles for the full document.

Database Lock to Final Analyses After the database has been locked, the following information should be incorporated into the CSR: source documents (listings, subject case report forms, etc.), summary tables, figures, graphs, and narratives. The results sections as well as the synopsis and the discussion-conclusion should be completed. Consistency between the methodology presented in the CSR *shell* and the results should be verified in detail, particularly when the CSR *shell* was written long before the CSR's completion. All CSR sections should also be cross-checked for consistency. For clarity, all tables, figures, listings, publications, and appendices should be referred to in the body of the document. The signatures of the sponsor's medical officer and coordinating investigator(s) responsible for the study should be collected at the CSR's completion.

Technical Issues Related to the CSR Content A CSR *shell* should be written prior to study completion and should present any changes made to the protocol (e.g., protocol amendment[s]) or the SAP during the course of the study. The information presented in the CSR *shell* may, therefore, require modifications prior to the CSR's completion.

The synopsis should be meticulously written. It should also accurately reflect what was written in other sections of the CSR, since this information will have been taken from other sections of the document. The synopsis should be revised any time a section has been modified.

The CSR team should identify which significant adverse events other than serious adverse events are to be included in the CSR. Because a narrative must be prepared for each of these events, they should be identified prior to study completion and planned appropriately.

When multiple authors are involved in the CSR's development, communication between authors is critical for retaining a consistent writing style. Study terms and verb tenses should be used in a consistent manner across document sections to facilitate comprehension of the final document. Verb tenses may be used within the CSR to differentiate what was planned from what was actually performed during the study, and what is presented in the CSR.

Conclusion Before initiating the development of a specific CSR, a CSR template should be in place within the company or institution. This template should be compliant with the ICH's E3 guideline and be adapted to the needs of the company or institution. The CSR template should be developed in coordination with the protocol template to facilitate the transfer of information from the protocol into the CSR. Finally, a well-formatted CSR template is essential when using an electronic document management system.

The CSR's development should begin during protocol development, since a quality protocol is essential to the development of a quality CSR. A well-written, well-organized, and comprehensive CSR may facilitate a regulatory agency's review process.

Writing an effective CSR is a team effort that must be based on strict timelines and roles and responsibilities that are clearly established at the beginning of the CSR development process. A quality CSR template and well-defined CSR development process facilitate the completion of a CSR. Finally, an electronic document management system expedites the writing of a CSR by allowing multiple authors to work simultaneously on a document. All of these conditions are essential for the rapid and efficient development of a quality CSR.

CHAPTER 16

Standard Data Presentations

By J. Steven Wilkinson, M.S.

The ability to quickly view and comprehend clinical data is at the heart of a quick and successful regulatory review and, hopefully, approval action by regulatory authorities. Data presentations include the tables, figures and listings that display the information gleaned from the clinical study process. These presentations primarily support the tables and conclusions provided in the clinical study report (CSR, see Chapter 16), but also provide a window into the analytical methods used, and support the basic principles of clinical research for efficacy and safety. These data presentations reveal the technical flow used in building the analysis, and can provide a chronology of reasoning to further support the CSR. Data presentations should maintain the same format and structure of the CSR to facilitate an integrated and natural review, and help present the case for the test article's (new drug, biologic or combination) approval. Additionally, the presentations must provide the elements that regulatory agencies require of clinical study submissions.

Data presentations provide a touchstone for all references to the clinical data gathered in a study. The ease with which data presentations can be reviewed, referenced, or more importantly cross-referenced, corresponds directly with the review speed and level of interpretation possible. Although integral to any CSR, new drug application (NDA)/biologics license application (BLA) data presentations represent the proof that the research was completed. They also play a central role in the CSR's ability to influence reviewer's opinions of the document. Generally, the CSR's descriptive results and conclusions are supported by tables and figures embedded in the text in the body of the report. These presentations should also be available in the appendices reflecting the larger body of data analyzed. The presentations should display the results of the entire analysis and will help draw a reviewer's attention to the same conclusions provided in the text. Basic listings are also provided to support the summary tables and figures with the raw data gathered during the study. Together, the tables, figures and listings should provide a reviewer with the complete picture of data capture and analysis.

There are two places in which a pharmaceutical sponsor displays clinical data—in the clinical trial's final report (see Chapter 16) and in the marketing application's clinical data section (see Chapter 8). Although the marketing application's clinical data section will contain far more data than will any individual clinical report, the format and content of these two data displays should be as similar as possible for reasons related to efficiency and other reasons discussed later in this chapter.

Programming Development In the creation of a study report, the data presentations represent an area in which one or two people work extremely hard to design, build and produce a section of a report that can greatly influence other sections. Data presentations represent an effort that can take many hours to complete, and in a team environment, those hours can quickly escalate if the effort is not properly managed. It is important that the analysis, programming, data management, and medical writing teams work together, with efforts coordinated to fit within the framework of all other reporting efforts. This framework can best be expressed through a proposed Table of Contents for the data presentations, and a style guide that coordinates with other report formats. The timing for building each section of the data presentations should also be considered during the planning stages. The sheer size of the report-building effort requires that these data presentations be built in close synergy with the data providers, statistical and medical team members, and the report writers. With study reports typically developed in sections by different personnel, active planning and management is required to coordinate these activities, and provide resources to minimize bottlenecks in any one area. The use of a standard set of data presentations for those tables, figures and listings that easily lend themselves to that approach provides a framework and guide that promotes overall efficiency, resource allocation and planning, and allows for a higher degree of coordination and teamwork.

As it has also become standard practice to supply study data with the CSR, the data presentation team has the additional concern of the structure of the data that are used and submitted. Recent efforts by the Clinical Data Interchange

Expediting Drug and Biologics Development

Standards Consortium (CDISC) are focused on establishing standards to address this issue, taking data structure from a company-based proprietary format to a more ubiquitous and common format. CDISC's Operational Data Standards (ODS) model addresses the collection and handling of data, while its Submission Data Standards (SDS) model describes the content, structure and attributes of data for the regulatory submission.

The full use of these standards will greatly ease presentation development. Until then, as these standards evolve and improve, the implementation introduces a problem in creating standard presentation programs. Data presentation members should be full team participants in any CDISC initiative, since they require a clear plan to manage these versions over time and over submissions. Though many of the issues and concerns described below are solved by using the CDISC standards, they provide a foundation of understanding for basic presentation concepts and must be addressed as review methods progress.

This chapter will help the reader understand how data presentations fit into the study report, provide a description of various challenges to this effort, and help formulate a standard structure and methodology for long-term use. As a means for accomplishing this, the chapter outlines a framework for programming development in an efficient and documented manner. International Conference on Harmonization (ICH) guidances and numbering conventions are presented as a practical example of a working standard.

Validated Display Development Before discussing data presentation development and standards, it is worth discussing the continually growing impact of electronic data collection and processing in clinical development. Currently, from data capture to submission and review, the entire process can be managed, controlled, reviewed and presented in a completely electronic mode. Today, auditors are looking as closely at procedures, training, and controls of the electronic tools as they have looked at the data in the past. To avoid auditing issues, one must consider development in a planned manner with fully characterized and documented processes.

In the tightly regulated arena of clinical development, Title 21 of the U.S. Code of Federal Regulations, Part 11 (21 CFR 11) demands that all manipulation of data be performed in a controlled manner using validated procedures and tools. Typically, development has focused on the creation of unique programs and data objects for each study report or submission. Although many people tend to feel that the validation requirements do not apply to something so distinct, many gains can derive not only from a review of the validation methodologies, but also in using many of these techniques as a means of standardization towards the overall compliance with 21 CFR 11.

Validation is achieved by using tested and workable procedures and following established methods that support the intended performance. As stated in 21CFR11, "validation of systems to ensure accuracy, reliability and consistent intended performance," is a core concept of successfully using and manipulating data electronically. The catch-phrase "intended performance" is significant for developing data presentations. As these programs tend to be unique to each study, developers tend to build for single execution. Without full validation, the ability to repeatedly provide desired results is placed that much more in doubt. With the use of standards, the reuse of previously validated program code, and adherence to previously successful practices, the programmer's ability to consistently create proper data presentations and comply with basic validation and 21 CFR 11 principles is enhanced.

Although the methodology and related documentation regarding how the programs are created and used are generally considered proprietary, more and more submissions include this information, along with the programs and development objects. This practice is encouraged for two reasons. First, the necessity of professional work is made even clearer when the programming team knows that not only the results, but also the methods and tools, will be submitted and available for examination by the regulatory authorities. This increases the team's attention to detail, adherence to standards, and conformity to all relevant requirements. Second, review time can be greatly minimized when the statistical reviewer can clearly see the paths that generated all data displays.

Practical Life Cycle Development All software must be created in an environment that addresses the user's requirements, and that does so in a consistent and auditable manner. The development of data presentations is no different. A common concept and planning tool in building software is the use of a so-called software development life cycle (SDLC). The use of an SDLC forces the stepwise evolution of each project, and ensures that documents are created as part of the process, rather than as an afterthought. This SDLC approach will greatly facilitate the adherence to standards and the development of a higher-quality product.

Although there are many approaches to, and versions of, an SDLC, the basic elements are: plan, design, build, test, implement, maintain and archive. While the use of an SDLC may seem impractical if considered for an individual study alone, stepping back and considering how the programs are used for integrated summaries, the eventual marketing application, and other pharmaceutical development programs, the impact can be better appreciated. The SDLC also provides the basic development structure that is essential for project documentation and supporting auditing activities. The use and active management of this structure then provides for easy tracking and status review of the presentation programs in development, allowing for better control and understanding of the development effort. Ultimately, these factors provide for greater confidence in, and awareness of, the programs and results.

The following is a brief introduction to a basic SDLC. This introduction can be used as a framework for a more comprehensive set of working procedures and a company-specific model.

Planning Planning should address the basic project management issues of timing, resources and costs. At a minimum, a schedule of assignments, tracking and oversight mechanisms, documentation activities, and test and validation methodologies should be described. As data presentations are developed to support and present the statistical analysis of study data, planning efforts begin with a solid draft protocol (see Chapter 20) and statistical analysis plan (SAP, see Chapter 18). Additionally, the study budget and timelines provide information for resource planning and management.

A crucial element of planning involves ensuring that the core project team is assigned and that it's members understand their roles and deliverables. Key participants in the development effort are the statistician, medical writer and programmers. Clinical research and data management personnel should be included as indicated, since clinicians are an intended end-user and the data managers are charged with providing the data in a compatible format. As with any team, a strong project manager is important. The project manager must know and enforce the long-term goals of the presentation standards discussed in this chapter, and understand the larger integration and submission requirements. The needs for study resources should always be carefully weighed against the planned marketing application submission as well as possible global submissions. The project manager should encourage the use of standards and force the team to continually review and consider long-term goals.

A standard SDLC development plan should be established to provide a template for the activities and documentation. This will establish and reinforce individual data presentation standards. An overall strategy for implementing and re-using a generic plan will greatly facilitate the tasks.

Designing It is during the design stage that the data standards are best identified and implemented. Typically, the result of the design phase is the creation of a set of requirements describing the data presentations. The study statistician and lead programmer can create the basic design based on the Statistical Analysis Plan (SAP) and a Tables Manual (see Chapter 18). The Tables Manual should describe the content, format and numbering of the data presentations. A standard presentation style guide describing formatting issues is also very helpful, and can be developed from the format and style issues described later in this chapter. Although the Tables Manual alone is sufficient to get the programming team going, a style guide will reduce the design requirements and speed development efforts.

At first, all efforts will be focused on the individual clinical study. The team should not lose sight of the long-term uses of the data presentation for planned summaries and integrated study submissions, however. Particular attention should be paid to the integration required for final submissions that represent the ultimate use of the data. If properly considered, the overall result will be the continual use of, and adherence to, standard programs, document templates and development tools.

Building and Testing The building and testing stage primarily involves the efforts of the programming staff. Testing should also involve an independent review phase, code execution, and duplication of results, and can be performed by independent programmers or a separate quality control group. This is a fundamental element of validating new code and its intended results. The documented, signed approval of code, resulting data presentations, and evidence of error correction efforts are not only essential to validation compliance, but can also be used as a staff training tool. Once approved, the code can be released for use (implementation). Subsequent changes that may be required should also be implemented in a documented manner, starting from the planning stage.

Maintaining and Archiving Once programs are implemented, all modifications must be well documented to display clear proof of product control and to suggest the continued successful and accurate execution of programs. These changes describe the evolution of the development effort, and can greatly reduce future duplication of effort.

Archiving not only includes the permanent storage of objects built and used, but also includes documenting and tracking later use. This documenting and tracking can prove extremely helpful in the integration of presentations in the various forms and uses of the clinical data. This is where the SDLC helps the individual study. The tracking can also be indispensable for subsequent integration efforts (NDA, IB, AR).

Expediting Drug and Biologics Development

Documenting Although good program development practices dictate self-documenting programs that are readable to the developers and other trained programmers, this is rarely sufficient for 21CFR11 compliance. Program use and methods must be understood by non-skilled and project-aware personnel as well. A well-implemented SDLC will contain templates and authorization documents that clearly show the overall project's evolution and status. This documentation should be provided in a Statistics Development Manual (SDM). The program documents will not only be available to guide interested parties, they will provide ready support for any possible audits and will provide future reference for training in the enforcement of standards.

Deviation from SDLC There are potential problems in using and adhering to a formal SDLC for clinical studies. One issue that requires consideration is the single-use nature of the programs. Most presentations have a singular purpose: Providing the displays required for one study alone. In other words, the displays may have minimal use elsewhere. Another problem is that the requirements and the analyses always seem to change. The reality of the study data also imposes changes that require near-instant re-coding, typically driven by study analyses changes based on real data. These changes are implemented "on-the-fly," and are made at the discretion of the statistician and the medical writers with very little planning. While this does not mean that the SDLC is not applicable to data displays, its implementation should be given more consideration within a company.

Electronic Presentation of Data More and more companies are providing submissions in an electronic format-as early as 2003, CDER reported that about 75% of all new NDAs were considered electronic filings to some extent, and that about 90% of those NDAs were entirely electronic. Under a December 2003 final rule, the agency required, for the first time, that a portion of the NDA-a new "content of labeling" section-be provided in electronic form in all cases.

In addition, the ICH E3 guidance mentions electronic formats as an option for any submission:

E3.PDF GUIDANCE FOR SECTION 11.4.2 - STATISTICAL/ ANALYTICAL ISSUES AND APPENDIX 16.1.9

" In the report of each controlled clinical study, there should be data listings. ... These data listings are necessary for the regulatory authority's statistical review, and the sponsor may be asked to supply these patient data listings in a computer-readable form."

This presents a formatting challenge, since the display media can affect the review in both positive and negative ways. On the plus side is the simple elimination of the bulk of paper. Even more helpful, electronic data filings allow for the generation of more varied and detailed presentations, with the computer providing advanced navigation and searching tools. The ability to quickly find, cross-reference, and use hyperlinks to show complex relationships, as well as to display multiple documents and/or even multiple versions of documents at once, can aid the review process significantly. Drawbacks for the developer include the significant extra effort required to build the advanced features into an ever-changing report, and uncertainty regarding whether the report(s) works in the unknown and uncontrolled reviewing environment. Reviewer equipment and capabilities for display can create issues such as limited viewing areas or only a partial ability to use some advanced reviewing techniques. In addition, the fact remains that some reviewers will always prefer paper, on which presentations must remain very clear.

In most cases, the development software provides a variety of output protocols. These protocols include the ability to generate HyperText Markup Language (HTML), Adobe's Portable Document Format (PDF), and eXtensible Markup Language (XML) output, which are available in most of the popular presentation tools. HTML is one of the standard Internet protocols. It allows instantaneous display of data to anyone privileged to have access to a company's web site. The FDA has requested the PDF protocol for submissions, although many of the standardization groups are moving towards XML as the technology of choice. Both allow for standardized formatting, hypertext linking, bookmarking and other electronic review techniques. The challenge for the developer is to ensure that displays are accurately provided using all protocols (HTML, PDF and XML), and that the subtle differences of each do not corrupt or detract from the intended presentation. Although currently built by programming integrators, this can be made more efficient by establishing workable standards for the initial development programmers in a format common to all display protocols.

It is worth noting that XML is becoming extremely popular as a presentation tool, not only for its formatting capabilities, but also for its machine and human readability, as well as its ability to transport data within the presentation. These features give a data presentation a broader range of use. The protocol allows reviewers to clearly see the source of the data, its manipulation, and its formatting into the eventual presentation. Reviewer validation of data formatting, summarization and derivation are apparent alongside the data. This makes the data readily available for validation or additional analysis as well. This technology could revolutionize the review of data, as its basic structure includes the framework for a comprehensive linking of listings, table displays, and data throughout and across reports. For developers, the capability for integrated analysis is made much easier, although it comes at the price of increased up-front planning. The complexity of this enhanced effort requires a much higher level of display development standardization. The early adoption of standards will provide the maximum returns over time.

Perhaps the most important point that can be made is that, for all of these reasons, efficiencies of development, review and use can be gained when standards are used. Each of the above DP uses represents a different end product, and may be used for differing studies and indications. Though there may be no constants in the review and approval process, the more that are attempted, the closer the process becomes to being standardized.

Standard Formatting As mentioned, the structure of the presentations should be consistent, readable, and clear. Most importantly, the presentations should assist and enhance the review. Established and enforced standards for the structural format will help achieve these imprecise goals. Decisions and ongoing attention are required at three levels of structure: (1) agreement on an organization and layout that meet regulatory standards; (2) consistency of display content; and (3) the use of a standard page format (font, orientation, numbering).

The ICH has addressed the organization of reports by providing a clear directive for report format and presentation in the guideline "STRUCTURE AND CONTENT OF CLINICAL STUDY REPORTS- E3." This guidance provides clear direction on the structure of a clinical study report. If this standard is used, decisions regarding display order become moot. Though deviations from the E3 guidance are sometimes required, there is just no compelling reason to not follow this clear format. When this format is employed, the order of the displays is clear, providing a numbering scheme required for report identification and compartmentalization, and allowing for accurate cross-referencing. This one issue will greatly enhance the ability to create data presentations and write the final study report with accurate cross-referencing. Not including data presentations that appear in the body of the text, the guidance separates the presentations into two sections: (1) additional tables, figures and graphs (Section 14); and (2) complete data listings of patient information (Appendix 16). The tables and figures should be sufficiently descriptive to stand alone, but require coordination with the tables and figures used within the study report (as described in Chapter 16). Within each section, there is a specific order of information for each data domain. A working Table of Contents is provided here, with examples provided later in the chapter.

Example Table of Contents of Standard Data Presentation

Table Number	Data Domain or Table title
Tables 14.1*	Demographic Data
Table 14.1.1	Summary of Subject Enrolled Status
Table 14.1.2	Summary of Demography By Treatment Group
Table 14.1.3	Demography Summary By Site - Test Article Group
Table 14.1.4	Demography Summary By Site - Control Group
Table 14.1.5	Demography Summary By Site - All Treatment Groups
Table 14.1.6	Supplemental Demography Summary By Site - Test Article Group
Table 14.1.7	Supplemental Demography Summary By Site - Control Group
Table 14.1.8	Supplemental Demography Summary By Site - All Treatment Groups
Table 14.1.9	Summary of Supplemental Demography By Treatment Group and Background Characteristics
Tables 14.2	Efficacy Data
Table 14.2.1	Number of Subjects Excluded from Efficacy-Evaluable Population
Table 14.2.2	Summary of Duration of Treatment Exposure
Table 14.2*****	Additional Efficacy Summary Displays
Tables 14.3	Safety Data
Tables 14.3.1	Displays of Adverse Events
Table 14.3.1.1	Summary of Treatment Emergent Adverse Events By Site - Test Article Group
Table 14.3.1.2	Summary of Treatment Emergent Adverse Events By Site - Control Group

–continued–

Table 14.3.1.3	Summary of Treatment Emergent Adverse Events By Site - All Treatment Groups
Table 14.3.1.	Summary of Treatment Emergent Adverse Events By Treatment Group
Table 14.3.1.5	Identification of Subjects with Treatment Emergent Adverse Events
Tables 14.3.2	Listings of Deaths, Other Serious and Significant Adverse Events
Table 14.3.2.1	Subject Listing of Deaths
Table 14.3.2.2	Subject Listing of Other Serious and Significant Adverse Events
Tables 14.3.3*****	Narratives of Deaths, Other Serious and Certain Other Significant Adverse Events
Table 14.3.3.1	Subject Listing of Serious and Related Adverse Events
Table 14.3.3.2	Subject Listing of Serious Adverse Events Narrations
Tables 14.3.4	Abnormal Laboratory Value Listing (Each Patient)
Table 14.3.4.1#	Treatment Emergent Abnormal Laboratory Values - Hematology (by Subject)
Table 14.3.4.2	Treatment Emergent Abnormal Laboratory Values - Clinical Chemistry (by Subject)
Table 14.3.4.3	Treatment Emergent Abnormal Laboratory Values - Urinalysis(by Subject)
Tables 14.3.5	Summary Abnormal Laboratory Results
Table 14.3.5.1	Summary of Laboratory Results - Hematology
Table 14.3.5.1 (transposed presentation)	Summary of Laboratory Results - Hematology
Table 14.3.5.2	Summary of Laboratory Results - Clinical Chemistry
Table 14.3.5.3	Summary of Laboratory Results - Urinalysis
Table 14.3.5.4	Summary of Laboratory Trends - Hematology
Table 14.3.5.5	Summary of Laboratory Trends - Clinical Chemistry
Table 14.3.5.6	Summary of Laboratory Trends - Urinalysis
Table 14.3.5.7	Summary of Laboratory Value Changes - Hematology
Table 14.3.5.8	Summary of Laboratory Value Changes - Clinical Chemistry
Table 14.3.5.9	Summary of Laboratory Value Changes - Urinalysis
Tables 14.4	Additional tables as needed
Table 14.4.1	Study Start and End Dates
Table 14.4.2	Summary of Vital Signs

* Shaded rows are standard or required as described in the ICH Guideline: Structure And Content Of Clinical Study Reports, E3. # Identical in format and presentation to Appendix 16.2.8, selecting only abnormal results that were considered treatment emergent.

Example Table of Contents of Standard Data Presentation Listings

Appendix Number	Data Domain or Appendix title
Appendix 16.2.1*	Discontinued patients
Appendix 16.2.1	Subject Listing of Premature Terminations
Appendix 16.2.2	Protocol deviations
Appendix 16.2.3	Patients excluded from the efficacy analysis
Appendix 16.2.3.2	Listing of Subjects, Visits, and Data Excluded from Effectiveness Analysis
Appendix 16.2.4	Demographic data
Appendix 16.2.4.1	Subject Listing of Demography
Appendix 16.2.4.2	Supplemental Demography Subject Listing
Appendix 16.2.5	Compliance and/or drug concentration data (if available)
Appendix 16.2.5.1	Subject Listing of Doses Administered

—continued—

Appendix 16.2.6**	Individual efficacy response data
Appendix 16.2.7	Adverse event listings (each patient)
Appendix 16.2.7.1	Treatment Emergent Adverse Event Subject Listing
Appendix 16.2.7.2	Verbatim to Preferred Term Coding for Adverse Events
Appendix 16.2.7.3	Subject Listing of Serious Adverse Events
Appendix 16.2.7.4	Subject Listing of Premature Terminations Due to an Adverse Event
Appendix 16.2.7.5	Subject Listing of Dose Reductions Due to an Adverse Event
Appendix 16.2.8	Listing of individual laboratory measurements by patient (when required by regulatory authorities)
Appendix 16.2.8.1.1	Clinical Laboratory Data Subject Listing - Hematology
Appendix 16.2.8.1.2	Clinical Laboratory Data Subject Listing - Hematology
Appendix 16.2.8.2	Clinical Laboratory Data Subject Listing - Serum Chemistry
Appendix 16.2.8.3	Clinical Laboratory Data Subject Listing - Urinalysis
Appendix 16.2.9	Additional listings as needed
Appendix 16.2.9.1	Subject Listing of Study Dates
Appendix 16.2.9.2	Vital Signs Subject Listing
Appendix 16.2.9.3.1	Subject Listing of Concomitant Medications
Appendix 16.2.9.3.2	Verbatim to Preferred Term Coding for Concomitant Medications
Appendix 16.2.9.4	Verbatim to Preferred Term Coding for Medical History
Appendix 16.2.9.5	Clinical Laboratory Test Normal Ranges

* Shaded rows are standard or required as described in the ICH Guideline: Structure And Content Of Clinical Study Reports, E3. ** Standard display examples are not available, or too numerous to present.

Consistent Display Content

The content for the CSR Appendix 16 data listings is clear-cut, as the sponsor should typically present all clinical information obtained from each study. Although some data may not be mentioned or used directly in the report, it is prudent to provide all data to support a level of openness with the reviewers. This simplifies the listing creation, since the programming staff can address listings early and shift the more complex effort involved in generating tables and figures that support the analysis to a later time. When standard CRFs and database designs are employed, the task of standard listing generation becomes extremely efficient because the standard listings can be reused.

This brings to light the design of the case report forms (CRF), and the role that programming and statistics personnel play in their creation. When this process is undertaken with planning and foresight, both groups, along with data management, are brought in to review and approve the CRF design before the CRFs are used. This is the time for the enforcement of any programming standards and the required reconsideration of the data's pertinence to the analysis and presentation. The overriding rule of data collection should be that the data collected must support the study objective and illustrate the drug's safety and efficacy. Another helpful rule is that all data collected should be analyzed in some pre-planned manner. If data do not meet these basic criteria, its collection should be questioned. Standards assist the enforcement of these rules by utilizing some simple comparisons. The data are either previously required by the standard report format and are specific to the study objectives, or they are being unnecessarily collected. Although arguments can be made to collect data for administrative, monitoring or educational objectives that may be important in their own right, the data are not needed for reporting purposes. While the data may have value for these peripheral reasons, their collection should be questioned against efficiency and basic study objectives. This issue goes to the heart of how and why clinical studies are preformed, with the implementation seemingly unique to each company. It is helpful to achieve consensus on this issue because it helps focus the project team on data that flow from design to submission, as opposed to transient data that are used for a singular or temporary purpose. Additional data capture can be distracting and require unnecessary handling and effort. When these rules of data collection are met, the data presented match those needed for the report, and additional CRF tabulations become unnecessary. As mentioned previously, a standard tables manual will help describe the basic data approved for report presentation. This manual should be provided to the project team for discussion and agreement on this issue, since this can represent significant work that can potentially affect data quality and/or delay submission.

Where listings are straightforward, tables and figures represent more of a challenge because they serve three functions: (1) they support study conclusions within the report; (2) they describe the actual analysis; and (3) they support regulatory requirements. The tables that display the data supporting the primary analysis(es) should be placed within the body of the report in direct support of conclusions. Although some of these tables stand on their own, others can be subsets of the more expansive tables provided in Section 14. In recognition of this, the development staff should be cognizant of the needs of the report author, while coordinating the tables required for Section 14.

Finally, regulatory requirements exist for summary tables to describe patient identification, status at termination, safety, and test article application and treatment. These requirements can clearly be seen in the tables identified in the ICH E3 guidance. As these are repeating requirements for all studies, the development staff can treat these as they would the basic listings by establishing standard templates and performing advanced programming as feasible.

Standard Presentation Format: Page Formatting

At a more granular level for the development staff is how the data will be formatted within each individual presentation. This can be achieved by establishing a standard style guide that describes page layout of the font, page layout, titles, headings and footers. Consideration should be given to the style used in the report versus the data presentations, although the objectives of these efforts clearly differ.

As previously mentioned, the numbering scheme should be agreed upon and carried forward using the same font and point-size for data presentation titles throughout the report. Other style points found in reports and presentations would be naming and terminology conventions, header and footer content and style, page numbering, the size and type of paper, and margin sizes. Font size may change within the presentations as a technique to provide as much similar data as possible on one page, but should not be so small that it becomes difficult to read. Landscape orientation is generally preferable for data presentations, since it allows for more information to be presented on a single page and should be consistent throughout.

As technology advances into non-paper displays, display standards are becoming more of an issue. While they provide a unique and powerful tool for reviews, the development of advanced interaction techniques demands a different set of skills and tools. In planning the layout, basic reporting formats such as margins should still address the most restrictive aspects of the tools used for review.

Finally, the amount of consistency within and between the data presentations should be considered. Different types of data may require different handling and presentation. The presentation of adverse event information is much different than that required by laboratory data, although the identification and sub-setting by patient number or treatment grouping should remain the same. An early decision is required on whether or not to subset displays by visit or study day, treatment grouping or site/patient grouping, or other demographic variables.

When the same content, format, and organization are used for the presentations in each report, uniformity develops among the presentations. Not only does each report contain the same presentations in the same order with the same numbering schema, but the presentations themselves resemble each other to a large extent. When evaluating an application, a reviewer will want to compare similar information among the different studies. The standard presentation order and numbering will allow the reviewer to quickly and easily locate the desired information. Once located, each presentation will display the same information in the same manner, which will allow the reviewer to focus on the data being displayed rather than forcing the reviewer to compare incongruent data presentations.

Following are examples of displays that are consistent with the ICH E3 guide and that have a consistent look and feel. These presentations can be used as the basis for a Tables Manual for all studies, and can be used as the target for standardized CRFs and data structures.

STANDARD TABLES AND FIGURES

The following listing comprises a suggested set of standard data presentations for a clinical study report (CSR). There will be many study-specific tables and figures in the CSR that will be in addition to this proposed list of standard tables and figures applicable to all CSRs. Following this list is a sample presentation format for each table and figure, including the appendices. These samples can be used either as templates or guides.

TABLES AND FIGURES RELATED TO STUDY PATIENTS

Figure 1   Study Design and Schedule of Assessments
Figure 2   Disposition of Patients
Figure 3   Flow Chart of Subjects Analyzed
Table 1.1   Summary of Subject Completion

TABLES, FIGURES AND GRAPHS REFERRED TO BUT
NOT INCLUDED IN THE TEXT

Table 14.1.1   Summary of Subject Enrolled Status
Table 14.1.2   Summary of Demography By Treatment Group
Table 14.1.3   Demography Summary By Site - Test Article Group
Table 14.1.4   Demography Summary By Site - Control Group
Table 14.1.5   Demography Summary By Site - All Treatment Groups
Table 14.1.6   Supplemental Demography Summary By Site - Test Article Group
Table 14.1.7   Supplemental Demography Summary By Site - Control group
Table 14.1.8   Supplemental Demography Summary By Site - All Treatment Groups
Table 14.1.9   Summary of Supplemental Demography By Treatment Group and Background Characteristics
Table 14.2.1   Number of Subjects Excluded from Efficacy - Evaluable Population
Table 14.2.2   Summary of Duration of Treatment Exposure
Table 14.3.1.1   Summary of Subjects with Treatment Emergent Adverse Events By Site - Test Article Group
Table 14.3.1.2   Summary of Subjects with Treatment Emergent Adverse Events By Site - Control Group
Table 14.3.1.3   Summary of Treatment Emergent Adverse Events By Site - All Treatment Groups
Table 14.3.1.4   Summary of Treatment Emergent Adverse Events By Treatment Group
Table 14.3.1.5   Identification of Subjects with Treatment Emergent Adverse Events
Table 14.3.2.1   Subject Listing of Deaths
Table 14.3.2.2   Subject Listing of Other Serious and Significant Adverse Events
Table 14.3.3.1   Subject Listing of Serious and Related Adverse Events
Table 14.3.3.2   Subject of Listing of Serious Adverse Events Narrations
Table 14.3.4.1   Treatment Emergent Abnormal Laboratory Values - Hematology
Table 14.3.4.2   Treatment Emergent Abnormal Laboratory Values - Serum Chemistry
Table 14.3.4.3   Treatment Emergent Abnormal Laboratory Values - Urinalysis
Table 14.3.5.1   Summary of Laboratory Results - Hematology
Table 14.3.5.2   Summary of Laboratory Results - Clinical Chemistry
Table 14.3.5.3   Summary of Laboratory Results - Urinalysis
Table 14.3.5.4   Summary of Laboratory Trends - Hematology
Table 14.3.5.5   Summary of Laboratory Trends - Clinical Chemistry
Table 14.3.5.6   Summary of Laboratory Trends - Urinalysis
Table 14.3.5.7   Summary of Laboratory Value Changes - Hematology
Table 14.3.5.8   Summary of Laboratory Value Changes - Clinical Chemistry
Table 14.3.5.9   Summary of Laboratory Value Changes - Urinalysis
Table 14.4.1   Study Start and End Dates
Table 14.4.2   Summary of Vital Signs

APPENDICES

Appendix 16.2.2   Subject Listing of Premature Terminations
Appendix 16.2.3.2   Listing of Subjects, Visits, and Date Excluded from Effectiveness Analysis

Appendix 16.2.4.1   Subject Listing of Demography

Appendix 16.2.4.2   Supplemental Demography Subject Listing

Appendix 16.2.5.1   Subject Listing of Doses Administered

Appendix 16.2.7.1   Treatment Emergent Adverse Event Subject Listing

Appendix 16.2.7.2   Verbatim to Preferred Term Coding for Adverse Events

Appendix 16.2.7.3   Subject Listing of Serious Adverse Events

Appendix 16.2.7.4   Subject Listing of Premature Terminations Due to an Adverse Event

Appendix 16.2.7.5   Subject Listing of Dose Reductions Due to an Adverse Event

Appendix 16.2.8.1   Clinical Laboratory Data Subject Listing - Hematology

Appendix 16.2.8.2.2   Clinical Laboratory Data Subject Listing - Hematology

Appendix 16.2.8.2   Clinical Laboratory Data Subject Listing - Serum Chemistry

Appendix 16.2.8.3   Clinical Laboratory Data Subject Listing - Urinalysis

Appendix 16.2.9.1   Subject Listing of Study Dates

Appendix 16.2.9.2   Vital Signs Subject Listing

Appendix 16.2.9.3.1   Subject Listing of Concomitant Medications

Appendix 16.2.9.3.2   Verbatim to Preferred Term Coding for Concomitant Medications

Appendix 16.2.9.4   Verbatim to Preferred Term Coding for Medical History

Appendix 16.2.9.5   Clinical Laboratory Test Normal Ranges

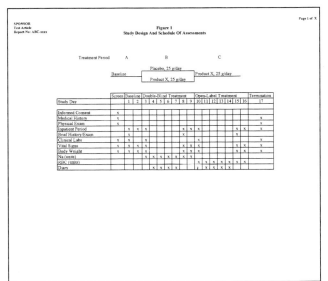

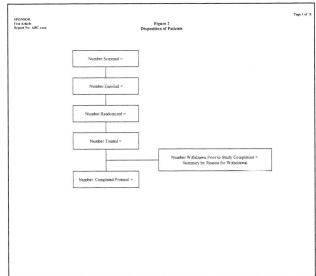

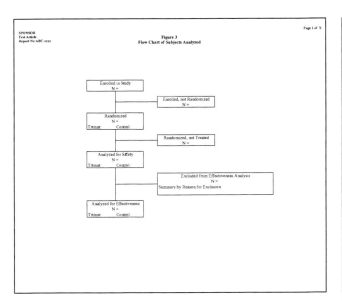

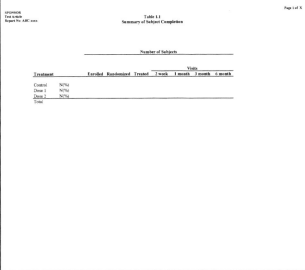

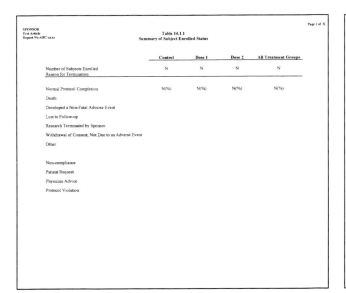

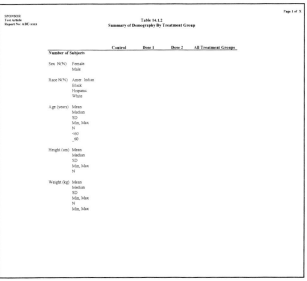

Expediting Drug and Biologics Development

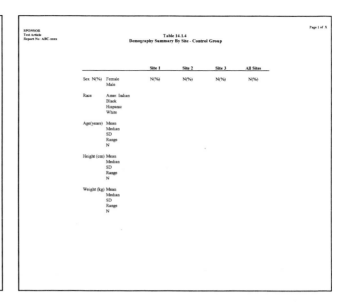

SPONSOR
Test Article
Report No:ABC-xxxx

Table 14.1.3
Demography Summary By Site - Test Article Group

		Site 1	Site 2	Site 3	All Sites
Sex N(%)	Female	N(%)	N(%)	N(%)	N(%)
	Male				
Race	Amer. Indian				
	Black				
	Hispanic				
	White				
Age (years)	Mean				
	Median				
	SD				
	Range				
	N				
Height (cm)	Mean				
	Median				
	SD				
	Range				
	N				
Weight (kg)	Mean				
	Median				
	SD				
	Range				
	N				

SPONSOR
Test Article
Report No: ABC-xxxx

Table 14.1.4
Demography Summary By Site - Control Group

		Site 1	Site 2	Site 3	All Sites
Sex N(%)	Female	N(%)	N(%)	N(%)	N(%)
	Male				
Race	Amer. Indian				
	Black				
	Hispanic				
	White				
Age(years)	Mean				
	Median				
	SD				
	Range				
	N				
Height (cm)	Mean				
	Median				
	SD				
	Range				
	N				
Weight (kg)	Mean				
	Median				
	SD				
	Range				
	N				

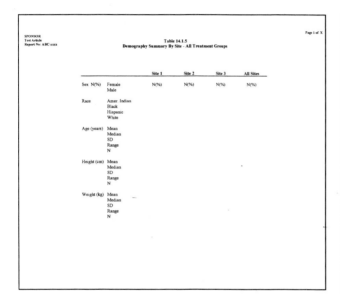

SPONSOR
Test Article
Report No: ABC-xxxx

Table 14.1.5
Demography Summary By Site - All Treatment Groups

		Site 1	Site 2	Site 3	All Sites
Sex N(%)	Female	N(%)	N(%)	N(%)	N(%)
	Male				
Race	Amer. Indian				
	Black				
	Hispanic				
	White				
Age (years)	Mean				
	Median				
	SD				
	Range				
	N				
Height (cm)	Mean				
	Median				
	SD				
	Range				
	N				
Weight (kg)	Mean				
	Median				
	SD				
	Range				
	N				

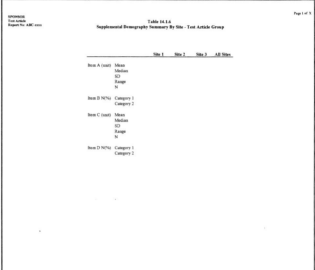

SPONSOR
Test Article
Report No: ABC-xxxx

Table 14.1.6
Supplemental Demography Summary By Site - Test Article Group

		Site 1	Site 2	Site 3	All Sites
Item A (unit)	Mean				
	Median				
	SD				
	Range				
	N				
Item B N(%)	Category 1				
	Category 2				
Item C (unit)	Mean				
	Median				
	SD				
	Range				
	N				
Item D N(%)	Category 1				
	Category 2				

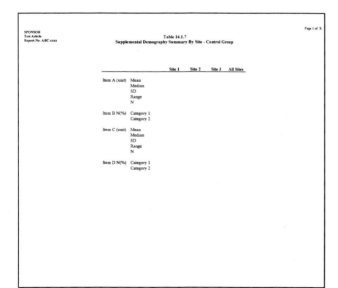

SPONSOR
Test Article
Report No: ABC-xxxx

Table 14.1.7
Supplemental Demography Summary By Site - Control Group

		Site 1	Site 2	Site 3	All Sites
Item A (unit)	Mean				
	Median				
	SD				
	Range				
	N				
Item B N(%)	Category 1				
	Category 2				
Item C (unit)	Mean				
	Median				
	SD				
	Range				
	N				
Item D N(%)	Category 1				
	Category 2				

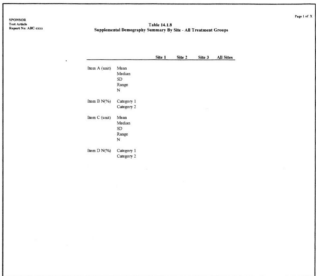

SPONSOR
Test Article
Report No: ABC-xxxx

Table 14.1.8
Supplemental Demography Summary By Site - All Treatment Groups

		Site 1	Site 2	Site 3	All Sites
Item A (unit)	Mean				
	Median				
	SD				
	Range				
	N				
Item B N(%)	Category 1				
	Category 2				
Item C (unit)	Mean				
	Median				
	SD				
	Range				
	N				
Item D N(%)	Category 1				
	Category 2				

SPONSOR
Test Article
Report No: ABC-xxxx

Page 1 of X

Table 14.1.9
Summary of Supplemental Demography By Treatment Group and Background Characteristics

		Control	Dose 1	Dose 2	All Treatment Groups
Number of Subjects					
Item A (unit)	Mean				
	Median				
	SD				
	Min, Max				
	N				
Item B N(%)	Category 1				
	Category 2				
Item C (unit)	Mean				
	Median				
	SD				
	Min, Max				
	N				
Item D N(%)	Category 1				
	Category 2				

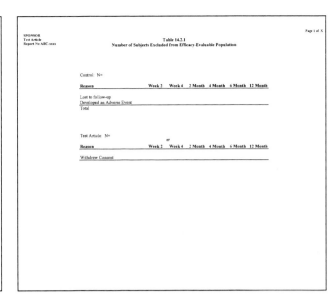

SPONSOR
Test Article
Report No: ABC-xxxx

Page 1 of X

Table 14.2.1
Number of Subjects Excluded from Efficacy-Evaluable Population

Control: N=

Reason	Week 2	Week 4	2 Month	4 Month	6 Month	12 Month
Lost to follow-up						
Developed an Adverse Event						
Total						

Test Article: N=

Reason	Week 2	Week 4	2 Month	4 Month	6 Month	12 Month
Withdrew Consent						

SPONSOR
Test Article
Report No: ABC-xxxx

Page 1 of X

Table 14.2.2
Summary of Duration of Treatment Exposure

p

Treatment	Less Than One Week	One Week To 30 Days	31 Days To 90 Days	91 Days To 180 Days	Total	Minimum	Mean	Median	Maximum
Control									
Test Article									

Time on Therapy (Days) spans Minimum, Mean, Median, Maximum.

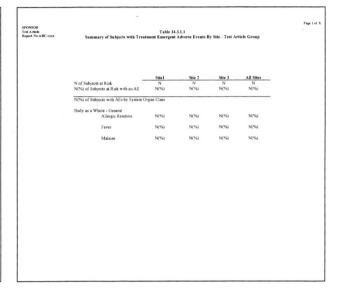

SPONSOR
Test Article
Report No: ABC-xxxx

Page 1 of X

Table 14.3.1.1
Summary of Subjects with Treatment Emergent Adverse Events By Site - Test Article Group

	Site 1	Site 2	Site 3	All Sites
N of Subjects at Risk	N	N	N	N
N(%) of Subjects at Risk with an AE	N(%)	N(%)	N(%)	N(%)
N(%) of Subjects with AEs by System Organ Class				
Body as a Whole - General				
Allergic Reaction	N(%)	N(%)	N(%)	N(%)
Fever	N(%)	N(%)	N(%)	N(%)
Malaise	N(%)	N(%)	N(%)	N(%)

SPONSOR
Test Article
Report No: ABC-xxxx

Page 1 of X

Table 14.3.1.2
Summary of Subjects with Treatment Emergent Adverse Events By Site - Control Group

	Site 1	Site 2	Site 3	All Sites
N of Subjects at Risk	N	N	N	N
N(%) of Subjects at Risk with an AE	N(%)	N(%)	N(%)	N(%)
N(%) of Subjects with AEs by System Organ Class				
Body as a Whole - General				
Allergic Reaction	N(%)	N(%)	N(%)	N(%)
Fever	N(%)	N(%)	N(%)	N(%)
Malaise	N(%)	N(%)	N(%)	N(%)

SPONSOR
Test Article
Report No: ABC-xxxx

Page 1 of X

Table 14.3.1.3
Summary of Treatment Emergent Adverse Events By Site - All Treatment Groups

	Site 1	Site 2	Site 3	All Sites
N of Subjects at Risk	N	N	N	N
N(%) of Subjects at Risk with an AE	N(%)	N(%)	N(%)	N(%)
N(%) of Subjects with AEs by System Organ Class				
Body as a Whole - General				
Allergic Reaction	N(%)	N(%)	N(%)	N(%)
Fever	N(%)	N(%)	N(%)	N(%)
Malaise	N(%)	N(%)	N(%)	N(%)

Expediting Drug and Biologics Development

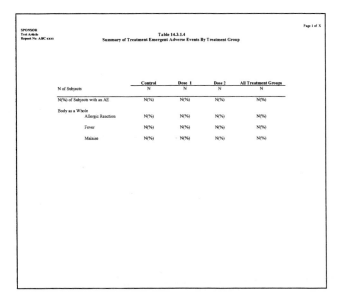

SPONSOR
Test Article
Report No: ABC-xxxx

Table 14.3.1.4
Summary of Treatment Emergent Adverse Events By Treatment Group

	Control	Dose 1	Dose 2	All Treatment Groups
N of Subjects	N	N	N	N
N(%) of Subjects with an AE	N(%)	N(%)	N(%)	N(%)
Body as a Whole				
Allergic Reaction	N(%)	N(%)	N(%)	N(%)
Fever	N(%)	N(%)	N(%)	N(%)
Malaise	N(%)	N(%)	N(%)	N(%)

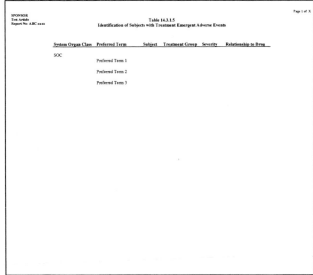

SPONSOR
Test Article
Report No: ABC-xxxx

Table 14.3.1.5
Identification of Subjects with Treatment Emergent Adverse Events

System Organ Class	Preferred Term	Subject	Treatment Group	Severity	Relationship to Drug
SOC					
	Preferred Term 1				
	Preferred Term 2				
	Preferred Term 3				

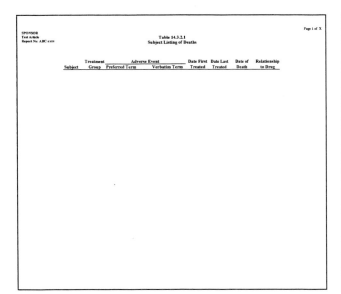

SPONSOR
Test Article
Report No: ABC-xxxx

Table 14.3.2.1
Subject Listing of Deaths

Subject	Treatment Group	Adverse Event Preferred Term	Verbatim Term	Date First Treated	Date Last Treated	Date of Death	Relationship to Drug

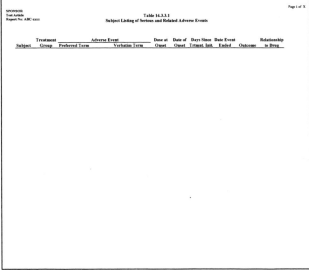

SPONSOR
Test Article
Report No: ABC-xxxx

Table 14.3.3.1
Subject Listing of Serious and Related Adverse Events

Subject	Treatment Group	Adverse Event Preferred Term	Verbatim Term	Dose at Onset	Date of Onset	Days Since Trtmnt. Init.	Date Event Ended	Outcome	Relationship to Drug

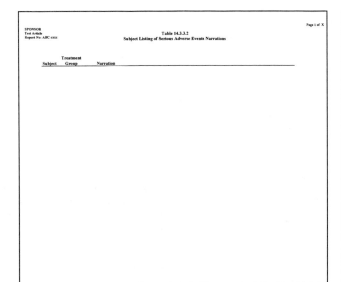

SPONSOR
Test Article
Report No: ABC-xxxx

Table 14.3.3.2
Subject Listing of Serious Adverse Events Narrations

Subject	Treatment Group	Narration

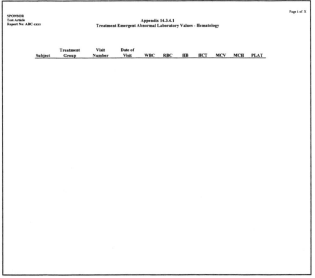

SPONSOR
Test Article
Report No: ABC-xxxx

Appendix 14.3.4.1
Treatment Emergent Abnormal Laboratory Values - Hematology

Subject	Treatment Group	Visit Number	Date of Visit	WBC	RBC	HB	HCT	MCV	MCH	PLAT

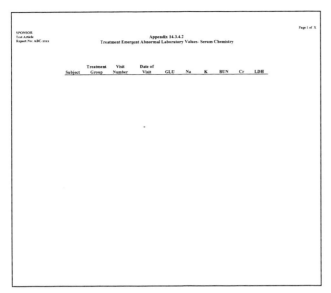

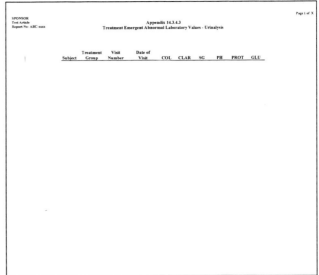

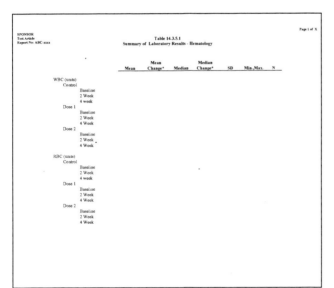

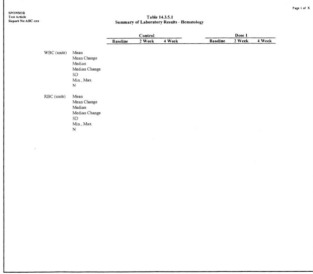

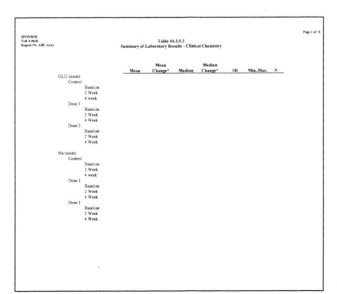

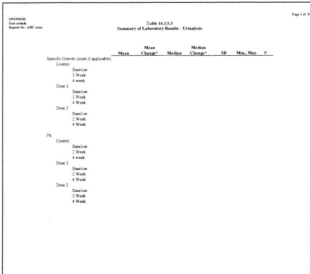

Expediting Drug and Biologics Development

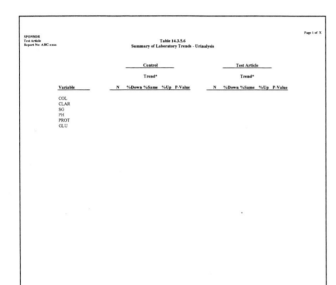

SPONSOR
Test Article
Report No: ABC-xxxx

Table 14.3.5.4
Summary of Laboratory Trends - Hematology

	Control					Test Article			
		Trend*					Trend*		
Variable	N	%Down	%Same	%Up	P-Value	N	%Down	%Same	%Up P-Value
WBC									
RBC									
HB									
HCT									
MCV									
MCH									
PLAT									
DIFF:									
POLY									
BAND									
LYMPH									
MONO									
EOS									
BASO									
ATY.LYM.									

SPONSOR
Test Article
Report No: ABC-xxxx

Page 1 of X

Table 14.3.5.5
Summary of Laboratory Trends - Clinical Chemistry

	Control					Test Article			
		Trend*					Trend*		
Variable	N	%Down	%Same	%Up	P-Value	N	%Down	%Same	%Up P-Value
GLU									
Na									
K									
BUN									
Cr									
LDH									

SPONSOR
Test Article
Report No: ABC-xxxx

Page 1 of X

Table 14.3.5.6
Summary of Laboratory Trends - Urinalysis

	Control					Test Article			
		Trend*					Trend*		
Variable	N	%Down	%Same	%Up	P-Value	N	%Down	%Same	%Up P-Value
COL									
CLAR									
SG									
PH									
PROT									
GLU									

SPONSOR
Test Article
Report No: ABC-xxxx

Page 1 of X

Table 14.3.5.7
Summary of Laboratory Value Changes - Hematology

	CONTROL					TEST ARTICLE				
		On Treatment					On Treatment			
Variable	Baseline	Low	Normal	High	Missing	Baseline	Low	Normal	High	Missing
WBC	Low					Low				
	Normal					Normal				
	High					High				
	Missing					Missing				
RBC	Low					Low				
	Normal					Normal				
	High					High				
	Missing					Missing				
HB	Low					Low				
	Normal					Normal				
	High					High				
	Missing					Missing				
HCT	Low					Low				
	Normal					Normal				
	High					High				
	Missing					Missing				

SPONSOR
Test Article
Report No: ABC-xxxx

Page 1 of X

Table 14.3.5.8
Summary of Laboratory Value Changes - Clinical Chemistry

	CONTROL					TEST ARTICLE				
		On Treatment					On Treatment			
Variable	Baseline	Low	Normal	High	Missing	Baseline	Low	Normal	High	Missing
Glucose	Low					Low				
	Normal					Normal				
	High					High				
	Missing					Missing				
Na	Low					Low				
	Normal					Normal				
	High					High				
	Missing					Missing				
K	Low					Low				
	Normal					Normal				
	High					High				
	Missing					Missing				
BUN	Low					Low				
	Normal					Normal				
	High					High				
	Missing					Missing				
Cr	Low					Low				
	Normal					Normal				
	High					High				
	Missing					Missing				

SPONSOR
Test Article
Report No: ABC-xxxx

Page 1 of X

Table 14.3.5.9
Summary of Laboratory Value Changes - Urinalysis

	CONTROL					TEST ARTICLE				
		On Treatment					On Treatment			
Variable	Baseline	Low	Normal	High	Missing	Baseline	Low	Normal	High	Missing
COL	Low					Low				
	Normal					Normal				
	High					High				
	Missing					Missing				
CLAR	Low					Low				
	Normal					Normal				
	High					High				
	Missing					Missing				
SG	Low					Low				
	Normal					Normal				
	High					High				
	Missing					Missing				
PH	Low					Low				
	Normal					Normal				
	High					High				
	Missing					Missing				
PROT	Low					Low				
	Normal					Normal				
	High					High				
	Missing					Missing				

SPONSOR
Test Article
Report No: ABC-xxx

Table 14.4.1
Study Start and End Dates

Page 1 of X

Investigator	First Patient Visit	Last Patient Visit

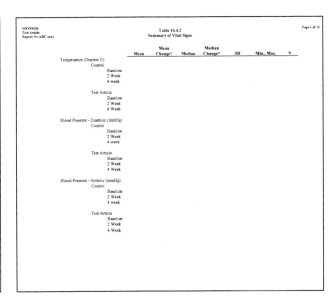

SPONSOR
Test Article
Report No: ABC-xxxx

Table 14.4.2
Summary of Vital Signs

Page 1 of X

	Mean	Mean Change*	Median	Median Change*	SD	Min., Max.	N
Temperature (Degrees C)							
Control							
Baseline							
2 Week							
4 week							
Test Article							
Baseline							
2 Week							
4 Week							
Blood Pressure - Diastolic (mmHg)							
Control							
Baseline							
2 Week							
4 week							
Test Article							
Baseline							
2 Week							
4 Week							
Blood Pressure - Systolic (mmHg)							
Control							
Baseline							
2 Week							
4 week							
Test Article							
Baseline							
2 Week							
4 Week							

SPONSOR
Test Article
Report No: ABC-xxxx

Appendix 16.2.2
Subject Listing of Premature Terminations

Page 1 of X

Subject	Treatment Group	Sex	Race	Age	Date of Last Visit	Duration of Treatment	Date Last Dose Received	Reason for Discontinuation

SPONSOR
Test Article
Report No: ABC-xxxx

Appendix 16.2.3.2
Listing of Subjects, Visits, and Data Excluded from Effectiveness Analysis

Page 1 of X

Treatment Group	Subject	Sex	Race	Age	Visit(s) Excluded	Data Excluded	Reason(s)
Test Article							
Control							

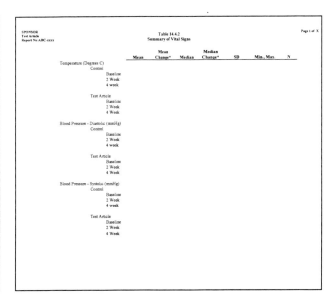

SPONSOR
Test Article
Report No: ABC-xxxx

Appendix 16.2.4.1
Subject Listing of Demography

Page 1 of X

Subject	Treatment Group	Age (yrs)	Sex	Race	Height (cm)	Weight (kg)	Concurrent Disease Preferred Term	Concurrent Disease Verbatim Term

SPONSOR
Test Article
Report No: ABC-xxxx

Table 14.4.2
Summary of Vital Signs

Page 1 of X

	Mean	Mean Change*	Median	Median Change*	SD	Min., Max.	N
Temperature (Degrees C)							
Control							
Baseline							
2 Week							
4 week							
Test Article							
Baseline							
2 Week							
4 Week							
Blood Pressure - Diastolic (mmHg)							
Control							
Baseline							
2 Week							
4 week							
Test Article							
Baseline							
2 Week							
4 Week							
Blood Pressure - Systolic (mmHg)							
Control							
Baseline							
2 Week							
4 week							
Test Article							
Baseline							
2 Week							
4 Week							

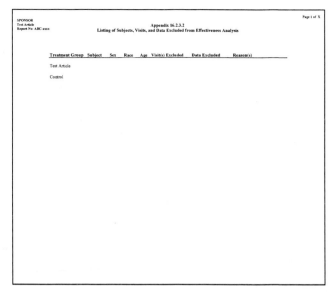

SPONSOR
Test Article
Report No: ABC-xxxx

Appendix 16.2.2
Subject Listing of Premature Terminations

Subject	Treatment Group	Sex	Race	Age	Date of Last Visit	Duration of Treatment	Date Last Dose Received	Reason for Discontinuation

SPONSOR
Test Article
Report No: ABC-xxxx

Appendix 16.2.3.2
Listing of Subjects, Visits, and Data Excluded from Effectiveness Analysis

Treatment Group	Subject	Sex	Race	Age	Visit(s) Excluded	Data Excluded	Reason(s)

Test Article

Control

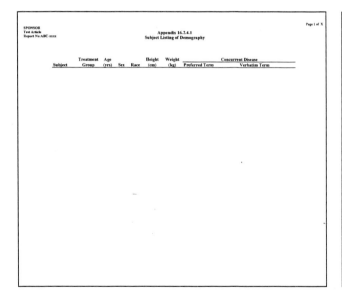

SPONSOR
Test Article
Report No: ABC-xxxx

Appendix 16.2.4.1
Subject Listing of Demography

Subject	Treatment Group	Age (yrs)	Sex	Race	Height (cm)	Weight (kg)	Concurrent Disease Preferred Term	Verbatim Term

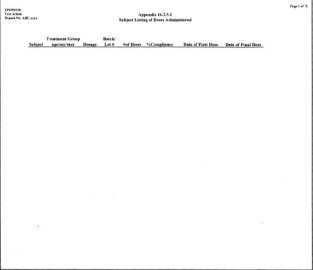

SPONSOR
Test Article
Report No: ABC-xxxx

Appendix 16.2.5.1
Subject Listing of Doses Administered

Subject	Treatment Group age/sex/race	Dosage	Batch/ Lot #	#of Doses	%Compliance	Date of First Dose	Date of Final Dose

SPONSOR
Test Article
Report No: ABC-xxxx

Appendix 16.2.7.1
Treatment Emergent Adverse Event Subject Listing

Subject=   Sex=   Race=   Age=   Weight=   Treatment Group=

Adverse Event Preferred Term	Verbatim Term	Dose at Onset	Date of Onset	Days Since Trtmnt. Init.	Date Ended	Severity	Causality	Outcome

SPONSOR
Test Article
Report No: ABC-xxxx

Appendix 16.2.7.2
Verbatim to Preferred Term Coding for Adverse Events

System Organ Class	Preferred Term	Verbatim Term

SPONSOR
Test Article
Report No: ABC-xxxx

Page 1 of X

Appendix 16.2.7.3
Subject Listing of Serious Adverse Events

Subject	Treatment Group	Adverse Event Preferred Term	Verbatim Term	Dose at Onset	Date of Onset	Days Since Trtmnt. Init.	Date Event Ended	Outcome	Relationship to Drug

SPONSOR
Test Article
Report No: ABC-xxxx

Page 1 of X

Appendix 16.2.7.4
Subject Listing of Premature Terminations Due to an Adverse Event

Subject	Treatment Group	Adverse Event Preferred Term	Verbatim Term	Date First Treated	Duration of Treatment	Date of Withdrawal	Severity	Relationship to Drug

SPONSOR
Test Article
Report No: ABC-xxxx

Page 1 of X

Appendix 16.2.7.5
Subject Listing of Dose Reductions Due to an Adverse Event

Subject	Treatment Group	Date First Treated	Date of Reduction	Original Dose	Reduced Dose	Reason for Dose Reduction

SPONSOR
Test Article
Report No: ABC-xxxx

Page 1 of X

Appendix 16.2.8.1
Clinical Laboratory Data Subject Listing - Hematology

Subject	Treatment Group	Visit Number	Date of Visit	WBC	RBC	HB	HCT	MCV	MCH	PLAT

SPONSOR
Test Article
Report No: ABC-xxxx

Page 1 of X

Appendix 16.2.8.2.2
Clinical Laboratory Data Subject Listing - Hematology

Subject	Treatment Group	Visit Number	Date of Visit	POLY	BAND	LYMPH	MONO	EOS	BASO	ATY.LYM.

SPONSOR
Test Article
Report No: ABC-xxxx

Page 1 of X

Appendix 16.2.8.2
Clinical Laboratory Data Subject Listing - Serum Chemistry

Subject	Treatment Group	Visit Number	Date of Visit	GLU	Na	K	BUN	Cr	LDH

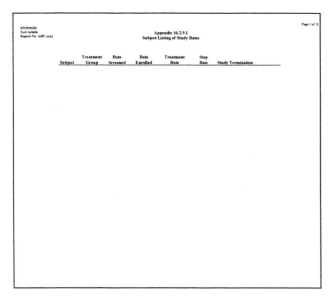

SPONSOR
Test Article
Report No: ABC-xxxx

Appendix 16.2.9.1
Subject Listing of Study Dates

Subject	Treatment Group	Date Screened	Date Enrolled	Treatment Date	Stop Date	Study Termination

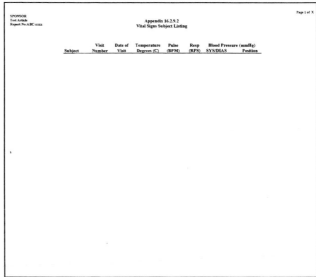

SPONSOR
Test Article
Report No: ABC-xxxx

Appendix 16.2.9.2
Vital Signs Subject Listing

Subject	Visit Number	Date of Visit	Temperature Degrees (C)	Pulse (BPM)	Resp (RPS)	Blood Pressure (mmHg) SYS/DIAS	Position

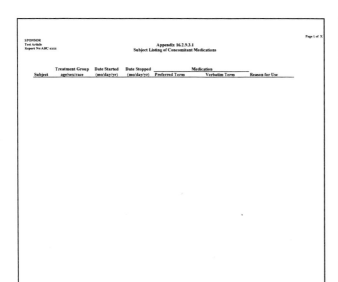

SPONSOR
Test Article
Report No:/ABC-xxxx

Appendix 16.2.9.3.1
Subject Listing of Concomitant Medications

Subject	Treatment Group age/sex/race	Date Started (mo/day/yr)	Date Stopped (mo/day/yr)	Medication Preferred Term	Verbatim Term	Reason for Use

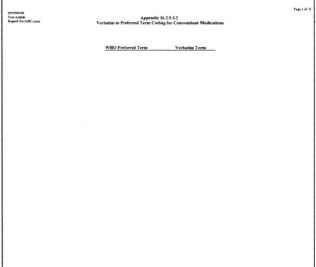

SPONSOR
Test Article
Report No: ABC-xxxx

Appendix 16.2.9.3.2
Verbatim to Preferred Term Coding for Concomitant Medications

WHO Preferred Term	Verbatim Term

SPONSOR
Test Article
Report No: ABC-xxxx

Appendix 16.2.9.4
Verbatim to Preferred Term Coding for Medical History

System Organ Class	MedDRA Preferred Term	Verbatim Term

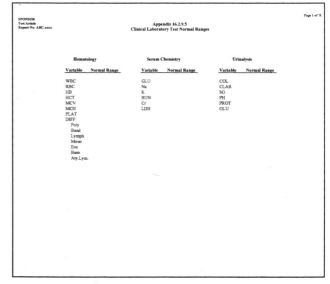

SPONSOR
Test Article
Report No: ABC-xxxx

Appendix 16.2.9.5
Clinical Laboratory Test Normal Ranges

Hematology		Serum Chemistry		Urinalysis	
Variable	Normal Range	Variable	Normal Range	Variable	Normal Range
WBC		GLU		COL	
RBC		Na		CLAR	
HB		K		SG	
HCT		BUN		PH	
MCV		Cr		PROT	
MCH		LDH		GLU	
PLAT					
DIFF:					
Poly					
Band					
Lymph					
Mono					
Eos					
Baso					
Aty.Lym.					

CHAPTER 17

Analysis Plans

by Antonis Koutsoukos, PhD and James Matcham, PhD, MSc, CStat.

The statistical analysis plan plays a number of important roles in ensuring the integrity of the results of any clinical trial. One of the more obvious roles that the analysis plan plays is in prospectively describing how a trial is to be analyzed. The highest level of scientific standards dictates that a clinical trial's analysis should be planned, and not conducted "on the fly." A second, less obvious, but equally important role for the analysis plan is that it dictates a certain discipline for the overall process when the plan is written in conjunction with a protocol and data collection tools. Viewed in this way, the analysis plan forms one of the "big three" documents at the start of every clinical trial. The smart clinical development team will finalize these three documents before starting any clinical trial.

In its own role, the analysis plan provides an anchor for what is being done, and the reason for why it is being done. It could be easily (and successfully) argued that, if the analysis of a particular variable is not in the analysis plan, that variable should not be in the protocol and should not be collected as part of the case record. Maintaining this philosophy will ensure that the protocols are always drafted with a well thought-out focus. Proper planning is essential when subjects are exposed to investigational products.

To further cement the importance of statistical planning prior to conducting clinical trials, the FDA has adopted the ICH guideline entitled, "Statistical Principles for Clinical Trials" (E9). The guidance provides recommendations regarding the statistical principles and methodology for conducting clinical trials designed to support marketing applications, and to promote the robustness of the results and conclusions drawn from these studies. Many in the drug development industry consider E9 to be a textbook within itself. This chapter focuses on the E9 guidance, and discusses issues that are essential in the statistical process of planning, analyzing and reporting clinical trials.

Study Planning: Protocol Development Statisticians should play an active role in the development of a protocol to ensure that it contains valid statistical design elements to meet the needs of the protocol and that valid statements adequately describe the anticipated analyses. The study objectives (primary and secondary) should be clearly stated in terms of specific endpoints or variables. Background information on the nature of the disease and its treatment, of the study treatment, and the practical constraints related to the availability of the patient population and resources should be considered in the study design and should be included in the protocol. Information on all preclinical and clinical studies should be provided. To the degree possible, the inclusion and exclusion criteria for the study population should mirror the treatment's intended use and be strictly followed.

Techniques used to avoid bias include randomization and blinding (masking). For randomized studies, details of the treatment assignments should be included. Methods of maintaining and breaking the blind in blinded studies, and reasons and methods of minimizing bias in unblinded studies, should be provided.

Information from which the sample size estimates are derived (usually from previous studies) and methods for the sample size determination, which should always be based on the primary endpoint of the study, should be clearly stated and referenced in the protocol. The selection of the primary endpoint must be based on experience gained in previous studies and the literature, and must be a reliable and objective measure of clinical activity, benefit, and relevance to the study population. Sometimes, one may use more than a single primary endpoint to design a study that covers a broad range of therapeutic effects. In this case, the primary hypotheses should be clearly stated with respect to these endpoints, and the effect on the type I error must be addressed. Appropriate adjustments of the type I error should be clearly written into the protocol. In some cases, a primary endpoint could be defined as the combination of other endpoints to create a so-called composite endpoint. This approach addresses multiplicity issues without requiring statistical adjustments for multiple endpoints. On the other hand, composite endpoints need to be validated to represent an objective measure of the treatment effect. Issues related to missing data from the individual components of a composite endpoint, and the subjectivity involved if these components represent rating scales (especially in non-blinded studies), need to be addressed prospectively.

Secondary endpoints are supportive variables related the secondary objectives of the study, and their selection should be based on the idea that they will play an important role in the interpretation of the study results. There should be a small number of secondary endpoints and they should be pre-specified in the protocol.

Formal or informal plans for any interim analysis used to compare treatments groups for either efficacy or safety need to be clearly stated in the protocol. Group-sequential designs are the most commonly used because of their practicality in assessing treatment effects at periodic intervals for accumulated data. There are a large number of statistical methods that control the overall type I error and provide specific rules for stopping a study for either efficacy (superior of inferior treatment) or safety; therefore, it is important to specify these methods in advanced. Although they need not be specified in the protocol, the staff involved in the interim analyses should always be assigned before any interim analysis takes place. In addition, personnel involved directly in the conduct of the study should not be aware of the results. An independent data monitoring committee could be used to evaluate the results of the interim analysis and make recommendations about continuation of the study. A statistician not involved in the conduct of the study should analyze the data.

The protocol should clearly define the primary analysis population (i.e., intent-to-treat or evaluable), or the per-protocol population, and details of the statistical methodology for analyzing the primary and secondary endpoints. The hypotheses to be tested together with the level of statistical significance to be used, an estimation of parameters, strategies and methods for handling missing data should be all clearly stated. Alternative ways of analyzing data should be described when assumptions underlying the statistical methods are violated. All variables collected in the study should be included in the protocol.

Statistical Analysis Plan The statistical analysis plan (SAP) details and documents the statistical aspects of a clinical trial or the planned analyses across clinical studies. The SAP documents prospective decisions for analysis made before the study begins, and expands on the statistical sections provided in the protocol. Details of the statistical methodology of analyzing all endpoints, definitions of endpoints and derivation rules, imputation methods, patient populations, and robustness/sensitivity analyses are included. All required tables, listings and graphs for the planned statistical analyses are included in the SAP. The SAP should also document analyses of clinical studies, such as meta-analyses, integrated summaries of efficacy and/or safety, and interim analyses. The SAP is written by a biostatistician, preferably the study statistician, and is reviewed and approved by a supervisory statistician and the clinical study team. For large clinical studies, the SAP may also need to be reviewed and approved by a separate review board and by the regulatory authorities.

An example of the content of an SAP is presented in an addendum entitled, "Statistical Analysis Plan Template," at the end of this chapter.

Statistical Process for the Analysis and Reporting of Clinical Trials This section provides some ideas regarding a standard statistical process for the analysis and reporting of clinical trials. This process could be used as the starting point in the planning for the analysis and reporting of any particular clinical trial. It includes the planning of statistical programming and analyses and reporting of results from an individual clinical trial. The section identifies the need for biostatistics department standards for endpoint definitions, dataset specifications, table shells and analysis methods. An established process will promote quality and efficiency in analyzing and reporting clinical trials, and in the completion of clinical study reports (CSRs) and electronic submissions to regulatory authorities.

Analysis Process Overview The main goal in the preparation for analysis should be to carry out as many tasks as possible, as early as possible, before the database is ready to be locked for analysis. This leaves the time after the database lock for running programs, interpreting analysis output, dealing with unexpected statistical issues and preparing the draft CSR. In this way, the time taken for the statistical analysis is minimized and, therefore, the time on the project critical path is also minimized.

Four critical periods are identified in the analysis process. The first period is defined as any time after the clinical trial protocol and statistical analysis plan have been completed but before the point of the database lock, and comprises activities that require little or no study data. During this time, all of the documents that specify the case report tabulation (CRT) datasets (analysis datasets), analysis methods, format of tables, listings and graphs, programming standards and directory structure conventions can be prepared.

The second period is defined as the period beginning four weeks before the database lock, and comprises activities that require nearly all study data. At this time, all trial data will be in the database, but will not be completely cleaned. This provides an opportunity for identifying protocol deviations and other issues that may impact the statistical analysis.

The third period is the planned analysis period, defined as beginning at the time of the database lock and finishing when all of the listings, tables and graphs identified in the statistical analysis plan have been generated, checked and interpreted. This includes presenting the main findings of the analysis to the clinical study team and identifying an agreed list of outstanding issues to be addressed in the unplanned analysis period.

The fourth period is the unplanned analysis period, which is defined as the period after the planned analysis period and during which all issues raised in the planned analysis period are addressed in an effort to complete the first draft of the CSR.

These four periods will be discussed in greater detail below.

Responsibilities Standards for many aspects of the statistics process should be generated within the biostatistics department to enable the statistical team to most efficiently prepare for the analysis and reporting of data from clinical trials. These standards can then be used across all teams (e.g., the statistical team within a clinical study team will not have to re-invent these standards every time a new project is started).

In addition to these more general standards, a statistical team within a clinical study team needs to generate standards specific to the clinical study team (e.g., standardizing the calculation of a specific endpoint across all studies within a submission). These standards can then be used across all studies that are being analyzed as part of a regulatory submission. Such standards will not have to be re-invented from one study to another.

The exhibit below shows the aspects of the statistical process for the analysis and reporting of data from clinical trials, which could be established in the biostatistics department standards related to demographics and safety.

Biostatistics Department Standards

Department	Standard
Biostatistics	Directory Structure
	Demography/Safety CRT Dataset Structures
	Demography/Safety Variable Definition Methods
	Demography/Safety Table/Graph/Listings Shells
	Demography/Safety Programming Code
	QC Standards
	Validation Documentation
	Programming Guidelines
	Programming Test Plans
	Program Indexing Method
Regulatory	Regulatory Style Guide
Safety	Safety Reporting Guidelines

CRT: Case Report Tabulation (analyses data sets or derived data sets)

The exhibit below lists the standards that could be defined within the biostatistics team of a clinical study team.

Clinical Study Team Biostatistics Standards

Standard

Efficacy Endpoint CRT Dataset Structures
Efficacy Variable Definitions
Efficacy Variable Definition Methods
Efficacy Endpoint Analysis Conventions
Efficacy Table/Graph/Listings Shells
Efficacy Endpoint Programming Code
Project Specific Safety Endpoints
Directory Structure Conventions

Expediting Drug and Biologics Development

When a new biostatistics team is formed within a clinical study team, it will be clear which aspects of standardization need to be addressed by the team and which aspects can be taken from the department standards.

First Period of Preparation The first preparation for the analysis and reporting of a clinical trial can be initiated as soon as the SAP is finalized (see exhibit below).

First Preparation Period based on a Final SAP

Table/Listing/Figure Shells
CRT Dataset Specifications

        CRT Programming
        PV Programming
        Patient Profile Programming

                Listing Programs
                Tables Programs
                Figures Programs

                        Testing

The SAP will contain a list of all the tables, listings and graphs that will represent the planned statistical analysis. Template shells for the tables, listings and graphs can then be generated beginning at any time. This process will be simplified if departmental and clinical study team standards are already in place. The specifications for the CRT datasets can also be completed at the same time. Again, this is simplified if department and clinical study team standards already exist.

Once all of the specifications are in place, the next step is to begin programming the CRT datasets, protocol violations and subject profile graphs. This programming should be carried out using standard validation document standards, which should include a standard level of testing (e.g., all test plans for CRT dataset programs should be similar). It is important that the directory structure be easily understood so that any staff can quickly and efficiently find files. A standard directory structure in use across all statistical functions would accomplish this.

As the CRT datasets are placed, the programming for the tables, listings and graphs can be put into place. Again, this should be carried out using standardized methods for validation and testing. This step involves a significant amount of programming, and involves all aspects of the data. To simplify this, standard methods for summarizing adverse events, demography, accountability, concomitant medications and laboratory parameters could be set by the biostatistics department. The existence of standard programs to create the relevant tables, listings and graphs could greatly reduce the time required to write and validate programs to summarize these data. For consistency within a submission, efficacy and project-specific safety endpoints should have standard definitions set and program code created. This again would greatly simplify the programming required for an individual study.

Upon the completion of programming for the tables, listings and graphs and upon the population of the clinical database with sufficient data to complete each table, listing or graph, a set of mock tables, listings and graphs can be produced. For blinded studies, these mock data presentations should be produced using dummy treatment assignments. These data presentations are useful as a final test of the SAS code, as a confirmation that the output matches table, listing and graph shells provided in the SAP, and as an aid in data review by the team.

Once all programming has been completed, indexed and validated, the programs should be tested as a unit. The programs should all be run in the correct order, perhaps in a batch job to ensure that, when the database is locked, there will be no unanticipated errors.

Second Period of Preparation Within four weeks in advance of the database lock, most of the clinical trial data will be in the database with only the last remaining data queries outstanding. This provides an opportunity to run the protocol violation programs, to discuss them within the clinical study team, and to prepare for the planned analysis period. The exhibit below outlines the activities in this period.

It is important at this stage to identify any protocol violations (PV) that may affect the planned analysis and adversely influence the results of the trial. Although the existence of particular PVs should have already been identified as they were reported, this is the point at which the extent of any particular PV will be come apparent.

Second Preparation Period

Run PV Programs

Review PVs with Clinical Study Team

                           Agree Communication Plan

                           Timetable for Analysis

                                                Database Lock

---

PV: protocol violations

In preparation for the planned analysis period, the clinical study team (if appropriate, with senior management) should agree upon the communication plan for the results of the study. In addition, a timetable for the planned analysis period should be given within the clinical study team. This ensures that all clinical study team members are informed as to when particular results will be available and when tables, graphs and listings will be made available to other groups (e.g., safety and medical writing).

Planned Analysis Once the database has been locked, the data transfer into SAS can begin. The exhibit below outlines the processes during this period.

The Planned Analysis Period

Data
Transfer

       Run Patient Profile
       Programs

       Run PVs Programs

       Run CRT Programs   Blinded Review

                            Update SAP

                            Unblind

                            Rerun CRT Programs

                            Run Accountability
                            Programs

                                                      Listings

                                                Accountability and Demography

                                              Efficacy

                                              Safety

                                                                Identify Unplanned
                                                                 Analyses

---

For studies for which the data management has been handled in-house, the data should be imported into SAS using a department-wide standard, validated method. For studies for which the data management has been outsourced, the data transfer into SAS should have been planned (and validated) in advance to promote an efficient start to the analysis.

After the data transfer, the programs that produce the CRTs, listings of protocol violations and subject profiles can be executed with dummy treatment codes in place. At that time, a blinded review of the data can occur according to a planned procedure. All assumptions for the important statistical analyses and protocol violations should be checked at this stage and an amendment to the SAP should be made, if necessary.

The "unblinding" process can then be undertaken, and the programs can be re-executed with the actual treatment codes in place. The planned analysis should then begin with the execution of the subject accountability programs. This is essential in order to define the number of subjects in each treatment at each stage of the study. Knowing these numbers will greatly enhance the ability to properly check all subsequent output.

Expediting Drug and Biologics Development

To get a feel for the data and to allow medical writing to compile the output into the CSR, the listings should be created and checked first. After that, the output for the accountability, demography, efficacy and safety sections can then be created and checked in quick succession.

Once the main efficacy and safety analyses have been completed, there should be a presentation of the main findings to the clinical study team. This will ensure that the results are being discussed and that issues are being carefully considered by other members of the clinical study team while the remaining planned analyses are taking place.

During the analysis, there may be several unexpected aspects of the results that will require further investigation. These should be listed and kept until the end of the planned analysis period so that they can be prioritized for the unplanned analysis period (see discussion below). Once the planned analysis has been completed, all program output should be indexed so that it can be located quickly, and CSR table insertion can proceed smoothly.

Unplanned Analysis The unplanned analysis period should begin with a clinical study team meeting in which the list of questions that require further investigation and that were identified during the planned analysis period can be discussed. The outcome of this meeting should be a list of tasks establishing a clear order of priority so that the statistical team can deploy to answer these questions according to the agreed upon timeline for the CRS completion. The clinical study team should be informed on the progress regarding these questions regularly.

Conclusions This chapter has explored the possibility of creating a single statistics process for the analysis and reporting of data from clinical trials, and has proposed what this process might look like. It has also proposed the responsibilities involved in providing standards for different aspects of the process. The benefits of a single statistics process will include a simple statement of best practice, simplified staff training, the possibility that SOPs can be written for analysis and reporting, a more structured approach to process improvement, improved quality through the creation of quality standards, increased efficiency, improved flexibility (i.e., quick reallocation of resources with little re-training), better resource predictability (i.e., through a standardized framework for metric collection), and lower and more precise budgets.

Overall, the implementation of a single statistics process will enable other groups within a company to understand the tasks and activities undertaken by the statistical group, and will result in an improved appreciation of what statisticians do in the analysis and reporting of data from clinical trials.

STATISTICAL ANALYSIS PLAN TEMPLATE

Table of Contents

1. INTRODUCTION 7
2. OBJECTIVES 7
3. STUDY DESIGN 7
4. STUDY ENDPOINTS AND COVARIATES 7
5. DEFINITIONS 8
6. ANALYSIS SUBSETS 9
   6.1   Data Subsets 9
   6.2   Interim Analyses 10
   6.3   Subgroup Analyses 10
   6.4   Post Hoc/Ad Hoc Analyses 10
7. INTERIM ANALYSIS AND EARLY STOPPING GUIDELINES 11
8. DATA SCREENING AND ACCEPTANCE 12
9. STATISTICAL METHODS OF ANALYSIS 13
   9.1   General Principles 13
   9.2   Subject Accountability, Demographic and Baseline Characteristics 14
   9.3   Safety Analyses 14
   9.4   Efficacy Analyses 14
   9.5   Pharmacokinetic or Pharmacokinetic/Pharmacodynamic Analysis 15
10. LIST OF PLANNED TABLES, FIGURES, LISTINGS, AND APPENDICES 15
11. PRIORITIZATION OF ANALYSES 15
12. LITERATURE CITATIONS(REFERENCES) 16

13. DATA NOT COVERED BY THIS PLAN 16

14. APPENDICES 16

1. INTRODUCTION: Include the purpose and scope of the SAP in the context of the purposes of the study and a summary of scientific rationale for the study. The protocol version/amendment(s) and dates to which the SAP applied should be included. Any other SAPs related to the study should be referenced. If the statistical section of the protocol/SAP has changed over time, these changes may be summarized.

2. OBJECTIVES: Include all objectives of the study exactly as they appear in the protocol. These objectives should be differentiated as primary or secondary.

3. STUDY DESIGN: Describe the number of treatment groups, number of centers/investigators, the randomization method, allocation ratio, level of blinding, sample size, planned power, type of control, phase, stratification variables (and categories), expected study duration, etc.

4. STUDY ENDPOINTS AND COVARIATES. List the study endpoints grouped as follows: safety; primary efficacy; secondary efficacy; quality of life (QOL); health economics (HE); and pharmacokinetic (PK) or pharmacokinetic/pharmacodynamic analysis (PK/PD). Endpoints should be listed as appropriate to the study design. QOL, HE, PK or PK/PD variables may be either the primary or secondary variables in a study and should be listed as such. Covariates, known prognostic factors or anticipated grouping variables (such as sex or age group) that would be used in the analysis should be listed. Those covariates that are pre-specified and those that were not pre-specified in the protocol should be identified.

5. DEFINITIONS: Definitions of the following should be included: study endpoints, analysis subsets, terms used to define endpoints or subsets, any element that improves the understanding of the SAP (e.g., reference or normal range), randomization and/or study enrollment day, Study day 1, study baseline, study completion, events that are tallied or used in time-to-event endpoints, and derived (calculated) variables. Methods used to calculate complex variables (e.g., quality of life measures, health economic measures, PK endpoints, and composite morbidity endpoints) should be provided. Reference quality-of-life and health-economic instruments that are described in the attachments.

6. ANALYSIS SUBSETS:

6.1 Data Subsets: This section identifies the primary analysis data set and planned subset analyses. If only an intent-to-treat (ITT) analysis is planned, then this should be stated. The intent-to-treat dataset should include all subjects as randomized-all subjects.

If there is a modified ITT group defined, the reasons for its use should be stated. A modified subset could be defined as all subjects in the ITT who received at least one treatment.

There could be an evaluable subset defined for efficacy or safety analyses. For safety analyses, this typically includes all subjects who received at least one dose of study drug. It should clearly specify how subjects who inadvertently received the incorrect drug or who received more than one type or dose of study drug will be analyzed. The criteria used to determine the efficacy, the PK or PK/PD, the QOL and/or health economics evaluable subsets of subjects must be stated. In addition, the criteria and the reasons used to exclude both subjects and/or individual data points from the analysis should be listed and documented.

6.2 Interim Analyses: List the criteria for including subjects in interim analyses—for example, if the timing of interim analysis is based on the proportion of planned enrollment, the number of subjects, the number of events, or some other factor.

Additional information related to interim analyses should be included in Section 7.

6.3 Subgroup Analyses: State the objectives and/or definitions for subgroups for exploratory and/or non-exploratory analyses (e.g., diabetic vs. non-diabetic subjects). List variables that will be summarized by sex, race, age or other groupings.

6.4 *Post Hoc/Ad Hoc* Analyses: If this SAP is developed or amended after some event, such as an interim breaking of the blind or examination of data in any manner or for any purpose, then this event should be identified. Endpoints, subsets, analysis or principles defined should be identified clearly as either those made prior to the event (*a priori*) or those made subsequent to that event (*post hoc*). Anticipated *ad hoc* analyses (e.g., those determined by the results of primary analyses) may also be listed.

7. INTERIM ANALYSIS AND EARLY STOPPING GUIDELINES For studies with planned interim analyses, the following items should be addressed in the SAP: rationale for planned interim analyses; number and timing of planned interim analyses; responsible people; access and distribution of results; handling of blinding and unblinding; procedures to ensure that no actions other than those specified by the interim analysis plan are taken; endpoints to be included in the planned interim analyses; planned statistical methods and adjustments; possible decisions and decision rules; and procedures that will be used to detect and document any changes in the conduct of the study, definitions of outcomes or derived variables, or methods of analysis which were the result of the interim analysis/analyses.

If interim analyses will be conducted for review by an internal or external data monitoring committee (DMC), the existence of, membership of, and charter for the DMC should be addressed or cross-referenced in the statistical analysis plan. A description of the data presented and any analyses done for the DMC should be outlined in the DMC charter and agreed to in advance by the DMC members. For interim analyses that are unplanned at the time the SAP is developed, a supplement to the SAP should be developed before the interim analysis is performed.

8. DATA SCREENING AND ACCEPTANCE This section should describe when and how data screening analyses will be done. Determine the protocol violations/deviations that may impact the analysis or interpretation of study results. List the variables that will be evaluated as part of the data acceptance procedure from data management.

Criteria for handling missing and incomplete data should be described. Methods to be used, such as examination of the frequency of missing data and determination of patterns in the missing data (if any), should be included. In addition, the conditions under which data will be imputed and carried over from previous measurement, and how missing dates be handled, should all be prospectively defined.

The methods to be used to check for the introduction of biases, and how outliers are to be identified and handled, should also be described in this section. Sources of bias to be considered include protocol violations, non-random or informative censoring, inadvertent breaking of the blind, interim analyses, administrative analyses, changes to the study conduct (e.g., changes in eligibility criteria, addition of centers, addition of countries, and other major protocol amendments) and results of procedural monitoring. Pre-planned assessments of data characteristics that affect the assumptions of the proposed statistical methodology should also be defined.

The source of data should be described (e.g., the clinical trials database), including if this is to be done internally (by the sponsor) or externally (by a consultant/contractor). Identify any external consultant/contractor. An identification of the planned application software (e.g., SAS, SPlus, Excel) and operating system software should be included.

9. STATISTICAL METHODS OF ANALYSIS Since this is usually the longest section of the SAP, a list of subsections is proposed.

9.1 General Principles: In this section, the defaults for the analyses are defined, such as the level of significance, one- vs. two-tail tests, adjustments for multiple comparisons, how multi-center data will be handled (separate tests, adjustment for center differences, assessment of treatment by center interactions, etc.), how centers with low recruitment would be pooled, and how data will be grouped or collapsed (e.g., age as a continuous variable vs. age groups as a discrete variable vs. age < 65 vs. (65 years as a binary variable). All statistical methods and hypotheses involving study endpoints or outcomes should be related to the study objectives.

9.2 Subject Accountability, Demographic and Baseline Characteristics: The planned assessment of subject accrual, disposition, eligibility, demographic and physical characteristics, disease characteristics of all appropriate subsets and hypotheses to be tested, if any, should be described.

9.3 Safety Analyses: This section should describe how safety information will be summarized (e.g., Will AEs be grouped/pooled? How will laboratory values be summarized? Will statistical comparisons of these summaries be made?). If coding standards will be applied, include this reference. If hypothesis testing or confidence intervals are used, they should be described here.

9.4 Efficacy Analyses: This section should describe the planned statistical analyses, and alternative methods if assumptions for the planned analyses are not met. Stratification variables at randomization, post-hoc stratification variables, covariates, and analysis models should be included.

All parameters to be estimated and whether confidence intervals will be calculated, together with the level of confidence (e.g., 95% confidence interval one sided or two sided), should be described. If hypothesis testing is used for any of the variables, the null and alternative hypotheses, the significance level(s) for specific analyses that differ from default (in Section 9.1) should be described.

9.5 Pharmacokinetic or Pharmacokinetic/Pharmacodynamic Analysis: This section should be written by the pharmacokineticist or clinical pharmacologist (a secondary author) whenever PK or PK/PD data will be modeled in a protocol. Endpoints should be listed in Section 4 and defined in Section 5. The type of PK model used (compartmental vs. non-compartmental) should be listed. Criteria for excluded subjects or observations should be listed. Again, all parameters to be estimated and whether confidence intervals will be calculated together with the level of confidence (e.g., 95% confidence interval one sided or two sided) should be described. If hypothesis testing is used for any of the variables, the null and alternative hypotheses and the significance level(s) for specific analyses that differ from default (in Section 9.1) should be described. The pharmacokineticists should provide the listings of tables and figures as well as table, listing, and figure shells.

10. LIST OF PLANNED TABLES, LISTINGS AND GRAPHS Lists of planned tables and figures should be included in this section. Standard tables should be used, as appropriate.

11. PRIORITIZATION OF ANALYSES For each analysis performed, there may be a need to review results from certain analyses earlier than others. For example, company decisions often rely on analyses involving primary efficacy endpoints and serious AEs as an aid in planning future trials. Phase I/II studies typically provide information needed to support Go/No Go decisions for additional Phase 2 or Phase 3 studies, and to aid in the design of those studies. Timely decisions and protocol development for these future studies depend on rapid extraction of this information after data from the current study are available. In these cases, define the subset of the analyses required for presentation to the clinical study team prior to completion of the full statistical report. A plan for these activities should be included here or as a separate document. If there is a separate document, it should be referenced here.

12. LITERATURE CITATIONS/REFERENCES This section should include literature citations and/or references that are used in the preparation of this statistical analysis plan.

13. DATA NOT COVERED BY THIS PLAN If there are data that are collected on case report forms and that will not be described or analyzed directly under this SAP, it is recommended that this be specified here.

14. APPENDICES A sample of shells for tables, listings and figures sufficient to illustrate common features (e.g., numbering, titles, subtitles, cross-references, footers) should be included here. A complete set of table, figure and listing shells should be completed and agreed upon by the team prior to the final analysis, in particular for pivotal studies. The contents for the data analysis files, including files containing derived (calculated) variables, could be part of this section. The protocol synopsis and the list of abbreviations could be included.

If the sample size/power analyses are not adequately described in a separate document (e.g., the protocol) that can be included by reference, a detailed description of sample size considerations and calculations, power curves, etc., should be included. References and/or values to be used as criteria for toxicity, abnormality, etc., including CTEA toxicity grades, laboratory "normal" ranges, and/or other reference levels, could be part of this section.

Quality-of-life forms/instruments and health economic forms/instruments, if applicable, should be included here. Details of PK or PK/PD methods for modeling should be provided by the pharmacokineticist or clinical pharmacologist and be part of this appendix.

CHAPTER 18

Data Capture

By Stephen A. Raymond, PhD, and Steven E. Linberg, PhD

Today, the art of capturing data in human clinical trials is in flux. The underlying technology is shifting from paper to electronic methods. This chapter will discuss each of these two primary methods. The chapter's first section addresses the emerging method—electronic data capture. Here, we will distinguish between two electronic approaches for initially capturing data, one relying on paper source documents (source data are later transcribed to electronic case report forms (eCRFs)), and the other relying on electronic source documents (eSource) (the initial data are captured electronically and parsed automatically to eCRFs). Each of these electronic data capture (EDC) methods contrasts with some of the historical practices that have evolved during the age dominated by paper methods. In addition to being covered in the second section of the chapter, the more traditional paper-based methods will be mentioned throughout the initial section to make it clear to those engaged in transitioning to electronic methods how EDC requires changes in established processes. In keeping with the central tenet of this book, the chapter begins with what researchers intend to keep as results (the deliverables) from clinical trials. It then considers how data capture methods can be designed and used to procure these intended results efficiently.

The chapter includes templates for traceability matrices, which are tools to document that requirements are met by electronic data capture systems. Key requirements for EDC systems include regulatory and guidance requirements. The chapter also provides templates for traditional case report forms, plus examples of suggested language for informed consent and protocols when electronic methods will be used to execute a clinical trial. While the primary focus of the chapter is at the level of a clinical trial, the issues involved and benefits of using eSource and Clinical Data Interchange Standards Consortium (CDISC) standards during clinical development are addressed as well. The viewpoint expressed is that of a technology provider/clinical researcher instructing a sponsor/clinical researcher in the best practices, risks and benefits of electronic methods for the capture of data in clinical trials.

Electronic Data Capture

Start with what you intend to deliver

Planning for capture through archiving and "reconstruction" of clinical trials

Trial Planning Data capture and management involve the gathering and the cleaning of data. Archiving involves the retention of the records of the trial with sufficient contextual information so that the results and data can be recovered and understood for years after the trial is completed.

What do you want at the end of the trial? While there are many possible goals, the objectives of conducting clinical research are fundamentally scientific: To determine the effects of therapeutic interventions (drugs, devices, new practices) and to assess the benefits and risks of such interventions. Unlike basic research, in which the standard of credibility is that someone else must be able to replicate the findings published by a scientist, clinical research is held to higher standards. The credibility of findings must be able to be established by audit. This means that the essential initial task in planning for data capture is to establish *requirements* for data capture. Requirements are the key to audit-ability, which is established by using suitable tests and records to document that the requirements of the trial's system were met. A reasonable set of deliverables for a clinical research trial includes the following:

- Reliable scientific conclusions (depend on trial design, logistics of execution, quality of data captured)
- Results and findings based on analysis (data, interpretation of the data, methods of interpretation)

- Clean, accurate and pertinent data about patients who have followed the protocol (data and the fully described processes both planned and followed to collect the data)
- Well-documented records of any exceptions, problems and surprises (the real world is usually surprising)
- All of the above elements in a standardized format, preserved for a "retention period" that may exceed 20 years so it can be audited, re-analyzed, re-audited and assessed years after the trial is over by: (1) regulatory authorities and auditors; and (2) future researchers for meta-analysis

Start planning capture requirements by considering the archive The archive of a study consists of ALL records that will be maintained. In executing complex operations such as a clinical trial, one cannot assume that common sense will prevail when the trial is over, and that someone will identify the necessary records and preserve them. Imagine a future encounter years after the trial is complete. Any record that an inspector or scientist would need to "reconstruct" the trial will probably NOT be available unless it was required at the outset to be part of the trial archive.

Archive Content: A Checklist

- Protocol, with amendments, including all versions used during the trial
- Requirements Specifications for data capture system (paper source, electronic patient diary (eDiary), EDC system, eSource devices)
- Requirements Specification for interim display of data during the trial and for any system used for data cleaning, analysis or monitoring
- Operational specification detailing who will be responsible for tasks, their identities, their authorities, and for documenting of their consent and training
- Important forms and lists: list of authorized users, documentation concerning electronic signatures and identity certification, training records
- Data Transfer Requirements Specifications for any transfer of clinical data between parties who have received or acted on trial data
- Trial system validation documents such as validation plan, executed test scripts, and validation reports pertaining to proof that the systems used for each of the requirements operated as intended
- History of Authorized User Roles and Privileges, as well as validation of any system used to capture and preserve this history. (Who was able to act on electronic records and what actions were they allowed to perform? How were privileges awarded and withdrawn over the course of the trial?)
- Copies of correspondence that provide documentation of decisions made regarding the trial (memos to file, if applicable)
- Meeting minutes, as appropriate.
- Trial change order documentation, if applicable
- Trial-specific help desk records
- System maintenance records
- Data Change Authorization Forms (DCF's), if applicable
- Database Lock Request
- Database Lock Verification Report
- Final Data Transfer
- Archive Request
- Archive Data Certification Plan
- Archive Data Certification Report
- And any other documents pertaining to the way the particular trial has been conducted that may be required to reconstruct and interpret the trial in the future.

Archive conventions: dimensions of archive quality.

Durability over time For electronic archives, both the storage media and the format must last a long time. For that reason, one should consider character-based formats for data, meta-data and documents. The ASCII character code is likely to be durable for centuries. It is so fundamental to the interactions of computers with human users, including programmers, that it is difficult to envision a scenario under which computers of the future will no longer rely on the ASCII code to represent written characters. By storing data as text characters, one is thus sensibly making such data permanently readable. Archivists today are settling on XML (eXtended Markup Language) as the convention for archiving the combination of words and data because, unlike HTML, it supports tags to identify data, data types, and other properties of character-based strings, not simply text or images.

Integrity of Source data The history of clinical research properly emphasizes the primacy of source data (records where individual data items are first recorded with an intent to make them permanent). When such source data are captured electronically, this tradition would best be respected if the data were preserved precisely as captured. This means that the information content and format should be preserved exactly. In contrast to paper source, where the physical paper binds the data fields to each other and to any signature or authorizations on the page, the physical uniqueness of the recording device(s) or playback devices is not an essential component of the record. With paper, the page itself is the sole technology for storing, revealing and maintaining the record. With an electronic system validated to make accurate copies of data records, the eSource character strings can carry within them markers of their own integrity, and the record content is thus freed from the device hardware or system. Thus, standardizing data formats for capturing data are a key to ensuring their ultimate recovery later. Given that many relational database applications rely on binary encoding that developers are constantly evolving, the copying of a relational database to durable media seems unlikely to constitute a durable or secure archive. Such electronic data "rots" in the sense that data stored by Version 1.0 of an application may not be processed properly or even accessed by Version 8.0 of the same application. Thus, an archive based on copying a set of records, each of which is protected by an ongoing, persistently testable method to detect or prevent alteration of the record is obviously preferable.

Minimize scanning and conversion This is one of the factors to consider in selecting or designing capture methods. Every step that converts records from one form to another (e.g., XML to PDF, paper to electronic scan) is in principle prone to error and must be validated. If one could capture the data in the same form as it would ultimately be archived, then the ideal of zero conversions could be attained.

Archive media considerations The media (disk, DVD, tape) and availability of any hardware and software required to view the media must last throughout the retention period. At this writing, one can purchase CD-ROM media warranted with an expected life in excess of 100 years at room temperature. Since it seems unlikely that CD-ROM drives will be ubiquitous in 100 years, archive planning should include a process to identify a time to retire the media and shift the content to an appropriate future substrate without alteration of archive content.

Regulatory requirements for the archive The archive should support any site audit of a trial by a regulatory authority. For an eClinical trial, an FDA guidance document ("Computerized Systems Used in Clinical Trials," or CSUCT: Section VI. System Features D. "Reconstruction of Study") specifies that the "FDA expects to be able to reconstruct a study. This applies not only to the data, but also how the data were obtained or managed." Hence, the archive should be presented in a way that makes it easy for an FDA inspector to reconstruct a study, and to assess the trustworthiness of the data by inspection of the validation records and the controls used to protect records from premature loss or destruction.

Requirements for EDC system "output" and deliverables

REQUIREMENTS EMERGING FROM THE SCIENTIFIC QUESTION OR OBJECTIVE:

Although these requirements will be apparent from the protocol, current practices for authoring protocols are still heavily influenced by constraints that paper-based technology has placed on trial execution over the past 60 years. It is probably worth examining the key scientific issue to be examined in the trial in light of new data capture technologies. The data requirements should emerge rationally from the hypotheses of the study and/or the observations that can be made to enhance the understanding of the health status of the participating subjects. In addition to items (data fields) collected on forms such as demographic information, adverse events, concomitant medications, physical exam, etc., the scientific purposes of the trial may require particular measurements and techniques. The case report form (CRF) identifies all the data to be collected for each subject according to the trial's protocol (CDISC Glossary Version 4.0, 2005). When "annotated," the CRF also can serve to specify the field names for each "item" to be collected. When EDC is used, the requirements for each "item" (CDISC ODM version 1.2) also include specifying format, variable types, string lengths, range limitations and other properties. In deciding what must be captured, protocol designers consider what they need to know about the trial subjects in order to resolve hypotheses. What would be useful observations to collect in order to provide compelling documentation that the conclusions of the trial are correct? Given prior observations and knowledge, what are the ideal sources for the information needed to address these questions?

Medical Instruments: For safety monitoring, trials usually include 12 lead EKG measurements. Additionally, images from Magnetic Resonance Imaging (MRI), Computed Axial Tomography (CAT) Scan, radiation maps, x-rays and the like may serve as source data. Readings of such images by radiologists summarize the radiographic findings in text form, and may also be part of the required trial data. Treadmill scores, joint evaluations, spirometric measures, vital signs and the like represent measures that are often entered by site personnel into the case histories of subjects participating in a trial. As with other data fields required for scientific and safety reasons, all the data to be collected in a trial are usually specified in the case report form.

Measuring devices: Direct physiological measuring sensors and devices exist. Planners should ask themselves if such measurements would make the trial more conclusive?

Subject self-reports: eDiaries support frequent, controlled capture of symptoms that can be used to track symptoms versus therapy. They also can capture perceived well-being, health status and quality of life assessments that are sometimes the key efficacy variables (e.g., for pain therapies). Even for therapies directed at imperceptible parameters (e.g., cholesterol, blood pressure), such quality of life data may yield findings that bear on the acceptability and utility of the drug.

Physicians, nurses, observers, caretakers: eSource methods can simplify data capture to the point that data of importance to the hypothesis can be considered for capture because logistical obstacles and difficulties historically present with paper methods may be avoided.

REQUIREMENTS EMERGING FROM THE TRIAL DESIGN AND ARCHITECTURE:

There exist implications for capture technologies based on the culture and customs of the specific subjects to be recruited. For example, immune unresponsive subjects may need special sterilization procedures for capture devices or of paper notes used as source documents. The system must embed or provide for the planned sequence of all measures (data to be captured) and planned study elements (processes, visits). Consider the benefits of using standardized protocol elements and models and of planning the archive to address emerging standards for electronic submission of reports to regulatory authorities (see section below).

REQUIREMENTS EMERGING FROM 21 CFR PART 11, PREDICATE RULES AND GUIDANCE

The "spirit of the regulations:" Trustworthiness, integrity, quality (ALCOA) Fundamentally, research conducted to guide medical decisions should be trustworthy. During the years of experience with paper methods, regulatory authorities working with clinical researchers have established "good practices," which are often enshrined in "guidance" documents and regulations with the aim of preventing research problems (fraud, sloppiness, undocumented claims, etc.) that have historically challenged the trustworthiness of such research. In developing its Part 11 (21 CFR Part 11) regulations, the FDA's goal was to "set forth the criteria under which the agency considers electronic records, electronic signatures, and handwritten signatures executed to electronic records to be trustworthy, reliable, and generally equivalent to paper records and handwritten signatures executed on paper."

In planning a trial, designers simply must be aware of current guidance and requirements, which may vary between countries and regions. The EU, Japan and the United States have harmonized GCP standards ("Guidance for Good Clinical Practice," E6) under the ICH initiative, and many national authorities appear to have security and privacy provisions that are similar to those set forth in 21 CFR 11, CSUCT and in HIPAA (Health Insurance Portability and Accountability Act)(see templates below). As noted in 1999 by Stan Woolen, then the director of the FDA's Office of Science and Research, the keys to data integrity are captured by the acronym ALCOA (data must be attributable, legible, contemporaneous, original, and accurate).

The same elements are also mentioned in the FDA's CSUCT. As noted in the introduction to CSUCT, "To be acceptable the data should meet certain fundamental elements of quality whether collected or recorded electronically or on paper. Data should be attributable, original, accurate, contemporaneous, and legible."

Standards Regulators and scientists who review clinical trial reports in determining whether therapies should be approved for marketing have bemoaned the lack of standardization in the capture, presentation and content of trial records. The variety of content, naming conventions, data formats, and the like, much of which is unrelated to data integrity or scientific objectives, makes it harder to establish good review practices, train reviewers, accomplish reviews quickly and consistently, and preserve results in ways that support ongoing use and access. It is also more difficult for regulators to communicate concerning trial details with sponsors and with others in the agency (Ref: Standard Data & eReview Tools; Presentation 40th Annual DIA meeting, Session 366 by Steve Wilson, June 16, 2004). Without unduly discouraging creativity in identifying better methods and processes, regulators have produced a string of industry guidance documents regarding submissions, including electronic submissions. Such standards are in flux, however; currently, eSubmissions are indexed hyperdocuments in Adobe Acrobat with SAS® datasets, although the FDA has also recently approved (July 21, 2004) the submission of data in XML formats for data and metadata in a CDISC standard (SDTM for Study Data Tabulation Model). Currently, CDISC and the FDA also are working with the pharmaceutical industry and others on standards for protocols, which will help EDC users implement trials more rapidly.

The "Letter of the regulations:"Specific regulatory requirements and trial requirements related to guidance documents A key requirement of 21 CFR 11 (for electronic records and signatures) is that any system used to act on electronic records that will be submitted to the agency be validated. Many excellent references on computer system validation exist. The FDA refers to an IEEE standard for device validation in its Guidance (ISO/IEC/IEEE 12207:1995 §3.35) (ISO is the International Organization for Standardization; IEC is the International Electrotechnical Commission; IEEE is the Institute of Electrical and Electronics Engineers).

In general, validation is the process through which the technology provider demonstrates that the system performs as required. Successful validation then involves testing each requirement against processes or actions of the system to document that the requirement is fulfilled. Usually, there is a validation plan describing how the requirements will be addressed and the documentation that will be provided. A matrix that shows the correspondence between each requirement and the tests/documentation that shows that the requirement has been successfully met "traces" requirements to relevant executed test scripts or other documentation, and is called a traceability matrix ("eClinical Trials, Planning & Implementation," Thomson Publishing, Centerwatch pg. 192, 2003). The exhibit below contains a sample traceability matrix that lists the individual requirements of 21 CFR 11 (dealing with validation in the example) and the compliance documentation that confirms that the system acts as required (the trial validation documentation in its entirety in this example). Traceability matrices can be quite detailed, and can have additional columns to make it easier for an auditor to assess the correspondence between requirements and test documents. For example, one column could be inserted to explain or expand the requirement, and another could be added to explain how the system operates to fulfill it.

Sample Traceability Matrix

Component of the Rule		Compliance Documentation
21 CFR 11.10 Controls for Closed Systems		
	Persons who use closed systems to create, modify, maintain, or transmit electronic records shall employ procedures and controls designed to ensure the authenticity, integrity, and, when appropriate, the confidentiality of electronic records, and to ensure that the signer cannot readily repudiate the signed record as not genuine. Such procedures and controls shall include the following:	SOPs, test documents, handwritten agreements, etc. See below.
(a)	Validation of systems to ensure accuracy, reliability, consistent intended performance, and the ability to discern invalid or altered records.	Trial Validation
(b)	The ability to generate accurate and complete copies of records in both human readable and electronic form suitable for inspection, review, and copying by the agency. Persons should contact the agency if there are any questions regarding the ability of the agency to perform such review and copying of the electronic records.	A test result
(c)	Protection of records to enable their accurate and ready retrieval throughout the records-retention period.	Trial System Security Trial System Backup & Restore Trial System Disaster Recovery Trial Archive

The validation documentation includes all the requirements and evidence that the system performs as intended. The idea is that an auditor should be able to have confidence in the system without having to test it. The annals of quality management also attest to the value of validation in supporting continued improvement of products—"Undocumented perfection is like magic; it can be admired, but it can't be trusted" (SA Raymond, in Kush et. al. Clinical Trials: Planning & Implementation, Thomson Publishing, Centerwatch, 2003).

Thus, the key to validation, which is required for electronic systems but would be a good practice for paper-based systems as well, is to have good documentation of requirements that lays out exactly what a system should do in fulfilling specific functionality. The extent to which the system is then exercised and documented tends to vary—more testing for aircraft, for example, than for printing presses—and determines the quality of the validation. Certain important requirements for

Expediting Drug and Biologics Development

EDC emerge from the letter of FDA regulations and guidance documents, and examples can be helpful in conveying the level of detail adopted in practice.

The exhibit below presents an example of a traceability matrix for 45 CFR Part 164 Subpart C - Security Standards for the Protection of Electronic Protected Health Information. The table is based on "Appendix A to Subpart C of 21 CFR 164-Security Standards: Matrix." Like Subpart C, the matrix is divided into three parts: Administrative Safeguards, Physical Safeguards, and Technical Safeguards. The matrix columns are as follows:

- *Standards*: The security standard quoted from 21 CFR 164, along with its section reference numbers
- *Section References*: The section identifies the paragraph references of standard's Implementation Specifications
- *Implementation Specifications*: Titles of the individual implementation specifications that support the Standard
- *Implementation Specification Details*: Text from 21 CFR 164 detailing how the Standard is to be put into practice
- *R/A (Required/Addressable)*: In 21 CFR 164, if an implementation specification is required, the word "Required" appears in parentheses after the title of the implementation specification. If an implementation specification is addressable, the word "Addressable" appears in parentheses after the title of the implementation specification. Refer to 164.306(d) for details regarding Addressable implementation specifications.
- *Evidence*: In the Evidence column, the Technology Provider using the matrix to document validation of their product would specify how it demonstrates that each implementation specification, Required and Addressable, has been fulfilled by the product or system. Such evidence may include reference to policies, SOPs, audit results or other such evidence of realization.

Traceability Matrix for 45 CFR Part 164 Subpart C-Security Standards for the Protection of Electronic Protected Health Information

(example using selected content and suggested layout
courtesy of R. LaFleur, PHT Corporation)

A. Administrative Safeguards						
Standards	Section References		Implementation Specifications	Implementation Specifications Details	R / A1	Evidence
21CFR164.308	21CFR164.308(a)(1)	(ii)	Implementation specifications:			
		(A)	Risk analysis	Conduct an accurate and thorough assessment of the potential risks and vulnerabilities to the confidentiality, integrity, and availability of electronic protected health information held by the covered entity.	R	
(a) A covered entity must, in accordance with [164.306]:		(B)	Risk management	Implement security measures sufficient to reduce risks and vulnerabilities to a reasonable and appropriate level to comply with [164.306(a)].	R	
(1)(i) Standard: Security management process.		(C)	Sanction policy	Apply appropriate sanctions against workforce members who fail to comply with the security policies and procedures of the covered entity.	R	
Implement policies and procedures to prevent, detect, contain, and correct security violations.		(D)	Information system activity review.	Implement procedures to regularly review records of information system activity, such as audit logs, access reports, and security incident tracking reports.	R	

–continued–

–continued–

Standards	Section References		Implementation Specifications	Implementation Specifications Details	R / A1	Evidence
21CFR164.308(a) (2) Standard: Assigned security responsibility. Identify the security official who is responsible for the development and implementation of the policies and procedures required by this subpart for the entity.			N/A	N/A	R	

1 R = Required; A = Addressable. See [21CFR164.306(d)].

The exhibit below provides another example of establishing requirements, clarifying the interpretation of the requirements and stating the approach to meeting the requirements, in this case concerning authorization and training of system users. Note that, since evidence is not provided—only requirements and approach are provided—the example is not a traceability matrix.

Requirements for Authorization and Training

> 21 CFR 11.10 requires the following:
> (d) Limiting system access to authorized individuals.
> (i) Determination that persons who develop, maintain, or use electronic record/electronic signature systems have the education, training, and experience to perform their assigned tasks.

We interpret the determination of authorized individuals to include identity certification, documentation of adequate training, and a request for system access. Such determination may initially be accomplished at the Investigator Meeting where records of identity and training can be collected for those users in attendance. Site and Sponsor staff assigned to the study after the initial training, and who require access to the system, may have their identities and training documented through a designated representative identified as the local point of contact for such certification. A signed record of these added certifications may then be sent to the technology provider for processing and possible approval.

Note that "persons who develop" systems are included in section (i). The comments in the Preamble to the Rule make it clear that the qualifications of personnel are a separate requirement from validation of the system, and that the requirement applies to vendors (contractors) as well as in-house developers. Maintaining training records is also expected (the comments say that "the agency believes that documentation of such training is also customary and not unreasonable.") The technology provider must, therefore, maintain training records for its employees, and document training of all users who conduct clinical trials and act on electronic records using any of the technology provider's products or services.

Courtesy R. LaFleur, PHT Corporation

SELECT DATA CAPTURE METHODS-PLANNING FOR EXECUTION, AVAILABLE TECHNOLOGIES IN EDC VS PAPER

Paper vs. Electronic Data Capture (EDC) Familiar paper methods of data capture rely on paper-based "source documents," which can be medical charts, clinical records associated with patient care, or a variety of other records (CDISC Glossary Version 4.0; ICH E6). The word "source" denotes that the document is the first point of capture for the data items pertinent to the trial, which are themselves transcribed from the source documents to paper CRFs. Typically, such transcription is manually accomplished by site personnel, and is therefore subject to transcription error as well as the possibility that the original source record itself is wrong, missing, illegible or illogical. To enhance the credibility of paper source data used in combination with paper CRFs, best practices usually include a provision for manual checking by "monitors," who physically visit the sites. The monitors compare the source documents, which are "maintained" on site, with each field transcribed to the CRF pages. They "resolve" differences with the investigator and site personnel, and prepare the study-specific CRFs for data entry. This monitoring process, while familiar, is a substantial burden associated with a paper-based data capture methodology.

EDC: Paper Source vs. Electronic Source Electronic data capture exists in two primary forms. In the first, which is most common today, the traditional method of capturing source data remains a task accomplished using paper. The transcription from paper source to CRFs, however, is accomplished via computerized forms called eCRFs (CDISC Glossary Version 4.0). Depending on the technology provider and the system used, the transcription of source data to eCRFs, while still an activity performed by site personnel, is assisted by edit checks that alert transcribers to missing fields and to fields with values that are out of reasonable range or are otherwise illogical. Illegible fields or improper formatting are prevented, assuming proper operation of the system. The principal advantage of this first type of EDC is that data are available for inspection and correction using computerized methods earlier than with paper CRFs, which are usually accumulated at sites and entered only following the monitoring process.

Alternatively, data capture may be accomplished electronically at the first instance of recording data pertinent to the study. Such electronic source data capture (eSource EDC) can support edit checks for completion and logic that operate at the time data are initially captured for the study. And when such eSource is used at sites that also record data on paper forms (in keeping with clinical practice or SOPs), the eSource records can serve as source data for the trial, provided that the protocol and planning documents set forth specifically the fields and records to be considered as source records (CSUCT and ICH E6). When eSource is used for the initial capture of trial data, then the manual transcription to eCRFs is replaced by automatic registration of data into storage systems, relational databases and/or electronic forms. The accuracy and integrity of this storage and representation of eSource is no longer a manual task, but must be assured through validation of the system that performs the task automatically.

ITEMS (DATA FIELDS), eCRF CONTENT AND DESIGN: DATA TO BE CAPTURED.

Protocol Standard Elements At this time, no standards have been established for protocol content (trial elements, design, practices). However, the ICH's GCP guideline (E6) includes many provisions that bear on protocol content as well as practices concerning the preparation and processes for treating records. In conjunction with the FDA, CDISC has undertaken an initiative to standardize protocol elements and to develop a standard model consistent with HL-7 models for electronic health records. The initiative has produced an initial document that establishes field names, explanations, attributes and definitions (The Standard Protocol Elements Version 1.0 Released for Comment in March 2004). Standards for data structure have been proposed in an operational data model that sets forth the XML schema for representing clinical trial data (CDISC Operational Data Model 1.2 January 2004). This standard supports the interchange of data across EDC and electronic data management applications from different vendors, and also can serve as a standard representation for archived trial data.

Field names and properties The standardization of field names and the data sets that group them is more advanced than for protocol elements. On July 21, 2004, the FDA announced that sponsors of clinical trials for drugs can use the CDISC Study Data Tabulation Model (SDTM) to submit clinical data in NDAs. This standard is targeted for submissions in XML, and stipulates how "observations" (interventions, events or findings) can be classified into datasets and standardized variable names. The standard is extensible (can be enlarged to accommodate variables that are specific to a particular trial and that are not part of a standards library), and also supports controlled terminologies for response options. For example, a variable describing dosing frequency is part of the "Interventions Observation Class" and has a name ("-DOSFRQ"), a qualifier variable ("Dosing Frequency per Interval"), and can use a pick list based on a controlled terminology (such as BID, TID, QID) to express the number of doses given per a specific interval.

The SDTM also sets forth similar standardized conventions for variables pertaining to demographics, inclusion and exclusion criteria, and "events" such as adverse events, findings, and timing. Although the standards have been established for submissions, it is reasonable in the interest of both clarity and efficiency (minimizing re-mappings) for trial designers to use the SDTM and ODM standards in specifying variable names and properties for capturing data initially in the same form that it will ultimately be submitted.

Direct capture of data from subjects "If you want to know what is happening to the patients, why not ask them?" (Dr. Bengt-Erik Wiholm, MD, Merck Research Labs). Subjects in clinical trials are, in fact, the sole authoritative source concerning symptom severity in a variety of diseases, such as chronic neuropathic pain, arthritic pain, angina, migraine headaches, fibromyalgia, sleeplessness, narcolepsy, and nausea, among many others. Subjects also can report most meaningfully concerning the impact of symptoms on their quality of life and the outcome of treatment (so-called patient-reported outcomes, or PRO). And it has proven useful to have subjects in clinical trials log their compliance with medication schedules for both the drugs under study and for concomitant medications. In principle, adverse event reporting can be made quicker and more interactive by using electronic methods, although existing regulatory concerns and legal liabilities make this a challenging area.

Electronic mobile technologies, including eDiaries, have many capabilities that trial planners can use to improve data capture and that provide insight into the health status of subjects as it changes during a clinical trial:

1. Dense Sampling - Selection of response options or ratings by touching is so easy that self-assessment can be done frequently without placing undue burden on subjects.

2. Real-Time Tracking - Data can be sent daily or even in real-time to a central server, where it can be represented in displays showing current values in relation to the history of the subject. This can support trial management for subject compliance with the protocol, and it can materially improve medical oversight.

3. Data Yield - Paper questionnaires are often not completed at all, completed at inappropriate times, and have missing, illegible or illogical fields. These nagging problems diminish the yield of analyzable fields in comparison to electronic capture methods.

4. Increased Precision of Self-Reported Efficacy and Safety Variables - Recent findings from controlled trials of methods of data capture show that the variance of key efficacy variables is lower when eDiary methods are used in comparison to paper. (Raymond SA, Pearson J. "Does Better Data From Electronic Patient Reported Outcomes (ePRO) Methodology Actually Improve Clinical Research? Results from a randomized trial comparing paper and ePRO diaries." ISOQOL 2004 Symposium Abstracts "Advancing Outcomes Research Methodology and Clinical Applications," Boston MA. 2004: 28)

5. Linkage to Measuring Devices - The literature shows that many subject-recorded measurements from devices, such as peak flow meters (asthma) and glucometers (diabetes), are faked. New methods of coupling such sensing devices to handheld devices now support verifiable, time-stamped records of physiological observations. This can increase the simplicity and yield of quality data.

REAL WORLD CONSTRAINTS

Budget For small, NIH-sponsored trials in which the investigator does much of the work in capturing data and analyzing it and in which the report will be evaluated against academic criteria for credibility (subject to the test of "repeatability") rather than audit-level documentation, paper methods remain less costly. However, the higher quality of eSource data and the capability of mobile capture methods to obtain trustworthy records directly from subjects as ePRO may be essential to derive key information regarding symptoms, attitudes, and psychological impact of treatments for pain, nausea and other "subjective" health conditions.

Access to patients The fundamental notion of a "visit" in clinical research is at least in part a solution to the problem of obtaining information from the subject. In between visits, the subject generally is not "observed" using paper methods. The structure of the exchange of information between physician, researcher and patient is strongly influenced by the limitations of paper. Questionnaires are built to obtain considerable information across a variety of health-related constructs simply because it takes advantage of the patient's availability and the relative sparseness of sampling. If reliable sampling can be accomplished hourly or daily, how would such data capture change? Historically, researchers and regulators have not put much credence in paper diaries due to data quality issues. With eDiaries, however, such issues are successfully addressed (Raymond & Ross, Applied Clinical Trials, 9:48-58, 2000, Hufford M, Shields A. Applied Clinical Trials, 11:48-59, 2002), and it becomes possible to obtain accurate tracking data over time. Such data can be used to investigate decision making and to test models for alcohol use (Tennen, DIA Presentation, April 4, 2005). Tracking key variables (pain intensity, relief, nausea for example) over time has only recently been employed using electronic methods (Schoenharting, Presentation at Advances in eClinical Conference, May 8, 2003 on tracking pain relief following a single injection to the knee in OA). The technology enables and supports research designs that rely on the subject's continued access to data capture appliances. Capturing and rating episodic events (headaches, periods of nausea, bowel movements, sexual encounters, etc.) are now possible, and trial designers have a means to gather highly resolved temporal records of symptom changes, attitudes and behaviors as they are influenced by therapeutic interventions. New designs that emerge from this capability can demonstrate efficacy even in the face of a large variation of symptom severity over the course of a day.

Expediting Drug and Biologics Development

Timing The familiarity of paper methods allows teams using paper to take advantage of certain well-known properties of paper to allow subjects to begin participating in trials before all the electronic systems have been validated. eClinical trials require more up-front planning (Kush et.al. Clinical Trials: Planning & Implementation, Thompson, Centerwatch, 2003), which can delay the enrollment of the first patient. On the other hand, more extensive planning and validation up front often detects and avoids problems that would be more expensive to fix in the midst of a trial, where the "flexibility" of paper methods may result in diminished scrutiny.

Operational planning and pre-deployment activities

Once the trial design issues, regulatory issues, and other planning have been addressed, there is usually a period of pre-trial operational planning, development and testing before commencing data capture. Several of the key steps are discussed below.

AUDIT AND QUALIFY TECHNOLOGY PROVIDERS

If the sponsor opts to employ electronic data capture, then the next operational step is to audit selected providers. At this writing, much of the responsibility for data integrity, conformance with 21 CFR 11 requirements, and elements of GCP rests with the sponsor. The sponsor can fulfill this responsibility by auditing providers of EDC systems to qualify such providers (e.g., as possessing the necessary quality management systems, validation processes).

Auditing for regulatory compliance As noted above, the requirements associated with 21 CFR 11, HIPAA and the CSUCT recommendations can be treated as requirements for EDC systems. Therefore, the systems can be audited by tracing each such requirement to the approach taken and tests performed to show that the system fulfills the requirement. Consistent with this book's thesis, such audits would be most useful if they focused on the deliverables (transferred data and archived trial data and documentation). Sponsors often rely on the audits to convey a sense of the provider's commitment to quality and to the sponsor's success in clinical trials.

The trial team EDC providers affect the ways sites, investigators and even sponsors fulfill their regulatory obligations. For example, sites have an obligation under 21 CFR 312.62b to prepare "accurate and complete" case histories and to protect such data against "premature loss and destruction." If the EDC provider will be supporting the sites in fulfilling these regulatory obligations by furnishing systems for data capture, data correction, access to data during the trial, and protection and security, then the investigators should be informed about how the provider can ensure that the investigator can fulfill these "predicate rule" obligations using the electronic system. The text below provides an example of how investigators can be so informed.

Informing investigators about how the EDC system supports them in carrying out their obligations with respect to patient histories and trial records.
[with permission from PHT Corporation]

[Technology Provider] product ensures that investigators meet their responsibilities concerning "Records and Reports" (ICH Guidelines for Good Clinical Practice E6 sections 2.10, 2.11, 4.9 and 8; and 21 CFR § 312.62)

In this trial you will be using [Technology Provider]'s EDC system to act on clinical research data. Depending on the requirements of the particular clinical trial and your role in it, such actions may include data capture, entry or transcription [preparing electronic records], data access and review, answering queries or commenting on data, preserving data, authorizing, editing data, approving or authenticating data, and tracking in an audit trial all such corrections and edits [maintaining electronic records] and retaining data and trial information at your site so that it can be accessed by regulatory inspectors or otherwise reviewed during the regulatory retention period [retaining electronic records].

Unless otherwise explicitly established, the investigators and their designated study nurses or other trained data specialists at the site (Investigator) control the content of electronic records (data values, entries, edits). This is in accord with the GCP guidelines and FDA predicate rules that stipulate it is the Investigators who have the responsibility to prepare, maintain and retain subject data.

In the several sections below, we summarize how [Technology Provider] ensures data integrity, security and privacy for elements of [Technology Provider]'s Product.

1. Entry, Transcription and/or Capture of Data in EDC Product

All EDC sessions are secure and encrypted. This is accomplished via industry standard SSL with 128 bit encryption. Data entry and capture actions will generally require two executions of your electronic signature, once to gain access to the trial and then the execution of the password at the completion of each "signing unit" (one or more forms for data entry done at one single continuous session and signed at one time). Study requirements will stipulate the data entry privileges by role. Each trial is validated to conform to these requirements. Unless otherwise expressly defined, only site personnel (Investigators and their designees) will be able (i.e., have privileges) to use the EDC product to act on data (enter, edit). Other system users such as monitors may use the EDC system to review and

---

–continued–

–continued–

query data, but not to enter or edit. The integrity and quality of data entered, captured or edited is supported by edit checks for any incomplete, missing, erroneous (inconsistent) and/or improperly formatted data.

2. Site Access and Review of Data

Data can be accessed and reviewed in the EDC product. The permissions on such review can be set so that only site personnel can see individually identifying health information captured in the study.

CONFIDENTIAL fields that have been specified during design to be hidden from other study personnel are supported. However, private information such as birthdates will usually be set to be viewable by Monitors and other study personnel. All such users of the EDC product will have undergone identity certification and will have signed an electronic signature agreement prior to issuance of access instructions. Thus, only bonafide study personnel will be able to access the eClinical Trial data via the web. All review sessions are secure using SSL with 128 bit encryption. Access and review is online only, and system controls and authority controls protect data integrity in ways that are fully compliant with FDA's 21 CFR Part 11 (Electronic Records; Electronic Signatures) and the Guidance on the Computer Systems Used In Clinical Trials.

3. Editing and audit trails

All edits, comments and other actions (e.g., approval, authentication) on data in eCRFs are automatically recorded in a computer generated and timestamped audit trail. Properly vetted users of the system can check the audit trail for particular forms, subjects or sites to review whomever made whatever changes or comments, when, and why. The full history of all data fields and comments is preserved throughout the trial and in the archive. The audit trail is also part of the archive (see below).

4. Security of All Subject Data and How Site personnel Maintain and Retain Data Locally

Site personnel ordinarily have access to review (and enter) any and all personally identifying information of subjects. HL7, the EU Privacy Directive and various other regulations on privacy in electronic commerce all apply to the personal health information gathered in clinical trials. Private data that might permit a person to derive the identity of a particular patient from routinely available information are specified in these regulations and must be removed from data prior to publication or unrestricted transfer. [Technology Provider]'s Product validation testing ensures that access to such data during a trial is restricted to study personnel according to the study plan and protocols. While this limits disclosure of private information, it nonetheless represents a disclosure that should be specifically described in the informed consent form. Formal informed waiver of any restrictions on the limited disclosure of such data and its transmission from the point of collection to the server ensures that electronic Clinical Trials will not violate known regulations concerning privacy. [Technology Provider] personnel who are not part of the study team do not have any access to data on study servers. Occasionally, for purposes of troubleshooting it may be necessary during the course of a study to directly access the database. [Technology Provider] procedures ensure that such access requires:

- the knowing collaboration of at least two people
- the approval of the site
- be for a limited time and for a disclosed purpose
- be fully documented.

[Technology Provider] maintains the system and security processes that ensure that the EDC product is available to sites and operates as intended during the trial so they can access data locally at any time. Furthermore, all [Technology Provider] personnel sign an agreement to respect and preserve the confidentiality of any private information that they may see in conjunction with servicing trials.

5. Access to Personal Identifying Data During the Trial and at Audit

Site personnel will have roles that will allow them to review and correct all subject data, including private data and signatures. The EDC product will support access at will via the Web during the trial, and the Archive CDROM will allow full review of the locked data during the retention period. The security and access control during the trial will derive from the encryption, firewall, server physical security, and password protection of [Technology Provider]'s Product. The Archive CD can be used by the Investigator and by FDA or other regulatory auditors to reconstruct the trial in compliance with regulations. For some trials private data in the archive may be visible only if a proper password is provided during use of the archive viewing tool. Under these conditions, the XML data in these private fields will be encrypted. Responsibility for security of the CD ROM Archive disk(s) will be transferred from [Technology Provider] to the Investigator upon receipt of the disk after the trial has been archived. [Technology Provider] will certify the authenticity and integrity of the data to the Investigator at the time the archive disk is created.

Another member of the trial team, the ethical committee or independent review board (IRB), has obligations before and during the trial to "assure the protection of the rights and welfare of human subjects." The data capture plans, including procedures at visits and any forms to be completed by subjects, are properly considered as part of the burdens to the subjects, and system providers can help IRBs by supporting online IRB access to such forms. Furthermore, the informed consent documents for each site may differ as regional needs are integrated into the forms. In some cases, several versions of the consent form are used during a trial as the review boards and investigators monitor the trial progress. Again, by providing access to trial information, particularly to data pertaining to patient safety and adverse events, the delays inherent in such monitoring can, in principle, be reduced.

The consent form (and HIPAA authorization) should include language describing any tasks to be required of subjects in a trial. The most common EDC task undertaken by subjects is the completion of a diary. The text below provides sample language for describing this task to subjects.

Sample Language for Informed Consent For a Trial Using an Electronic Diary to Capture Data from Subjects (with permission from PHT Corporation)

GENERAL: You will be asked to make daily reports about how you are feeling, and about taking your medications. Your study nurse will assign an electronic diary for you to use in making these reports. It is important that you answer the questions in the diary each day as carefully as you can. You will sign each report so your doctor can make sure that it is genuine. You will be asked to send reports each day by connecting your electronic diary to your telephone. Such data transmissions will use toll-free lines and will not result in telephone charges to you. All the data that you provide in these diaries will be held as confidential. Only your doctor and the study nurse will be able to review your signed reports. When the results of the study are analyzed, your diary data will be used as part of the analysis, but it will not contain your name. Such data may be seen by scientists and other analysts who will be working on this study, but it will not be accessible except for identified members of the study staff.

If you have questions about the use of the electronic diary that requires contact with the Help Desk, any personal information that you provide will be kept confidential and will not be shared with any third party.

PUBLICATION OF DIARY DATA: In this study, the data compiled on all the study subjects such as yourself will be combined into reports that may be published. Any published data will be anonymous, which means that the publication will not reveal your name, birth date or other identifying information.

Increasingly, and with continued FDA encouragement to do so, sponsors involve the FDA reviewers responsible for the IND review (i.e., necessary for the initiation of clinical trials in the United States) in the planning of clinical trials. EDC technology providers can assist in making the case to these FDA reviewers that the clinical trial systems planned for use are designed to promote data integrity, to support investigator actions on electronic records, and to conform with relevant requirements for eSignatures.

OPERATIONAL PREPARATIONS FOR TRIAL EXECUTION

Operational steps that must be accomplished after planning and selecting the technology provider but before initiating data capture from a trial subject include the use of a trial designer to develop the data capture application configured for the specific trial. Usually, this design is undertaken using an EDC design application that supports the detailed specification of each item to be captured, the grouping of items into sections and forms, and the implementation of a system of data capture devices, web and/or database server(s) to run the application that the study staff will use to capture, review and correct the trial data. For EDC systems, the protocol and requirements documents, with due consideration for available standards, will have established the intended content and operation of the data capture system. In contrast to paper methods, which demand only that the design and printing of a paper CRF incorporating protocol-mandated content be accomplished prior to enrolling the first trial subject, the fully operational EDC system, including any inspection and validation testing, must precede active enrollment. Such distinctions between paper and EDC methods (i.e., in the extent of preparation prior to initiating trial execution) are now well known. Despite the early-stage advantages of paper-based systems, it seems clear that the additional pre-planning required for electronic methods, including the implementation of logic checks, offers many benefits (e.g., detecting and preventing problems).

Testing, traceability and other pre-deployment activities Usability and beta testing are valuable methods for ensuring not only that the EDC system operates as intended, but that the planned operation fits sensibly into the real-world environment in which the trial will operate. Given the pressure to initiate the trial at the earliest possible time, there is a natural tension between accommodating the time necessary for user testing and the need to begin the trial. While user testing is rather common for EDC methods, it is rare with paper CRFs; therefore, process problems often emerge during paper-based trial start-up. Often, these problems include amendments to the site instructions regarding the processing of subjects and completing the CRFs. User testing of EDC systems can turn up similar problems. The difference is that amending the EDC system usually requires a change to the design of software or hardware and this, in turn, triggers a re-validation. Even apparently minor changes (e.g., deleting a visit) can have consequences for system operation that are difficult to anticipate. Such validation can be time consuming, and can add to the delays and costs associated with EDC. With experience, sponsors that adopt EDC accelerate the schedule of user testing and anticipate the time demands associated with performing a full validation.

Archiving test documentation The final requirements documents, traceability matrix, and executed test scripts must be completed before the "deployment" of a validated system. Further, it is helpful to perform an internal audit of the validation documentation to ensure that any deficiencies in the documentation are caught early and that any gaps in validation itself are identified. It is particularly important, given the reliance on EDC for data content, that system operation, timestamp accuracy, and data transport accuracy be tested in substantial detail.

Record capture, review (pre-deployment activities) With EDC, particularly eSource, there will be an availability of real-time data that can be used in enrollment management, medication compliance, and protocol adherence remotely via the web. Preparing for this post-deployment benefit is an essential aspect of pre-deployment planning, which should be performed at a level of detail that may surprise sponsors. For example, tracking enrollment can be accomplished by counting each new subject who advances from assessment for participation to participation in the trial. The event that usually constitutes enrollment is the execution and signing of the informed consent form by the subject or subject representative. How will this event be captured? An excellent, but still rare, way to capture the event is to provide the subject with a way to review the consent form and sign it using a traditional handwritten signature linked to an electronic version of the form. Alternatively, enrollment tracking can be marked by other events that occur on the same day and near the same time. One such event is the assignment to the patient of an eDiary, which can also provide additional data confirming the training of both patient and site personnel. The plan for displaying enrollment will establish the content and appearance of interim reports intended to be available on the web for those who will track and manage site performance. These displays may show the number of subjects who have enrolled, those who are currently active, those who have completed the protocol, those who withdrew early, and those who failed to meet inclusion, exclusion or randomization criteria. It is extremely important to stipulate exactly how each category of enrollment will be defined so that any disparities with alternative tracking of enrollment, such as by examination of paper logs at the site, can be easily understood. This will support the detection of meaningful problems with enrollment tracking from apparent disparities that can be expected from the differences in operational definitions.

Medication compliance is another area that can be more carefully tracked and, thus, more tightly managed with EDC than with paper methods. As with enrollment, the expectations concerning the schedule for the administration/consumption of the study drug should be defined exactly, and explained on the data summary or review report. As with other aspects of the system, such reports must be validated, especially if they will serve as the basis for decisions regarding the prosecution of the trial or the management of subjects. However, the EDC system should be designed so that changes or improvements to displays of interim data do not require re-validation of the system.

Key trial metrics that can be made available from EDC data should be contemplated prior to deployment and should be built into interim reports. These might include measures of query resolution time, fields resulting in an unusually high level of queries, screening activity at different sites, total participants at various sites together with the number of instances of the system's use or the use of particular reports, among others. A common feature in the design of interim reports should be a legend that explains in detail how each variable shown in the report is defined in terms of the trial data.

Trial Execution Post Deployment: *How EDC can be leveraged during a trial to improve trial management and scientific results.*

Once the trial is deployed, users will begin to operate the EDC system. The particulars of who will serve on the study team and what they will do will generally be part of the requirements documents, site contracts, and protocols. Generally, the first data that the EDC system will capture following deployment are the logins and agreements of study staff.

USER AND SUBJECT TRAINING, QUALIFICATION

Regulations require that users of EDC systems be properly authorized (including that they be identified, trained and properly qualified) for the roles they fulfill in conducting the trial. An EDC system will provide a technical infrastructure for capturing such data, and the inclusion of regulatory requirements in the EDC system requirements will ensure that all users are identified and authorized.

Roles and responsibilities in the trial The data captured will include data on the roles and responsibilities (privileges to act on electronic records) for each participant. As these roles and privileges change, and as new staff are recruited to the trial and prior staff cease to have active responsibilities, this key administrative data will be updated. Given the FDA CSUCT guidance's provisions concerning the reconstruction of a trial (section VI A), it would be both possible and desirable to generate a table showing the full history of the roles, responsibilities and privileges for each person who was ever recorded as part of the study staff. Thus, an auditor or regulatory inspector could determine who was able to act on electronic records at any time during the trial, and look at the signatures and actions on such records for consistency.

Likewise, EDC training and training documentation can be embedded in the EDC system. Forms and training documents can record who has read them, when and whether they acknowledge (or even demonstrate) mastery of the EDC system, and their understanding of any agreements under which they operate (e.g., that they will be held accountable for any actions on electronic records under their digital signature or other electronic signature).

Expediting Drug and Biologics Development

Passwords, access controls, signatures Federal regulations require that digital signatures (comprised of an ID that can be publicly known and a password that is known only to the user) must be unique. Thus, such "signatures" are often used to provide EDC system access to users who will review data as well as those who may act upon trial records in other ways (e.g., edit, approve, reject, comment). Given its concern over the possibility that, over time, a password may become compromised (i.e., used by another person), the FDA required (21 CFR 11.300 (b)) that digital signatures based on identification codes in combination with passwords be "periodically checked, recalled or revised." Therefore, many EDC systems require the periodic changing of passwords. Ironically, however, it appears from interviews with users of such systems that the burden of maintaining numerous passwords in human memory alone is great enough that many users either write down passwords or work out a system that allows them to easily change to a new version of a familiar password at each change interval. Such habits clearly thwart the intention of the provision.

An alternative approach, called the "forever password," may be worth promoting. The idea is that, by supporting the "checking" of all uses of a signature, possibly by providing a summary similar to the ones generated by credit card companies, EDC system users could inspect the summary and check for any un-remembered or inappropriate uses that might indicate that the password had become compromised. The benefit of such a system is that an individual could invest the energy in developing a truly proper password and protect it carefully from disclosure as a way to avoid the need to change it.

A clear feature of EDC systems that rely on login IDs and passwords is that electronic records may be "signed" using a digital signature for which there is no predicate rule requiring a signature.

Site monitoring by sponsors Patient screening activity can be revealed by capturing data on the evaluation of potential subjects, including the reasons that possible study subjects were rejected. Such data can then be used to quantify and forecast the impact that modifying inclusion/exclusion criteria could have on recruitment. By capturing such data through EDC systems, it is possible to monitor remotely (over the web) the relative performance of sites in assessing subjects for a trial.

Monitors are charged with verifying that the investigators follow the approved protocol and amendments, if any, and that the investigators document subject suitability and the completion of informed consent. With EDC systems that reflect the protocol and capture data concerning subject suitability and consent, much of this task can be facilitated by remote reports. In principle, this can make visits to the site more productive.

Since sponsors are often concerned with enrollment rates, EDC systems, by providing timely enrollment data, have offered benefits in supporting the tighter control of recruitment interventions and in managing sites that are high or low enrollers.

Subjects also must comply with the protocol, especially in terms of following the visit schedule, adhering to medication schedules and completing diaries and questionnaires. By enabling subjects to enter data as eSource on mobile data capture appliances such as eDiaries and handheld devices at sites, patient compliance can be tracked daily and used by sites to manage subjects. Technology providers are finding that active site management through daily diaries can raise completion compliance by 10% to 20% over the 75-85% compliance levels obtained without active management. Sponsors find that ongoing confirmation that subjects are complying with schedules during a trial (or not) provides essential information for intervention decisions.

Sponsors may also be interested in data queries, data management and cleaning activity, which can reveal CRF data items that are particularly ambiguous or difficult. Again, midcourse corrections can be undertaken earlier and with a clearer rationale than might otherwise be the case with paper-based systems.

System monitoring and changes A validation principle is that the EDC system continue to operate as intended for the duration of the trial. While the initial testing can confirm an expectancy in this regard, some degree of ongoing system monitoring regarding the proper operation of servers, client machines, handhelds, phones, medical devices and measuring devices will clearly be required. Documenting such monitoring can establish evidence that the EDC system, together with any handheld devices, kept accurate timestamps and properly updated any timezone definition changes that might have occurred during a trial.

System issues may arise because of faulty operation or because of ambiguous questions, poorly performing questionnaires and assessments, the need to escalate a dose, or changes to retain subjects who find it difficult or uncomfortable to comply with a planned provision of the protocol. Thus, it is essential that an EDC system support protocol amendments and be capable of incorporating essential changes to trial procedures that are embedded in the system. Therefore, trial change procedures can be part of the initial requirements and be a tested capability of the system. Each change should itself be documented, archived and subjected to the appropriate audits and approvals by an IRB. A properly planned EDC trial can support protocol versioning and record IRB approvals that will trigger the roll out of any change on a site-by-site basis.

Clinical Research Associates and trial monitoring EDC systems that support eSource data capture for most or all of the trial data offer the most significant benefits for monitors. As mentioned, the burden of field-by-field source document verification in such cases shifts from a manual task of examining documents for consistency (paper source matches paper CRF matches printout of the database) to one that is automated. The validation of the system's capability to accurately capture and store data as captured is the essential guarantee that data in the system are accurate. Therefore, monitors can engage in more substantial review of sites for procedures, authenticity of patients and the like. Note, however, that the burden of field checking persists for EDC systems that rely on paper source, since the transcription of source data to eCRFs is vulnerable to error and must be checked manually (ICH E6 section 5.18.4 (m) (i)).

EDC systems can include forms that monitors use to prepare monitoring reports. If the system is used to examine and check eCRFs against source, at least it can help document the work for the report, which simplifies the monitor's workload a bit. In cases in which eSource is used, the monitoring report can include text summaries and procedural judgments that are useful in ascertaining the credibility and professionalism of the site and in checking for signs of fraud or other misconduct.

Investigator performance with EDC systems can be monitored remotely by examining data pertaining to enrollment and by examining the progress of subjects through the scheduled events of the trial. Although monitoring does change with EDC (Carpenter, J: "21CFR11 Compliance at Investigator Sites" ACT, July 2003 pp35-40), with forethought the process can be made more effective and less burdensome (Raymond, Presentation at DIA ePRO Conference, Washington, October 30, 2003).

With EDC systems, issues of interest to monitors can be programmed into the system so that alerts are triggered algorithmically, supporting a rapid examination of issues that might otherwise linger until the next monitoring visit.

With paper, the archived data are vulnerable to loss, rot and dissipation. Similar risks pertain to electronic data for which the method of archiving has not been shown to fulfill the requirements for reconstruction over a retention period of 15 to 20 years. eSource and EDC that relies on SDTM or an XML-equivalent to assure that data are captured in archival format can support dynamic archiving that will permit sponsors and monitors to examine the archive as it accumulated during the trial. The examination could be accomplished with the FDA standard archive or submission review tools (Steve Wilson, Session 366 DM, 40th annual DIA Meeting, Washington, June 16, 2003), and a high degree of confidence can be gained in the archive's integrity long before the trial is completed. Users can effectively debug the archive and assess content for completeness, regulatory compliance and "reconstruction" as the trial progresses.

Trial completion: *EDC supports interim data assessment and correction and should result in delivery of analyzable data on LPO*

Data transfers When the sponsor will analyze captured data using a different system than the data capture system used during the trial, there is usually a transfer of data from the technology provider to the sponsor. As mentioned early in this chapter, such a transfer should have been specified in the detailed requirements documents, tested, validated, and possibly used throughout the trial. Thus, at trial completion, a final transfer should be easy to make in keeping with an established schedule or on demand.

eSource certification process and validation When data have been captured as eSource and in a format suitable for archiving and submission, the final archive of such data (as corrected using the system during the trial, including the necessary XML to include the audit trail and to prove that the data have been protected against tampering) can be created as a simple COPY action. Validating accurate copies through computer operating systems to archival media is simple, and should continue to be supported as long as electronic records continue to be widely used. Thus, the continued viability of the archive can be supported over decades simply by copying the data, metadata and necessary documentation as XML records onto appropriate storage media as preferred storage methods evolve.

Multiple trials and the Sequence of clinical drug development

THE CASE FOR eSOURCE AND eDIARIES IN PHASE 2 TRIALS.

Phase 2 decisions concerning safety and efficacy mean the most. If made incorrectly, a sponsor may wind up prosecuting an ineffective or dangerous therapy OR, alternatively, failing to develop an effective and safe therapy. Since the decision is made based on a modest number of subjects, it seems obvious that it would be useful to obtain as much information from each subject as possible. Thus, in Phase 2, it seems clear that relying on eSource to provide early and sensitive assessments makes sense. Sponsors want to avoid missing a key observation that could lead the preclinical team to modify the drug or procedure so as to rescue or preserve therapeutic benefit. The BEST data must inform these decisions, and the most sensitive, accurate and revealing methods should be used for Phase 2 trials.

EDC APPROACHES CAN BE TRANSFERRED TO PHASE 3 AND 4

Program efficiencies can be harvested if the questionnaires, variables, outcomes and methods are consistent across a sequence of trials. Furthermore, standards across an organization can support sponsor and regulatory agency meta analysis from the archives. In principle, the long-term benefits of clinical research findings are reduced unnecessarily when the sponsor neglects to capture and store the records in repositories that support reconstruction over lengthy periods. The distinction should be drawn between warehouses, which expedite the examination of several trials, and repositories, which keep data reliably in an open, standardized format so that they can be recovered. Typically, speed of analysis is not a requirement for a repository, which fulfills the critical but modest goal of providing the means to be able to retrieve data to attempt a meta analysis. It is much cheaper simply to maintain data in an archival repository than to settle on a proprietary tool designed for rapid analysis and assume that such a tool will continue to support files that were built and saved using early versions of the system.

Traditional Paper CRFs

The following recommendations and guidance comprise best practices that have been established over more than 50 years of performing clinical research studies using paper CRFs. Many of these practices continue to apply to eCRF and EDC systems as well as to paper-based methods.

General Guidance Consider adopting a standard format for the header information as early in the CRF development process as possible. Information that a CRF header might feature include the subject's initials, subject identification (SID), and the date the information on the page was captured for the CRF. Having both the subject initials and SID will be useful whenever one of the two is entered incorrectly, which can be a common occurrence. The SID is usually formatted so that the first two digits represent the site and the last three digits indicate the subject's number at that site.

In designing the case report forms, the sponsor's main goal should be to make the forms as user-friendly as possible, while still providing for the collection of all necessary information. If the necessary data are not gathered, the all-important analysis cannot be conducted. The design that is chosen for each form can have a significant impact on the accuracy of the data that are collected and/or entered into the clinical database. Simplicity and clarity are the keys to case report form design.

Directions provided on the CRF pages should be clear and concise. Site personnel will not always reference a study procedures manual or the protocol on CRF completion issues. Therefore, CRFs that provide brief, straightforward directions contribute to data accuracy and overall site efficiency by highlighting sensitive or confusing areas.

The sponsor should divide complex questions into several smaller questions, and should avoid leading questions that permit multiple responses. Instead of offering a general comment field, the sponsor should provide possible actions that should be taken and should ask the site to indicate the primary reason(s) that apply. While general, non-directed responses cannot be analyzed easily, predefined responses can be grouped and analyzed efficiently. If all possible responses cannot be anticipated, the sponsor should specify the most likely responses and provide an "other" category along with limited space for a response. If this option is chosen, monitors must pay special attention to ensure that the reasons written under the "other" category would not be more appropriately captured under one of the predefined responses.

The CRF should pose a question only once. As a general note of caution, the manner in which you ask certain questions can have profound consequences. For example, CRFs that request a particular piece of information twice will all too often lead to two different answers. Although requesting certain information multiple times may seem to provide a quality control check, it seldom works that way in practice. When the sponsor is interested in a piece of information, it should request it once and then check the data against the site's source documents and records.

Wherever appropriate, it is a good idea to incorporate checkboxes for answers to CRF questions. If specific baseline conditions are important for the analysis, for instance, they can be identified with a checkbox, thereby minimizing the likelihood that the condition might be overlooked. Doing so also facilitates the grouping of conditions, significantly decreasing or eliminating the need for coding the conditions.

Be consistent in the placement of response fields. For instance, make an effort to place the response to the right or the left of the question consistently, and avoid alternating between the two. Ideally, all checkboxes should be placed to the left of the responses to which they correspond.

Make an effort to list the predetermined responses in a meaningful order, and attempt to employ this order consistently. If the site must provide more information to answer a question, consider listing the answers so that the additional information follows the appropriate response (see exhibit below). If an affirmative response requires that additional information be provided, the CRF will flow better if the "no" response is listed first, followed by the "yes" response and then a "please specify" section.

ABC Pharmaceuticals

MEDICATIONS LOG
Screening Phase through Termination

NOTE: *Please PRINT using BLUE ink.*

Page #

COMPOUND NAME	
ABC Comp	
PROTOCOL NUMBER	IND NUMBER
ABC1234	XX,XXX

SUBJECT INITIALS

First Middle Last

SUBJECT IDENTIFICATION NUMBER

Were any medications administered? ☐ ₂No ☐ ₁Yes. If Yes, record below:

NAME OF DRUG	REASON FOR USE	START DATE	END DATE
		Day Month Year ☐ ₁Prior to CTM ☐ ₂After 1st CTM Dose	Day Month Year ☐ ₁Ongoing
		Day Month Year ☐ ₁Prior to CTM ☐ ₂After 1st CTM Dose	Day Month Year ☐ ₁Ongoing
		Day Month Year ☐ ₁Prior to CTM ☐ ₂After 1st CTM Dose	Day Month Year ☐ ₁Ongoing
		Day Month Year ☐ ₁Prior to CTM ☐ ₂After 1st CTM Dose	Day Month Year ☐ ₁Ongoing
		Day Month Year ☐ ₁Prior to CTM ☐ ₂After 1st CTM Dose	Day Month Year ☐ ₁Ongoing
		Day Month Year ☐ ₁Prior to CTM ☐ ₂After 1st CTM Dose	Day Month Year ☐ ₁Ongoing
		Day Month Year ☐ ₁Prior to CTM ☐ ₂After 1st CTM Dose	Day Month Year ☐ ₁Ongoing
		Day Month Year ☐ ₁Prior to CTM ☐ ₂After 1st CTM Dose	Day Month Year ☐ ₁Ongoing

Although they seem to be straightforward elements of the CRF, the date and time fields often trigger an inappropriately large number of problems. Simple details like units of conversion can also represent significant problem areas. One proactive approach is to begin CRF design with the most common sources of discrepancies in mind. Sponsors genuinely interested in site efficiency, data quality, and other important factors should immediately abandon the philosophy reflected by those who state, "I pay these investigators a lot of money to do this trial, so they should enter data in whatever format I choose." Such chest-thumping will not promote the desired results, regardless of who is paying the bills.

Consider the study's timeframe in attempting to collect date-related information. If data are to be collected for a certain number of hours after dosing, keep in mind that the clock may pass midnight. If it does, collecting the date change may or may not be necessary, depending on the form's design. Date changes do not always occur only at the end of 12- or 24-hour collections. If the subject was dosed at 8:00 a.m. and data must be collected 18 hours after dosing, a date change will occur. If all subjects are not being dosed at the same time of day, the date changes may occur at different intervals. When this is the case, dates may have to be collected at every interval. As an alternative, the sponsor may choose to collect only the initial date and time on the CRF, and allow its database to calculate the date change. If the database will track the date, there may not be any justification for attempting to collect the date change on the CRF (and invite the unnecessary problems that this can cause).

Expediting Drug and Biologics Development

It is imperative that dates be collected in a consistent format. If date formats change from page to page, errors can easily be made at the site and then be overlooked during monitoring and data entry. Although some inconsistencies can be detected through electronic validation, the sponsor should not rely exclusively on automated checks. Take a situation in which a study is conducted from June through October. If a validation check is developed to verify that the dates occurred within that timeframe, it would not detect transpositions of 08-09-XX and 09-08-XX. To further promote accurate date collection, sponsors should use an alphanumeric date format (09-AUG-XX) rather than a completely numeric format (08-09-XX).

Geography must also be considered when selecting a date format. In the United States, for example, 08-09-XX is most often interpreted as August 9. In Europe, however, it would represent September 8. Typically, a date variable should be collected in the format that is most familiar to the personnel completing the forms. The international format is becoming increasingly common in the United States, and its use in CRFs is encouraged. It is suggested that the data be collected in three separate fields: (1) a two-digit numeric for the day; (2) a three-letter alpha for the month; and (3) a two-digit numeric for the year (e.g., 18MAY99). The bottom line is to get it right in the CRF.

Sponsors should approach CRF design not only with the data transcriber in mind, but the person responsible for entering the data into the company's computer database as well. While the primary goal is to make sure that the correct data are captured on the CRFs, it is also extremely important that the sponsor do everything possible to ensure that the data are accurately transferred into the database.

There are two general ways in which the CRF booklet can be formatted—by visit or by type of data. Experience indicates that study personnel find it easier to enter data by visit, since they do not have to flip through a number of pages to enter the data for a particular visit. On the other hand, the sponsor's database is likely to be organized and grouped by variables, such as body weights across visits. This fact sometimes pressures CRF designers to format CRF pages across multiple visits, an approach called "log style."

Since the goal is to have accurate data entered onto the CRFs and into the sponsor's database, the method that yields the fewest data transcription errors at the study site is generally the best option. In practice, however, methods that address both issues have proven to be the most appropriate for site personnel and the most reliable with respect to site-related transcription errors and data entry by the sponsor. By limiting the use of log-style CRF pages, data from completed visits may be harvested from the site upon their completion (as opposed to the subject's completion of the trial). If logs are used in a limited fashion, they can be harvested at each monitoring visit as well. Simply enter all of the data available at that time on the CRF. When additional data become available later, the missing information can be entered and the revised page can be forwarded for processing. This allows the data management process to begin earlier, which helps minimize related demands during the time-critical trial-completion period.

Certain standard CRF pages, such as the medications log and the adverse events form, are best formatted in log style so they can be used across the entire study, regardless of whether they are collected in a single entry per page or multiple-entry format. This practice is intended to prevent the problems often encountered when an entry continues across more than one visit. When a singular occurrence of an adverse event or medication is recorded in only one place in a CRF booklet, there is less opportunity for discrepancies that must be resolved either during or at the end of the trial. An adverse event or medication should only be repeated on the CRF if it is a true reoccurrence of that same adverse event or medication, and if the form's format and content dictate the additional entry. Consider nausea, for example. One bout of nausea spanning more than one visit would be recorded only once, with start and stop dates that define the occurrence. If the event resolved but then reoccurred at a later date, it should then be considered a new event and be recorded a second time. Alternatively, the AE page could have a checkbox to indicate that the event is "intermittent," eliminating the need for an additional entry. Similarly, a concomitant medication page could include a checkbox to indicate "PRN."

An alternative method (that is not recommended but is often practiced) involves recording continuing adverse events and concomitant medications separately on a new CRF page at every visit. This method is almost certain to cause confusion, however. Data entry personnel may enter the same event multiple times when, in reality, it is only one event that has continued over multiple visits. When the same data are entered multiple times, there are significantly more opportunities for database errors and data inconsistencies.

In addition, if the verbatim text used to describe the event is not the same for the two entries of the same event, they are difficult to link unless a numbering system is used. If a numbering system is used, this system comprises another item to be monitored and reviewed. Adopting a system in which someone must examine the CRFs to ensure that the dates are continuous simply invites trouble. If an event spans two or more visits, what start and stop dates and times are used to describe the same event over time on the individual forms? While there are numerous ways to address that question, the bottom line is that, in practice, it causes confusion. In turn, confusion results in discrepancies and discrepancies result in lost time and wasted resources.

It is worth noting that key presentations of adverse events in final reports and marketing applications (NDAs) are usually summaries, and customarily list the total number and percent of subjects who experienced at least one occurrence of any particular event, not the total number of events including multiple occurrences in individual subjects. Generally, a subject does not appear more than once in any summary listing for a single adverse event.

The data collected on the CRFs should be transcribed from source documents at the investigational site. Although these source documents will generally include study notebooks, patient charts and laboratory printouts, any document that accurately reflects a subject's treatment course may be used. The CRF design should permit the direct transcription of data from the source documents. For example, a CRF should ideally allow the transcriber to record data in the same units used on the source document (with a checkbox to indicate the unit used). If this unit is not the one to be used in the sponsor's report, the conversion should be made by the sponsor's computer, rather than during the transcription stage at the study site. If the units are pre-defined as choices on the CRF page, data management can default the units in the database, which minimizes the need to enter defaulted data. Keep in mind that computers generally do not make calculation errors, but that humans do. Many collection and transcription errors can be avoided through the use of thoughtfully planned, well-organized, and clearly labeled CRFs.

As mentioned, the sponsor's data management staff must also be considered in CRF design. A sponsor's data management team is responsible for entering the data from the CRFs into the clinical database and for ensuring the accuracy of the entered data. Many simple CRF design features can significantly speed data entry and reduce data entry errors without adversely affecting the collection of data. Foremost among these is the use of checkboxes (as mentioned above) on the CRFs. If specific data are of interest, prompt for them. For instance, if the use of specific classes of concomitant medication will be analyzed and presented rather than specific medications, the different classes can be prompted with a yes/no checkbox reply. The alternative would require coding and the subsequent classification of handwritten medication names, something that would be significantly less efficient than the checkbox approach.

Another strategy that can aid the data entry process is the use of preprinted code numbers on CRFs for those items that would typically employ a codelist. If the data entry process involves a coding system instead of the entry of actual values—as is often the case when multiple choices are available for a response—then having the code printed on the CRF speeds the data entry process. If a data entry staffer must reference a list in the system or on the entry screen, his or her flow of entry will be broken and slowed, promoting entry errors.

In the early stage of CRF development, a form can undergo many changes. To keep track of these changes, sponsors should include version dates, version numbers and revision numbers (01-FEB-98 version 1.05). When extensive changes are made to a particular CRF page, the version date and number should be updated (09-FEB-98 version 2.00). Small changes or corrections to a page will be reflected in the revision date and number (09-FEB-98 version 2.01). Once a form reaches the late stages of development, the number of changes will drop significantly. Even when a form has been "finalized," revisions may be made as the development philosophies change.

Standard Case Report Forms Two general types of CRFs are used in clinical trials—standard CRFs and study-specific CRFs. The sponsor should develop a set of standard CRFs as early as possible, ideally prior to the start of the first clinical trial. These standard case report forms will then be made part of the CRF packet for every clinical trial conducted by a particular sponsor—ideally across product lines, but at a minimum across all trials for a specific product. The information that will be captured on these forms will be a function of many of the standard data presentations. Obviously, the idea at this point is to standardize CRF pages as much as possible. This approach avoids "reinventing the wheel" every time a study is initiated, and eliminates the likelihood that important data or information will be omitted. At a minimum, standard CRFs generally comprise the following pages:

> Demographic Data (see exhibit below);
> Medical History (see exhibit below);
> Inclusion Criteria (see exhibit below);
> Medications Log (see exhibit below)
> Laboratory collections/results (see exhibit below)
> Adverse Events (see exhibit below)
> Completion/Termination (see exhibit below)

Demography CRF: As is evident in the standard demography data CFR, the demography CRF page contains a field to capture the date on which the informed consent was signed as well as sample demography information. Although recording

Expediting Drug and Biologics Development

Form 1: Demographic Data

ABC Pharmaceuticals

DEMOGRAPHIC DATA

SCREENING PHASE

Page #

COMPOUND NAME	
ABC Comp	
PROTOCOL NUMBER	IND NUMBER
ABC1234	XX-XXX

NOTE: *Please PRINT using BLUE ink.*

SUBJECT INITIALS — First Middle Last

SUBJECT IDENTIFICATION NUMBER

DATE — Day Month Year

INFORMED CONSENT

Informed Consent Form must be signed prior to initiation of any Screening Period assessments.

Date Informed Consent Form was signed: Day Month Year

DEMOGRAPHIC DATA

DATE OF BIRTH: Day Month Year

SEX: ☐ Male   ☐ Female

ETHNICITY:
☐ White
☐ Black
☐ Hispanic
☐ Asian
☐ Other, specify _____

Form 2: Medical History/Physical Examination

ABC Pharmaceuticals

MEDICAL HISTORY/PHYSICAL EXAMINATION

Page #

COMPOUND NAME	
ABC Comp	
PROTOCOL NUMBER	IND NUMBER
ABC1234	XX-XXX

NOTE: *Please PRINT using BLUE ink.*

SUBJECT INITIALS — First Middle Last

SUBJECT IDENTIFICATION NUMBER

DATE — Day Month Year

Does the subject have a current disease or condition (including allergies and abnormalities)?   ☐ No   ☐ Yes. If Yes, specify below.

Check all body systems examined:
☐ General Appearance   ☐ Abdomen   ☐ Ears, Nose, Throat   ☐ Genitalia
☐ Skin   ☐ Musculoskeletal   ☐ Eyes   ☐ Lymph Nodes
☐ Cardiovascular   ☐ Rectal   ☐ Chest/Lungs   ☐ Psychiatric Status

Disease, Abnormality, Condition or Allergy	Diagnosis Date (MO/YR)	ICD-9 Codes

Form 3: Inclusion Criteria

ABC Pharmaceuticals

INCLUSION CRITERIA

Page #

COMPOUND NAME	
ABC Comp	
PROTOCOL NUMBER	IND NUMBER
ABC1234	XX-XXX

NOTE: *Please PRINT using BLUE ink.*

SUBJECT INITIALS — First Middle Last

SUBJECT IDENTIFICATION NUMBER

DATE — Day Month Year

INCLUSION CRITERIA

For a patient to be considered eligible for this study, Questions 1 through 5 must be answered Yes.

		No	Yes
1.	Criteria one	STOP	
2.	Criteria two	STOP	
3.	Criteria three	STOP	
4.	Criteria four	STOP	
5.	Criteria five	STOP	

Use same format for Exclusion Criteria

Form 4: Medications Log

ABC Pharmaceuticals

MEDICATIONS LOG

Screening Phase through Termination

Page #

COMPOUND NAME	
ABC Comp	
PROTOCOL NUMBER	IND NUMBER
ABC1234	XX-XXX

NOTE: *Please PRINT using BLUE ink.*

SUBJECT INITIALS — First Middle Last

SUBJECT IDENTIFICATION NUMBER

Were any medications administered?   ☐ No   ☐ Yes. If Yes, record below.

NAME OF DRUG	REASON FOR USE	START DATE			END DATE		
		Day	Month	Year	Day	Month	Year
		☐ Prior to CTM		☐ After 1st CTM Dose		☐ Ongoing	

Form 1 (top left):

ABC Pharmaceuticals
CLINICAL CHEMISTRY
Treatment Period
Study Day X

COMPOUND NAME — ABC Comp
PROTOCOL NUMBER — ABC1234
IND NUMBER — XX,XXX
Page #

NOTE: Please PRINT using BLUE ink.

SUBJECT INITIALS (First Middle Last) SUBJECT IDENTIFICATION NUMBER

CLINICAL CHEMISTRY

Date sample collected: Day Month Year   Time sample collected: (0000-2359)

TEST/MEASUREMENT	VALUE	UNITS	Specify Units (if different)	Is result clinically significant?
Lab Parameter 1		A/B		No / Yes
Lab Parameter 2		XXXX/Y		No / Yes
Lab Parameter 3		A/B		No / Yes
Lab Parameter 4		A/B		No / Yes
Lab Parameter 5		A/B		No / Yes
Lab Parameter 6		XXXX/Y		No / Yes
Lab Parameter 7		XXXX/Y		No / Yes
Lab Parameter 8		XXXX/Y		No / Yes

Form 2 (top right):

ABC Pharmaceuticals
CLINICAL CHEMISTRY
Treatment Period
Study Day X

COMPOUND NAME — ABC Comp
PROTOCOL NUMBER — ABC1234
IND NUMBER — XX,XXX
Page #

NOTE: Please PRINT using BLUE ink.

SUBJECT INITIALS (First Middle Last) SUBJECT IDENTIFICATION NUMBER

CLINICAL CHEMISTRY

Was the sample collected? No / Yes   If Yes, record collection below.

Date sample collected: Day Month Year

Accession number:

Form 3 (bottom left):

ABC Pharmaceuticals
ADVERSE EVENTS LOG
Screening/Baseline Period through Post-treatment Follow-up Period

COMPOUND NAME — ABC Comp
PROTOCOL NUMBER — ABC1234
IND NUMBER — XX,XXX
Page #

NOTE: Please PRINT using BLUE ink.

SUBJECT INITIALS (First Middle Last) SUBJECT IDENTIFICATION NUMBER

Were any adverse events observed or reported since CTM administered? No / Yes If Yes, record below.

DESCRIPTION OF SINGLE ADVERSE EXPERIENCE:

ONSET DATE AND TIME	END DATE AND TIME	SERIOUSNESS (Regulatory definition)*
Day Month Year (0000-2359) Unknown	Day Month Year Continuing (0000-2359) Unknown	Check (✓) all that apply: Death † (see below); Life-threatening (immediate risk of death) † (see below); Requires or prolongs inpatient hospitalization † (see below); Persistent or significant disability/incapacity † (see below); A congenital anomaly/birth defect † (see below); Other events that required medical or surgical intervention to prevent one of the above outcomes † (see below); None of the above (Not Serious)

SEVERITY	ACTION(S) TAKEN*	
Check (✓) one. Mild; Moderate; Severe	Check (✓) all that apply: None; Drug Therapy Administered†; Nondrug Therapy Administered†; CTM Dosage Changed; CTM Interrupted; CTM Discontinued	†CONTACT MEDICAL MONITOR IMMEDIATELY

CAUSALITY*	OUTCOME*
Check (✓) one. None; Possible; Probable; Definite	Check (✓) one. Recovered; Recovered with sequelae; Not yet recovered; Fatal; Resulted in Termination; Unknown

* Refer to back of page for definitions of Seriousness, Severity, Relationship to Study Drug, and Outcome.
†Specify drug treatment administered by recording medication(s) in the Medications History Log section of the CRF.
‡Specific details should be recorded in the Comments Log section of the CRF.

Form 4 (bottom right):

ABC Pharmaceuticals
TERMINATION RECORD

COMPOUND NAME — ABC Comp
PROTOCOL NUMBER — ABC1234
IND NUMBER — XX,XXX
Page #

NOTE: Please PRINT using BLUE ink.

SUBJECT INITIALS (First Middle Last) SUBJECT IDENTIFICATION NUMBER DATE Day Month Year

Characterize the subject's termination from the study: (Check (✓) the primary reason only)

- Normal Completion
- Adverse event, regardless of association with the test article
- Withdrawal of Consent
- Lack of effectiveness
- Protocol violation/Research terminated by Sponsor
- Death
- Lost to follow-up
- Other

I certify that I have examined all case report forms for this subject and found them to be complete and accurate.

Investigator's Signature   Day Month Year

the date on which the consent was signed is not recommended unless the sponsor plans to use it in the analysis or the database, various sponsors continue to capture such information. In the exhibit, note the formatting of the date fields, the use of check boxes, and the use of code numbers as subscripts adjacent to boxes with entries that will be coded in the database. Remember that this is just an example and could contain a variety of different information. The key is to try to keep it consistent throughout a particular drug's development.

Medical History CRF: A subject's medical history and data on the subject's baseline signs and symptoms are virtually always captured. This information can be collected in a number of ways, depending on how they are to be analyzed and/or presented in the clinical study report. Medical history, physical examination results, and baseline signs and symptoms can be recorded either separately or together on the same form.

The sample medical history/physical examination CRF presents a simple form for collecting all medical history, physical examination and baseline signs and symptoms data. Some find this particular sample to be evolutionary; others find it to be revolutionary. Think carefully about the end result of the information to be collected and the simplicity of this form becomes apparent. This format provides for the collection of all the information on a subject's baseline status on a single page (and its continuation, if necessary). Because the format also minimizes the opportunities for discrepancies, it has been used quite successfully.

Since we are talking about history and pre-study physical findings, only month and year are captured. Codes may or may not be used, depending on whether or not the information will be analyzed.

If more than one form is used to collect medical history, physical findings, and baseline signs and symptoms at screening and baseline, it is likely that data will be duplicated. The determining factor on which form(s) should be used will be the manner in which the data are to be displayed in the final report summaries and listings.

Inclusion/Exclusion CRF: Some forms may be standard in format only, such as inclusion and exclusion criteria and laboratory collections or results. While these forms may vary in content from study to study, their basic format can remain the same. Often, it is not necessary for the sponsor to capture inclusion and exclusion criteria in the clinical database, unless the criteria drive a listing of inclusion—and exclusion—criteria violators. Although some sponsors prefer to have these data in the database to show that the subjects met the criteria, the data must be monitored, entered, validated and reported if they are collected.

Medication Log: When the sponsor is considering what data must be collected regarding concomitant medications, it should consider whether dose, route and frequency information are truly necessary (refer to the analysis plan for the study). The exhibit provides a sample medications log CRF that captures almost all types of related data. While such a thorough data capture may be necessary for some drugs, it will generally not be useful for most concomitant medications or most studies.

Some drugs are dosed on a sliding scale and may change daily. To capture these data, the sponsor would have to list the drug multiple times on the CRF. In turn, the CRF would have to capture an entry of each dose or a range so that the highest and lowest dose can be captured. This approach creates more transcription, monitoring, data entry and validation efforts, which are often not reflected in the final report. Alternatively, sponsors can decide not to collect dose information or to collect the total daily dose.

Route of administration is another variable that can have multiple responses. Some patients may be receiving a drug via multiple routes. Again, either the information must be indicated multiple times on the CRF, or the database must be adjusted to accommodate these multiple responses. Detailed data may not be useful because responses like these are not easily analyzed unless they are grouped. Again, by collecting only the information necessary for reporting, the sponsor avoids having to monitor, enter, validate or report extraneous data, thereby saving time and money. The sample medications log CRF proposes a straightforward alternative.

Clinical Laboratory Data: Laboratory data, such as hematology, clinical chemistry and urinalysis data, are time-consuming to enter and reconcile. Although they are best captured electronically, they can be transcribed onto a CRF (see sample clinical chemistry CRFs) or entered into the database directly from the laboratory report. If data are collected electronically, they can be uploaded directly into the clinical database. This method eliminates data entry errors as well as errors due to illegible handwriting. To support the process of matching up electronic lab data to hand-entered data in the database, the sponsor must place on the CRF pages unique sample identifiers that can be compared to the electronic lab file.

Typically, laboratory data are collected a number of times throughout a study for each subject. To verify that the correct electronic data were received for each subject, the sponsor must establish, at the minimum, a sample identifier and the date that the lab sample was drawn. All laboratories assign a unique number to each laboratory sample for identification purposes. When this number and the collection date are collected on the CRF page (see exhibits), the identification number can be entered into the clinical database, which will streamline the electronic data upload.

Laboratory data that are transcribed onto the CRF are not subject to such problems, since the CRF will identify the subject and the date of the draw, and will provide the parameter and the result. However, laboratory data that are manually collected must be carefully scrutinized to ensure accurate transcription and data entry, a process that is time consuming for the site and for the data management team as well.

Because it is so labor intensive, entering the laboratory data directly from the laboratory reports is the least desirable of these three methods. Generally, laboratory parameters are not collected consistently, and may not be listed in the same order across sites or even from one sample to the next.

Adverse Event CRF: The sample adverse event (AE) CRF is one of the most important CRF pages. Along with the CRF pages that collect the primary effectiveness data, these pages collect the information that is the most crucial to a product's approval. The AE CRF is also a focal point for another reason: It generally results in the most discrepancies.

As is true for the other CRFs, the data requested on the AE CRF should be guided by the content of the desired output—in this case, the safety summaries and listings. Obviously, the AE CRF page must have a description of an adverse event. This (verbatim) text describing the AE is usually coded to a preferred term using a standard dictionary, such as Medical Drug Regulatory Activities (MedDRA). (Previously, this also included Coding Symbols Thesaurus of Adverse Reaction Terms (COSTART) and the World Health Organization Adverse Reaction Terminology (WHOART)). Dates of AE onset and termination provide information on whether or not an event is "treatment emergent," and help assign the AE to a more specific segment of a trial, if necessary.

The proposed AE CRF collects only one AE on a page. An advantage to collecting just one event per page is that the AE CRF page can be harvested as soon as that AE—rather than a cohort of events—resolves. Site and data management personnel have found these forms to be extremely user friendly. The majority of the form utilizes checkboxes—the only area in which the site has the opportunity to write text is in describing the adverse event. This format also allows the site to complete the form without having to reference a list for coded responses. In addition, it permits the site to review all of the allowed responses easily before checking the appropriate one. The form provides for easy data entry by data management personnel as well, since all entries are coded on the form. Although a disadvantage to this form is that it requires many AE pages per patient for some studies, it still works well in practice.

Quite often, a sponsor will require that a study closeout physical examination be completed at the end of the trial and that, for this examination, the site complete another CRF page similar to the one used for the physical conducted at the beginning of the trial. Comparisons of pre- and post-study physical examinations may indicate the existence of an adverse event. If no AE is recorded on the AE CRF, considerable time can be invested in attempts to formally reconcile differences between these two physicals and the AE CRFs. Alternatively, the sponsor can ask the investigator to compare the two examinations (without using a second physical examination page), and to enter any changes discovered in the final physical exam on the adverse event CRF. The primary rationale for conducting the exit physical examination is to identify adverse events. Any detrimental change in the subject's condition is, by definition, an adverse event. There is no need to collect the actual physical examination data unless it will be analyzed and presented in some other way.

Termination CRF: A study completion/termination form is usually the last CRF in the study packet. This is an appropriate place to capture information that will classify the subject into one of the primary subgroups under which the summary data are sorted. This makes it an ideal form for the use of checkboxes. The fields within which the reason for termination will be captured should be a function of the final report templates that will present the same information. This page is also an appropriate place for the investigator's signature to certify that the information in the entire packet meets his or her approval. CRF changes dated after the date associated with the investigator's signature will require a subsequent re-approval by the investigator.

Comment Fields: Generally, comment fields and other areas in which the investigator can make random, free-form notes are not recommended. If these fields contain information useful to the trial, this information probably belongs elsewhere on that form or on another CRF. The sponsor is then left with the task of moving the data from the comment field to the more appropriate location on the forms. If no other location in the entire set of CRFs accommodates the text in the comment field, either the sponsor did not want it for the analysis or neglected to include it. More often than not, it is the former. Experience has shown that avoiding the use of comment fields by providing an alternative method for collecting that information eliminates a whole host of problems.

Study-specific Case Report Forms Quite often, study-specific CRFs are not designed until after the study protocol has been drafted and, in some instances, finalized. The disadvantage of this approach is that the sponsor does not have the benefit of an outlined strategy for the data collection. In such cases, what was thought to be a detailed procedures section in the protocol often turns out to be missing several key aspects, necessitating a change in the protocol at a point that produces a delay in the trial's initiation.

By starting with an analysis plan and using it to plan backwards, the traditional approach is replaced with a more efficient and manageable process for CRF development and implementation. In our proposed approach to clinical development, the precise data needed for the analysis and presentation will first be defined in the analysis plan. Based upon the analysis plan, the CRFs can be designed to capture only the data that are necessary for the analysis, thus avoiding the collection of unnecessary data. All too often, vast amounts of unused data are collected and entered into the clinical database, wasting precious time and money.

The draft CRFs then serve as an outline for the procedures section of the protocol, resulting in fewer omissions of necessary data and facilitating the writing of the protocol's procedures section. As revisions are made to draft CRFs, the procedures section within the protocol must be updated to reflect any changes that may affect CRF completion. Therefore, the CRFs should be based upon the analysis plan rather than the study protocol, and the procedures in the protocol should be based on the CRFs and should be used as a means of generating the pre-specified data for analysis and presentation in the study's final report—and eventually the NDA.

Increasingly, drug development is a race to the finish line. With some forethought and planning in the CRF development process, the efficient capture of quality data will help speed the drug sponsor to that finish line.

CHAPTER 19

The Clinical Protocol

by Steven E. Linberg, Ph.D., Bao-Van Tran, M.S., and Matthew R. Dauphin, M.S.

The protocols of every study conducted and included in a marketing application establish the foundation upon which the entire clinical and statistical sections of a marketing application rest. With so much at stake, it is imperative that each study protocol be carefully planned and well written. The front-end time and planning necessary to design and write a sound protocol is well worth the investment. It is ironic that many people working in clinical development hastily plan and write protocols, yet carefully analyze data and write final reports. If the protocol is poor, the study will be poor. No subsequent analysis or report will be able to salvage it. If a poorly developed protocol happens to be for a trial critical to the development program, it may prevent the trial from providing pivotal support for an anticipated claim.

Given the importance the protocol has in the overall scheme of product development and given that every protocol places the subject at some degree of risk, the clinical developer should make every effort to ensure that each and every protocol provides the necessary support for the results of the trial. The protocol, as discussed in this chapter and in the protocol template guide provided, is derived from many sources. In addition to being a companion document to the clinical study report, the protocol derives a good deal of its content from federal regulations, as referenced throughout this chapter and the protocol template guide.

Beginning the Protocol Development Process Before the writing of a protocol outline even begins, a good amount of up-front work should be completed. The first step in this process should be to convene what is called a "protocol strategy meeting." The protocol strategy meeting is an internal company meeting that involves representatives from all disciplines involved in clinical research. Participants should include the study director, medical monitor, statistician, data manager, and one or more potential investigators serving as medical consultants, plus representatives from regulatory affairs and marketing. Inviting potential investigators to this meeting will help promote the development of a protocol that is practical and avoid unnecessary delays at a later date. These investigators also can help the sponsor defend the protocol at the investigators' meeting.

The protocol strategy meeting is likely to last all day. Discussion topics should include the study's objectives, variables, design, study population, inclusion/exclusion criteria, primary and important secondary analyses, anticipated data displays (tables and figures), and basic study procedures.

The product of this protocol strategy meeting will be an abbreviated clinical analysis plan on which the protocol will be based. The abbreviated clinical analysis plan (sometimes called a "study concept document") will clearly describe the study objectives, variables (what and when), trial design, study procedures (at least in the form of a "time and events chart"), as well as preliminary information on the intended study population (preliminary inclusion and exclusion criteria). It will also describe the anticipated analyses and data displays, randomization methods, anticipated trial duration, number of sites, and sometimes even the estimated cost.

Once the clinical analysis plan has been drafted, several sections can be lifted directly from it for inclusion in the protocol. The clinical analysis plan will also serve as the basis for determining the content of the draft case report form content, which will be used to drive much of the procedures described in the protocol.

As discussed in the chapter on final study reports, it is strongly recommended that each sponsor adopt a standard template for the final study report format and content. Once the format and content of the final study report have been determined, the protocol can be designed to generate the information necessary to meet the study objectives. So, while protocols and final study reports are individual documents that stand alone and must meet separate content requirements, they should be designed so that the protocol will support the final report. Coordinating the protocol and final study report will provide the reviewer with a sense of the planning, organization and professionalism that went into the studies, and will highlight how well the studies were conducted. The efforts made in planning the protocol will maximize the value of the final result, including the planned integration of a group of studies into the marketing application.

Standard Protocol Content As stated, the protocol and final study report are intended to be companion documents that contain much of the same information. A protocol states how a study is to be conducted and provides the methodology for obtaining pre-determined information for the analysis and final study report of a clinical trial. The final study report states exactly how well the protocol was followed, and presents the results of the study. In fact, much of the final study report's content can be derived from the protocol, reinforcing the support that the protocol provides for the final study report and facilitating the process of writing the final study report, which saves time by allowing the author to copy much of the information from the protocol directly into the report.

Recognizing the importance of the protocol, the FDA has made a significant effort to explain what information must be included within the document. The minimum criteria are specified in 21 CFR 312.23(a)(6)(iii), which states that any study protocol must contain the following elements:

(a) A statement of the objectives and purpose of the study.

(b) The name and address and a statement of the qualifications (curriculum vitae or other statement of qualifications) of each investigator, and the name of each subinvestigator (e.g., research fellow, resident) working under the supervision of the investigator; the name and address of the research facilities to be used; and the name and address of each reviewing institutional review board.

(c) The criteria for patient selection and for exclusion of patients and an estimate of the number of patients to be studied.

(d) A description of the design of the study, including the type of control group to be used, if any, and a description of the methods to be used to minimize bias on the part of subjects, investigators, or analysts.

(e) The method for determining the dose(s) to be administered, the planned maximum dosage, and the duration of individual patient exposure to the drug.

(f) A description of the observations and measurements to be made to fulfill the objectives of the study.

(g) A description of clinical procedures, laboratory tests, or other measures to be taken to monitor the effects of the drug in human subjects and to minimize risks.

The criteria listed above represent the minimum FDA requirements for a protocol that exposes subjects to a test article in clinical trials (similar guidance is provided in Section 6 of the ICH's E6 guidelines entitled, "Good Clinical Practice," and in the ICH's E8 guideline entitled, "General Considerations for Clinical Trials). However, a protocol that meets only these minimum requirements may not be able to provide "substantial evidence" of safety and effectiveness in support of a marketing application. Therefore, the FDA has established a higher standard that so-called "pivotal trials, which are those that will be most critical in providing the "substantial evidence" necessary to establish a new product's safety and effectiveness, must meet. As such, the Federal Food, Drug and Cosmetic Act defines substantial evidence as "evidence consisting of adequate and well-controlled investigations..." The criteria for adequate and well-controlled status are defined in 21 CFR 314.126(b) as follows:

(1) There is a clear statement of the objectives of the investigation and a summary of the proposed or actual methods of analysis in the protocol for the study and in the report of its results. In addition, the protocol should contain a description of the proposed methods of analysis, and the study report should contain a description of the methods of analysis ultimately used. If the protocol does not contain a description of the proposed methods of analysis, the study report should describe how the methods used were selected.

(2) The study employs a design that permits a valid comparison with a control to provide a quantitative assessment of drug effect. The protocol for the study and report of results should describe the study design precisely; for example, duration of treatment periods, whether treatments are parallel, sequential, or crossover, and whether the sample size is predetermined or based upon some interim analysis. Generally, the following types of controls are recognized:

(i) Placebo concurrent control. The test drug is compared with an inactive preparation designed to resemble the test drug to the degree possible. A placebo-controlled study may include additional treatment groups, such as an active treatment control or a dose-comparison control, and usually includes randomization and blinding of patients or investigators, or both.

(ii) Dose-comparison concurrent control. At least two doses of the drug are compared. A dose-comparison study may include additional treatment groups, such as a placebo control or active control group. Dose-comparison trials usually include randomization and blinding of patients or investigators, or both

(iii) No treatment concurrent control. When objective measurements of effectiveness are available and placebo effect is negligible, the test drug is compared with no treatment. No treatment concurrent control trials usually include randomization.

(iv) Active treatment concurrent control. The test drug is compared with known effective therapy—for example, when the condition treated is such that administration of placebo or no treatment would be contrary to the interest of the patient. However, an active treatment study may include additional treatment groups, such as a placebo control or a dose-comparison control. Active treatment trials usually include randomization and blinding of patients or investigators, or both. If the trial's intent is to show similarity of the test and control drugs, the report of the study should assess the study's ability to detect a difference between treatments. Similarity of test drug and active control can mean either that both drugs were effective or that neither was effective. The analysis of the study should explain why the drugs should be considered effective in the study—for example, by reference to results in previous placebo-controlled studies of the active control drug.

(v) Historical control. The results of treatment with the test drug are compared with experience historically derived from the adequately documented natural history of the disease or condition, or from the results of active treatment, in comparable patients or populations. Because historical control populations usually cannot be as well assessed with respect to pertinent variables as can concurrent control populations, historical control designs are usually reserved for special circumstances. Historical controls are most appropriate for certain studies of diseases with high and predictable mortality (e.g., certain malignancies), and studies in which the effect of the drug is self-evident (e.g., general anesthetics, drug metabolism).

(3) The method of selection of subjects provides adequate assurance that they have the disease or condition being studied, or evidence of susceptibility and exposure to the condition against which prophylaxis is directed.

(4) The method of assigning patients to treatment and control groups minimizes bias and is intended to assure comparability of the groups with respect to pertinent variables such as age, sex, severity of disease, duration of disease, and use of drugs or therapy other than the test drug. The protocol for the study and the report of its results should describe how subjects were assigned to groups. Ordinarily, in a concurrently controlled study, assignment is by randomization, with or without stratification.

(5) Adequate measures are taken to minimize bias on the part of the subjects, observers, and analysts of the data. The protocol and report of the study should describe the procedures used to accomplish this (e.g., blinding).

(6) The methods for assessing subjects' responses are well-defined and reliable. The protocol for the study and the report of results should explain the variables measured, the methods of observation, and criteria used to assess response.

(7) There is an analysis of the study results adequate to assess the effects of the drug. The report of the study should describe the results and the analytic methods used to evaluate them, including any appropriate statistical methods. The analysis should assess, among other things, the comparability of test and control groups with respect to pertinent variables, and the effects of any interim data analyses performed.

Further guidance on the standards for providing substantial evidence of effectiveness and the adequacy of clinical investigations is provided in the FDA guidance entitled, "Providing Clinical Evidence of Effectiveness for Human Drug and Biological Products."

Protocol Content Considerations The argument is often made that early Phase 1 studies need only be designed to meet the minimum requirements for submission and review, as required by 21 CFR 312. According to this argument, it is assumed that the developer will "save money" by conducting a preliminary trial to simply get a look at what the product can do before initiating full-scale clinical development. In many cases, however, this type of approach wastes money rather than saves it, and presents an unacceptable risk-to-benefit ratio. Even if the sponsor's goal is to gain only preliminary evidence of the product's effectiveness, the process of protocol development should be no less rigorous, and the additional expense of conducting a well-planned trial that exceeds minimum standards is generally modest and may be well worth the investment. By designing and conducting a Phase 1 study that satisfies as many of the criteria for an adequate and well-controlled trial as possible, the protocol developer is practicing the best science possible and can be assured that the data more accurately reflect the product's true profile.

Regarding the risk-to-benefit ratio, a trial that places subjects at risk yet cannot provide accurate and dependable results should not be conducted. Any trial lacking the potential to significantly expand the scientific knowledge base regarding a product places subjects at undue risk. Having made this statement, it is important to note that, in some cases, an adequate and well-controlled trial may simply not be feasible early in Phase 1. As a general rule, however, all trials in a development program should be designed to meet or exceed as many of the criteria necessary for an "adequate and well-controlled" study as possible.

Standard Protocol Format The content required of all protocols should be contained in a standard format. The purpose of a standard format should be to present the required elements of the protocol in an easily readable, user-friendly manner. Information should be divided into sections and subsections, with logical groupings of related information clearly identified through the use of indicative headings (see the protocol template guide at the end of this chapter). Ideally, the protocol's general format will be coordinated with that of the final study report template. Wherever possible, the information that is contained in both the final study report and the protocol should be contained in similarly numbered sections and subsections, and under the same headings, within both documents. Most of the other information in the protocol is also used in some form within the final study report. The use of similar formatting in the final study report and the protocol enhances and emphasizes the shared content of the documents, and is an indication of the planning involved throughout the design, conduct and report of a clinical trial.

The major structural elements contained in the standard protocol format and final study report are discussed briefly below and are featured in the protocol template at the end of the chapter.

Title Page The protocol title page should contain administrative information about the protocol. At a minimum, the protocol title page should include the following elements (as applicable): study title and protocol identification number; protocol version number and date; name of the product under investigation; sponsor name and address; CRO name and address; and name and affiliation of the principal or coordinating investigator.

Table of Contents The table of contents' (TOC) main purpose is to provide a listing of, and a location for, the protocol's sections and subsections. Ideally, the TOC will be generated automatically by the word-processing software. As is evident in the TOC within the protocol template at the end of this chapter, all sections and subsections are neatly organized in a coherent, logical sequence. Related information is grouped within sections and subsections under indicative headings.

While the overall standard format should be utilized for every protocol, each protocol will vary considerably in the content of certain sections due to the trial's study-specific details. Therefore, the numbering scheme selected for the protocol allows for compartmentalization of information and flexibility within the established format. For example, Section 3.6 contains a description of the procedures to be followed during each study visit. While the number of visits and procedures will change from study to study, any number of subsections can be added to the section by numbering them 3.6.1, 3.6.2, 3.6.3, etc. In this way, there is flexibility within the protocol without having to change the overall numbering scheme, thereby maintaining the format's integrity.

Body of the Text The body of the protocol should contain all of the information required by federal regulations, recommended by relevant FDA guidances and policies, and encouraged by the developer's final study report template. It is the authors' responsibility to ensure that each topic is covered in such a manner that all regulatory requirements are met, and that an investigator and the members of his or her staff can clearly understand and comply with the instructions given.

Protocol Summary After the body of the text has been written, the authors should prepare a brief high-level summary of the study's major characteristics. A protocol summary is an effective way to familiarize reviewers and potential investigators with the study plan in a few pages. For instance, the FDA, which is well aware of the benefit of a protocol summary, has requested that a protocol cover sheet be attached to each protocol included in a marketing application and that this sheet include many of the same study characteristics included in the summary advocated here.

While a protocol summary can be arranged in any number of ways, the information included in the summary should be consistent across all summaries. The recommended protocol summary contains the following elements: (1) the title of the study (identical to the title page) and protocol number; (2) the clinical phase; (3) the name, medical specialty, institutional affiliation and address of the principal investigator; (4) the period of the trial (projected dates of enrollment of first subject to completion of last subject); (5) study objectives; (6) study variables; (7) study design; (8) inclusion criteria; (9) exclusion criteria; (10) number of subjects to be enrolled, then listed for each test article, along with a description of the test article(s); (11) the dosage form, route of administration and dose regimen; (12) the duration of therapy; and (13) any reference product and its dosing regimen.

For a multi-center study, the investigator description should state "multi-center," and a list of investigators should be added after the summary. The protocol summary is usually placed immediately before the table of contents.

As part of the protocol summary, it is advisable to include a study flow chart incorporating a time and events table to illustrate the study design. If possible, the study flow chart should be contained on one page. An example of a study flow chart is included in the protocol template at the end of the chapter. The study flow chart should illustrate the periods of the study (e.g., baseline placebo, double-blind, open-label) in chronological order. The time and events table should illustrate the major measurements or assessments to be made or procedures to be followed at each division within the study (e.g., screen, baseline, study day #). All of the measurements/procedures on this table should be consistent with the procedures section of the protocol.

Standard Protocol Template For each protocol to conform to the standard protocol's format and content, the previously mentioned elements should be combined into a standard protocol template to be used as a tool by any primary protocol author. In this case, there is a further contributor to the proposed standard format and content. The ICH's E3 guideline, which defines the format and content of the clinical study report (CSR), was used to help format the standard protocol. In that way, many parts of the CSR are a simple cut-and-paste from the protocol. The ability to simply move content from the protocol to the report saves time and reduces errors. It may make the organization of the protocol a bit less than optimal, but that disadvantage is more than made up for by efficiency gains.

The standard protocol template is a full protocol outline comprising prompts for all of the content identified above, organized in a clear, easily-readable format. The standard protocol template also dictates the stylistic guidelines for the protocol, ensuring that the protocol's visual elements are consistent with the sponsor's image. The template should be used in drafting each new protocol. The use of a standard protocol template will provide the following benefits:

1. Following a standard template provides the best assurance that no details will be overlooked and no sections will be omitted. The protocol is a document that addresses every element of how a study is to be carried out in extremely specific detail. This detail is essential to ensure uniform compliance with the requirements of the protocol. However, the protocol should not be so specifically devised as to make its implementation difficult on a practical and operational basis. Details that are unnecessarily restrictive may lead to protocol violations or significantly impede enrollment in, and the conduct of, the trial. The end result should be a realistic but detailed document that can be understood and implemented by the investigator and his or her staff during the clinical study. The use of a standard protocol template facilitates the organization of this necessary information into a consistent format, resulting in a detailed, complete and professional-looking protocol.

2. Since the standard template will be used for every protocol, the authors of each new protocol need only follow the prompts set forth by the adopted format and content of the template. Without a standard format or content, the authors of each new protocol would have to decide upon the information that should be included in the protocol and then develop some format to accommodate this information. In essence, the authors of each new protocol would have to "reinvent the wheel." The use of a standard template frees the authors from format and content considerations, allowing them to focus their efforts on designing a safe and efficient protocol.

3. Many protocol sections contain information that is vital to the information's ultimate utility in supporting a marketing application. As stated, the protocol is the document that establishes the data's credibility and the ultimate conclusions of the trial. The use of reliable and generally accepted methods and procedures in the protocol will provide a strong foundation upon which to make conclusions about the clinical trial's success. Employing a standard protocol template can significantly contribute to the protocol's ability to support the conclusions of the trial by ensuring that every protocol will contain the following: elements associated with "good science," such as blinding and randomization; safety features, such as definitions of adverse events and procedures for reporting serious adverse events; and quality control issues, such as data collection and monitoring. The result is that each protocol developed from the standard template will employ the same sound methods, thereby maximizing both the safety of the subjects participating in the trials and the validity of the results.

4. Establishing uniformity in format and content makes the jobs of study personnel and FDA reviewers much easier. The use of a standard protocol template ensures that the format and content of

each protocol are very similar. Information contained in a particular section or subsection in one protocol will be contained in the same place in every other protocol. This arrangement enables a reader to employ a methodical approach to finding information quickly and easily among any number of protocols and, therefore, can be of particular benefit during the FDA review process. While FDA reviewers will look at each study used in support of an NDA/BLA individually, they will also look across trials, particularly at those of similar design. The use of a standard protocol template will facilitate these comparisons and aid the reviewer in evaluating any clinical program.

A standard protocol template, presented as an annotated protocol template, is provided at the end of this chapter. It is helpful if the body of the text contains a brief description of the information needed in each section and subsection when designing the standard protocol template. Such descriptive text prompts the authors with content cues for drafting their own protocols, and enables them to be certain that all necessary information has been addressed. The content cues in the protocol template also include references to federal regulations, where appropriate, to indicate information that is specifically called for by the FDA. Additional protocol elements have also been included as content cues to provide essential support for the final report. These content clues can easily be removed when drafting any study protocol.

Finally, sample protocol text is included in the protocol template guide as italicized text. The italicized text represents standard protocol language and, therefore, "modularizes" the protocol template. The protocol author may therefore retain, remove, or expand on this language for any study protocol.

Drafting an Individual Study Protocol After the template's table of contents, body, and summary have been designed and adopted, the developer is ready to begin writing protocols for the anticipated clinical trials. Since the key elements of a protocol are the clinical and statistical design features, the clinical monitor and the statistician should collaborate as its primary authors. The clinical monitor and statistician can combine their individual areas of expertise to develop a protocol based upon sound clinical procedures and analytical methods.

If the protocol template has been designed correctly, the authors need only follow the content cues of each section and subsection and fill in the necessary information. When writing the protocol, the authors must keep the protocol's purpose in mind. The protocol is a means for generating pre-defined information for the analysis and final report of a clinical trial. This information will have been identified based upon the anticipated content of the marketing application, the anticipated content of the final study report, the clinical analysis plan and the case report forms. The entire process of planning works backward to the protocol. The protocol is designed to provide all of the pre-defined information, which is then collected, analyzed and presented in a predetermined manner. If planned properly, the entire process can run smoothly and efficiently, saving a great deal of time and money.

Conclusion In the philosophy of clinical development advocated in this text, the protocol is crucial in establishing a proper foundation for the conduct of the study and its analysis and reporting. The study objectives and, in particular, the study variables must be clearly defined to eliminate any ambiguity or misinterpretation. The procedures and methods must be operationally practical and the protocol must adequately describe the manner in which the study is to be conducted. Finally, the statistical methods and analysis section must predefine the crucial analyses to be conducted at the study's completion in order to evaluate safety and effectiveness. By clearly defining all of these elements in the protocol, the study will be conducted in a proper manner, and the final result of the trial will be free from criticism relating to bias or data manipulation. The protocol is crucial in establishing the foundation for the results and conclusions of individual trials and, ultimately, those reached in the marketing application.

TITLE PAGE

The format for study titles is: (Acute, Long-term, Single Dose, etc.) (randomized, if applicable) (controlled, open, dose-response, etc.) (study of [drug] versus [placebo and/or comparative drug] for number of days or weeks) in patients with (disease or condition). Capitalize only first letter and proper names. The title should be in bold face and centered at the top of the title page.

PROTOCOL NUMBER: (The protocol number assigned, ABC-###)

PROTOCOL DATE: (The date the protocol is issued. The date may float when in the drafting stage and become fixed when the protocol is finalized.)

(INVESTIGATIONAL) PRODUCT:

SPONSOR: (Name)

(Address)

(COORDINATING) INVESTIGATOR: (If applicable)
(Name of Principal Coordinating Investigator)
(Medical Specialty)
(Affiliation)
(Address)
(If multicenter, state Multicenter)

CRO: (If applicable)
(Name)
(Address)

Medical Monitor:

(signature)	(signature)
Name:	Name:
Title:	Title:
Affiliation:	Affiliation:
Address:	Address:
Phone No:	Phone No:

Statistician:

(The following confidentiality statement should be centered at the bottom of the title page)

This document is a confidential communication of company/institution. Acceptance of this document constitutes the agreement by the recipient that no unpublished information contained herein will be published or disclosed without the prior written approval of company/institution, except that this document may be disclosed to appropriate institutional review boards/ethical committees so long as they are requested to maintain its confidentiality.

Protocol No: ABC-### **Page 2**
Effective Date: January 9, 2006

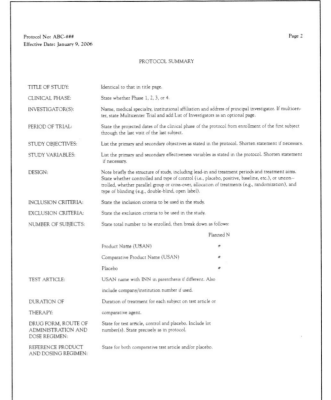

PROTOCOL SUMMARY

TITLE OF STUDY: Identical to that in title page.

CLINICAL PHASE: State whether Phase 1, 2, 3, or 4.

INVESTIGATOR(S): Name, medical specialty, institutional affiliation and address of principal investigator. If multicenter, state Multicenter Trial and add List of Investigators as an optional page.

PERIOD OF TRIAL: State the projected dates of the clinical phase of the protocol from enrollment of the first subject through the last visit of the last subject.

STUDY OBJECTIVES: List the primary and secondary objectives as stated in the protocol. Shorten statement if necessary.

STUDY VARIABLES: List the primary and secondary effectiveness variables as stated in the protocol. Shorten statement if necessary.

DESIGN: Note briefly the structure of study, including lead-in and treatment periods and treatment aims. State whether controlled and type of control (i.e., placebo, positive, baseline, etc.), or uncontrolled, whether parallel group or cross-over, allocation of treatments (e.g., randomization), and type of blinding (e.g., double-blind, open label).

INCLUSION CRITERIA: State the inclusion criteria to be used in the study.

EXCLUSION CRITERIA: State the exclusion criteria to be used in the study.

NUMBER OF SUBJECTS: State total number to be enrolled, then break down as follows:

	Planned N
Product Name (USAN)	#
Comparative Product Name (USAN)	#
Placebo	#

TEST ARTICLE: USAN name with INN in parenthesis if different. Also include company/institution number if used.

DURATION OF THERAPY: Duration of treatment for each subject on test article or comparative agent.

DRUG FORM, ROUTE OF ADMINISTRATION AND DOSE REGIMEN: State for test article, control and placebo. Include lot number(s). State precisely as in protocol.

REFERENCE PRODUCT AND DOSING REGIMEN: State for both comparative test article and/or placebo.

Protocol No: ABC-### **Page 3**
Effective Date: January 9, 2006

STUDY FLOW CHART / TIME AND EVENTS SCHEDULE

Provide a Study Flow Chart/Time and Events Schedule here that shows the design of the study, the doses given, the timing of clinic visits, and the measurements made at each visit.

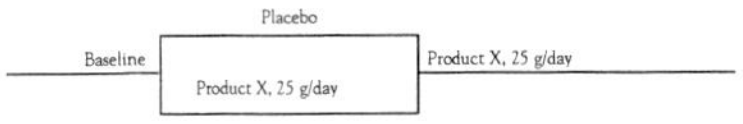

	Screen	Baseline	Double-Blind Treatment							Open-Label Treatment							Termination
Study Day		1	1	2	3	4	5	6	7	8	9	10	11	12	13	14	15
Visit		1	1					2	2	2					3	3	4
Informed Consent	x																
Medical History	x																x
Physical Exam	x																x
Inpatient Period		x	x					x	x	x					x	x	x
Brief History/Exam		x						x							x		
Clinical Labs	x	x	x							x							x
Vital Signs	x	x	x					x	x	x					x	x	x
Double-Blind Study Meds			x	x	x	x	x	x	x								
Open-Label Study Meds										x	x	x	x	x	x	x	
Adverse Events			x	x	x	x	x	x	x	x	x	x	x	x	x	x	x
Diary				x	x	x	x				x	x	x	x			

The following language should be included to ensure that the status of each subject is evaluated in a standard manner across all sites.

Definitions that can be used in describing the status of subjects in a trial are as follows:

"Screened" subjects are those who receive the initial history, physical and laboratory examinations to determine whether they meet the inclusion and exclusion criteria.

"Enrolled" subjects are those who are screened and have undergone some intervention as a part of the trial, such as a baseline evaluation. A randomized subject is automatically enrolled. [Note: The time at which a subject should actually be considered "enrolled" should be clearly stated in the protocol].

"Randomized" subjects are those who are assigned to a treatment group. This may occur, for instance, at the end of a lead-in period or at the time of enrollment, depending upon the design of the study.

Protocol No: ABC-### **Page 4**
Effective Date: January 9, 2006

TABLE OF CONTENTS

LIST OF ABBREVIATIONS AND DEFINITION OF TERMS 6
ETHICS 77
1.0 INTRODUCTION 11
2.0 STUDY OBJECTIVES 11
2.1 Primary Objective 12
2.2 Secondary Objective(s) 12
3.0 INVESTIGATIONAL PLAN 12
3.1 Overall Study Design and Plan - Description 12
3.2 Discussion of Study Design, Including the Choice of Control Groups 13
3.2.1 Justification of Design Type 13
3.2.2 Choice of Controls/Comparators 14
3.3 Selection of Study Population 15
3.3.1 Inclusion Criteria 15
3.3.2 Exclusion Criteria 15
3.3.3 Removal of Subjects From Therapy or Assessment 16
3.4 Treatments 16
3.4.1 Treatments Administered 16
3.4.2 Identity of Investigational Product(s) 17
3.4.3 Method of Assigning Subjects to Treatment Groups 17
3.4.4 Selection of Doses in the Study 17
3.4.5 Selection and Timing of Dose for Each Subject 17
3.4.6 Blinding 18
3.4.7 Prior and Concomitant Therapy 19
3.4.8 Treatment Compliance 19
3.4.9 Clinical Supplies Accountability 19
3.5 Efficacy and Safety Variables 19
3.5.1 Efficacy and Safety Measurements Assessed 19
3.5.1.1 Efficacy Evaluations 19
3.5.1.2 Safety Evaluations 20
3.5.2 Appropriateness of Measurements 23
3.5.3 Efficacy and Safety Variables 23
3.5.3.1 Primary Efficacy Variable 24
3.5.3.2 Secondary Efficacy Variables 24
3.5.3.1 Safety Variables 25
3.5.4 Drug Concentration Measurements 25
3.6 Study Procedures 25
3.6.1 Screening 26
3.6.2 Baseline 26
3.6.3 Visit 1 26
3.6.4 Visit 2 26
3.6.5 End of Study/Early Termination 26
3.6.6 Follow-up 26
3.7 Data Quality Assurance 27
3.7.1 Clinical Procedures 27
3.7.2 Monitoring 27
3.7.3 Data Handling 28
3.7.4 Review of Original Subject Records 28
4.0 ANALYTICAL AND STATISTICAL EVALUATION PLAN 28
4.1 General Statistical Issues/Information 28
4.1.1 Sample Size 28
4.1.2 Missing Value Handling and Subject Evaluability 28
4.1.3 Group Comparability at Baseline 29
4.1.4 Interim Analysis and Stopping Rules 29
4.1.5 Statistical Adjustments for Multiple Endpoints 29
4.1.6 Approach to Multicenter Analysis 29
4.2 Analyses Addressing the Primary Study Objective 29
4.2.1 Primary Analysis 29
4.2.2 Supplemental Analyses 29
4.3 Analyses Addressing Secondary Study Objective(s) 30
4.4 Subgroup Analyses 30
4.5 Safety Analyses 30
4.5.1 Analyses Addressing Adverse Events 30
4.5.2 Analyses of Clinical Laboratory Data 31
5.0 REFERENCES 31
6.0 APPENDICES 32

Protocol No: ABC-### Page 5
Effective Date: January 9, 2006

LIST OF ABBREVIATIONS AND DEFINITION OF TERMS

ICH/FDA require that any abbreviations used, as well as the definitions of unusual or specialized terms or measurement units referred to in the protocol, be listed up-front. An abbreviated term should be written in full upon its first appearance in the text, with the abbreviation indicated in parentheses. Wherever feasible, a sponsor should adopt a uniform glossary of abbreviations and definitions for a particular project and rely on conventional designations. This will prevent the use of multiple abbreviations for the same term appearing in different protocols for a particular project. In addition, overuse of abbreviations should be avoided.

It is recommended that this section immediately follow the Table of Contents, with the list of abbreviations presented first followed by the definition of any unusual or specialized terms. The following are examples of abbreviations commonly referred to in the study protocol:

ADR	adverse drug reaction
AE	adverse event
AUC	area under the curve
CFR	Code of Federal Regulations
Cmax	maximum concentration
CRA	clinical research associate
CRF	case report form
CRO	contract research organization
FDA	United States Food and Drug Administration
GCP	Good Clinical Practice
GMP	Good Manufacturing Practices
HIPAA	Health Insurance Portability and Accountability
ICH	International Conference on Harmonization
IEC	independent ethics committee
IND	investigational new drug application
IRB	institutional review board
ITT	intent-to-treat
IVRS	interactive voice response system
NOAEL	no observable adverse event level
PP	per protocol
QA	quality assurance
QC	quality control
SAE	serious adverse event
SAP	statistical analysis plan
Tmax	time to maximum concentration
WOCP	women of childbearing potential

Protocol No: ABC-### Page 6
Effective Date: January 9, 2006

ETHICS

Ethical Principles. Ethical Principles;

State the following:

This study will be conducted in accordance with Title 21 of the Code of Federal Regulations (or the Declaration of Helsinki and the laws of (country), if applicable).

This statement must then be followed by an explanation of how the research will conform to the ethical principles in 21 CFR and/or the Declaration of Helsinki. Ordinarily, the following explanation should suffice:

Specifically, this study is based on adequately performed laboratory and animal experimentation; the study will be conducted under a protocol reviewed by an institutional review board (or independent ethics committee or review committee); the study is to be conducted by scientifically and medically qualified persons; the benefits of the study are in proportion to the risks; the rights and welfare of the subjects will be respected; the physicians conducting the study will ensure that the potential hazards do not outweigh the potential benefits; the results to be reported will be accurate; subjects will give their informed consent and will be competent to do so and not under duress; and the ethical principles in Title 21 of the Code of Federal Regulations (or the Declaration of Helsinki, if applicable) will be complied with.

Any additional explanations of the ethical standards to be used, as required by local law, should be included here.

Informed Consent. Informed Consent;

State the following if the study is conducted in the U.S.:

This study will be conducted in full compliance with the informed consent regulations in 21 CFR 50. Refer to Appendix 6.2 for reference to 21 CFR 50 Protection of Human Subjects, Subpart B Informed Consent of Human Subjects.

State the following if the study is conducted outside of the U.S.:

Informed consent will be given by all subjects in this study in accordance with the Declaration of Helsinki (and the laws of (country), if appropriate).

Briefly describe the informed consent procedures to be used, including who will discuss the study with the subjects, what information will be given to the subjects (written or verbal), whether written informed consent is to be obtained and, if not, how consent will be obtained and documented. The following statements can be used for any study:

The investigator is responsible for obtaining written informed consent from potential subjects prior to performing any trial tests or assessments required by the protocol. If a potential subject is unable to provide written informed consent, the investigator or his/her designee should fully inform the subject's legally acceptable representative of the pertinent aspects of the study and obtain written informed consent from the representative.

If a potential subject or the subject's legally acceptable representative is unable to read, an impartial witness should be present during the informed consent process. The impartial witness is to sign and date the informed consent form acknowledging that the subject has been accurately informed of the pertinent aspects of the study and has freely consented to participate in the study.

A copy of the signed and dated informed consent form will be given to the subject or the subject's legally acceptable representative. The investigator will retain the original informed consent form with the site's copy of the case report form(s).

The consent form must contain a full explanation of the possible advantages, risks, alternate treatment options, and availability of treatment in the case of injury, in accordance with 21 CFR 50.25 Elements of informed consent (or ICH E6 Section 4.8.10). The consent form should also indicate that, by signature, the subject, or where appropriate, legal guardian, permits access to relevant medical records by the sponsor and by representatives of the FDA (or applicable regulatory authority).

Furthermore, the informed consent form should include, when applicable, elements related to the use and disclosure of protected health information in accordance with 45 CFR 164 Security and Privacy, Subpart E Privacy of Individually Identifiable Health Information (45 CFR 164.508(c) Implementation specifications: Core elements and requirements).

The following statements are sufficient to explain sponsor/IRB (or IEC) approval and FDA submission of the informed consent form:

The sponsor must review and approve the informed consent form prior to its submission to the IRB (or IEC). The investigator must subsequently receive written approval from the IRB (or IEC) prior to the initiation of the study. Should the approved informed consent form be modified during the course of a study, the investigator must obtain written IRB (or IEC) approval prior to the informed consent form's use.

Protocol No: ABC-### Page 7
Effective Date: January 9, 2006

The sponsor will submit a copy of the initial IRB- (or IEC-) and sponsor-approved consent form to the FDA (or applicable regulatory authority) and will maintain copies of revised consent forms which have been reviewed and approved by the IRB (or IEC).

Refer the reader to Appendix 6.2, which contains 21 CFR 50.

Institutional Review Board/Independent Ethics Committee. Institutional Review Board/Ethical Committee;

State the following if the study is conducted in the U.S.:

This study will be conducted in full compliance with the Institutional review board regulations in 21 CFR 56.

State the following if the study is conducted outside of the U.S.:

This study will be reviewed by an Independent Ethics Committee (or Review Committee, as appropriate) in accordance with the Declaration of Helsinki (and the laws of (country), if appropriate).

Continue to state the following:

This protocol will not be initiated unless it has been reviewed and has received written approval by, and remains open to continuing review by, an IRB (or IEC) meeting the requirements of 21 CFR 56 (or the Declaration of Helsinki).

Briefly summarize that the IRB (or IEC) shall review and have the authority to approve, require modification to (to secure approval), or disapprove the protocol. The IRB (or IEC) shall notify the investigator and the institution in writing of its decision. The IRB (or IEC) shall require that the information given to subjects as part of the informed consent is in accordance with 21 CFR 50.25 (or ICH E6 Section 4.8.10). The IRB (or IEC) shall conduct continuing reviews of the protocol at intervals appropriate to the degree of risk, but not less than once per year.

Briefly summarize that the IRB (or IEC) is to retain all relevant trial records for a minimum of three years after the trial's completion and make them available to a regulatory authority upon request. Copies of all reports to and correspondence between the investigator and the IRB (or IEC) must be provided to the sponsor. Furthermore, at the completion or early termination of the trial, the investigator should promptly (i.e., within 90 days) provide a final report to the IRB (or IEC). Finally, if the IRB (or IEC) terminates or suspends its approval of a trial, the investigator should promptly inform the sponsor with a written explanation of the termination or suspension.

Continue to state the following:

Any change or revision in a Phase 1 protocol that significantly affects the safety of the subjects, or change in a Phase 2 or 3 protocol that significantly affects the safety of the subjects, the scope of the investigation, or the scientific quality of the trial must be approved by the sponsor and the IRB (or IEC) prior to implementation. However, any protocol change intended to eliminate an apparent immediate hazard to the subject or protocol change that involves administrative or logistical aspects of the trial may be implemented immediately if the FDA (or applicable regulatory authority) is subsequently notified of the amendment by the sponsor and the IRB (or IEC) is promptly informed by the investigator. [21 CFR 312.30 (b); ICH E6 Section 4.5.2]

It is the investigator's obligation to maintain an IRB correspondence file, and to make this file available for review by the sponsor's representatives as part of the trial monitoring process. [21 CFR 56.115] Additionally, the investigator should submit written progress reports of a trial's status annually to the IRB (or IEC), or more frequently, as the IRB (or IEC) requests. [ICH E6 Section 4.10.2]

The following statement commonly refers to Phase 1 protocols included in the investigational new drug application (IND). Sponsors may interpret the regulations differently for Phase 2 or Phase 3, multicenter studies:

The sponsor will submit a copy of the initial IRB approval document to the FDA and will maintain records of the continuing review of the protocol by the IRB. [21 CFR 312.23(a)(1)(iv)]

Protocol No: ABC-### Page 8
Effective Date: January 9, 2006

1.0 INTRODUCTION

The Introduction section is meant to provide a brief background summary on the disease or indication for which the test article is being developed. One-half page is usually sufficient for providing a review of the disease. The following is an example of an introductory paragraph that could be used for a product to treat asthma:

Asthma is a chronic inflammatory disorder of the airways characterized by reversible airflow obstruction due to airway inflammation, bronchial smooth muscle spasm, and increased mucus secretion. More than 100 million people worldwide have asthma, with an estimated 14.6 million people, including 5 million children, affected in the United States. Since 1982, the overall incidence of asthma has increased 46%. However, the incidence in children under the age of 18 has increased 80%. There has been an alarming increase in asthma mortality over the past decade. According to the Centers for Disease Control and Prevention, the death rate due to the illness rose 61% between 1982 and 1994, bringing the annual toll to nearly 7,000 deaths in the United States; most of them among the elderly. Asthma clearly represents a significant medical condition that requires improved therapies.

The review of the disease or indication should be followed by the rationale in support of using the test article in clinical trials. One-half page is usually sufficient for providing the rationale for the study. The following paragraph is an example of a rationale:

Although numerous therapies for asthma are available, inhaled glucocorticoids are a first-line therapy for chronic asthma. Glucocorticoids attenuate bronchial inflammation and responsiveness to various trigger factors, improve the patient's status, and reduce the number of asthma attacks. The most recent guidelines on the management of asthma, the Global Initiative on Asthma and the National Asthma Education and Prevention Program, suggest that inhaled glucocorticoids are the primary long-term preventative or controller medication for persistent asthma. Inhaled glucocorticoids have been available in Europe, Canada, and the United States for a number of years and have been extensively studied.

In the following sections, continue to provide background information to place the trial in context within the clinical program and indicate any special features or aims of the trial.

Now it's your turn.

2.0 STUDY OBJECTIVES

The Study Objectives section is meant to provide a high-level summary of the primary and secondary objectives of the study.

Ideally, this section will be copied directly from the clinical analysis plan. [Note: Reference Chapter 19: Analysis Plans, for additional information].

2.1 Primary Objective

State the primary objective of the study [21 CFR 312.23(a)(6)(iii)(a)]. The primary objective is usually concerned with the evaluation of effectiveness. All adequate and well-controlled trials give a clear statement of the objectives of the investigation to eliminate any confusion about the primary analysis [21 CFR 314.126(b)(1)]. The following statement could be used to state a hypothetical primary objective:

The primary objective of this study is to determine the effect of 25 μg of Product X, by a single intravenous injection on infection rate over a 52-week period in subjects undergoing chronic peritoneal dialysis.

2.2 Secondary Objective(s)

List secondary objectives numerically (e.g., 2.2.1, 2.2.2, 2.2.3, etc.). These objectives are usually concerned with the evaluation of secondary questions regarding effectiveness, safety variables, and subgroup hypotheses [21 CFR 312.23(a)(6)(iii)(a) and 314.126(b)(1)]. The following statement could be used to state a hypothetical secondary objective:

The secondary objective of this study is to evaluate the long-term safety of Product X in the treatment of subjects undergoing chronic peritoneal dialysis.

3.0 INVESTIGATIONAL PLAN

The Investigational Plan section must be written in considerable detail so that a reader can understand exactly how the study is to be conducted. This section is usually the longest section in the protocol; the information included is more extensive than in published medical papers. Ideally, sections 3.1 to 3.3 will be copied directly from the clinical analysis plan. [Note: Reference Chapter 19: Analysis Plans, for additional information].

3.1 Overall Study Design and Plan - Description

Describe the basic design of the study (i.e., parallel-group, cross-over, sequential, matched-pair, or other); the specific treatments (test article, placebo and control article) and doses compared; the degree of blinding (e.g., open, double-blind, single-blind); any randomization methods; the sequence and duration of study periods, including, as appropriate, any previous therapy withdrawal period, the baseline placebo lead-in period, the treatment period, and any post-treatment withdrawal and observation periods. Note the timing of clinic visits and measurements [21 CFR 312.23(a)(6)(iii)(d) and 314.126(b)(2), (4) and (5)].

The trial design should be comprehensively illustrated in the Study Flow Chart/Time and Events Schedule attached to the Protocol Summary and reference to it should be made in this section.

The following language should be included to ensure that the status of each subject is evaluated in a standard manner across all sites.

Protocol No: ABC-### Page 9
Effective Date: January 9, 2006

Definitions to be used in describing the status of subjects in a trial are as follows:

> *"Screened" subjects are those who receive the initial history, physical and laboratory examinations to determine whether they meet the inclusion and exclusion criteria.*
>
> *"Enrolled" subjects are those who are screened and have undergone some intervention as a part of the trial, such as a baseline evaluation. A randomized subject is automatically enrolled. [Note: The time at which a subject should actually be considered "enrolled" should be clearly stated in the protocol].*
>
> *"Randomized" subjects are those who are assigned to a treatment group. This may occur, for instance, at the end of a lead-in period or at the time of enrollment, depending upon the design of the study.*

3.2 Discussion of Study Design, Including the Choice of Control Groups
Clearly and concisely summarize the rationale used by the sponsor in designing the study. Design elements meriting discussion are indicated in the subsections below. Note that no description is required directly under Section 3.2; descriptions are required beginning with Section 3.2.1.

3.2.1 Justification of Design Type
State the rationale for selection of the trial design and comparison group(s). All adequate and well-controlled trials use a design that permits a comparison with a control to provide a quantitative assessment of drug (or biologic) effect [21 CFR 314.126(b)(2)]. Specific design features that should be commented upon in this section include: 1) the method used for assigning subjects to a particular treatment or control group, 2) the method used for blinding of treatment assignments, 3) the duration of study periods, including any lead-in or washout periods, and 4) the rationale for design. Sound reasoning that stable baselines are likely to be achieved prior to intervention should be provided and that steady-state effects of the test article are to be achieved. Discuss any recognized benefits and problems associated with the design type in terms of the disease state or study population under evaluation. For example, for a crossover design, there should be consideration of the likelihood of spontaneous change in baseline characteristics during the study and the need (or lack thereof) for re-establishment of baseline values between treatment periods. Alternatively, one might describe how residual effects were estimated and shown to be inconsequential.

3.2.2 Choice of Controls/Comparators
Specify the reason for the use of specific control and/or comparator treatments [21 CFR 314.126(b)(2)]. For example, a placebo control is typically used to establish the magnitude of change in clinical endpoints that occur spontaneously during the treatment period. State the type of control as: (1) placebo concurrent control; (2) dose-comparison concurrent control; (3) no-treatment concurrent control: (4) active or positive-treatment concurrent control; or (5) historical control. Reference may also be made to the FDA Clinical Investigator Information Sheet dealing with 'Placebo Controlled and Active Controlled Drug Study Designs.' If the trial uses a positive or active control, this section should defend the appropriateness of the active control and the regimen employed (e.g., by citation of regulatory approval of the drug or literature support of effectiveness). State also whether the trial was intended to show a difference or similarity between treatments. If it was the latter, caution is urged. Generally speaking, you cannot prove two products are equivalent, you can only fail to show a difference. Even though an approved drug was used as an active control, there is no assurance that the active control worked in the trial in question. Careful consideration should be given to an excellent article by Dr. Robert Temple of the FDA, "Government Viewpoint of Clinical Trials" with regard to the use of a positive-control trial (Drug Information Journal, January/June 1982; pp. 10-17).

Known or potential problems associated with the study design or control group chosen, should be discussed in light of the specific disease and therapies being studied. For a crossover design, for example, there should be consideration, among other things, of the likelihood of spontaneous change in the disease and of carry-over effects of treatment during the study. [ICH E3]

If efficacy was to be demonstrated by showing equivalence, i.e. the absence of a specified degree of inferiority of the new treatment compared to an established treatment, problems associated with such study designs should be addressed. Specifically there should be provided a basis for considering the study capable of distinguishing active from inactive therapy. Support may be provided by an analysis of previous studies similar to the present study with respect to important design characteristics (patient selection, study endpoints, duration, dose of active control, concomitant therapy etc.) showing a consistent ability todemonstrate superiority of the active control to placebo. How to assess the ability of the present study to distinguish effective from ineffective therapy should also be discussed. For example, it may be possible to identify a treatment response (based on past studies) that would clearly distinguish between the treated population and an untreated group. Such a response could be the change of a measure from baseline or some other specified outcome like healing rate or survival rate. Attainment of such a response would support the expectation that the study could have distinguished the active drug from an inactive drug. There should also be a discussion of the degree of inferiority of the therapy (often referred to as the delta value) the study was intended to show was not exceeded. [ICH E3]

If the trial is historically controlled, special discussion and comparison with other studies taken from the literature are necessary. This discussion should state how the particular control study was selected, what other historical experiences were examined (if any) and how their results compared to the particular control used. Because of the known limitations of historical controls (e.g., the difficulty of assuring com-

Protocol No: ABC-### Page 10
Effective Date: January 9, 2006

parability of treated groups; inability to blind investigators to treatment), regulatory acceptance of historically controlled trials is likely only in the case of an obviously effective new treatment for a serious disease.

3.3 Selection of Study Population
Explain the selection of subjects sharing specific characteristics and/or histories, along with the justification for the use of special or unusual exclusion or inclusion criteria. The specific selection criteria used to enroll subjects into the study typically pertain to primary/secondary diagnoses, including specific disease requirements (e.g., particular results of a diagnostic test or rating scale; treatment failure or success on prior therapy); demographic characteristics, presence or absence of concurrent diseases or medical conditions and use of concomitant medications [21 CFR 312.23(a)(6)(iii)(c) and 314.126(b)(3)]. Care should be taken to thoughtfully define the study population in order to achieve desired results without bias, and to be selective so as not to confound one's data while not being too restrictive in the enrollment of subjects.

3.3.1 Inclusion Criteria
State, in a list format, the criteria required to qualify, or include, the appropriate population of potential subjects for the study. If there were additional criteria for randomization or entry into the active treatment phase, these should be adequately described. The following statement could be used to state a hypothetical inclusion criterion:

- *After 4 weeks of placebo administration in the run-in period, subjects were considered eligible for entry into the double-blind treatment period if their trough (21 to 27 hours post-dose) sitting diastolic blood pressure was between 95 and 114 mm Hg and did not differ by more than 7 mm Hg when measured on two separate occasions more than 1 week apart.*

3.3.2 Exclusion Criteria
State, in a list format, the criteria required to exclude an inappropriate population of potential subjects from the study. In addition to any study-specific exclusion criteria, the following standard exclusion criteria are generally appropriate, and recommended, for every protocol:

- *Any condition that, in the judgment of the investigator, would place a subject at undue risk, or potentially compromise the results or interpretation of the study.*
- *Administration of any investigational test article within 30 days preceding the first dose of study drug. Test article is defined as any material (placebo or drug) dispensed under the provisions of a protocol. (This criterion is dropped when one protocol leads into another with the same test article, such as when patients in a short-term controlled study are rolled over into a long-term open study.)*

3.3.3 Removal of Subjects From Therapy or Assessment
Describe any predetermined reasons for removing subjects from study treatment, along with the nature and duration of any planned follow-up observations in those subjects. Typical reasons for withdrawal from the study include the following: development of intolerable adverse events, major protocol violations, lack of therapeutic response, non-compliance with the treatment regimen or assessment schedule, consideration of discontinuation as advisable by the investigator, or in the subject's best interest. State whether subjects were fully aware of their right to terminate participation in the study at any time without penalty by providing the following standard section in all protocols:

A subject may end his or her participation in a study at any time. If a subject withdraws, the investigator is to make a reasonable effort to determine the reason for the subject's withdrawal from the study and to complete termination procedures, as described in Section 3.6. Telephone calls, registered letters, and offers of transportation to the investigational site are considered reasonable effort.

If there are pre-determined criteria for removing a randomized subject from any of the analyses, such as due to a violation of one or more specific, major entry criteria, these should be clearly stated.

3.4 Treatments

3.4.1 Treatments Administered
List the specific test articles that will be used, including the active test article, placebo, comparative agent(s) and any pharmacological tools used in clinical pharmacology studies. Discuss the route, mode of administration, dose, dosage schedule, and planned duration of administration for each treatment [21 CFR 312.23(a)(6)(iii)(e) and 314.126(b)(5)]. The timing of dosing in relation to meals should be described, if specified.

List/describe the instructions to the investigator/subject for the use of the test article (e.g., "Administer two tablets in the morning with food."). Include any restrictions or preferences (e.g., use of non-dominant arm) in the delivery of the test article to the subject.

3.4.2 Identity of Investigational Product(s)
Describe the appearance, shape, smell, and taste of the clinical supplies and the extent to which the test drug(s) and control or comparator drugs are distinguishable from one another. In the event that a commercially-available product is used as a control or comparator treatment, any modification from the marketed product should be noted. If appropriate, describe any measures taken to assure that the bioavailability of any commercial product is unaltered.

The formula identification and batch numbers for each test article are typically summarized in tabular fashion along with the USAN generic name (with brand name in parentheses) and the name of the manufacturer. A listing of active and inactive ingredients for each test arti-

Protocol No: ABC-### Page 11
Effective Date: January 9, 2006

cle (e.g., copies of package inserts for commercially-available products) could be included in, and reference should be made to, Appendix 6.3.

Include information on how the test articles are supplied and packaged, including descriptions of the containers (e.g., 3 ml glass vial sealed with a 13 mm gray butyl rubber stopper and aluminum seals), and the use of any tear-off labels. Reproduce the text on the label, complete with any cautions or special instructions regarding storage. Indicate any special instructions regarding handling or storage (e.g., store in a 4°C refrigerator in a secured area). If a certificate of analysis is included, it should be referred to here, along with its location (probably in Appendix 6.3).

If applicable, procedures for re-supply should be described.

3.4.3 Method of Assigning Subjects to Treatment Groups
Include information on how subjects will be assigned to a particular treatment group [21 CFR 314.126(b)(4)] (e.g., randomized in equal proportions; stratified based on gender and then randomized; randomized using a 2:1 ratio) as well as the assignment/use and format of subject identifiers (e.g., screening and/or randomization numbers). If randomization is not used, explain how the technique chosen will guard against systematic selection bias.

3.4.4 Selection of Doses in the Study
List the doses or dose ranges for all treatments to be used in the study, and describe the basis for choosing them (e.g., prior experience in humans, animal data).

3.4.5 Selection and Timing of Dose for Each Subject
It is imperative that the procedures used to determine the dose of study medication for each subject are adequately described and consistent across all study centers. These can include a fixed dose/drug regimen, a specified titration schedule (e.g., forced dose titration after specified duration of treatment) or a response-determined procedure (e.g., dose titrated upwards at specific intervals until a specified endpoint such as intolerance, therapeutic response, or maximum allowable dose was achieved).

3.4.6 Blinding
State which of the participants in the study (i.e., subject, investigator, research nurse, study coordinator, personnel involved in monitoring study, data entry personnel) are blinded to the identity of the study treatment and who has access to the subject codes [21 CFR 314.126(b)(5)]. Describe how drugs are packaged to maintain the blind (e.g., how bottles are labeled, whether the double-dummy technique is needed, etc.). Indicate also the planned time at which blinding codes will be broken (e.g., "Blinding was maintained until the study was completed, the data file was verified, and the final trial database was locked."). Describe the procedures to be followed and who should be contacted in the event that the blind is broken earlier than planned.

The following statements are applicable to, and should be used in every randomized, blinded protocol:

The treatment code for an individual patient is not to be broken during the trial, except in the case of a medical emergency where knowledge of the treatment group is necessary to properly evaluate and treat the patient. Care must be taken to prevent "spurious" breaking of the blind to satisfy curiosity in a situation where knowledge of the treatment group would have no bearing on the treatment of the patient. In all circumstances where the blind is broken by the investigational site personnel, the clinical investigator must notify the medical monitor within 24 hours.

Where patients are returned to standard therapy at the end of a trial, the blind should not be broken for individual patients as they complete the trial, merely as a matter of curiosity. However, in certain trials, patients are maintained on open-label, long-term therapy for safety monitoring after the original trial is over and unblinding may be necessary at that time. Describe the procedure for unblinding in this case.

If there is a central committee with access to unblinded data, procedures used to maintain the integrity of the study blind need to be described. Also explain the procedures used to preserve the blind in the event of interim analyses.

If the protocol allows the investigator to remain unblinded (e.g., single-blind design), describe the method for shielding the investigator from the blinded participants (e.g., subject). In the event that blinding is imperfect because of obvious drug effects (e.g., dry mouth, injection site reactions, changes in laboratory data), the difficulty should be identified and implications discussed. Describe attempts to manage the problem (e.g., have key endpoint measurements done by blinded observers or use objective methods).

3.4.7 Prior and Concomitant Therapy
Detail which drugs are allowed before or during the study and how their use is recorded. List any specific concomitant drugs or therapies that are disallowed during the study, and any washout periods that are required for forbidden medications. If the effect(s) of concomitant therapies on endpoint measurements is(are) evaluated, the method(s) used should be detailed in this section.

3.4.8 Treatment Compliance
Specify the method for assessing compliance with dosing regimens (e.g., pill count, measurement of drug concentrations in blood, plasma, urine or saliva), as well as drug accountability record-keeping procedures. If appropriate, state the level of non-compliance required to exclude either a subject or his/her data at a particular visit from the analysis. State also any decision rule for dropping subjects from the trial because of poor compliance.

Protocol No: ABC-### Page 12
Effective Date: January 9, 2006

3.4.9 Clinical Supplies Accountability
Describe the record keeping procedures required by both the FDA and the sponsor. Reference may be made to the FDA Clinical Investigator Information Sheet entitled "Required Recordkeeping in Clinical Investigations." It should be stated that clinical investigators are required to maintain records pertaining to the test articles received from the sponsor, the date the test articles were received, and the disposition of the test articles (e.g., their use by the subjects, or if unused, the return of the test article to the sponsor or other mutually agreed upon disposition or destruction). Describe the audit trail in place for tracking the test article from the sponsor to the investigator, to the subjects, and the return of unused supplies to the sponsor.

3.5 Efficacy and Safety Variables
A study variable is a measurement made under specified conditions that is considered to reflect the response of the subject to a study treatment. Variables are typically divided into those considered to reflect the effectiveness of the study drug in the desired indication and those that are relevant to the safety and tolerability of the study drug in the population under investigation. The criteria for efficacy, Section 3.6.1.1, and safety, Section 3.6.1.2, can be referenced in Chapter 19: Analysis Plans. Note that no description is required directly under Section 3.6; descriptions are required beginning with Section 3.6.1.1.

3.5.1 Efficacy and Safety Measurements Assessed

3.5.1.1 Efficacy Evaluations
Describe the various assessments used to evaluate the efficacy of the study treatment(s), including the measurement methods and/or instruments. This section is generally organized into sub-sections according to evaluation type (e.g., hourly pain assessments, use of supplemental analgesics, overall assessments of study medication; numbered as 3.6.1.1.1, 3.6.1.1.2, etc.). Where subjective rating scales or questionnaires are used, describe them in detail, including precise definitions of any categorical responses such as good, fair, poor. Provide any references to published literature pertaining to the reliability and validity of all measurement tools.

3.5.1.2 Safety Evaluations
Describe any safety variables and the time points for the analyses. If any of the safety variables are not widely used or generally accepted, state why they were selected and, if appropriate, state why other more obvious alternatives were not used. If appropriate, provide an explanation for the choice of variables and their relevance to the disease process under investigation and the study population. This section is typically divided into subsections describing each safety variable.

3.5.1.2.1 Clinical Laboratory Tests
List by category each of the safety laboratory tests to be performed (i.e., hematology, clinical chemistry, urinalysis). It is helpful to list the specific sub-panels for each safety laboratory test (e.g., WBC, RBC, platelets, etc.) to aid in the determination of core laboratory specifications. In addition, provide the procedure and timing of sample collection along with the identity of the facility used in analyzing the samples. The timing of the sample collection should be in accordance with the Study Flow Chart/Time and Events Schedule. A tabular format is usually helpful. Specify the criteria used in defining clinically significant laboratory abnormalities. If possible, identify the core laboratory facilities to be used in this section.

3.5.1.2.2 Adverse Events
Note: 21 CFR 312.32 refers to adverse events (AEs) as adverse drug experiences and ICH refers to them as adverse events. These terms are considered to be equivalent and the authors have chosen to use ICH terminology in this text.

Define the sponsor's system for recording and classifying adverse events. The content of this section is largely driven by the sponsor's standard operating procedure for adverse events and, as such, is likely to be applicable to most clinical studies. The following wording from ICH Guidance E2A and 21 CFR 312.32 may be used:

An adverse event is defined in as any untoward medical occurrence in a patient or clinical investigation subject administered a pharmaceutical (drug or biologic) product and which does not necessarily have to have a causal relationship with this treatment. An adverse event can, therefore, be any unfavorable and unintended sign (including an abnormal laboratory finding, for example), symptom, or disease temporally associated with the use of a medicinal product, whether or not considered related to the medicinal product. This definition includes intercurrent illnesses, injury (including accidental injury), exacerbation of a pre-existing condition, and an adverse event occurring as a result of product withdrawal, abuse, or over dosage. These treatment-emergent adverse events include those events that are reported during the active treatment period which were either not present prior to the onset of active treatment (i.e., during baseline or lead-in periods) or worsened in severity during the active treatment period.

Note: the sponsor may expand the AE reporting period to include a timeframe exceeding conclusion of active treatment (e.g., 30 days following the discontinuation of the study drug).

An adverse event is considered serious if it results in death, is life-threatening, requires inpatient hospitalization or prolongation of inpatient hospitalization, results in persistent or significant disability/incapacity, or is a congenital anomaly/birth defect. Important medical events that may not result in death, be life-threatening or require hospitalization may be considered a serious adverse event if they may jeopardize the patient or subject and/or may require medical or surgical intervention to prevent one of the outcomes listed above.

Protocol No: ABC-### Page 13
Effective Date: January 9, 2006

This definition encompasses the FDA definition of a "serious adverse drug experience" [21 CFR 312.32]. If the trial is conducted in the US, it should further be stated:

Investigators are instructed to immediately report any serious or unexpected adverse events to the sponsor, and the sponsor is obligated to report any serious unexpected adverse events to the FDA, according to 21 CFR 312.32.

Most companies collect information on the date of onset, severity or intensity, relationship to study treatment, date of resolution (if resolved), and any measures taken and follow-up results for each adverse event. Specify any criteria provided to the investigator for rating adverse event severity and causal relationship to study treatment.

Adverse Event Recording
For most protocols the following standard paragraphs are applicable:

Adverse events are intended to be volunteered by subjects or observed by the investigator. So as to not bias the collection of adverse events, the investigator or his/her designee should ask the subject how he/she has been feeling since the last study visit. All adverse events are to be recorded on appropriate case report form pages. A checklist to elicit adverse events, such as vaccine reactogenicity, may be used in any study. The investigator is instructed to report any serious adverse event immediately to the sponsor (preferably on a serious adverse event reporting form). Case report forms on all adverse events will be collected at periodic monitoring visits.

The case report forms for non-serious adverse events will be reviewed by the medical monitor, who will review each event for severity and causality. In the case of serious adverse events, the classification for causality will be manually decided by the Drug Safety Committee of the sponsor. The clinical investigator may be consulted on factual matters but will not officially participate in classifying adverse events for either severity or causality.

The classification of adverse events occurring during double-blind periods will be done on a blinded basis, i.e., the classifier (medical monitor or Drug Safety Committee) will not be aware of the treatment group to which the subject was assigned. In the case of serious adverse events, unblinding will occur after classification to permit a decision on whether or not the adverse event needs to be reported to the FDA as a written report or a telephone report, as indicated in 21 CFR 312.32.

Laboratory Abnormalities as Adverse Events
For most protocols, the following standard paragraphs are applicable:

The clinical investigator will review any abnormal laboratory changes and, if such changes are significant and additional action is taken (e.g., adding a treatment such as a potassium supplement, reducing the dose or stopping the drug), report the laboratory abnormality as an adverse event on an adverse event case report form page.

In addition, all laboratory values will be evaluated at the end of the study, according to the following procedure, to identify any additional laboratory changes sufficiently large to be considered adverse events. All laboratory values for each subject will be screened by the computer against the normal ranges adopted for the trial. High values out of the normal range for the trial will be flagged with an 'H' and low values with an 'L' in the listing of all laboratory data. All laboratory values will also be screened against a wider set of limits designed to identify laboratory abnormalities of potential clinical concern. Values outside these limits will be flagged with an asterisk in the listing of all laboratory data.

The subject listing will then be reviewed by the medical monitor on a blinded basis to determine whether, when taken in context, the identified values should be considered adverse events. The intent of this review is to exclude isolated spurious values, probable laboratory errors, borderline abnormals, random variation and abnormal values that are disease-related or unchanged from baseline. For each of the remaining values beyond the limits of potential clinical concern, a judgment will be made as to whether or not the value should be considered an adverse event. The clinical investigator may be consulted on factual matters relating to the potential clinical severity of the abnormal laboratory finding. Any such events will then be entered onto adverse event case report form pages and classified for severity and causality like other adverse events.

Serious Adverse Event Reporting
For most protocols, the following standard paragraphs are applicable:

Any serious adverse event must be reported to the (company/institution) within one business day by telephone. Reports of serious adverse events should be directed to the medical monitor listed on the front page of the protocol. The chairman of the Institutional review board at the study site must also be notified within one business day. In addition to the completion of a serious adverse event reporting form (if applicable), all serious adverse events must also be recorded on an adverse event CRF page.

An initial written report of any serious adverse event will be submitted by the investigator to the sponsor and to the Institutional review board, within three business days of the occurrence of the adverse event. Any necessary follow-up reports will be submitted within a reasonable time thereafter.

The follow-up report will give full details of the experience, including an assessment of the relationship to the test article(s) and will be sent to the sponsor promptly. Serious adverse events will be reported promptly to the FDA by the sponsor in accordance with 21 CFR 312.32. When contacting the sponsor regarding adverse experiences, site personnel should be prepared to provide as much of the following information as is available at the time:

(1) Subject's initials and subject number;

Protocol No: ABC-### Page 14
Effective Date: January 9, 2006

(2) Investigator's name and center number;
(3) Protocol title and number;
(4) Subject's date of birth, gender, and race;
(5) Test article(s), date(s) of administration, if blinded, please indicate;
(6) Concomitant medication(s): dose, route, duration of treatment, date of last dose;
(7) Information regarding the adverse event:
  (i) description;
  (ii) dates the event began and ended;
  (iii) whether the experience resulted in death or was life-threatening;
  (iv) whether hospitalization was required or prolonged;
  (v) any treatment(s) required;
  (vi) outcome(s) of treatment(s); and
  (vii) Investigator's determination of relationship to the test article(s).

3.5.2 Appropriateness of Measurements
The reliability, accuracy, and relevance of any measurements not considered to be standard for the condition being studied should be documented. Any surrogate endpoints should also be justified (e.g., by reference to clinical data, publications, guidelines, or previous actions by regulatory authorities).

3.5.3 Efficacy and Safety Variables
In the sections below, define each primary and secondary efficacy variable to be evaluated in the study, along with any methods used to compute these variables [21 CFR 312.23(a)(6)(iii)(f), (g) and 314.126(b)(6)]. An efficacy variable is a measurement made under carefully specified conditions that is considered to reflect the response of an individual to treatment. An effectiveness variable may be a change from baseline of a continuous variable such as an antibody titer, or the achievement of a categorical response such as "improved" or "not improved."

Also define any safety variables for the study.

All adequate and well-controlled trials must use methods of assessment of subjects' responses that are well defined and reliable. The protocol should explain the variables measured, the methods of observation, and the criteria used to assess response [21 CFR 314.126(b)(6)]. It is particularly important to specify any definitions used in characterizing outcome (e.g., criteria used in assigning cause of death). This is especially necessary for multicenter studies to assure that similar criteria are applied at each investigational site. Furthermore, the use of any central committee (e.g., a data and safety monitoring board) to review and adjudicate outcomes must be clearly described. Note that no description is required directly under Section 3.6.3; descriptions are required beginning with Section 3.6.3.1.

3.5.3.1 Primary Efficacy Variable
The primary efficacy variable(s) is directly related to the primary objective of the study, as stated in Section 2.0, and is the variable that is compared between the test/investigational drug group and the control or comparator treatment group(s) with the intent of providing the most credible evidence of effectiveness. This variable is also typically the one used in estimating the sample size needed for the study. The rationale for selecting a particular efficacy variable may be necessary if it is not a widely used or generally accepted standard. The rationale for selecting a primary variable may also be needed if it is a surrogate endpoint, an endpoint that is not a true determination of effectiveness, however, is historically accepted as an efficacy measurement (e.g., viral load in HIV trials). If the primary variable is a categorical response to treatment (e.g., poor, fair, good, or excellent), precise definitions of each response term must be provided. If a large number of measurements are made to assess effectiveness, state which response or pattern of responses will be taken as the primary effectiveness variable. The advantage of a precise, detailed statement of the primary effectiveness variable in the protocol is that it enhances the credibility of the final result of the trial. A primary variable is particularly vulnerable to criticism if: 1) it was selected retrospectively after completion of the study, 2) it appears inconsistent with other studies, or 3) it appears to have been arbitrarily chosen. If retrospective modification is required, careful justification must be provided.

3.5.3.2 Secondary Efficacy Variables
All variables that provide supplementary support of the effectiveness of the investigational treatment are considered secondary efficacy variables. Secondary efficacy variables include responses at time points other than those specified in the primary analysis, categorical responses (e.g., the need for rescue medication use) in instances where the primary variable is a continuous response, and responses in certain subject subgroups. If the methods chosen to measure a secondary efficacy variable(s) are not widely used or generally accepted, state why they were used. If there were no secondary efficacy variables, that should be stated here.

Protocol No: ABC-### Page 15
Effective Date: January 9, 2006

3.5.3.1 Safety Variables
List any additional safety tests or variables to be evaluated, along with the timing of these evaluations and any criteria used for defining a clinically significant change. Examples of other safety variables include vital sign measurements, electrocardiograms and physical examinations.

3.5.4 Drug Concentration Measurements
If applicable to the study, list specific drug and/or metabolite concentrations to be measured, including sample collection methods and sampling times (particularly in relation to the timing of drug administration). Identify the laboratory analyzing the samples and provide a brief description of the analytical method used, including reference to internal assay validation documentation. Define the pharmacokinetic variables to be assessed (e.g., area under the plasma concentration-time curve, elimination half-life). Detailed descriptions of the analytical and pharmacokinetic procedures, along with data listings and analytical results, are typically located in an appendix.

3.6 Study Procedures
This section should begin with the following statement:

All subjects must give their informed consent in accordance with the informed consent regulations in Title 21 of the Code of Federal Regulations, Part 50 or, if the trial is conducted outside the United States, in accordance with the Declaration of Helsinki and the laws of (country).

This section can benefit from a presentation of a comprehensive flow chart of procedures conducted/performed at each visit. Refer the reader to the Study Flow Chart/Time and Events Schedule preceding the Table of Contents.

A narrative description of the various evaluations performed at each visit, representative of the Study Flow Chart/Time and Events Schedule, should be presented. State for each clinic visit (or appropriate sequence of visits) exactly what measurements are to be made, what test articles and test article doses are to be administered, what laboratory tests are to be done, what compliance checks are to be made, and what instructions are to be given to the subject, in accordance with the Study Flow Chart/Time and Events Schedule [21 CFR 312.23(a)(6)(iii)(g)].

3.6.1 Screening
Clearly outline the procedures and assessments to be performed during the screening process. Additionally, clearly describe the specific timing/duration of the Screening period in relation to the Baseline visit and what actions should be taken upon determining subject eligibility and/or non-eligibility.

3.6.2 Baseline
Clearly outline the procedures and assessments to be performed as part of the Baseline visit. Indicate the individual responsible for the measurements, as well as the equipment and technique(s) used (e.g., "Blood pressure was measured in subjects by the investigator after five minutes in a sitting position using a standard mercury sphygmomanometer.").

3.6.3 Visit 1
Clearly outline the procedures and assessments as in the preceding Study Procedures subsections.

3.6.4 Visit 2
Clearly outline the procedures and assessments as in the preceding Study Procedures subsections. Continue to outline the procedures/assessments of all subsequent visits. Should such procedures/assessments be consistent from visit to visit, group such visits as applicable (e.g., Visit 2 through Visit 4).

3.6.5 End of Study/Early Termination
Indicate the procedures and assessments to be followed if a subject completes, withdraws, or is terminated from the study. Additionally, explain that should a subject discontinue the study early, the appropriate end of study procedures should be performed, whenever possible.

3.6.6 Follow-up
Indicate the procedures and assessments to be performed at the Follow-up visit, when applicable. Indicate the specific timing of the Follow-up visit in relation to the End of Study/Early Termination visit. Additionally, explain that should a subject discontinue the study early, the appropriate follow-up procedures should be performed, whenever possible.

3.7 Data Quality Assurance
Describe in detail the steps to be taken and the quality assurance and quality control systems that will be implemented to assure the accuracy and reliability of the data collected. This should include steps taken at the investigational site and/or by the sponsor to ensure the use of standard terminology and accurate, consistent and complete data collection, such as training sessions, instruction manuals, site monitoring, cross-checking of case report forms against source documents, use of centralized laboratories and data audits.

3.7.1 Clinical Procedures
The following paragraphs are sufficient to describe the recording of data on paper case report forms:

Protocol No: ABC-### Page 16
Effective Date: January 9, 2006

Data generated under the protocol will be collected on case report forms (CRFs) supplied by the sponsor. CRFs are to be completed using a black or dark blue pen. Corrections are to be made by placing a single, thin line through the incorrect entry so that the data will not be obscured. The correct entry is then to be written next to it, along with the date and the initials of the person who made the corrections. The investigator is responsible for the accuracy of the data transcribed on the forms.

Should electronic CRFs be utilized in lieu of traditional paper CRFs, procedures for recording data in that format should be described. Any statements regarding compliance with 21 CFR 11 should also be made.

The following paragraphs are applicable when either paper or electronic CRF methods are being utilized.

Completed CRFs must be ready and available for on-site review by the sponsor or their designated representative within 14 days of a subject's termination from the trial.

Steps taken to ensure accurate, complete and reliable data will begin with pre-study reviews of the protocol design and procedures with the principal investigator and his or her study coordinator who will then review these procedures with his/her staff.

3.7.2 Monitoring
Clinical monitoring visits to the investigational site will be conducted by the sponsor's personnel or their representative, as required. To ensure that the investigator and his or her staff understand and accept their defined responsibilities, the clinical monitor will maintain regular correspondence with the site and may be present during the course of the study to verify the acceptability of the facilities, compliance with the investigational plan and relevant FDA regulations, and the maintenance of complete records. Clinical monitoring will include review and resolution of missing or inconsistent results and source document checks (i.e., comparison of submitted study results to original reports) to assure the accuracy of the reported data. [21 CFR 312.50 and 312.56]

3.7.3 Data Handling
All data will be manually entered into the computerized file and independently verified to be 100% correct by either the sponsor or their representative.

3.7.4 Review of Original Subject Records
Original subject records (source documents) will be audited or reviewed during the course of monitoring to verify the accuracy of the case report forms. This audit or review will be conducted according to (company/institution) monitoring guidelines.

4.0 ANALYTICAL AND STATISTICAL EVALUATION PLAN
The Analytical and Statistical Evaluation Plan section is meant to provide a detailed description of the general statistical approach for the study [21 CFR 314.126(b)(1) and (7)]. Ideally, this section will be copied directly from the clinical analysis plan. [Note: Reference Chapter 19: Analysis Plans, for additional information].

4.1 General Statistical Issues/Information

4.1.1 Sample Size
Present information on the method used for determining the number of subjects to be enrolled in the study. State the planned sample size and give the statistical justification for the sample size calculation. If previous data or assumptions were made in the calculations, reference, summarize, or detail these as appropriate. For studies that did not utilize a formal sample size calculation, justify the number of subjects enrolled in terms of supporting conclusions regarding therapeutic effect. Address power considerations.

4.1.2 Missing Value Handling and Subject Evaluability
Provide a "bullet" style presentation of the rules for excluding subject data from analysis. Each rule should be accompanied by a justification for its use.

Exclusion criteria should be as consistent as possible across studies in a project to avoid the impression that the criteria were selected on a study-by-study basis to favor desired outcomes.

4.1.3 Group Comparability at Baseline
If the study is a multiple group study, provide a discussion of how group comparability at baseline will be established.

4.1.4 Interim Analysis and Stopping Rules
If any interim analyses are planned during the course of the study, detail the methods of analysis planned and the time point at which the analysis will be performed. Also, describe the methodology that will be used to statistically adjust for these analyses. If no statistical penalty will be incurred, provide a rationale.

4.1.5 Statistical Adjustments for Multiple Endpoints
If more than one variable will be analyzed for addressing the primary study objective, provide a description of the procedure used to maintain a specified, overall type I error rate. If no multiple comparison/simultaneous inference procedure will be used, provide a rationale.

Protocol No: ABC-###   Page 17
Effective Date: January 9, 2006

4.1.6 Approach to Multicenter Analysis
Describe the general approaches to be taken to incorporate the center as a factor in the analysis and briefly describe how estimates of treatment effect will be obtained across centers.

4.2 Analyses Addressing the Primary Study Objective
Begin this section with a restatement of the primary objective.

4.2.1 Primary Analysis
Typically in the analysis of a study, one analysis of the primary variable is used to provide the degree of significance used to evaluate test article effectiveness. Describe, in non-technical terms, the planned analysis here.

4.2.2 Supplemental Analyses
Describe additional analyses to be performed on the primary variable here. If, for example, an analysis of covariance will be used for the primary analysis, but preliminary analyses and analyses based on ranks will also be done, describe them briefly and justify their use.

4.3 Analyses Addressing Secondary Study Objective(s)
Information in this section may be broken into subsections for each secondary effectiveness variable as appropriate.

State each secondary variable and describe, in general terms, the statistical methods planned in their evaluation.

4.4 Subgroup Analyses
If the size of the study permits, relevant demographic or baseline value-defined subgroups should be examined for unusually large or small responses and the results presented, e.g. comparison of effects by severity groups, by age, sex or race or by history of prior treatment with a test article of the same class. The analyses are not intended to "salvage" an otherwise non-supportive study, but to suggest hypotheses worth examining in other studies or to help in refining labeling information, subject selection, dose selection, etc. Describe here the analytic methods planned to evaluate subgroup responses.

4.5 Safety Analyses

4.5.1 Analyses Addressing Adverse Events
The following statements are applicable to most studies:

Safety analysis will be undertaken on all patients randomized.

Adverse experience data will be listed individually and summarized by body system and preferred terms within a body system for each treatment group. Serious and/or unexpected AEs will also be discussed on a case-by-case basis. For the tabulation of AEs by body system, a patient will be counted only once in a given body system. For example, a patient reporting 'nausea and diarrhea' will be reported as one patient, but the symptoms will be listed as two separate AEs within the class. Therefore, the total number of AEs reported within a body system may exceed the number of patients within the body system reporting AEs.

Each AE (based on preferred terminology) will be only counted once for a given patient. If the same AE occurred on multiple occasions, the highest severity will be assumed. Thus, patients are not counted multiple times in a given numerator in the calculation of reaction rates for a specific AE. Also, if two or more AEs are reported as a unit, the individual terms will be reported as separate events. For example, if a patient reported 'nausea and vomiting,' the terms 'nausea' and 'vomiting' will be reported as individual AEs.

The total number of AEs reported within body systems between each of the treatment groups and the control group will be compared using Fisher's exact test.

Changes in pulse rate, systolic and diastolic blood pressure, weight, and respiratory rate will be compared within each group and among groups using analysis of variance procedures.

Depending upon the sample size, the more common adverse events that may be drug related should be examined for a dose, duration or demographic relationship or other analyses such as standard life-table methods.

4.5.2 Analyses of Clinical Laboratory Data
For most studies, this evaluation can be described in standard paragraphs as follows:

For hematology and serum chemistry tests, the mean, mean change, median, median change and range of all values for each test, for each treatment group at baseline, and for the final 'on therapy' value will be printed in a summary table. A second table ('shift table') will be made showing, for each laboratory variable, the percentage of subjects in each treatment group whose values decreased, stayed the same or increased between the baseline or pre-treatment period and the end of the study. A third table will be prepared displaying the numbers of subjects in each treatment group who had values below, within and above the normal range at baseline and at the final visit.

These tables will then be reviewed by the clinical monitor to evaluate whether any significant trends in laboratory values occurred. The clinical monitor will also review the urinalysis data by inspecting the laboratory data tabulations, but no summary tables of these data will be prepared.

Protocol No: ABC-###   Page 18
Effective Date: January 9, 2006

In the case of long-term studies or studies in which special evaluations were done, the above standard description should be modified as necessary.

5.0 REFERENCES
The References section should include a proper bibliographical listing of all published material referenced in the protocol. This section should begin a new page.

6.0 APPENDICES
6.1 Investigators, Facilities, Qualifications and IRBs [21 CFR 312.23(a)(6)(iii)(b)]

6.2 Title 21 of the Code of Federal Regulations, Section 50, or Declaration of Helsinki

6.3 Pharmaceutical Ingredients and Quality [21 CFR 314.126(d)]

6.4 Case Report Forms

6.5 Additional Information

Protocol No: ABC-###   Page 19
Effective Date: January 9, 2006

6.1 Investigators, Facilities, Qualifications and IRBs [21 CFR 312.23(a)(6)(iii)(b)]
Attach here a list of all investigators who are involved in the study. Also attach a Curriculum Vitae for the principal investigator and each sub-investigator. This information should include the name of the institution(s) where the investigator(s) work, along with contact information such as addresses and phone numbers.

Names and addresses of the Institutional Review Board(s) should be listed for each site.

Names and addresses of any clinical laboratories that are involved in supplying data for the trial should be listed.

Protocol No: ABC-###   Page 20
Effective Date: January 9, 2006

6.2 Subpart B - Informed Consent of Human Subjects
§ 50.20 General requirements for informed consent.

Except as provided in § 50.23, no investigator may involve a human being as a subject in research covered by these regulations unless the investigator has obtained the legally effective informed consent of the subject or the subject's legally authorized representative. An investigator shall seek such consent only under circumstances that provide the prospective subject or the representative sufficient opportunity to consider whether or not to participate and that minimize the possibility of coercion or undue influence. The information that is given to the subject or the representative shall be in language understandable to the subject or the representative. No informed consent, whether oral or written, may include any exculpatory language through which the subject or the representative is made to waive or appear to waive any of the subject's legal rights, or releases or appears to release the investigator, the sponsor, the institution, or its agents from liability for negligence.

§ 50.21 Effective date.

The requirements for informed consent set out in this part apply to all human subjects entering a clinical investigation that commences on or after July 27, 1981.

§ 50.23 Exception from general requirements.

(a) The obtaining of informed consent shall be deemed feasible unless, before use of the test article (except as provided in paragraph (b) of this section), both the investigator and a physician who is not otherwise participating in the clinical investigation certify in writing all of the following:

(1) The human subject is confronted by a life-threatening situation necessitating the use of the test article.

(2) Informed consent cannot be obtained from the subject because of an inability to communicate with, or obtain legally effective consent from, the subject.

(3) Time is not sufficient to obtain consent from the subject's legal representative.

(4) There is available no alternative method of approved or generally recognized therapy that provides an equal or greater likelihood of saving the life of the subject.

(b) If immediate use of the test article is, in the investigator's opinion, required to preserve the life of the subject, and time is not sufficient to obtain the independent determination required in paragraph (a) of this section in advance of using the test article, the determinations of the clinical investigator shall be made and, within 5 working days after the use of the article, be reviewed and evaluated in writing by a physician who is not participating in the clinical investigation.

(c) The documentation required in paragraph (a) or (b) of this section shall be submitted to the IRB within 5 working days after the use of the test article.

(d)(1) The Commissioner may also determine that obtaining informed consent is not feasible when the Assistant Secretary of Defense (Health Affairs) requests such a determination in connection with the use of an investigational drug (including an antibiotic or biological product) in a specific protocol under an investigational new drug application (IND) sponsored by the Department of Defense (DOD). DOD's request for a determination that obtaining informed consent from military personnel is not feasible must be limited to a specific military operation involving combat or the immediate threat of combat. The request must also include a written justification supporting the conclusions of the physician(s) responsible for the medical care of the military personnel involved and the investigator(s) identified in the IND that a military combat exigency exists because of special military combat (actual or threatened) circumstances in which, in order to facilitate the accomplishment of the military mission, preservation of the health of the individual and the safety of other personnel require that a particular treatment be provided to a specified group of military personnel, without regard to what might be any individual's personal preference for no treatment or for some alternative treatment. The written request must also include a statement that a duly constituted institutional review board has reviewed and approved the use of the investigational drug without informed consent. The Commissioner may find that informed consent is not feasible only when withholding treatment would be contrary to the best interests of military personnel and there is no available satisfactory alternative therapy.

(2) In reaching a determination under paragraph (d)(1) of this section that obtaining informed consent is not feasible and withholding treatment would be contrary to the best interests of military personnel, the Commissioner will review the request submitted under paragraph (d)(1) of this section and take into account all pertinent factors, including, but not limited to:

(i) The extent and strength of the evidence of the safety and effectiveness of the investigational drug for the intended use;

(ii) The context in which the drug will be administered, e.g., whether it is intended for use in a battlefield or hospital setting or whether it will be self-administered or will be administered by a health professional;

(iii) The nature of the disease or condition for which the preventive or therapeutic treatment is intended; and

(iv) The nature of the information to be provided to the recipients of the drug concerning the potential benefits and risks of taking or not taking the drug.

(3) The Commissioner may request a recommendation from appropriate experts before reaching a determination on a request submitted under paragraph (d)(l) of this section.

(4) A determination by the Commissioner that obtaining informed consent is not feasible and withholding treatment would be contrary to the best interests of military personnel will expire at the end of 1 year, unless renewed at DOD's request, or when the specific military operation creating the need for the use of the investigational drug has ended, whichever is earlier. The Commissioner may also revoke this determination based on changed circumstances.

§ 50.25 Elements of informed consent.

(a) Basic elements of informed consent. In seeking informed consent, the following information shall be provided to each subject:

(1) A statement that the study involves research, an explanation of the purposes of the research and the expected duration of the subject's participation, a description of the procedures to be followed, and identification of any procedures which are experimental.

(2) A description of any reasonably foreseeable risks or discomforts to the subject.

(3) A description of any benefits to the subject or to others which may reasonably be expected from the research.

(4) A disclosure of appropriate alternative procedures or courses of treatment, if any, that might be advantageous to the subject.

(5) A statement describing the extent, if any, to which confidentiality of records identifying the subject will be maintained and that notes the possibility that the Food and Drug Administration may inspect the records.

(6) For research involving more than minimal risk, an explanation as to whether any compensation and an explanation as to whether any medical treatments are available if injury occurs and, if so, what they consist of, or where further information may be obtained.

(7) An explanation of whom to contact for answers to pertinent questions about the research and research subjects' rights, and whom to contact in the event of a research-related injury to the subject.

(8) A statement that participation is voluntary, that refusal to participate will involve no penalty or loss of benefits to which the subject is otherwise entitled, and that the subject may discontinue without penalty or loss of benefits to which the subject is otherwise entitled.

(b) Additional elements of informed consent. When appropriate, one or more of the following elements of information shall also be provided to each subject:

(1) A statement that the particular treatment or procedure may involve risks to the subject (or to the embryo or fetus, if the subject is or may become pregnant) which are currently unforeseeable.

(2) Anticipated circumstances under which the subject's participation may be terminated by the investigator without regard to the subject's consent.

(3) Any additional costs to the subject that may result from participation in the research.

(4) The consequences of a subject's decision to withdraw from the research and procedures for orderly termination of participation by the subject.

(5) A statement that significant new findings developed during the course of the research which may relate to the subject's willingness to continue participation will be provided to the subject.

(6) The approximate number of subjects involved in the study.

(c) The informed consent requirements in these regulations are not intended to preempt any applicable Federal, State, or local laws which require additional information to be disclosed for informed consent to be legally effective.

(d) Nothing in these regulations is intended to limit the authority of a physician to provide emergency medical care to the extent the physician is permitted to do so under applicable Federal, State, or local law.

§50.27 Documentation of informed consent.

(a) Except as provided in § 56.109(c), informed consent shall be documented by the use of a written consent form approved by the IRB and signed by the subject or the subject's legally authorized representative. A copy shall be given to the person signing the form.

(b) Except as provided in § 56.109(c), the consent form may be either of the following:

(1) A written consent document that embodies the elements of informed consent required by § 50.25. This form may be read to the subject or the subject's legally authorized representative, but, in any event, the investigator shall give either the subject or the representative adequate opportunity to read it before it is signed.

(2) A short form written consent document stating that the elements of informed consent required by § 50.25 have been presented orally to the subject or the subject's legally authorized representative. When this method is used, there shall be a witness to the oral presentation. Also, the IRB shall approve a written summary of what is to be said to the subject or the representative. Only the short form itself is to be signed by the subject or the representative. However, the witness shall sign both the short form and a copy of the summary, and the person actually obtaining the consent shall sign a copy of the summary. A copy of the summary shall be given to the subject or the representative in addition to a copy of the short form.

6.3 Pharmaceutical Ingredients and Quality [21 CFR 314.126(d)]

For an investigation to be considered adequate for approval of a new drug, it is required that the test drug be standardized as to identity, strength, quality, purity, and dosage form to give significance to the results of the investigation.

6.4 Case Report Forms

Attach a blank copy of the case report forms, patient diaries, or electronic data collection tools used in the trial.

Protocol No: ABC-###   Page 25
Effective Date: January 9, 2006

6.5 Additional Information
As indicated.

CHAPTER 20

Informed Consent and IRB Review

By Paul W. Goebel, Jr., C.I.P., and Janet C. Donnelly, C.I.P.

This chapter describes the philosophy and procedures to be followed by the sponsor, the institutional review board (IRB) and the clinical investigator in assuring the accuracy and integrity of the informed consent document and the informed consent interview process. FDA regulations and guidance documents[1,2] outline the agency's expectations for obtaining the informed consent of subjects involved in clinical research[3] and the composition and operations of IRBs[4]. The regulations and guidances clearly assign primary responsibility for the protection of human subjects involved in clinical research to the study's IRB and clinical investigator. However, the investigational new drug (IND) regulations also mention sponsor responsibilities. Title 21 of the Code of Federal Regulations (21 CFR) Part 312.23(a)(1)(iv) requires "a commitment [from the sponsor] that an IRB that complies with the requirements set forth in 21 CFR Part 56 will be responsible for the initial and continuing review and approval of each of the studies ...." Further, 21 CFR 312.56(b) requires a sponsor "... who discovers that an investigator is not complying with the signed agreement ... or other applicable parts [of the FDA regulations, including the IRB and informed consent regulations] promptly either secure compliance or discontinue shipments of the drug."

Accordingly, it is not uncommon for sponsors to conduct on-site audits of IRBs to ensure their compliance with the relevant regulations and guidance pertaining to IRB operations and recordkeeping. As the voluntary IRB accreditation process takes hold in the United States (through the Association for the Accreditation of Human Research Protections Programs), sponsors are expected to rely increasingly on this accreditation for assurance that an IRB's basic operations comply with FDA requirements. On-site audits would then be limited to assuring the adequate review of the studies of interest.

Despite the fact that the failings of an IRB generally are considered to be outside a sponsor's control, they certainly can jeopardize the sponsor's use of trial data in a marketing application. Although the FDA has seldom disqualified study data solely on the basis of inadequate IRB review and informed consent, the questionable protection of study subjects has resulted in marketing approval delays as FDA concerns were resolved. In some cases, the inadequate human subject protection has been a factor in FDA decisions to exclude data from certain clinical site(s) in reviewing pending marketing applications. Sponsors should make every reasonable effort to ensure that all the factors within their control and knowledge comply with current good clinical practice (GCP) standards and take a proactive stance in avoiding other problems.

Who Should Prepare the Initial Draft of the Informed Consent Document? The source of the initial draft of the informed consent form-specifically, whether the sponsor or investigator should prepare it-is a topic that generates considerable controversy and discussion. When the regulations were written in 1981, most clinical research was performed in academic medical centers. The protocol and the informed consent form were written by the clinical investigator, who was an expert in the disease or condition under study. The expansion of clinical research outside the academic medical centers has changed this dynamic. Today, however, much of the expertise regarding the condition being studied in clinical trials is far more likely to rest with the clinical and medical professionals employed by a clinical study's sponsoring company. Therefore, the protocol, investigator's brochure and draft informed consent document are often written by the sponsor, which then hires qualified clinicians to serve as clinical investigators for the study.

One can strongly argue, however, that the investigator has a more unbiased interest in the subject's safety, and therefore is in a better position to draft a balanced and protective document. While that may be true, there are many other factors that are in play for commercially sponsored studies and that generally take precedence. First, the clinical investigator is often involved late in the process, and is expected to get the necessary documents to the IRB as quickly as possible. Presenting the clinical investigator with an accurate and complete first draft of the informed consent document accelerates the IRB approval process (see discussion of IRB review of multi-site studies below).

A possible exception involves Phase 1 studies conducted at contract research laboratories that specialize in such trials. In this case, the study site may have extensive "boilerplate" text that is applicable to most or all of their procedures. This text may have been approved by an IRB for similar and previously conducted studies. When this is the case, the IRB would already have a high level of understanding of the risks and benefits of similar studies, and will have reviewed and approved an informed consent document that can be used for the new study, likely with only a few changes.

Regardless of the reason, a sponsor's failure to review and approve informed consent documents prior to IRB review ultimately will delay the initiation of a trial in at least half of all cases. The idea is to anticipate potential problems and avoid surprises and duplication of effort at every opportunity.

Perhaps the most persuasive argument, however, is that, compared to specialists on a sponsor's clinical development team, many clinical investigators are not as well versed in the regulatory aspects of informed consent. Composing a sample informed consent document that adequately and accurately conveys all required information and is written in a style that is readable by and understandable to those without a higher-level reading ability involves a skillful blending of medical and scientific knowledge about the study, familiarity with regulatory requirements, knowledge regarding the conduct of clinical trials, and the ability to compose accurate and easily readable documents. The preparation of a well-written consent document generally requires the contributions of more than one person. A word of caution, however: A sample [model] informed consent document that is not well written is not beneficial. Misleading, coercive or unclear wording placed in a model consent document by the sponsor tends to remain in all copies until it is removed by the IRB. The process of correcting unsatisfactory wording in the informed consent form is one of the IRB's most time-consuming duties, and may result in considerable delay in completion of the IRB's review.

The sponsor-employed clinical scientist in charge of the study should have overall responsibility for the informed consent form's drafting and final content. The clinical scientist or a designated clinical research associate (CRA)/clinical monitor should draft a sample informed consent document that fulfills all the requirements of 21 CFR 50. Their work should be examined by other qualified professionals, ideally regulatory affairs personnel. The informed consent checklist (see attachment at end of chapter) provides a convenient reference that identifies all of the informed consent elements. This checklist also contains the elements of informed consent found in the ICH's Good Clinical Practice (GCP) E6 guidance document (www.ich.org).

The Preparation of the Informed Consent Document Once the informed consent document is drafted, the appropriate regulatory affairs specialist should review the sample informed consent document and forward any comments to the author of the draft. All comments that are considered essential should be noted as such. All other comments, although they may not represent mandatory changes, should receive adequate consideration from a regulatory perspective. For example, suggested changes often involve address the use of language indicating that the clinical trial involves research. The draft informed consent may clearly state that the clinical trial is "investigational" or a "study," and describe the study using every word but the term "research." Although it may be clear to all involved in the development project that the consent form's text implies very strongly that the study involves "research," because the term is not used, it may well trigger what ultimately degenerates into a heated discussion that could have been avoided if that one word had been included in the first place. This is what expedites the work: Anticipating the common problem areas and eliminating them before they occur. Only after all issues have been resolved should the clinical scientist or CRA forward a copy of the sponsor-approved sample informed consent document to the investigator.

The Clinical Investigator's Review of the Draft Informed Consent Document In the development of the informed consent document, the clinical investigator will play one of three possible roles. He/she may elect to use the document provided by the sponsor as is, which is clearly the best option from the sponsor's perspective when a well-written document has been prepared. More commonly, the investigator will opt to modify the draft, a revised version of which he/she should forward for sponsor for review before providing it to the IRB. Alternatively, the investigator may create an entirely original document, something that may be a cause of concern for the sponsor. Unfortunately, not every investigator can quickly prepare an informed consent document that complies with all relevant federal regulations. The sponsor should make it clear that, if the investigator opts to draft an informed consent document, he/she should forward a copy of the proposed document for sponsor review before submitting it to the IRB. To facilitate this, the sponsor should commit to a 24-hour (or less) turnaround for the document.

The sponsor's clinical and regulatory staff should compare the sponsor's sample informed consent document to the investigator's proposed informed consent document. The sponsor should then transmit the document to the investigator with any suggested or required changes in writing. Assuming that the changes are accepted, the investigator should make the changes and forward the revised informed consent document with the protocol to the IRB for review and approval. The IRB should either approve the package or request specific changes. If the IRB requests that additional changes be made, the investigator should make the requested changes and forward this to the sponsor for review. Again, a 24-hour turn-around (or less) is imperative. The clinical scientist or CRA can then finalize the "IND package" and then forward to the regulatory affairs group for a final compliance review and submission to the FDA. Although this process sounds involved, it is worth noting that some IRBs have required changes that are not consistent with federal regulations, triggering another round of corrections and delays. A careful sponsor review of any and every change to the original draft will be an investment that will pay off in the long run.

When the term is intended to be all-inclusive, the consent document should refer to study participants as "subjects" or "study subjects" rather than "patients."[5] A healthy volunteer agrees to participate in a trial for reasons other than medical reasons, and therefore receives no direct health benefit from participating. A subject is an individual who participates in a clinical trial, either as a recipient of the investigational product or as a control. It is best to avoid calling a research subject a patient because the individual may not be receiving the standard therapy that would be administered in the practice of medicine. [6]

An adequate and well-written consent document has a solid chance of receiving IRB approval with the addition of only site-specific information, such as contact information. In such cases, IRB approval is accomplished at the same meeting as the initial review. On the other hand, even when all of the required elements are adequately covered, sample consents that contain unexplained medical or scientific jargon or are otherwise difficult to read may trigger an IRB request for revision or, worse, a marked up document with all of the unacceptable passages clearly highlighted, but no clear indication of what changes the IRB is requesting. Since many IRBs meet only once a month, an IRB request for revisions in the consent document will result in at least a 30-day delay in IRB approval.

In the end, it is preferable for the sponsor to prepare an initial draft of a sample informed consent document that contains all of the elements required by the regulations. Ultimately, it is more efficient for the clinical investigator to modify an existing, well-written document than to create a completely new document.

IRB Review of the Research Project Before an IRB can approve a clinical study, it must determine that the study meets all of the seven criteria listed in the FDA regulations (e.g., risks to subjects are minimized and are reasonable in relation to anticipated benefits, subject selection is equitable, informed consent will be sought).[7] If some or all of the subjects are likely to be vulnerable to coercion or undue influence, the IRB must assure that additional safeguards have been included in the study to protect the rights and welfare of those subjects. Although the FDA's regulations and guidance documents do not specify the additional safeguards that might be implemented, it does specify examples of vulnerable subjects[8]: children, prisoners, pregnant women, handicapped or mentally disabled persons, or economically or educationally disadvantaged persons. If the sponsor anticipates that such individuals may be enrolled in the study, it should consider that implementing appropriate additional safeguards in the original study plan will likely speed IRB approval.

The IRB Approval Letter The IRB must notify the clinical investigator and the institution in writing of its decision to approve, request modifications in, or disapprove the study.[9] The approval letter should positively identify the study so that it is clear which protocol and which version of that protocol is being approved. In the letter, it is appropriate to include the exact name of the study, IRB review number, protocol number, revision number and revision date. The IRB's written procedures should outline the format for such letters. In the past, it was not uncommon for the sponsor to reject the IRB's first approval letter when the letter did not include the complete identification of the study (i.e., the protocol version, protocol number and any other specific identification). Today, most IRBs are aware that complete and specific identification of the protocol is required. The sponsor should do its part by clearly indicating the name and all of the identification numbers on the protocol and on any correspondence with the clinical investigator and the IRB. In advance, the sponsor can also emphasize to the clinical investigator that complete study-identifying information should be included on any correspondence. It is important that any revisions of ongoing studies be completely identified so that the version control may be easily transferred to the approval letter.

Sponsors seeking rapid IRB approval should accept the IRB's standard approval letter format if it is minimally acceptable, and resist the temptation to insist on special wording in the letter. Customizing each approval letter can delay the IRB approval process. Sponsors should also resist asking the IRB for special letters acknowledging the receipt or review of adverse event reports and other documents that are not required by the regulations. While each individual letter might not add significantly to the IRB administrator's duties, the cumulative effect can be considerable, particularly given that most IRBs do not have a large administrative staff.

Pediatric Studies The FDA Modernization Act of 1997 required the FDA to consult with experts in pediatric research to develop, prioritize and publish a list of approved drugs for which additional pediatric information may produce health benefits in the pediatric population. This consultation resulted in the publication, on March 25, 1998, of a draft list of approximately 400 drugs for which pediatric labeling should be developed.[10] On December 2, 1998, the FDA published a final rule requiring pediatric labeling for drugs that meet one of the following criteria: (1) the drug product represents an improvement over standard therapy for children; (2) the drug is prescribed at least 50,000 times per year; (3) the drug belongs to a class or for a use for which additional therapeutic options for children are needed.[11]

This series of events—and the more recent Best Pharmaceuticals for Children Act (January 4, 2002[12]) and the Pediatric Research Equity Act of 2003[13]—led to a significant increase in drug research studies being performed in children of all ages. The FDA's regulations regarding the IRB review of and informed consent for research conducted in children were not changed at that time. In 2001,[14] however, the FDA adopted Subpart D of the DHHS regulations,[15] which provide for additional safeguards for children in clinical investigations.[16] The FDA adopted the DHHS regulations largely as is, except for those passages that conflicted with the FDA's regulations. For example, the FDA did not adopt the DHHS provision for the parental waiver of informed consent.[17]

Subpart D requires that IRBs find and document the level of risk to the children at the time it approves pediatric studies. The IRB must also find and document whether assent will be solicited from the children and, if so, whether and how it should be documented. The IRB should also determine whether the permission of one parent or both parents will be required in a study.

Minorities and Women of Child-Bearing Potential In 1993, the FDA published a guidance document reversing a 1977 policy stating that women of childbearing potential should not be included in clinical studies.[18] In 1998, the agency issued a final rule requiring sponsors to tabulate, in IND and NDA annual reports, the number of subjects enrolled according to age group, gender, and race.[19]

Since the FDA does not enforce guidance documents or proposed regulations, what is their significance for study sponsors? There are two points at which delays and confusion could arise if the protocol excludes women and minorities:

(1) If an IRB is aware of the guidance documents it may request justification of the exclusion. Furthermore, IRBs at academic medical centers that have a FederalWide Assurance (FWA) or Multiple Project Assurance (MPA) from the Department of Health and Human Services (DHHS)[20] may be required to adhere to the National Institutes of Health (NIH) guidelines on the inclusion of women and minorities in studies.[21]

(2) The FDA reviewing division may request scientific justification for the exclusion of women and minorities. Even if lack of such data does not result in a denial of marketing approval, it may cause a significant delay in obtaining IRB or marketing approval. Unless there is a compelling scientific or medical reason to exclude women and minorities, the sponsor should seriously consider their inclusion.

IRB Review of Multi-Site Studies When sponsors undertake studies that are to be conducted at multiple and separate locations, the prototype informed consent document prepared by the sponsor becomes an important element of consistency. While it is possible for the clinical investigators at the various sites to compose all of the wording in the informed consent document independently, it is appropriate for the sponsor to provide a draft consent document. Centrally prepared wording for the product-specific portions of the consent offers the advantage of initial consistency. The accuracy and completeness of the information in the initial draft consent form is very important, since any shortcomings tend to be perpetuated at the various study sites.

The Sponsor's File Copy The sponsor's files should include a copy of the final, IRB-approved informed consent document for each investigator/study site until the study report is archived at the very end of the trial. At that time, a copy of the final informed consent form for each site should be placed in the documentation section of the appropriate final report of the study.

Direct Communication Between Sponsors and IRBs As is true in any situation, direct communication generally is preferable to communication that involves a third party. When complicated issues must be resolved, the IRB and the sponsor may decide that it is better to communicate with each other directly rather than through the clinical investigator. Formal information/communication, however, generally should flow from the sponsor to the clinical investigator to the IRB. This is important because it helps maintain a line of communication between the clinical investigator and the IRB, and also because the clinical investigator should be aware of issues as they are addressed. Many IRBs will bring issues directly to the sponsor in the interest of efficiency. The FDA realizes that such direct communication may be the most rapid and efficient means of addressing problems. Clinical investigators should promptly report serious and unexpected adverse events directly to the responsible IRB, and should send progress reports directly to that IRB rather than waiting for a summary prepared by the sponsor.

Sponsor Access to IRB Written Procedures, Minutes and Membership Rosters FDA regulations do not require public or sponsor access to IRB records. However, the FDA does not prohibit the sponsor from requesting IRB records or the IRB from disclosing them. IRB minutes may contain proprietary information that is regarded as confidential. Some states have so-called "sunshine" laws that could be interpreted as requiring the disclosure of certain IRB records.

All IRBs that review FDA-regulated studies should be willing to provide sponsors with assurance that they are organized and operate according to the 21 CFR 50 and 21 CFR 56 regulations. The documents that many IRBs will provide to sponsors include written operating procedures, membership roster, a roster showing the qualifications of members but omitting the names, standard consent paragraphs that the IRB prefers to use, the dates of previous FDA inspections, any post-inspection correspondence from the FDA, and an OHRP-issued federalwide assurance (FWA) or multiple project assurance (MPA) number (note: The absence of an FWA/MPA number does not mean that the IRB is substandard. The OHRP negotiates an assurance with research sites that perform studies with DHHS grant money or that are performed by DHHS employees. IRBs that are not part of institutions that perform such research generally will not have an assurance number. However, any IRB that is named as the IRB of record in an assurance must register with OHRP and receive an OHRP registration number.)

The IRB should provide enough information to permit the sponsor to evaluate the board's state of compliance. Some sponsors routinely audit the IRBs that review their research projects.

Certificates of Confidentiality In January 1997, DHHS granted all Public Health Service agencies, including the FDA, the authority to issue Certificates of Confidentiality, as outlined in section 301 of the Public Health Service Act. Certificates of Confidentiality are issued to protect identifiable research information from forced disclosure. They allow the investigator and others who have access to research records to refuse to disclose identifying information on research participants in any civil, criminal, administrative, legislative, or other proceeding, whether at the federal, state, or local level. Certificates of Confidentiality may be granted for studies involving the collection of information that, if disclosed, could have adverse consequences for subjects or damage their financial standing, employability, insurability, or reputation. The certificates help assure confidentiality and privacy by protecting against forced disclosure of the study subject's identity.

The FDA can issue a Certificate of Confidentiality to sponsors of research projects conducted under an IND or Investigational Device Exemption (for devices). [22] For research that is not conducted under an IND or IDE, the FDA will refer applicants to the NIH's certificates of confidentiality office. [23]

Certificates can be used for biomedical, behavioral, clinical or other types of research considered sensitive. Research is regarded to be sensitive if the disclosure of identifying information could have adverse consequences for subjects or damage their financial standing, employability, insurability, or reputation. Examples of sensitive research activities include, but are not limited to, the collection of genetic information, information on psychological well-being of subjects, and information on subjects' sexual attitudes, preferences or practices, data on substance abuse or other illegal risk behaviors. Studies in which subjects may be involved in litigation related to exposures under study (e.g., breast implants, environmental or occupational exposures) would also qualify.

Certificates of Confidentiality are not intended to take the place of appropriate data security or clear data protection policies and procedures, which are essential for the protection of research participants' privacy. Researchers should implement an adequate process to safeguard research data and findings that indicate the identity of study subjects from access by unauthorized individuals.

IRB Approval A Certificate of Confidentiality will not be issued to an applicant that is conducting clinical research unless the project has obtained IRB approval. The approving IRB must be in compliance with applicable federal requirements.

Informed Consent When a researcher obtains a Certificate of Confidentiality, the research subjects must be told about the protections afforded by the certificate and any exceptions to that protection. That information should be included in the informed consent form. The following statement provides an example of the explanation that can be included in the informed consent document:

> "We have obtained a Certificate of Confidentiality from the Food and Drug Administration (FDA). The purpose of this Certificate is to prevent the forced disclose of information that may identify you, even by a court subpoena, in any federal, state, or local civil, criminal, administrative, legislative, or other proceedings. The Certificate cannot prevent authorized agents of the FDA from receiving the information necessary to perform their official duties.

Expediting Drug and Biologics Development

A Certificate of Confidentiality does not prevent you or persons you authorize from voluntarily releasing information about you. If you authorize disclosure of your research information to an insurer, employer, or other person, then the Certificate will not prevent uch release."

The researchers should include language, such as the following, if they intend to make voluntary disclosures about such areas as child abuse, a subject's intent to hurt him/herself or others, or other voluntary disclosures:

"The Certificate of Confidentiality does not prevent the researchers from disclosing voluntarily, without your consent, information that would identify you as a participant in the research project under the following circumstances: [Here, the researchers should identify the conditions under which voluntary disclosure would be made. If no voluntary disclosures will be made, the researchers should so state.]"

International Conference on Harmonization (ICH) Some sponsors are asking IRBs to certify that they are organized and operating under procedures consistent with the ICH's good clinical practice (GCP) guidelines (E6). The rationale for this request is that the sponsor intends to submit the study data to the European Union or to Japan for marketing approval.

The FDA published the ICH's E6 guideline in 1997.[24] The document was published as official guidance and not as a regulation. The FDA neither requires IRBs to provide nor prohibits IRBs from providing assurance to the sponsor concerning their compliance with the ICH guidelines.

References

[1] FDA Information Sheets for Institutional Review Boards and Clinical Investigators

[2] ICH Good Clinical Practice Guidance, E-6

[3] 21 CFR 50, Protection of Human Subjects of Research

[4] 21 CFR 56, Institutional Review Boards

[5] Levine, R.J., Ethics and Regulation of Clinical Research, Yale, Second Edition (1986), page 8.

[6] Chambers, G.K., Fairbarn, M.S., Clinical Trial Design, Applied Clinical Trials, Volume 7, Number 9, Page 60, September 1998

[7] 21 CFR 56.111(a)

[8] 21 CFR 56.111(b)

[9] 21 CFR 56.109(e)

[10] http://www.fda.gov/bbs/topics/NEWS/NEW00629.html

[11] Regulations Requiring Manufacturers to Assess the Safety and Effectiveness of New Drugs and Biological Products in Pediatric Patients; Final Rule 63 FR 66631, December 2, 1998: http://www.fda.gov/ohrms/dockets/98fr/120298c.pdf .

[12] http://www.fda.gov/cder/pediatric/index.htm#bpca

[13] http://www.fda.gov/cder/pediatric/index.htm#prea

[14] 66 FR 20598, April 24, 2001

[15] 45 CFR 46.401 through 409

[16] 21 CFR 50.50 through 50.56

[17] 45 CFR 46.408(c)

[18] Guideline for the Study and Evaluation of Gender Differences in the Clinical Evaluation of Drugs, 58 FR 39406, July 22, 1993

[19] Investigational New Drug Applications and New Drug Applications, 63 FR 6854, February 11, 1998 (final rule)

[20] OHRP Approved Assurances Database: http://ohrp.cit.nih.gov/search/asearch.asp#ASUR

[21] NIH Guidelines on the Inclusion of Women and Minorities as Subjects in Clinical Research; Notice, 59 FR 14508, March 28, 1994

[22] FDA contacts for Certificates of Confidentiality: Drugs: Julie Unger, DSI (301/827-1685) Biologics: Pat Holobaugh (301/827-6347); Devices: Marsha Melvin (301/594-1190)

[23] http://grants.nih.gov/grants/policy/coc/index.htm

[24] 62 FR 25691, May 9, 1997.

FDA/ICH Informed Consent Checklist

Protocol No:________

Investigator:____________________

This list references the relevant sections of both the FDA informed consent regulations and the ICH GCP guidance (E6). The ICH guidance does not contain all of the detail found in the FDA's part 50 regulations. In several places, however, the ICH guidance contains the provision, "to ensure compliance with applicable regulatory requirements." The specific FDA elements are regarded to be "applicable regulatory requirements."

Basic Elements of Informed Consent

(These eight elements are required for all informed consent forms that must meet FDA requirements.)

Basic Element 1 21 CFR 50.25(a)(1) ICH 4.8.10(a), (b), (c), (d), (f), (s)

YES NO

___ ___ A clear statement that the study involves research. (The word "research" should be used.)

___ ___ A clear explanation of the purposes of the research. (Should include determination of safety and effectiveness, when true.)

___ ___ The expected duration of the subject's participation (e.g., number of days, number of visits, number of cycles, overnight stay or hospitalization required).

___ ___ A clear description of the procedures to be followed. How many needlesticks per visit, other discomforts. (Verify procedures with protocol.)

___ ___ An identification of any procedures which are experimental, including diagnostic testing procedures required only for study purposes.

(A time vs. event chart is recommended for studies that involve multiple visits or other complicated arrangements. Most protocols contain a chart that can be simplified and included in the consent document. Most study subjects can easily understand what will be done at each visit from such a chart. A chart can take the place of many lines of dense prose.)

ICH 4.8.10(c) (specific requirement)

___ ___ How randomization will be accomplished.

ICH 4.8.10(d) (specific requirement)

___ ___ Any invasive procedures should be outlined.

Basic Element 2 21 CFR 50.25(a)(2) ICH 4.8.10(g)

YES NO

___ ___ A clear description of any reasonably foreseeable risks or discomforts to the subject. This should include a description of those risks which might be attributable to the test article, and a description of those risks which might be attributable to any of the procedures described in the protocol that a reasonable person would want to know about. Discomforts, such as number of needle-sticks, should be explained, but should not be situated or worded so as to lead readers to believe they are the most serious risks, when such is not the case.

(When standard hospital procedures are being performed as part of the study, the standard hospital consent may be used and referenced in the informed consent document. Examples include certain x-rays, NMR.)

Basic Element 3 21 CFR 50.25(a)(3) ICH 4.8.10(h)

YES NO

___ ___ A clear description of any benefits to the subject or to others which may reasonably be expected from the research. The possibility of cure or favorable medical outcome should not be presented with a greater chance of certainty than can be supported by what is known about the test article, as outlined in the protocol. If there are no anticipated medical benefits to the subject, this should be explained in the informed consent document.

ICH 4.8.10(k) (Specific requirement)

___ ___ Although not a medical benefit, any payment to the subject for participation in the study should be outlined in the consent.

Basic Element 4 21 CFR 50.25(a)(4) ICH 4.8.10(i)

YES NO

___ ___ A disclosure of appropriate alternative procedures or courses of treatment, if any, that might be advantageous to the subject. Any clear advantages or disadvantages of the alternatives should be listed. An alternative such as surgery may be listed without further explanation. Available classes of drugs may usually be listed rather than specific drugs (e.g., calcium channel blocker, beta blocker).

ICH 4.8.10(i) (Specific requirement)

___ ___ The important potential benefits and risks of alternative procedures or courses of treatment must be disclosed.

Basic Element 5 21 CFR 50.25(a)(5) ICH 4.8.10(n)

YES NO

___ ___ A clear statement describing the extent, if any, to which confidentiality of records identifying the subject will be maintained and, in the case of FDA regulated research, that notes the possibility that the FDA may inspect the records. All entities anticipated to have access to the records should be named. If the sponsor or agents of the sponsor, such as the contract research organization, monitor and auditor, anticipate needing access to the study or medical records containing the personal identifying information of the study subjects, the consent should specifically include such permission. This eliminates the need to re-contact subjects to obtain consent at a later date if there is a need for access.

ICH 4.8.10(n)

___ ___ that the subject is authorizing access to original medical records by the monitor, auditor, IRB and regulatory authorities by signing the informed consent form.

ICH 4.8.10(o)

___ ___ requires records identifying the subject to be kept confidential and not be made publicly available to the extent permitted by the applicable laws and/or regulations. If the results of the trial are published, the subject's identity will remain confidential.

Basic Element 6 21 CFR 50.25(a)(6) ICH 4.8.10(j)

YES NO

___ ___ A clear explanation as to whether any compensation is available if injury occurs, and what it consists of, or whom to contact for information. (This element must be met for studies that impart greater than minimal risk. All studies conducted under an IND or IDE are regarded to impart greater than minimal risk to the subjects. ICH has no such qualifier.)

___ ___ A clear explanation as to whether any medical treatments are available if injury occurs, and what they consist of, or a description of where additional information may be obtained (more than minimal risk studies).

(Compensation refers to payment for lost work time or payment for medical services to treat study-related injuries. Medical treatment refers to access to medical services. Access can be pre-arranged at a specific location or there can be a general instruction to go to the study site, an emergency room or to the subject's private physician.)

Basic Element 7 21 CFR 50.25(a)(7) ICH 4.8.10(q)

YES NO

___ ___ An explanation of whom to contact for answers to pertinent questions about the research (usually the clinical investigator).

___ ___ An explanation of whom to contact for answers to pertinent questions about research subjects' rights (usually the IRB office.).

___ ___ An explanation of whom to contact for answers to pertinent questions in the event of a research related injury (usually the clinical investigator).

(Most medical schools/institutions/IRBs will have prepared standardized wording for this element.) (FDA requires each of the three components to be outlined, because it is just as important to know why someone may need to be contacted as whom to contact.)

Basic Element 8 21 CFR 50.25(a)(8) ICH 4.8.10(m)

YES NO

___ ___ A statement that participation is voluntary. (The word "voluntary" should be used.)

___ ___ A clear statement that refusal to participate will involve no penalty or loss of any benefits to which the subject is otherwise entitled.

___ ___ A clear statement that the subject may discontinue participation at any time without penalty or loss of benefits to which the subject is otherwise entitled.

Additional Elements of Informed Consent

Each of these elements should be included when it is appropriate to the study
The ICH guidance does not differentiate between basic and additional elements.

Additional Element 1 21 CFR 50.25(b)(1)

YES NO NA

___ ___ ___ A statement that the investigational procedure or exposure to the investigational drug may involve risks to the subject (or to the embryo or fetus, if the subject is or may become pregnant) which are currently unforeseeable.

Additional Element 2 21 CFR 50.25(b)(2) ICH 4.8.10(r)

YES NO NA

___ ___ ___ A statement of anticipated circumstances under which the subject's participation may be terminated by the investigator without regard to the subject's consent. (It is not sufficient to state "your doctor will explain the possibilities to you." Examples of appropriate statements: "Your participation will be ended if tests show you are not responding to the drug." "You do not follow the instructions of the study staff."

Additional Element 3 21 CFR 50.25(b)(3) ICH 4.8.10(l)

YES NO NA

___ ___ ___ Any additional costs to the subject that may result from participation in the research. (These may include cost of administering the drug, cost of tests or procedures that would not be performed under standard treatment. Subjects in studies conducted under an IND should not be charged for investigational drugs unless the study is under a treatment protocol or prior FDA permission has been obtained, see 21 CFR 312.7.)

Additional Element 4 21 CFR 50.25(b)(4)

YES NO NA

___ ___ ___ The consequences of a subject's decision to withdraw from the research and the procedures for orderly termination of participation by the subject. (The subjects should be warned if sudden withdrawal from the study drug might adversely affect their health.)

Additional Element 5 21 CFR 50.25(b)(5) ICH 4.8.10(p), 4.8.2

YES NO NA

___ ___ ___ A statement that significant new findings developed during the course of the research which may relate to the subject's willingness to continue participation will be provided to the subject or legally authorized representative. (Such a statement would generally not apply if the study is a single-dose study for which there is no time for new findings to develop during the subject's participation).

Additional Element 6 21 CFR 50.25(b)(6) ICH 4.8.10(t)

YES NO NA

___ ___ ___ The approximate number of subjects (and sites) involved in the study.

(The number of subjects who had previously been given the drug may be important if the subjects were among the first to be given the drug [phase 1 or phase 2] or if many thousands had already been given the same dose).

Additional ICH Element ICH 4.8.10(e)

YES NO NA

___ ___ ___ The responsibilities of the study subject should be explained in both the informed consent discussion and the written informed consent form.

Additional ICH Element ICH 4.8.12

YES NO NA

___ ___ ___ When permission of a subject is provided by an authorized representative, the subject should be informed about the trial to the extent they are capable of understanding and, if capable, should assent, sign and date the written informed consent. This provision applies to both children and adults (e.g., those with dementia so severe that they are judged not capable of deciding for themselves). (ICH does not specifically require preparation of a simplified version of the informed consent document (assent document), just an oral explanation and a signature on the informed consent document). However, ICH does allow for "applicable regulatory requirements."

General Requirements

YES NO Language (mandatory):

21 CFR 50.20 ICH 4.8.6

___ ___ 1. Translation of the informed consent form. (The consent should be translated if it is anticipated the consent interview will be conducted in another language. A translator may be used to facilitate conversation, but routine ad-hoc translation is inappropriate. If the prospective study subject does not understand English, provision would also have to be made for a translator to be present during the study visits. Investigators are cautioned against using family members of the subjects as translators. Experience has shown that accurate translation is not always their highest priority.)

ICH 4.8.4

___ ___ 2. The consent document should avoid exculpatory language. Exculpatory language is defined in the regulations as language that would result in:

(i) waived legal rights (or the appearance of waiver of rights) of the study subject; (ii) release from liability for negligence (or the appearance of release from liability for negligence) of the investigator, sponsor, institution or others conducting the study.

This standard is broader in scope that the strict legal meaning of exculpatory.

Documentation of informed consent

YES NO

21 CFR 50.27(a)

___ ___ Subject/representative signature/date (dated signature of study subject is required by the FDA regulation) (it is good practice for all signatures to be dated by the persons as they sign).

ICH 4.8.11

___ ___ The subject must receive a signed and dated copy of the written informed consent form prior to participation in the trial.

21 CFR 50.27(b)(1).

When the subject has the opportunity to read the informed consent document, FDA requires only one signature—the subject or legally authorized representative

ICH 4.8.8

The written informed consent form should be signed and dated by the subject and by the person who conducted the informed consent discussion.

21 CFR 50.27(b)(2)

FDA requires three signatures when the subject or legally authorized representative does not have an opportunity to read the informed consent document: (1) the subject or the legally authorized representative; (2) a witness (witness to the entire oral presentation, not just the signature) and (3) person conducting the consent interview (cannot be the same person as the witness). The regulation also appears to require preparation of a "short form" consent and a written narrative of the information that will be presented orally. However, use of three signatures on the "long form" consent document is commonly used as an alternative to the short form and written narrative.

ICH 4.8.9

An impartial witness is required for those who are unable to read or cannot decide for themselves. By signing the consent form, the witness attests that the information in the consent form and any other written information was accurately explained to, and apparently understood by, the subject or the subject's legally acceptable representative, and that informed consent was freely given by the subject or the subject's legally acceptable representative. (ICH has no provision for a "short form" and narrative.)

(FDA does not require the clinical investigator to sign the informed consent document. The sponsor or the IRB could impose such a requirement on its own authority. When the clinical investigator is required to sign the consent, the explanation should be consistent with what the investigator is in a position to know. For example, if the investigator is not present during the consent interview, he/she could not know and should not be asked to certify "All of the items in the informed consent document were clearly explained and the subject appeared to understand them and willingly agreed to participate.")

(The sponsor, investigator and IRB should agree on how many signatures will be required and what each of the signatures signifies. For example, if persons who cannot consent for themselves will not be entered into the study, there may be no need for a witness signature block.)

[signature]

______________________ __________
[clinical scientist name] Date

[signature]

______________________ __________
[regulatory affairs specialist name] Date

CHAPTER 21

Clinical Trial Operations

By Angela Fleming

There is an enormous amount of activity that comprises the successful conduct and outcome of a clinical trial. These activities frequently fall under several general categories, including protocols, informed consent and IRB review, data capture, data management, monitoring, data analysis, report writing, trial financing, reports to senior management, among many others. As a separate discipline, the so-called "clinical trial operations" traditionally oversee how all of these activities are managed to promote a seamless process.

Generally, a clinical trial has two key leaders who work in a highly integrated partnership. One of these leaders is the team member with control over day-to-day medical/scientific issues in a trial, and with overall leadership of the clinical trial team. That person is most frequently someone with a medical, or doctoral-level scientific, degree, and is employed within a company's medical or clinical research department(s). This individual's overall role on the project team may be to serve as a project leader in smaller projects, or he/she may report to the project leader in large projects that comprise many simultaneous clinical trials. The clinical investigator generally is this person's key contact at the clinical site.

The second of these two key leaders for a clinical trial is the clinical trial manager, or clinical research manager (CRM). Although the two terms are interchangeable, CRM will be the preferred term in this chapter. The operational person on the clinical trial team, the CRM handles day-to-day operational issues. The CRM's main contact at the investigational site is the study coordinator. This chapter will focus on the role of a CRM within the framework of a clinical study.

Protocol Planning The first and most critical element that will guide a study's direction is the clinical protocol. It is important for the CRM to participate in the initial strategy meeting that should represent the first step in protocol creation. During this process, it is important that the CRM review the emerging protocol outline with a particular focus on the inclusion and exclusion (I/E) criteria and the clinical procedures and assessments that will take place during the study. The CRM should ask such pertinent questions as:
  - "How will this affect enrollment?"
  - "How does all of this fit into the clinical setting and daily routines of inpatient or outpatient care?"
  - "Are the inclusion and exclusion criteria written such that deviations will not be permitted (good idea), or referred to the medical/scientific leader (bad idea)?"
  - "How will any unintended deviations from the inclusion and exclusion criteria and procedures be handled?"
  - "Are all procedures clearly described?"

It is critical that reviewers from other disciplines, such as medical, regulatory affairs, nonclinical, statistics, and data management, participate in the strategy meeting and provide input to the protocol. It might also be very helpful to have marketing represented, although most never think to involve them at the early stages. It is a mistake to forget about marketing and the important role that this group should play in the direction of clinical research. This is not to say that marketing drives the discussion, but it is always a good idea to gain their input. It is easy to forget that the product must be sold when development is successful from a clinical/regulatory perspective.

Site Selection Once a protocol has been finalized, site selection is the next step in the process. FDA regulations at 21 CFR 312.53 state that a sponsor shall select only investigators qualified by training and experience as appropriate experts to investigate the drug. To comply with this regulation, the CRM must find sites that can and will validate their expertise and ability to conduct clinical studies according to these regulations, as well as the good clinical practice standards spelled out in the ICH's GCP guidance (E6).

The experience of study site personnel and the time that a study site's team can provide before, during and after a study can be the difference between success and failure. The potential sites must have a qualified physician-investigator, an experienced staff that can dedicate the time to properly conduct the study, and the appropriate patient population.

So where do you begin the process of identifying the perfect site? There are many sources of potentially good investigators and sites. There are various directories that list physicians, including those maintained by many medical associations. It is worth joining a relevant medical association just to get the membership directory. Known "performers" from previous studies are kept in a log by every good company (and CRM). A search of the medical literature to see who is publishing in a particular area is a great source of information. Others on the study team, including the medical/scientific leader and the clinical research associates (CRAs) assigned to the project, are all likely to have useful insights and suggestions. There are also a particular field's "thought leaders," who can add great value to a study, particularly in the development and defense of a protocol and, subsequently, in dealing with other investigators who may want to modify the protocol.

Once the CRM has chosen a list of sites to contact and has detected initial interest from the sites, the CRM forwards a Confidential Disclosure Agreement (CDA) before sending any confidential information to the sites. (Alternatively, when time is tight, another option is to send the CDA with the confidential information, such as the protocol outline, with prior verbal agreement that the investigator will sign the CDA prior to reading any confidential material.) Once the CDA is signed, the protocol can be sent to the investigator for review and discussion.

To assist in gathering the information necessary to determine whether the sites meet the necessary qualifications for the study, the CRM can forward investigator questionnaires for completion by the sites. Information on areas such as medical specialty, size and type of patient population, research experience (including the experience of the study coordinator), and the available facilities and equipment are critical to help the sponsor focus on the most appropriate sites. The sponsor should also assess factors such as an investigator's motivation, the site's organization, and the personalities of the study staff. The company should also ensure that the investigator is not listed on the FDA's so-called "black list" due to a compliance problem in another study. This list of disqualified and restricted investigators can be reviewed on the FDA's website.

An evaluation visit is another early-stage activity that can produce in-depth information about the site. Nothing else can replace the value of a face-to-face meeting with the individuals with whom you might be collaborating. An evaluation visit aids in understanding how well a site may perform, and what a site may be able to contribute to the study. A clinical research associate usually makes this visit, which is documented through a report that is subsequently reviewed by a CRM to assure that the site is able to conduct the study. This information, along with the site's preliminary qualifications, should be distributed to the project leader or study director (or to the sponsor if a CRO is involved) with the site-related recommendation.

Keep in mind that this can be a lengthy process and that, in some cases, a good CRM's instinct about a site can be all that is needed. Remember that unanswered phone calls and/or the absence of return calls could mean that the site is either inattentive or overloaded with work, and that your study could suffer.

Regulatory Documents Once the study sites are chosen, important regulatory documents (see discussion below) must be collected and maintained by the site as well as in a central repository by the sponsor (e.g., the drug company) and/or the CRO. This task can be a lengthy process and, in some cases, it may be the site's study coordinator alone who is gathering these documents for the sponsor. Some sites have a regulatory department and are better able to collect and forward necessary regulatory documents.

It is imperative that a sponsor obtains all of the regulatory forms from each site before shipping the test article (also called the study drug, clinical test material, and FDA-used term "test article) to the sites. The following documents must be collected from the sites:

- Form FDA 1572-Statement of the Investigator. Signed by the principal investigator (PI), this form states they the investigator will conduct the clinical study according to the clinical protocol. Please note that this document may be revised throughout the study as new personnel are added or removed from the study. Historically, maintaining this form is troublesome and prone to mistakes. Omitting a sub-investigator or a central clinical laboratory are common errors. Others include listing only one center when an investigator practices at two different centers and will be screening patients from both centers. Others include the failure to list multiple IRB committees—such as an ethics committee or a human rights committee—when they are both used at a single institution. If the study calls for an ECG and for a cardiologist to interpret the results, the cardiologist should also be named on this form.
- The investigator must submit the protocol to the IRB and, if applicable, to other relevant reviewing bodies (i.e., ethics committee or human rights committee), if any, to obtain approval to initi-

ate the study at that medical institution or center. An IRB letter stating that the site may begin participating is usually sent to the investigator. That letter documents the approval date, renewal timelines and the approval of the informed consent document, and will also remind the investigator that all adverse events must be reported in a timely manner. Many times, the IRB will request periodic status reports.

- To ensure patient safety, an approved (stamped by the IRB) informed consent document that specifies the patient's rights, study procedures, compensation and contact personnel (if questions arise) is also necessary. Under the Health Insurance Portability and Accountability Act (HIPAA), if a patient's protected health information (PHI), which is individually identifiable health information, is to be used or disclosed for research purposes, the subject must now grant his/her written permission through a formal authorization of this use or disclosure. When both an informed consent form and HIPAA authorization are required in a study, the two forms may be combined into a single form or presented for the subject's signature separately. This authorization procedure and document is designed to give patients more control over the use and release of their health records. Obviously, in any study, certain medical history must be collected and, during the study, medical records must be reviewed by monitors to validate data. The authorization process allows the patient to permit study personnel to access his/her study-related records.

- A list of the IRB members and/or the members' backgrounds is also collected. Alternatively, an IRB letter establishing that the board complies with 21 CFR 50 and 56 can serve as a substitute. Also remember that, if the investigator is a member of the IRB, the sponsor must obtain a letter stating that he/she abstained from voting on the protocol.

- Information on the investigator is also needed to complete the Form FDA 1572. This information is usually captured in the curriculum vitae (CV) for all principal and sub-investigators. A CV ensures that the investigator maintains an affiliation with the investigational site, confirms the investigator's medical specialty, and documents the investigator's research experience. It is fairly common for sponsors to receive outdated CVs that list a previous hospital or clinic's name rather than the current and relevant institution. CVs should be updated regularly.

- Financial Disclosures. The investigator's financial interests (e.g., a proprietary interest in the product being investigator or the sponsoring company) are considered when the FDA evaluates the clinical data collected by the investigator. According to 21 CFR 54, all participating investigators must document financial interests relevant to the study, including any proprietary interest in the product or equity interest in the sponsor. If such a financial interest exists, the sponsor must disclose that information to the FDA. The FDA has the right to evaluate the disclosed information to determine the possible impact of that financial interest on the reliability of the study.

- Laboratory certifications must be kept current at each study site. Two certifications are collected and maintained in the regulatory files: a CLIA (Clinical Laboratory Improvement Amendments) Certificate and the College of American Pathologists (CAP) Accreditation are necessary when the site's laboratory will be analyzing any samples that are collected for the study. This is also true in cases in which a specialty laboratory performs magnetic resonance imaging (MRI) scans or electrocardiograms (ECG's) for the study. If a central laboratory is used for all of the sites, the central lab's certifications must be sent to all participating sites for the sites' files. Normal ranges are also collected to ensure that the lower and upper limits of a particular value as well as the units of measure are noted. These ranges assist in building the study database, in ensuring that the values obtained are within the expected ranges, and in ensuring safety parameters (i.e., when there are critical high and low values that may have to be recorded as adverse events).

If, after reviewing these documents, the CRM finds that they are in order, he/she usually will ask the project team's regulatory affairs representative to review the documents and approve the release of the test article to the clinical site. With this approval, a site initiation visit may be scheduled.

Investigator Meetings It is usually within the pre-study timeframe that the sponsor schedules an investigator meeting, during which all of the key personnel who will be participating in the study will be in the same room. The investigator meeting is a means for getting the key personnel involved with the study (generally the principal investigator and the study coordinator from each site) all on the same page simultaneously. Generally, the protocol is presented in complete detail, with particular attention to procedures and safety. Following that, one effective approach involves dividing the large group into smaller discussion groups (e.g., a break-out meeting for investigators to discuss investigator obligations, a separate study coordinator meeting to discuss study procedures and case report form completion). This enables each group to concentrate on its assigned responsibilities, and allows discussions between personnel at the different sites (e.g., to share ideas or thoughts on enrolling patients). The connection made at the investigator meetings is the key to opening up communication.

Case Report Forms Ideally, case report form (CRF) design (either paper or electronic) will take place while the protocol is being developed, and will be finalized when the protocol is finalized. The CRFs should be a procedural mirror of the clinical protocol. Data on all of the evaluations, procedures and assessments should be captured on these forms. CRF development is vital to the study in that the CRF must capture all of the protocol-identified data. It is important that the CRM assist in the CFR design to ensure that the CRF will accommodate all of the data that must be captured. A general rule of thumb: If you are not planning to analyze it, do not capture it in the CFR. If you believe a specific data point must be captured, plan to do something with it.

Study Procedures Manual The study procedures manual (SPM) is a companion document to the protocol. The SPM offers more detailed guidance to the study personnel by providing additional information and clarification about the procedures and assessments that are to be conducted in the clinical study. It provides clinical and administrative details regarding how the study should be conducted to ensure compliance with the protocol and GCP principles. The SPM should clearly define how screening procedures should be documented, how source documents or worksheets should be completed, what randomization procedures should be followed, how adverse events (AEs) and serious adverse events (SAEs) should be reported, and how CRFs should be completed. It is recommended that the SPM also detail the following: study roles and responsibilities (who does what), along with study contact information (whom to contact, and for what reasons); regulatory procedures (record keeping, record retention, etc.); an explanation of monitoring responsibilities (what the monitor will do before, during and after the study at various visits); a time and events chart (identical to the one in the protocol); informed consent procedures (obtain consent prior to any invasive tests, etc.); test article information (labeling, storage information, preparation, etc.); prohibited medications, if applicable; procedures for collecting laboratory samples; study-specific procedures (x-rays, ECG's, MRI's, etc.); adverse event, and serious adverse event reporting procedures; instructions for completing CRFs; and samples of any study-specific forms that a site is required to complete (screening logs, patient identification logs, time and events checklist, etc.).

Pharmacy Binder Another document that can complement the protocol is a pharmacy binder. As the name implies, this document is intended for the pharmacist and pharmacy staff at the investigational site, and should contain information such as drug accountability records, drug dispensing records, drug re-order and return information, test article preparation worksheets, and any contact information specific for pharmacist.

Monitoring Plan The sponsor's monitoring plan is an internal document that is meant for distribution primarily among the monitoring staff. When the clinical study is initiated and finally underway, the CRAs will be busy conducting monitoring visits at the sites. The CRAs will monitor the sites to assess their performance and compliance with the regulations and to audit case report forms. A monitoring plan is a document that coordinates and assists the monitors while they are working in the field (at the investigator sites). The monitoring plan should contain guidance and information that the CRA should familiarize him/herself with before the monitoring process begins. The document should provide applicable standard operating procedures as well as study-specific instructions. The monitoring plan should explain how each type of monitoring visit should be carried out, and also provide guidance to the CRA on how issues that will arise in the field should be handled. The plan should describe procedures for the protection and safety of human subjects and that will ensure that the study data are accurate, complete and verifiable. Sample contents include the following: monitor overview (number of sites, patients, general introduction to the study); site assignments with monitor information (who goes where, contact information); breakdown of monitoring visits (monitoring report timing and requirements, etc.); tools available to the monitor (project team teleconferences, face-to-face project team meetings, edit logs for use at the sites, etc.); and quality control checks.

Discrepancies and Queries Once CRFs are available for data entry (if paper CRFs are used) or once the electronic data arrive from the sites, a data review of some type must be performed. Every CRM should become familiar with the data that arrive from the sites, beginning with the very first transmissions. Many problems can be spotted and avoided at this point.

The initial data review involves a quick check for accurate monitoring and to validate that the data make sense. Electronic edit checks will eventually be performed and data discrepancies will be issued if needed. Some of the issues that electronic edit checks can address include, but are not limited to: ensuring that start dates come before end dates; ensuring that medical history and concomitant medications match up; ensuring that adverse events and serious adverse events are properly documented; ensuring that laboratory values are within normal ranges; ensuring that missing and null data points are identified; and ensuring that correct patient identifiers are provided.

If a data query or discrepancy must be issued, the query or discrepancy should be written clearly to explain the uncertainty with the data. The query or discrepancy is then sent to the respective CRA or directly to the site, depending on internal standard operating procedures (SOPs). The CRA and/or the site will then resolve the query by providing the correct data or an explanation of why the data are correct. The resolved data (on an edited CRF or other form) are sent back to data management for revision in the database, if necessary.

A low number of data queries is, in part, a function of effective monitoring. Working closely with the CRAs in the field is one of the most important functions that a CRM can do in promoting the efficient conduct of a study.

CHAPTER 22

Clinical Monitoring

By Natalia Owen, M.S., CCRA

Clinical research associates (CRA), also referred to as study monitors, play a key role in the conduct of a clinical trial by overseeing its progress at the various study site(s). Generally possessing a health care or science background (e.g., nurse, technologist or pharmacist), a CRA is not expected to be qualified to diagnose or treat the disease/condition for which the investigational product is being studied, but will be expected to have a level of familiarity with the commonly used concepts, practices and procedures within a particular field.

The CRA should be an active member of the project team, and usually is assigned to a clinical research manager, who will oversee any number of CRAs. The CRA and clinical research manager (or clinical trial manager) should work closely together to ensure that all site visits are conducted in an efficient and productive manner, and that all of the CRA's findings are appropriately communicated to the rest of the project team (e.g., project lead, data management). Because the clinical research manager may also have access to site-related information that will require the CRA's follow-up, an open line of communication between these two individuals is imperative.

So what exactly does a CRA do? The goals of clinical monitoring are to protect the rights and well-being of human subjects, to ensure that the trial data are complete, accurate, and can be verified with source documents, and to ensure that the trial is conducted, recorded, and reported in accordance with the protocol, standard operating procedures (SOPs), and good clinical practice standards and applicable regulatory requirements. The CRA accomplishes these goals by serving as the principal line of communication between the sponsor and the site, conducting visits to the investigators' sites, and reporting the findings from such visits to the sponsor/CRO.

The sections below highlight and discuss the various types of site visits that comprise the CRA's work before, during, and after a clinical study.

Site Selection Visits: Background Information for Site Selection Visits Given the large number of clinics, hospitals, and academic institutions available throughout the United States, a sponsor/CRO must determine which sites will participate in their clinical trial. This decision is a critical factor in determining a clinical trial's success, since the selected sites will enroll eligible patients to keep the sponsor's timelines moving forward and data to support the safety and efficacy of the investigational product. It is also the sponsor's obligation to select qualified investigators who possess adequate expertise and resources to conduct the trial. Depending on the sponsor's SOPs, a CRA may or may not assist with identifying sites to participate in a clinical trial.

Today, there are more resources to identify potential sites than ever—Internet-based searches, computerized searches, previous business relationships, physicians listings, telephone listings, professional networks, medical societies, investigator-selection services, medical journals and/or abstracts, and directories. A company should use caution if it decides to pursue a site based on a previous business relationship. If a site is referred from a sales person within the company, for example, is there a strong correlation between the physician being an adequate investigator and an adequate business person? There is not in many cases.

Once a list has been compiled, identified physicians should be screened to ensure that they are not on the FDA's disqualified or restricted lists. The FDA's Office of Regulatory Affairs publishes, on the agency's website, lists of those physicians who have been cited for severe non-compliance and, because of this, have been disqualified or restricted (e.g., limited to certain types of studies or under certain supervision) from participating in FDA-regulated clinical trials.

After determining an investigator's eligibility, the sponsor should make an initial contact to determine if there is an interest on the investigator's part to participate in the clinical trial. It may be useful to provide the potential investigator with a corporate fact sheet in addition to a description of the proposed trial's overall approach. Information provided to the site should be general (e.g., type of patients being recruited or total number of sites), and discussions with the site and investigator should be limited until a confidentiality disclosure agreement (CDA) has been signed. Once the site's interest has been established, a CDA has been forwarded, signed, and received, and general study-related materials have been forwarded to the site, the sponsor should ensure that the CRO conducts a sufficient, preliminary site screening.

Some companies will provide the investigator with a questionnaire that asks both general and study-specific questions regarding the investigator's ability to conduct a clinical trial at his/her site (e.g., determining if the investigator has a study coordinator or if the investigator has access to the study population). Having the investigator provide a curriculum vita is an excellent way for the sponsor to determine his/her level of experience. Once the appropriate factors have been assessed and the sponsor/CRO feels that the investigator could contribute to the trial, the CRA will then be responsible for contacting the site to schedule a site selection visit (SSV).

Site Selection Visit: Preparation Consistent with the sponsor's SOPs, the CRA should confirm the date and time of the visit, and should provide the site with verbal or written notification of this visit. Ideally, the CRA should provide the investigator with an agenda that details the topics to be covered, the estimated time to be spent on each topic area, required resources (e.g., meeting room), and which site personnel should attend (see exhibit below).

Site Selection Visit Notification Letter

<Date Letter Sent to Site (MM/DD/YYYY)>

<Principal Investigator's or Primary Contact's Full Name>
<Address 1>
<Address 2>
<City, State Zip>

Re: <Study Name>

Dr. <Last Name> or Ms./Mr. <Primary Contact's Last Name>:

This correspondence serves as confirmation that a Site Selection Visit (SSV) will be conducted on <Date of Visit> at <Time of Visit (a.m./p.m.)>. This visit will be conducted at <Location for SSV>, and should last for approximately <Number of Hours to Conduct SSV> hours. During the conduct of the SSV, please note the following topics to be covered and which study staff personnel will need to be present:

Subject	Approximate Time Required	Attendee(s) Required (e.g., Principal Investigator or Study Coordinator)
Investigational Product Overview		
Investigator's Brochure and Protocol		
Subject Population		
Site Staffing Requirements, Time, Training and Experience		
Adequacy of Facilities		
Monitoring Requirements & Activities		
Institutional Review Board (IRB) Requirements		
Financial Aspects and General Responsibilities of Potential Investigators		

Should you have any questions or concerns regarding the conduct of the SSV, please do not hesitate to contact me at <Enter Your Phone Number>. We look forward to the potential of working with you on this important research study.

Regards,
<Full Name>
<Sponsor/CRO Name>
<Job Title>
<Phone Number>
<Email Address>

Cc: Study Files

To prepare for the visit, the CRA should become extremely familiar with the protocol to be in a position to answer questions during the SSV. During the visit, a CRA will be introduced to a fair number of site personnel (e.g., pharmacist(s), nursing staff, and physicians). Generally, it will be the CRA's responsibility to provide a study overview to these individuals (the CRA may be accompanied by another project team member, such as the project leader), which will be impossible if he/she is not aware of the drug's dose, route of administration, or the duration of post-treatment follow-up. The CRA should be familiar with the investigator's brochure, which is a compilation of the clinical and non-clinical data on the investigational product(s) and which will facilitate an understanding of why and how the study is being conducted. The CRA should also review the applicable regulatory requirements and the sponsor's template for the SSV report that must be completed after the site visit. Some CRAs will bring a blank copy of the report to complete as the visit progresses and will use these notes to facilitate the development of the report at a later date.

Site Selection Visite: Conduct During the SSV, the CRA's goal is to provide and obtain enough information to allow the sponsor to determine the site's level of interest and ability to participate in the clinical trial. The areas that should be addressed during the visit include: the investigator's qualifications and experience; the protocol (e.g., What are the eligibility criteria? How long are patients followed after their enrollment?); a summary of the investigator's brochure (e.g., What are some of the known risks?); the subject population (e.g., Does the site have adequate access to the subject population for the trial?); site staffing requirements, time, training and experience (e.g., How many other clinical trials are being conducted at the site, and will this impact enrollment activities for the trial?); the adequacy of facilities (e.g., Is there a freezer to store laboratory samples?); monitoring requirements and activities (e.g., Where do routine monitoring visits take place at the site?); IRB requirements (e.g., Has the IRB ever been audited by a regulatory authority?); financial aspects of the clinical trial (e.g., Will the investigator provide a budget or will the sponsor need to provide a template for their completion?); and general responsibilities of potential investigator (e.g., Who will be obtaining informed consent?)

One item, in particular, that the CRA should not discuss with the site at this time is compensation—specifically, per-patient reimbursement. Due to certain factors, such as demographics (urban versus suburban facilities), academic versus non-academic institutions, and a site's reputation, there is some variation in the amount that sites are compensated. If the investigator or study coordinator is interested in knowing more about this, it is best for the CRA to defer these issues to a clinical research manager or a similar sponsor representative.

At the conclusion of the visit, the CRA should discuss with the investigator the sponsor's timeline for providing a decision regarding the site's participation in the clinical trial, and be sure that all questions pertaining to the study and the site's qualifications have been answered. In the follow-up letter to the site, the CRA should provide responses to questions that could not be answered at the conclusion of the visit.

Site Selection Visit: Follow-up After the visit, the CRA is responsible for documenting his or her relevant findings in a SSV report. A monitoring report should include the date the visit was conducted, the name of the CRA who conducted the visit, the site that was visited, the name of the investigator and any other individuals who were contacted, a summary of the information reviewed, any significant findings or facts, and any recommended actions taken or to be taken. This report should be reviewed and finalized with a sponsor representative within the timeline specified in the sponsor's SOPs.

This report will assist the sponsor in determining whether a site/investigator can/should be selected to participate in the clinical trial. In addition, the CRA should prepare for the site a SSV follow-up letter that details the information that was covered and that clarifies any unanswered questions that may have arisen during the visit (e.g., protocol-specific questions). The sponsor will not necessarily notify the site whether it has been selected for the trial at the time of the follow-up letter, in which case the follow-up letter should be sent to the site in accordance with the timelines specified in the sponsor's SOPs.

Once a site has been selected and so notified, the sponsor and investigator will begin to collect and submit the applicable documentation. A site cannot be initiated or receive investigational product until it has received IRB approval for the study protocol, the informed consent form, and any other documents as specified by the site's IRB. In addition, the site must also provide certain documentation to the sponsor, some of which is required by FDA regulations and some of which may be required by the sponsor's SOPs. These documents include: the Form FDA 1572-Statement of Investigator; Form FDA 3454-Certification: Financial Interest and Arrangements of Clinical Investigators; Form FDA 3455-Disclosure: Financial Interest and Arrangements of Clinical Investigators; a letter of indemnification; a signed protocol and amendments; Curriculum vitae and/or other relevant documents evidencing qualifications for the principal investigator, subinvestigator(s), and study coordinator(s); compensation agreement and/or budget agreement; IRB membership roster or assurance number; IRB approval of other documents, as specified by the site's IRB (e.g., case report forms or subject recruitment materials); certification or accreditation of the medical, laboratory or technical facility to be used by the site; and normal value(s)/range(s) for medical, laboratory or technical procedures included in the protocol

The unavailability of some of these items may not preclude the site from being initiated (e.g., the site faxes the IRB approval for the protocol and informed consent form, but the original has not yet been received by the sponsor), in which case it becomes the CRA's responsibility to ensure that the applicable, original documents are collected and provided to the sponsor during the next site visit.

After participating sites have been selected, the sponsor must assign a CRA for each selected site. Ideally, the CRA will be assigned to sites that are within a reasonable distance from the CRA's location, since many CRAs function in a regional capacity today.

The Site Initiation Visit: Background Information for Site Initiation Visit After the sponsor receives the required documents detailed above and IRB approval of the applicable documents, but before activating a site for enrollment, the sponsor will begin appropriate training at the selected sites. In some cases, when the planned trial involves a large number or sites, the sponsor may elect to conduct an "investigators meeting," to which it will invite appropriate staff and investigators from many or all sites, rather than individual site initiation visits (depending on the number and locations of sites, it may be necessary to conduct a few investigators meetings). Generally, an investigator's meeting covers the same material as a SIV, but will save the sponsor time and money and permit the sponsor to activate a large number of sites for patient enrollment in a shorter timeframe. When an investigators meeting is conducted, the sponsor may decide that only the lead CRA for the project will attend this meeting.

When an SIV is to be conducted, it is critical that the CRAs be aware of all the information that must be conveyed to the sites (e.g., medical monitor's contact information, preparation and administration of the investigational product, timeline for first routine monitoring visit). The intent of the SIV is to provide sufficient training so that the site is able to successfully implement the applicable aspects of the protocol. Given this goal, the sponsor may elect to have a training session for the CRAs to promote the consistent dissemination of information to the sites.

Site Initiation Visit: Preparation Once the sites have been selected and assigned, the CRA should introduce him/herself to the site, specifically to the study coordinator. Establishing a good rapport with the study coordinator is essential, since the coordinator will be the primary site contact person with whom the CRA will be visiting during the all-important routine monitoring visits. During this initial interaction, the CRA should attempt to confirm a date and time to conduct the SIV. The SIV itself should be conducted according to the sponsor's SOPs and applicable regulatory requirements.

Once the SIV's date and time have been confirmed, the CRA should provide the site with verbal or written notification of the visit in accordance with the sponsor's SOPs. Again, to assist with coordination efforts, the CRA should provide an agenda that specifies the topics to be covered, the estimated time to be spent on each item, necessary resources (e.g., projection screen for the protocol presentation), and an indication of which study staff should attend. Generally, the CRA should attempt to conduct a review of the protocol with the principal investigator, subinvestigators, and other relevant study staff during the lunch hour, since this is when schedules tend to be the most open.

Preparation is critical to the SIV's success. The CRA should thoroughly review applicable sections of the investigator's brochure (e.g., safety profile, metabolism and excretion of the investigational product, etc.), the protocol, the case report forms, the study procedures manual (an optional aide that the sponsor creates for the site and that provides source document worksheets, forms, and detailed explanations of procedures, such as randomization, the investigational product's preparation, and documentation of serious adverse events), the template for the SIV report, applicable regulatory requirements and guidelines (e.g., 21CFR 312 Subpart D, 21CFR 50, 21CFR 56, ICH GCP), and any other sponsor-recommended materials (e.g., a sponsor-established website that outlines the procedures for completing and submitting electronic case report forms).

During an ongoing clinical study, one of the CRA's principal tasks will be the verification of source documents against the case report forms. The ICH's GCP guideline (E6) defines source documents as original documents, data and records (e.g., hospital records, office charts, laboratory reports, memoranda, subject's diaries, recorded data from automated instruments, photographic negatives, x-rays, records maintained in the pharmacy, laboratory or medico-technical departments involved with the study). A sponsor will often provide source document worksheets for a site, thereby giving the site a central location for recording their study-related findings (e.g., baseline temperature and blood pressures). If a sponsor does not provide these worksheets, the CRA might want to determine if creating such a document would be useful to the study coordinator. The CRA should be sure to coordinate this intent with the project team, as a similar form could have already been created by another CRA for use by the site. Providing such documents to record a large amount of data will assist the coordinator with transcribing data to the case report forms, and will expedite the CRA's comparison of source documents to the case report forms during the routine monitoring visits. If there are detailed explanations or procedures, such as the preparation of laboratory samples or the investigational product, the CRA should determine if a visual aide would facilitate educating the relevant study staff.

Site Initiation Visit: Conduct In conducting the SIV, the CRA should feel confident, upon his/her departure from the site and the resolution of any outstanding issues, that the site could be activated for enrollment and would be able to implement the protocol without difficulty. Depending on the study's complexity, an SIV can last between four and six hours, particularly if all of the following materials and procedures are reviewed with the applicable study staff:

- relevant highlights from the investigator's brochure
- the study protocol (e.g., time and events schedule, inclusion/exclusion criteria, randomization procedures, decoding procedures for blinded trials, core laboratory or radiology procedures, sample labeling of the investigational product)
- storage, handling, preparation and administration of investigational product
- investigational product and ancillary supplies storage, shipment and return, accountability, and record-keeping requirements
- case report form (CRF) completion
- data clarification request (DCR) procedures
- source documentation requirements
- study procedures manual or the review of any worksheets and forms that the site must complete and/or submit to the sponsor (e.g., study staff signature log (see exhibit below) to document the signatures and initials of the study personnel who will be authorized to make entries and/or corrections to the CRFs)
- documenting and reporting adverse events and serious adverse events
- the process for obtaining and documenting informed consent and the authorization for the use and disclosure of protected health information prior to the subject's participation in the trial (as specified in 21 CFR 50, 21 CFR 56, 45 CFR 160, and 45 CFR 164
- the investigator's regulatory obligations, as specified in 21 CFR 312 Subpart D and other applicable regulatory requirements. While the investigator can authorize qualified study staff to execute some study-related tasks, these delegated tasks must be documented. The sponsor may provide ask

Study Staff Signature Log

Please complete an entry (printed name, signature and position held) for each study site staff member who is participating in this study.

Printed Name	Signature	Position (PI, SC, SI)

the investigator to complete a sponsor-provided Study Staff Responsibilities Form (see exhibit below) or similar document that specifies all of the investigator's obligations and allows the investigator to identify the various roles of the site's study team members (e.g., the pharmacist is responsible for dispensing the investigational product). Despite the existence of such a document, the investigator will still be held accountable in cases of protocol noncompliance or the violation of applicable regulatory requirements.

- IRB review and approval procedures (as specified in 21 CFR 56)
- monitoring visit requirements (e.g., procedures, documentation, roles, frequency)
- unresolved items from the SSV

Study Staff Responsibilities Form

Complete and verify this form during the Site Initiation Visit, using the following abbreviations: Principal Investigator = PI Other = Specify Subinvestigator = SI Not applicable = N/A Study Coordinator = SC	Study Name: Enter Name of Protocol> Primary Investigator: Enter Full Name> Enter Site Number:

Delegated/Shared Responsibility	Responsible Participant(s)
Submit the protocol, Informed Consent and Patient Authorization Form, and other documents that are required by the Institutional Review Board (IRB) for approval.	
Inform the IRB of protocol amendments, as applicable.	
Provide guidance and training to the Subinvestigators and other study site personnel on proper conduct of the study.	
Prepare, administer, and maintain accountability of investigational product and ancillary supplies, as stated in the protocol.	
Obtain signed consent from each study subject.	
Complete and fax Screening Log to Sponsor, as applicable.	
Conduct and document assessments for each subject's screening and enrollment.	
Collect, prepare, and ship biological samples, as stated in the protocol.	
Conduct and document assessments for subjects post-enrollment through study completion.	
Collect and document adverse events.	
Report serious adverse events to Sponsor and IRB, as applicable.	
Complete subjects' Case Report Forms (CRFs).	
Review and sign off on CRFs (only PI and/or SI).	
CoCoordinate site visits and related activities with the Clinical Research Associate.	
Review and resolve Data Clarification Requests (DCRs).	
Return to the sponsor or dispose of investigational product and ancillary supplies, as stated in the protocol.	
Submit Final Study Report to Sponsor and IRB, as applicable.	

I have reviewed this document, and agree to the designated party(ies) assigned to each responsibility. I understand that this document does not remove my responsibilities as Investigator, as defined in the Investigator Agreement and applicable regulatory requirements.

_____ _____
Principal Investigator's Printed Name Principal Investigator's Signature and Date

The CRA should be sure to review the organization of the site's regulatory files with the study coordinator and other relevant study staff. The regulatory study files generally are maintained in a sponsor-provided binder and within a delineated format for filing applicable correspondence and documents. The CRA should emphasize that maintaining the site's regulatory files will demonstrate compliance with GCP and the applicable regulatory requirements, and will assist in the trial's successful management by the investigator, sponsor, and CRA. It is also worth noting that these regulatory files might be audited by the sponsor's independent auditor and/or the regulatory authorities to ensure the validity and integrity of the data collected in the study.

At the SIV's conclusion, the CRA should sign a Monitoring Log (provided to the site by the sponsor) to document that the visit was conducted, retrieve a photocopy for the sponsor, and review any outstanding investigator or study staff issues. This is particularly critical if any of these issues would prevent the site from being activated to enrollment (e.g., the pharmacy does not have a required, dedicated fax line to receive randomization information for a blinded trial). With the investigator and study staff, the CRA should review the timeline for the next monitoring visit, and should review the timelines for submitting any forms to the sponsor (e.g., weekly submission of a Screening Log). Before leaving the site, the CRA should ensure that the investigator and study coordinator have the CRA's contact information in case study-related questions or concerns arise.

Site Initiation Visit: Follow-up As he/she is for the SIV, the CRA is responsible for documenting his or her relevant findings in an SIV report. The monitoring report should include the date of the visit, the name of the CRA who conducted the visit, the site that was visited, the name of the investigator and any other individuals that were contacted, a summary of the information reviewed, any significant findings or facts, and any recommended actions taken or to be taken. This report should be reviewed and finalized with a sponsor representative within a timeline specified in the sponsor's SOPs. It is worth noting that the ICH GCP guideline recommends that a photocopy of this report also be provided to the site as documentation of the procedures that were reviewed with the investigator and study staff personnel.

The CRA should prepare an SIV follow-up letter that details the information that was covered, clarifies any unanswered questions, and addresses any issues that require follow-up by either the study site (e.g., purchasing a freezer to store laboratory samples) or the sponsor/CRO (e.g., providing the site with laminated copies of inclusion/exclusion criteria for the physicians to carry with them for screening purposes). The timeline for the next monitoring visit should be provided in the follow-up letter as well (see exhibit below). Finally, it may be beneficial for the CRA to remind the site of any documents that must be submitted to the sponsor on a regular basis (e.g., weekly submission of a Screening Log).

Site Initiation Visit Follow-up Letter

<Date Letter Sent to Site (MM/DD/YYYY)>

<Principal Investigator's or Primary Contact's Full Name>
<Address 1>
<Address 2>
<City, State Zip>

Re: <Study Name>

Dr. <Last Name> or Ms./Mr. <Primary Contact's Last Name>:

A Site Initiation Visit (SIV) was conducted by <Name(s) and Role(s) of Employee(s) Who Conducted SIV> on <Date(s) of Visit> at <Location for SIV>. During the conduct of the SIV, the following topics were covered:
- Protocol and applicable sections of the Investigator's Brochure
- Preparation and administration of investigational product
- Investigational product and ancillary supplies storage, shipment, accountability, and record-keeping requirements
- Collection, preparation, and shipment of biological samples
- Case Report Form (CRF) completion
- Data Clarification Request (DCR) procedure
- Source documentation requirements
- Documenting and reporting of Adverse Events (AE) and Serious Adverse Events (SAEs)
- Obtaining informed consent and documentation requirements, as specified in 21CFR 50
- The applicable regulatory requirements and sponsor requirements, as specified in 21 CFR 312 Subpart D
- IRB review and approval procedures, as specified in 21 CFR 56
- Site Binder organization and maintenance
- Monitoring visit requirements (procedure, documentation, roles, and frequency)
- Unresolved items from the Site Selection Visit[bullet ends]

Use the following text if questions were raised that required follow-up (otherwise delete):
The following information provides answers to those questions that were raised during the SIV:
- <Enter Question>
  <Provide Answer>
- <Enter Question>
  <Provide Answer>

Use the following text, if the site is being activated for enrollment for the study (otherwise delete):
Based on the successful conduct of the visit, we are pleased to inform you that, effective <Enter Date of Activation>, your site has been authorized to begin screening activities for enrollment in the aforementioned study.

–continued–

Although the issues will not prevent your site from being activated to enrollment, please note the following items that will require follow-up: **(delete this section if there are no follow-up issues for the Sponsor/CRO or the site)**

- <Enter Item>
- <Enter Item>
- <Enter Item>
- <Enter Item>

Once a subject has been enrolled, the clinical research associate (CRA) assigned to your site, <Enter Name of CRA>, will contact you to determine a monitoring visit date. Please note that the first Periodic Site Visit for your site is scheduled to take place after enrollment of the first <Enter Number of Subject(s)> subjects at your facility.

Should you have any questions or concerns regarding the conduct of the SIV or any other study-related questions, please do not hesitate to contact me at <Enter Your Phone Number> or <Enter Clinical Research Manager's Name>, Clinical Research Manager, at <Enter CRM's Phone Number>.

We look forward to working with you on this important study.

Use the following closing and signature format:

Regards,

Full Name
Company
Title
Phone Number
Email Address

Cc: Sponsor/CRO's Study Files, <Enter Additional Study Staff Personnel to Copy (otherwise delete)>

Periodic Site Visits: Background Information for Periodic Site Visits Once a site has been initiated, the sponsor must "patiently" wait for the site to enroll subjects. Unfortunately, this can be a frustrating period for the sponsor, since there are timelines and budgets to maintain and since the sites' success in enrolling subjects is a key to meeting development timelines. It is helpful to the project team if the CRA maintains regular correspondence with the site, through which it can inquire about screening and enrollment activities and provide updates to the project team. It is also important that the project team acknowledges the CRA as the point of contact with the site, as this will prevent unnecessary communication from other project team members and will keep the site from being inundated with multiple contacts regarding the same study. If a CRA is traveling excessively, the team should assign an individual to ensure that updates from the site are obtained in a reasonable timeframe.

When enrollment activities begin at a site, the CRA will conduct a periodic site visit (PSV), or routine monitoring visit, consistent with the protocol, the sponsor's SOPs, GCP, and applicable regulatory requirements. Regardless of the monitoring visit timelines that are specified in an individual protocol, the CRA must visit the site frequently enough to assess the following: the continued acceptability of the facilities for the purposes of the study; the site's adherence to the protocol; the investigator/site's compliance with the applicable regulatory requirements; that any protocol changes have been reported to the sponsor and have been approved by the IRB; that accurate, complete, and current records are being maintained; and that accurate, complete, and timely reports are being submitted to the sponsor and IRB.

The PSV is the most frequent type of visit that a CRA conducts at a site and is the visit through which data are verified and retrieved for delivery to the sponsor. Through technological advances that are permitting data to be captured and transmitted electronically, however, it is becoming possible to obtain data from study sites without a formal site visit (see chapter on electronic data capture).

Periodic Site Visit: Preparation When a CRA is responsible for multiple sites (or even multiple projects with multiple sites), it is important that the CRA track enrollment activities at each site in an effort to prioritize the periodic site visits (PSVs) that should occur first. The CRA should consider the CRF submission requirements for the study (i.e., either partial or entire CRFs are being submitted to the sponsor), since this will also determine the priority for conducting a PSV at a particular site. Proper planning by the CRA will save the sponsor both time and money. If a CRA visits a site two days prior to a subject's completion date, for example, the CRA will have to conduct another PSV to retrieve the subject's data. With proper planning, however, the CRA could have altered his/her original plans to visit the site after the patient was off study, thereby eliminating the need for the subsequent visit. For this and many other reasons, organization and communication within the project team is important for ensuring efficient clinical trial conduct.

Since good, productive trial sites are often recruited to participate in a number of other studies, the CRA should coordinate the PSV date(s) with the study coordinator well in advance. Because some sites limit the number of days that a CRA can conduct the visit, the CRA must consider such factors in determining the goals that can be met by the end of a visit.

Consistent with the sponsor's SOPs, the CRA should, after confirming the visit date(s) and objectives with the site and project team (in particular, the clinical research manager), provide the site with verbal or written notification of the visit. A visit notification should be provided to the site in a timely manner, to permit the site to adequately prepare for the upcoming visit. The CRA might want to specify the goals for the visit (e.g., resolve all outstanding data queries, retrieve case report forms for Subject XX) as well as the site staff who should be available to the CRA and the amount of time required for the meeting(s) (e.g., principal investigator for 20 minutes, pharmacist for 10 minutes). Generally, it is useful for the CRA to identify in the letter the subjects' medical records that must be available for review during the visit. Depending on the site and the nature of the study (e.g., inpatient study), the site may have to request and obtain the charts from a centralized medical records department, a process that could take several days.

To prepare for the PSV, the CRA should review the protocol, applicable sections of the investigator's brochure (e.g., expected adverse events), case report forms, the Study Procedures Manual, previous trip reports that were completed for the site (the reports should provide an overview of the site's conduct during the study, and should identify any outstanding issues that must be addressed during the next visit), the template for the PSV report, the sponsor's SOPs, applicable regulatory requirements and guidelines (e.g., 21 CFR 312 Subpart D, 21 CFR 50, 21 CFR 56, and ICH GCP), and any other relevant materials identified by the sponsor.

Since the CRA will be handling a large number of documents for submission to the sponsor, he/she should plan for the PSV as if they were locked in a room with limited access to resources and supplies. While this is not an exhaustive list, the CRA should consider bringing some or all of the following items: writing tablet or notebook, blue or black pens; highlighter(s); paper clips and/or binder clips; small stapler; calculator and/or conversion tools; adhesive flags and/or notepads to identify issues or data discrepancies; case report form (CRF) Edit Logs (or a similar document that will be used to document those discrepancies that were noted during the review of the source documents and case report forms); extra pages or photocopies of any frequently used form(s) that might be needed during the conduct of the site visit (e.g., a study-specific fax transmittal form); a pocket-sized medical dictionary and/or drug handbook (often times, the site will have these, but it is always better to be prepared); and a pocket-sized handbook of selected regulations and guidance documents for drug studies.

For those sites with outstanding issues, the CRA might want to consider creating a list to provide to the study coordinator at the beginning of the PSV (this list should be similar to the objectives that are specified in the notification letter to the site). This will enable the CRA to review the source documents and case report forms (or other necessary aspects of the visit) while the study coordinator is addressing the outstanding items.

Periodic Site Visit: Conduct The PSV's main objective is to determine if the site (investigator and study staff personnel) is conducting the study in accordance with the protocol, the sponsor's SOPs, GCP standards, and applicable regulatory requirements.

The sponsor must assure that the data to be submitted to the FDA in support of the investigational product are accurate and complete. The CRA accomplishes this by reviewing individual subject records and other supporting documents with the case report forms (or other reports prepared by the investigator for submission to the sponsor). Some sites will provide the CRA with so-called "shadow charts," which are photocopies of some or all of the subject's records. The CRA should be sure to verify this information with the subject's original records, since it is possible that some pages will be omitted and could substantiate documentation in the subject's CRF.

For the reasons mentioned above and in accordance with the protocol and the sponsor's specifications, the CRA should compare a representative number of subject records and other supporting documents to determine that: (1) informed consent and authorization for the use and disclosure of public health information have been obtained prior to the subject's participation in the study, and have been documented in accordance with regulatory requirements; (2) the investigator is enrolling only eligible subjects; (3) the information documented in the CRFs is complete, accurate, legible, and consistent with the source documents; (4) all data have been properly documented, and there are no missing items (e.g., such as the development of an intercurrent illness); (5) missed visits are noted in the source documents; and (6) ample documentation in the source documents has been provided for subjects who failed to complete the study (i.e., withdrawals, dropouts or deaths).

In comparing the source documents with the CRFs (and other relevant reports), the CRA should document any discrepancies on a CRF Edit Log (or similar document used to record noted discrepancies) and review the Edit Log(s) with the investigator (this is generally done toward the end of the PSV). The investigator or other authorized study staff personnel will be responsible for making changes, additions or corrections to the data. If the investigator authorizes another study staff member to make changes to the data (e.g., study coordinator), the documentation of this authorization should be made available for the CRA. Under no circumstances should the CRA make changes to a site's data. The person making the change should do so by drawing a single line through the incorrect data (i.e., the previously entered data should remain visible), writing the correct information, and then initialing and dating the change.

Once the data have been reviewed and all changes have been finalized, the investigator will provide his or her signature on the CRF as an acknowledgment that the data being submitted are accurate and complete. The CRA should ensure that the investigator did not sign and date the CRF prior to the date of the PSV, since any changes made subsequent to the date of the investigator's signature could be questioned during a sponsor or FDA audit. The CRA is then responsible for ensuring that the original CRFs are submitted to the sponsor in a timely manner, and that copies of the CRFs are retained at the site (if the CRFs are not personally delivered by the CRA, they can be forwarded using a courier service, since such a shipment can be tracked).

The monitoring of electronic records should be conducted in a similar manner, as explained above. When data are submitted to the sponsor/CRO through electronic means, an in-house CRA usually will be responsible for verifying that the data are accurate and complete. Those issues that cannot be resolved in-house can be addressed either through electronically issued data queries to the site or by the CRA during the next PSV.

In addition to ensuring the site's compliance with the protocol and applicable regulatory requirements and verifying the source documents with the CRFs (and other relevant reports), the CRA is also responsible for the following:

- Assessing the continued acceptability of the site and study staff and facility.
- Assessing drug accountability (this should not be done if the CRA is "blinded"). This includes reviewing receipt documents, assessing the use and disposition of the investigational product and ancillary supplies, ensuring that the investigational product was administered only to those subjects enrolled in the study, ensuring that the current investigational product and ancillary supplies are adequate, and verifying the storage conditions and security for the investigational product and ancillary supplies.
- Verifying the collection, preparation, storage and shipping procedures for any biological samples that were drawn for enrolled subjects.
- Determining if all adverse events and serious adverse events are appropriately documented and, if necessary, reported to the IRB (acknowledgment by the IRB depends on the site's IRB requirements).
- Ensuring that the necessary documentation has been submitted to the IRB for continuing approval of the protocol, the informed consent and authorization form, and any other study-related documents as required by the site's IRB.
- Reporting the site's subject recruitment rate.
- Ensuring resolution of outstanding data queries for subject data (the original, resolved queries should be retrieved for the sponsor/CRO, and photocopies should be left with the site).
- Determining whether the investigator and study staff are maintaining their regulatory files for the study.
- Reporting any deviations from the protocol, the sponsor's SOPs, GCP standards, or applicable regulatory requirements with the investigator. These deviations should be discussed, and appropriate actions for preventing their recurrence should be implemented.

Before leaving the site, the CRA should sign the Monitoring Log to document the visit, and should retrieve a photocopy for the sponsor. The CRA should also meet with the investigator to discuss the status of the study at the site. The results of the visit, any noted protocol violations, issues regarding enrollment (e.g., ineligible subject enrolled, slow enrollment rate), overall enrollment for the study, or other study-related concerns are all relevant areas that the CRA should address with the investigator. If there are any conference calls or meetings related to the study, the CRA should ensure that the investigator and study staff are appropriately notified of these events. During these calls or meetings, the sponsor generally will present study-wide (i.e., including all sites) updates and findings.

Periodic Site Visit: Follow-up As he/she is for the SIV and SSVs, the CRA is responsible for documenting the relevant findings in a PSV report consistent with the sponsor's SOPs. The report should include the date of the visit, the name of the CRA who conducted the visit, the site that was visited, the name of the investigator and any other individuals that were contacted, a summary of the information reviewed (including the numbers of the subjects whose CRFs were reviewed and/or retrieved for submission to the sponsor), any significant findings, facts, deviations, or deficiencies, and any recommended actions taken or to be taken. This report should be reviewed and finalized with a sponsor representative within a timeline specified in the sponsor's SOPs.

The CRA should also prepare a PSV follow-up letter that detail the information that was covered, any protocol violations and the actions taken or to be taken to prevent their recurrence, clarifications on any unanswered questions, and any issues that require follow-up by either the study site (e.g., resolving a drug accountability discrepancy) or the sponsor (e.g., providing the site with additional CRFs). The follow-up letter should also provide the timeline for the next monitoring visit as well.

An important consideration for the CRA is ensuring that PSV trip reports and follow-up letters are completed in a timely manner. While this obviously is applicable to all site visits and all timelines will be specified in the sponsor's SOPs, it is easy for the CRA to fall behind in completing these reports simply due to the number of PSVs that can take place during the conduct of the study (i.e., especially if the CRA is assigned to multiple high-enrolling sites and multiple projects). The CRA should remember that the PSV reports are the project team's primary means for determining a site's compliance with the protocol, sponsor's SOPs, GCP standards, and applicable regulatory requirements. If the CRA becomes overburdened by the demands of the study(ies), he/she should inform the clinical research manager or appropriate sponsor representative. Many times, there is another CRA on the same project with less-demanding responsibilities (i.e., assigned sites are not enrolling any subjects), and this CRA can assist with the site visits and trip reports, or even assume responsibility for some of the busier CRA's sites.

Termination Site Visits:Background Information for Termination Site Visits The study's enrollment has been successfully completed. All CRFs are in-house. At least in terms of the site's interaction with the sponsor, the study is in its final stages. While this is the ideal scenario (i.e., the successful completion of a trial), there actually are a number of scenarios in which the sponsor will seek to discontinue a study site's participation in a clinical trial. Other potential reasons why a sponsor would seek to discontinue, or "terminate," a site's participation include the following:

- Low enrollment rates: The site is actively screening patients, but those subjects are not meeting the subject eligibility requirements established in the protocol.
- Lack of interest by a participating site: If a sponsor sets a limit to the number of participating sites in a trial, it can gain access to another site that may be more interested and qualified by terminating an existing site that shows little interest in the study (i.e., no contributions to subject enrollment).
- Severe non-compliance with the protocol, the sponsor SOPs, GCP or applicable regulatory requirements, thereby jeopardizing a subject's safety in the trial.
- Unacceptable conditions at a participating facility. Although the site was found to be acceptable for the study initially, it is possible that essential equipment or staffing needs are not being provided for the study.
- Early termination by the sponsor/CRO: The sponsor/CRO and/or regulatory authority(ies) determine that the current trial or the investigational product is not safe and/or effective and, for this reason, must discontinue the site's participation.

Whatever the reason(s) for a site being discontinued, or terminated, from a study, the CRA or appropriate sponsor representative should communicate the reason(s) for the action directly to the investigator. If the reasons for terminating a study are other than a sponsor's decision or normal study completion, the investigator will sometimes object to the termination. In some cases (e.g., if the investigator is likely to be an asset for future studies), the sponsor may opt to provide the investigator an opportunity to address the issue that is the basis for the proposed termination. Specifically, the sponsor and investigator may negotiate a timeline within which the investigator must address the issue and, therefore, remain active under the study. If the investigator fails to meet this timeline, the sponsor will have ample reason to proceed with terminating the site. In other situations, an investigator may be extremely understanding and may accept the sponsor's decision to terminate the site's participation. As with most trial-related issues, the discussion should be well-documented, and the appropriate correspondence should be forwarded to the investigator for retention in the study files.

Termination Site Visit: Preparation Consistent with the sponsor's SOPs, the CRA should confirm the date and time of the Termination Site Visit (TSV), and should provide the site with verbal or written notification of this visit. As he/she did with the PSV notification letter, the CRA should provide the correspondence in a timely manner so that the site can adequately prepare for the TSV. The CRA might want to specify the goals for the visit (e.g., resolve all outstanding data queries, retrieve photocopies of applicable correspondence from the site's regulatory files) as well as the individuals who the CRA plans to meet with during the visit and the amount of time required for the meeting(s) (e.g., principal investigator for 30 minutes, pharmacist for 20 minutes).

To ensure a successful TSV, the CRA should review the protocol (e.g., timeline for following up on any site-specific SAEs), any PSV reports that list the outstanding issues for the site and/or the sponsor, the sponsor's template for the TSV report, the sponsor's SOPs (e.g., publication policy), GCP standards, and the applicable regulatory requirements. The CRA should also confer with appropriate members of the project team to ensure that there are no additional outstanding issues that were not covered in the PSV reports. Often, the clinical research manager will obtain this information from the other members of the project team, and can forward these requests to the CRA for resolution. The CRA also should be aware of the status of any outstanding data queries or CRFs. Ideally, all original CRFs will have been retrieved during the PSVs, thus allowing any necessary data queries to be generated and issued to the site prior to its termination from the study.

Termination Site Visit: Conduct Depending on the number of subjects enrolled at a site and the site's status, the TSV should usually be the shortest of the site visits that the CRA conducts. The main objectives of the TSV are to ensure that records for enrolled subjects are available (informed consent forms, source documents, CRFs, and data queries), the site's regulatory binder is complete and accurate, investigational product accountability issues have been reconciled, and the investigator is aware of his/her continuing responsibilities with regard to the study. To achieve these objectives, the CRA is responsible for the following during the TSV: (1) ensuring the investigator/site's continued compliance with the protocol, sponsor SOPs, GCP standards, and the applicable regulatory requirements; (2) ensuring that the original, signed informed consent forms and authorizations for the use and disclosure of protected health information are present for all enrolled subjects; (3) ensuring that copies of CRFs and photocopies of resolved Edit Logs, if applicable, are present for all enrolled subjects (original CRFs should be maintained by the sponsor); (4) verifying the source documents with any outstanding CRFs, reviewing any corrections to be made with the investigator or authorized study staff, and retrieving the original CRFs for submission to the sponsor; (5) ensuring that all serious adverse events have been appropriately reported to the sponsor and IRB; (6) resolving any outstanding data queries for submission to the sponsor (original, resolved data queries should be returned to the sponsor, and photocopies of the resolved queries should be retained at the site); (7) assessing the accountability of the investigational product, which includes used or unused product located at the site, any erroneously discarded product, and used or unused product that was returned to the sponsor, and providing the site with instructions for returning investigational product (used or unused) to the sponsor or for disposing investigational product (used or unused); (8) verifying the status of any remaining biological samples and, if applicable, forwarding the samples to the appropriate location for processing and analysis; (9) providing the site with instructions for the return or destruction of any unused ancillary supplies that were provided for the study (e.g., CRF notebooks, syringes, saline bags); and (10) determining the status of the site's regulatory files and ensuring that all essential documents are present.

Before leaving the site, the CRA should sign the Monitoring Log to document the visit and should retrieve a photocopy for the sponsor. The CRA should also meet with the investigator to discuss the study, any future studies that the sponsor might conduct with the investigational product, and the investigator's continuing responsibilities under 21CFR 312 Subpart D, GCP standards, and the sponsor's SOPs. Specific points of discussion include the following:

Final Study Report: An investigator must provide the IRB with an adequate report shortly after the completion his/her participation in the study (the timeline is generally determined by the sponsor's SOPs). This report, sometimes provided as a template by the sponsor or IRB, must provide a summary of the trial's outcome and the overall enrollment status of the site (e.g., number of subjects enrolled across all sites, number of subjects enrolled at the site, number of serious adverse events at the site). A photocopy of this report and an acknowledgment by the IRB (if applicable) should be provided to the sponsor.

Audit: An investigator, upon request from any properly authorized FDA officer or employee, must permit such an officer or employee to access, copy and verify any records or reports that were made by the investigator and that related to the clinical investigation that was/is being conducted. Generally, a sponsor will ask that the investigator contact the company if the agency makes such a request. In many cases, the sponsor can provide resources and guidance to help ensure that the site is adequately prepared for the audit.

Recordkeeping requirements: An investigator must retain records for a period of two years following the date a marketing application is approved for the drug for the indication for which it is being investigated or, if no application is to be filed or if the application is not approved for such indication, until two years after the investigation is discontinued and the FDA is so notified.

Transfer of responsibility: If an investigator leaves a site, the sponsor and IRB should be notified in writing. This notification should identify the person(s) who will assume study responsibility for the duration of the recordkeeping requirements.

Publication policy: Many sponsors establish their own standards regarding an investigator's use and disclosure of study-related data in any publication (e.g., journal article). These requirements should be made clear to the investigator.

Serious adverse events: Consistent with the sponsor's SOPs and/or protocol, the investigator may be required to track subjects' serious adverse events until they have resolved or for a period of time after the administration of the last dose of the investigational product. If these dates occur after a site's termination, the CRA should ensure that the investigator is aware of his/her responsibility for reporting such data to the sponsor.

Termination Site Visit: Follow-up As he/she did for all previous site visits, the CRA should document his/her relevant findings in a Termination Site Visit report consistent with the sponsor's SOPs. The report should include the date the visit was conducted, the name of the CRA who conducted the visit, the site that was visited, the name of the investigator and any other individuals who were contacted, a summary of the information reviewed, any significant findings or facts, and any recommended actions taken or to be taken. This report should be reviewed and finalized with a sponsor representative according to a timeline specified in the sponsor's SOPs.

The CRA should also prepare a TSV follow-up letter that details the information that was covered, clarifies any unanswered questions, and addresses any issues that require follow-up by either the study site or the sponsor. For documentation purposes, the CRA should also consider briefly restating the investigator's continuing responsibilities with regard to the study.

It is important that the CRA and other project team members ensure that any outstanding issues are resolved by the site. Many times, the sites will inadvertently forget to submit a final study report to the IRB or to return investigational supplies to the sponsor (e.g., investigational IV pumps). Once all outstanding issues have been resolved, the CRA might want to provide the site with written correspondence stating that all outstanding issues have been resolved and that the site has been successfully terminated from participation in the study.

Site Interactions Since they are critical site contacts for CRAs, study coordinators were asked for their perspectives regarding CRAs and monitoring-related roles and responsibilities. The study coordinators who were approached work with CRAs every two to four weeks, and are quite familiar with site/monitor dynamics. These coordinators offered the following:

- Qualities that the study coordinators appreciated most in their CRAs included supportive approaches, an ability to provide direction and to negotiate changes, and a sense of humor. The study coordinators felt that some CRAs were inflexible, and that this quality made the coordinators' jobs more difficult.
- The study coordinators felt that all of the CRAs with whom they have worked were extremely familiar with the protocol, GCP standards, and applicable regulatory requirements, and were always well prepared to conduct the site visit. There were no differences noted between those CRAs who were employed directly by a sponsor/CRO or were contracted by the sponsor/CRO.
- According to the study coordinators, the greatest challenge facing CRAs was establishing a working relationship with the coordinator and investigator.
- Having all documents readily available and starting a meeting early in the morning were among the ways that the coordinators felt CRAs could promote an efficient SIV.
- When asked what approaches would make the conduct of a PSV more fluid, the study coordinators stated that presenting a "plan of attack" for the duration of the visit and asking the coordinators to stop in periodically would be most beneficial.
- The study coordinators stated that the most useful tools their CRAs had provided to them to assist with the conduct of the study were temperature conversion charts, source document worksheets, and calendars/logs to document upcoming subject visit dates.
- The most frustrating aspect of a PSV for the study coordinators is the length of time involved in the visit. The study coordinators stated that, in their view, two days should be allotted for a PSV. Also, the study coordinators estimated that investigators spend a maximum of 30 minutes with the CRA at the conclusion of a PSV.

CHAPTER 23

An Integrated Approach to Data Management

By Peg Regan and Christine VerStraate

Obviously, each day that a product is delayed in getting to market can translate into millions of dollars in loss of sales and patent opportunity for a drug or biologic. This fact, along with the level of competition in the market today, demands that every aspect of the clinical research process be examined for possible process improvement.

Data management's (DM) role within the clinical research process is often overlooked and oversimplified. Often times, it is generalized as "data processing," and therefore reliant on high levels of transactional processing to make improvements in the overall clinical timeline. Those companies truly interested in improving efficiencies and quality, and in reducing the cost of the clinical trials process, can benefit greatly from fully understanding how process improvements in data management can affect their business.

Consistent with the approach advocated in this book, this chapter will examine the practical application of an integrated approach that incorporates the use of a multi-disciplinary team and well-defined procedures to the data management process, from requirements analysis to study start-up through production data management and submission. The overall benefits and key advantages of applying this approach to the data management process will be discussed in relation to reduced cycle time, increased accuracy and efficiency, and ultimately the overall reduction in time and cost for a successful submission. Anyone working in the clinical development process, particularly those within the data management function, will benefit by incorporating and applying these approaches to their everyday work and practices.

An Integrated Approach to Data Management The concept of an integrated approach to data management relies on the use of multi-disciplinary teams spanning clinical development, project management, biostatistics, medical writing, data management, and the study investigators to design a study that is based upon final analysis requirements and that will be used in the submission of a trial. This process begins with the protocol strategy meeting, at which the clinical project team defines the content of the final report, standard data presentations and the analysis requirements. The draft analysis plan then supports the design of the CRFs, and the CRFs then support the procedures section of the protocol. This is the basis for significant improvements in the quality of the clinical trial as well as the data management process.

The Role of Data Management in the Clinical Trials Process To provide a context for the discussion of data management's role, the following table presents the high-level phases, process, and general roles and responsibilities throughout the clinical trials process.

Phase	Process	Roles & Responsibilities
Study Requirements Analysis	Data Management Requirements	The study analyst's role within the data management team is to work with the clinical team to ensure data management requirements are understood and properly documented as defined by the analysis planning and final protocol. This is initiated in the protocol strategy meeting. Draft CRFs are produced.
	CRF Design	The study analyst will work with the CRF designer to design and develop the final CRFs based upon the protocol and draft CRF requirements.
	Database Requirements Definition	The study analyst will work with the technical database designer to define database requirements for data collection, edit checks, coding, tracking, as well as analysis and reporting.
	Review & Approval	The study analyst will review all requirements documents and final CRF design with the clinical team to obtain approval prior to the technical study start-up phase.

–continued–

Expediting Drug and Biologics Development

–continued–

Phase	Process	Roles & Responsibilities
Technical Study Start-up	Design & Build	The database designer will proceed to design and build the clinical database according to specifications as defined by the requirements documents and CRF design. Database elements will be tested during this phase to ensure the database functions as specified.
	Validation	The validation analyst will plan, script, execute and summarize the validation of the clinical database system to ensure all requirements are met and the database meets the goals of the integrated approach to study design.
	Documentation & Change Control	Upon successful completion of the validation process, the technical project manager is responsible for ensuring that all technical documenttion is complete and the study database and documentation are placed under change control prior to releasing the clinical database for production study management.
Production Study Management	1st CRF In-house	The production phase of DM starts with the receipt of the first CRF in-house for processing.
	CRF logging/tracking	Logging of all CRFs. Key information /metrics are obtained in this process. Tracking all CRFs by visit/page throughout the DM process.
	Data entry/cleaning	The data specialist role will perform single or double data entry of all CRFs as well as discrepancy management of identified manual and electronic edit checks. These need to be resolved either in-house or through communication by the clinical monitor with the site.
	Managing external data	The data specialist or data manager will manage the uploading and cleaning of all external data needs for a specific study. This includes the management of outside vendors (i.e., central labs, PK labs, etc.) to coordinate the data requirements for a successful transmission and loading of external data. In addition, it includes the cleaning of all external data based on the study requirements.
	Medical Coding	The data manager will utilize the clinical database system to perform auto-encoding, which maps preferred-to-verbatim terms as well as a manual review process for those that do not have a direct match. This includes coding of adverse events, concomitant medications. Medical histories are sometimes coded pending the study requirements.
	Reporting/Transferring of Data	The data manager provides a variety of study/data reports on an ongoing basis to provide overall /detailed status of the production /processing process. The data manager also works closely with the biostatistician to ensure that he/she has access to review and transfer data on an on-going/as needed basis to support analysis and safety reporting.
	Study Close-Out/Quality Control (QC)	Once all the data have been received and the DM team has completed all close out steps, the database is deemed frozen. The DM team then completes the defined QC process, which involves a manual review of a percentage of patients/CRFs against the database to determine overall error rate. Upon the completion of a successful QC, the database is then locked, preventing any further activity to the database. Upon completion of successful QC, the statistician can then pull the final set of data to support his/her already programmed tables/listings ensuring a quick turnaround of a final analysis and report.

Using the concept of a multi-disciplinary team within and across the data management process requires key roles to impact process improvement:

- The study analyst's role is key in ensuring that the study requirements are properly defined, resulting in clearly documented requirements to support the design and implementation of an efficient and effective study database.
- The technical team is responsible for designing, implementing, validating and delivering the electronic clinical study database as defined by the requirements.
- The data management team is responsible for supporting the production study conduct to ensure that the clinical data are accurately collected and cleaned to support the final analysis, final report and, ultimately, the NDA/BLA submission.

Practical Application The use of the integrated approach, which is based upon the notion of designing the clinical protocol and CRF to support the analysis and reporting aspects of the study, greatly improves the technical study start-up process and resulting quality of the study database. This multi-disciplinary team approach includes the technical DM representatives that will ultimately be responsible to design, implement, validate, and maintain change control over the clinical study database, as well representatives of all the "users" of the resulting clinical database and data, including data managers, data specialists, statisticians, medical writers, clinicians, and study investigators.

This approach leads to higher quality study databases as well as fully knowledgeable data management staff that can support the study conduct throughout the processing phase to analysis and submission. The following sections describe the practical application of an integrated team approach in developing optimal clinical databases.

A clinical database is defined as an electronic system that provides the necessary functionality to support the entry, storage, tracking, coding, cleaning, analysis and reporting of electronic data for a specific clinical trial. The use of a documented development process or lifecycle is fundamental to the process of creating a quality clinical database. The use of an integrated team approach to carry out the development lifecycle is fundamental to the development of an *optimal* clinical database.

Generally, the process requires the accurate translation of a paper CRF into a robust electronic database. The traditional method of designing clinical databases has proven to be problematic with respect to the accurate translation of study requirements between clinical and technical staff. As a result, the production study database often must undergo many changes throughout the production phase of data management, reducing the overall quality of the data and ability of the study team to rely upon the clinical database and data.

Study Requirements Analysis The integrated approach to analysis is the basis of the philosophy behind optimal database design. As described above, this multi-disciplinary team approach is carried through the analysis of all requirements of the clinical database, also starting from the data presentations or analysis requirements and working backwards to add the other necessary database elements to ensure the entire data management (study conduct) process requirements are defined for the development of an optimal clinical database.

Initial Protocol Strategy Meeting The key role of DM in the initial protocol strategy meeting is to gather and obtain an understanding of the data that are to be collected in the planned data presentations and data analysis. Working from an outline of the data analysis plan as well as input from the project team, DM will develop a set of draft CRFs. The draft CRFs provide key input to the procedures section of the protocol.

Using an integrated approach to analysis, the DM team participates in the initial protocol strategy meeting in support of draft CRF design from a technical perspective, as well as the additional requirements gathering processes carried out below. Just as the integrated approach utilizes the notion of knowing what the end result must be before defining the protocol, the DM team also must understand what the end result of the clinical database must be before they design the system. The study analyst and technical designer benefit from the opportunity to discover and gather key information that can later be translated into optimized design approaches to support the development of a database driven by the same principles and goals of the multi-disciplinary study team—to design a clinical database that supports the data presentations, collection, cleaning, and reporting needs as required to conduct the *optimal* clinical trial.

Database Design Requirements As discussed above, the basis for clinical database design requirements lies within the design of the CRF. Therefore, the role of the technical DM staff within the integrated approach is to provide insight and expertise in designing optimal databases as input to the design of the paper CRF. This approach then ensures that the foundation of database design requirements has a basis in good database design. Often times, these are simply layout requirements or ease of translation that can improve the interpretation and translation from paper to electronic CRF. Additional database design requirements are gathered to support overall study conduct that spans beyond the data collection and cleaning requirements. Examples of this may require the use of extended clinical systems to support workflow for CRF logging and tracking, medical coding, and loading of external data.

Programming Requirements Programming or edit check requirements are driven by the analysis/protocol requirements to ensure adherence to study conduct. These requirements are traditionally written by clinical team members and are later delivered to technical staff for implementation. The pitfall of this approach/process is in the translation of clinical study requirements based upon the paper CRF to functional requirements based upon the clinical database. This results in an extremely high rate of misinterpretation and subsequent implementation of edit checks that do not meet the study requirements. This process can be extremely time consuming, since it typically results in many iterations between the requirements definition and technical implementation phases, and is mostly driven by trial and error. This just doesn't work.

Expediting Drug and Biologics Development

This process can be greatly improved by incorporating standardization of the *format* or structure of the requirement statements themselves. If you have ever developed edit checks for a clinical trial, you must be aware of how the same edit check requirement can be stated in a seemingly unlimited number of ways. Therefore, the key to improving this process is to limit the variety of requirements statements through the development of clear, consistent, and reusable requirements statements "formats." This does not mean the development of standard edit check requirements per se, but the process or manner in which a requirement is stated.

For example, the most common edit check requirement is to "check for missing values." Assuming the value is a patient's age, this can be stated in many ways, including the following: (1) age must be present; (2) age cannot be empty; (3) age must be between 18 and 65 years and must be present; or (4) date of birth and date of drug administration must be present. All of these somehow require that age is not blank. However, they are stated in: (1) the positive; (2) the negative; (3) in combination with other requirements; or (4) implied through the check against dependent variables.

This may seem quite understandable from the world of clinical review, but the translation to database language can be quite different depending upon the way that the requirement is stated. Requirements stated inconsistently within and across studies results in longer analysis time, erroneous interpretations, lower quality databases, and more study changes. This is often the result of a disjointed study design team and inefficient processes with few controls. The impact of this seemingly simple process on the overall time to submission is quite astounding.

Yet, a simple process improvement can go a long way. Utilizing the clinical project team to develop standard conventions for stating requirements consistently across all edit check statements is the first step. With this, the translation of consistently stated edit check requirements formats can easily be understood and efficiently translated into consistent edit check programs. This along with the use of an integrated team that understands the goals and supports this process can greatly improve the quality of a clinical database design and, ultimately, the data.

Data Analysis / Reporting Requirements Perhaps the most important aspect of the study requirements is the need to review, extract and report on study data accurately, efficiently, and *consistently* throughout the duration of a clinical trial. Carrying through with the approach of working backward from the analysis plan to the protocol design, the integrated approach to study database design includes the specification and implementation of analysis requirements that ensure that the access, view, and organization of the data within the clinical database are available, accurate, and consistent throughout the clinical trial.

The traditional method of supporting the analysis requirements of a study typically relies on the development of an annotated CRF (aCRF), which is used to map the data stored in the database tables to the paper CRF. The production of the aCRF can be tedious and error-prone, since it may require a non-technical staff member to translate and transcribe database element names onto the paper CRF. This aCRF is then given to the statistical team to develop analysis tables as extracts from the clinical database, based purely on the manual transcription of a clinical database design to a paper CRF. It is quickly apparent that this process and resulting analyses can become difficult and out of synch with the database as study changes occur.

The ultimate benefit of an integrated approach to analysis is the addition of analysis requirements in the clinical database design and implementation. The database is then designed to support the ease of translation or view of the planned analyses and data presentations throughout the trial. The results of databases designed to support the intended presentation of results using a validated, compliant and controlled process/system can dramatically improve the quality, efficiency, and compliance of a regulatory submission.

Requirements of an Optimal Clinical Database

The list below comprises specific requirements documents that must be generated from the integrated analysis phase of a study. This list includes only those documents required for the study database implementation.

Requirements Document	Process Description	Database Design Elements
Analysis & Reporting Requirements	This document is produced from the analysis plan and input from the statistical team to document the database "views" required to support review, analysis, and reporting directly from the study database.	These requirements are designed to enable the statistical team to perform analysis directly from the study database.

–continued–

–continued–

Requirements Document	Process Description	Database Design Elements
Database Design Requirements	The final CRF becomes the basis of the design of the "data collection" elements of the study database. Standard database elements as well as design conventions are incorporated as requirements to the database design process.	The database tables and entry screens are designed and implemented to support the accurate entry and storage of study data as per documented and approved requirements.
Additional Database Design (Configuration) Requirements	This requirements document is an addition to the Final CRF, and may be generated from several sources to document the database design requirements to support logging, tracking, coding, and cleaning of the study data.	The study database is configured to include the integration of other systems and/or database functionality to support the extended workflow requirements such as lab loading, tracking, etc.
Edit Check Requirements	This document is used to record the protocol rules as statements that reference the final CRF and final protocol document.	The database designer must translate the clinical requirements into database language and implement them as automated edit checks.

The Review & Approval Process The review and approval process is quite straightforward if, of course, the development process follows a rigorous lifecycle that includes well-defined requirements in a form that can be traced throughout the study database design and implementation process. The review and approval of the requirements documents is key to supporting the subsequent implementation, validation, and change control procedures used to ensure compliance throughout the management of the study data.

The review and approval of study requirements documents also takes on an integrated team approach. Based upon the idea that both clinical and technical experts from the data management team are involved in the analysis phase of the study, the reviewers essentially become the sub-team members assigned to complete the specific phase or document to support the quality management of the study data. The approver of all requirements documents may be identified as the person who has responsibility for the design of the study protocol. The review and approval process can dramatically improve the quality of requirements and therefore the quality of the clinical database.

Technical Study Start-up

Technical study start-up can be defined as the design and implementation process used to translate study requirements into an electronic system, better known as the study database. The key to the design and implementation of an optimal study database continues with the philosophy of a team approach in meeting the requirements of all aspects of the study conduct. If the requirements documentation above is accurate and complete, the process of design and implementation becomes quite straightforward.

Design & Build Using a validated and documented process for study database development, the technical team begins by documenting the design specifications of each database element as defined by the approved requirements documents above. The design specification document must provide a mapping back to each of the related requirements to ensure that all requirements will be met with the implementation and that validation can be accurately performed and documented for the final production study database. An integrated technical team conducts internal reviews and approves all design specifications prior to proceeding with the implementation phase of the database elements.

Just as the design specifications are driven through the requirements statements, the implementation process is now driven by the design specifications. Here, the technical team translates the design specifications into the clinical database elements using technical database systems and integrated development tools. The implementation process is governed by good programming practices, coding standards, and development guidelines to ensure consistency across study databases and to ensure that future maintenance or changes can be performed in a controlled, compliant manner.

Each of the database elements defined in the requirements and design documents are implemented first as a separate unit. Each unit is then tested by the technical developer to verify that it performs as expected, and as stated in the requirements and design documents. This process will iterate between development and verification until the developer is satisfied that the database element is implemented as specified. Once all elements of the clinical database have been implemented, the final integration testing must be conducted prior to release to production use.

Validation Often times, validation is viewed as the final phase of database design, and as a process that begins upon the completion of the design and implementation above. However, the proven method of validation requires that the process begin early in the analysis phase as well.

Expediting Drug and Biologics Development

The validation process must answer the following questions in order to determine the completeness and accuracy of the requirements as well as database design and implementation:

1. "Was the study database designed and implemented correctly?"
2. "Was the correct system implemented?"

Question 1 refers to the notion of ensuring that the system was implemented according to functional requirements, as documented and approved. Question 2 refers to the notion of ensuring that the system meets the study workflow (study conduct) requirements in production use, which may or may not have been documented accurately in the functional requirements. Nevertheless, the validation of the study database must result in an acceptable answer to the above questions.

The validation process can be quite time consuming if it is not well planned and defined from the beginning. Study database validation includes the planning, scripting, and execution of specified test cases, and an analysis of the overall results to determine the answers to the above questions. Using the integrated approach places the responsibility of ensuring the quality of the study database on all team members, from requirements definition through design and implementation. The validation analyst's role on the team is to ensure that the study is implemented, documented, and tested according to the study requirements. This use of the integrated team approach in study validation can result in a significant reduction in technical start-up time, and improvements in the quality of the clinical database and resulting data.

Documentation & Change Control The level of documentation required to support an optimal clinical database must ensure that the study requirements, database design, implementation, validation, as well as change control procedures are accurately represented and auditable from the start of a study through to database lock and submission. The use of a rigorous development lifecycle and robust standard operating procedures to support the study start-up process is fundamental to the successful production and maintenance of clinical database documentation.

In addition, a rigorous change control process must be utilized to ensure that changes to the clinical database follow the proper procedures. In turn, this will ensure that the database maintains its validated state and that the clinical data are not compromised as a result of changes occurring during the production phase of a trial. Another key element to documentation and change control includes the use of version control of all study-related documentation. This includes all documentation as defined above for the study start-up process, as well as the production process for requesting and implementing study changes. This level of documentation, together with the audit trail of the clinical data, provides the traceable map back through the history of a trial. Without it, the picture can become quite distorted and questionable to those outside the process.

Production Study Data Management

The integrated approach to the design and development of an optimal clinical database ensures that all requirements of the study design and conduct are met, procedures are documented, databases are validated, and processes to manage database changes are in place for the production study management phase to begin. As the production phase begins, however, the integrated process must continue to ensure quality and compliance. The production DM processes below present the good practices that can and must be incorporated into the integrated DM procedures in order to use *and maintain* a quality clinical database/data.

Study Change Procedures The integrated approach to analysis and the overall implementation process of an optimal clinical database strives to minimize the need for study database changes. It is unreasonable, however, to expect that any study will proceed without change simply due to the ongoing review and analysis of the data that occurs throughout the production phase. Therefore, one must assume changes will occur. This can often cause the study database and potentially the data to be compromised if documented, predictable processes are not utilized and enforced.

Good practices in study change procedures continue to use the integrated team approach to first understand the need for study changes as a team, and to ensure that the change is communicated effectively to the technical team for implementation as well as the clinical team for changes in functionality. As mentioned above, the rigorous change control procedures govern the actual implementation. However, it is imperative that the production DM process includes well-defined procedures to define, request, review and approve study changes to a production database. In addition, these practices must ensure that communications to the broader study team are delivered, received, and documented effectively.

Communication Channels As described above, the risk of implementing study changes relates to the database design and performance, but possibly more importantly, to the understanding of the study team members who are using the clinical database to enter, clean, track, analyze and report on study data. Therefore, adequate communication channels to all clinical study team members must be available as a part of the production study management process. The advantage of using an integrated team from the start provides a vehicle through which to review and approve the study changes (i.e., in integrated team meetings). Formal signatures and/or other, less formal procedures can greatly improve this aspect of study change management. Some options include the use of electronic study management tools and communications databases, and even web-based training sessions to communicate and demonstrate the options, impacts, and final changes once they are implemented to the database. Without adequate communications channels, the time and effort to maintain a quality clinical trial is increased dramatically.

Data Processing For data entry, perhaps the most important factor in an optimal database design is the translation or mapping of the paper CRF to the eCRF of the clinical database. As discussed above, the integrated approach to the design of a quality CRF provides and ensures that this requirement is met. Another very important requirement of a quality CRF design is to ensure study questions are easily understood by the investigator sites. The integrated team approach ensures the implementation of these primary requirements as the basis for good CRF design. This translates into significant improvements in the quality of the data collection process overall. The benefits of these good practices are also evident in the speed of entry, error rate, the numbers of queries, and overall database performance.

Data Cleaning As mentioned above, the data cleaning process can be quite intensive if (1) requirements were not fully understood, (2) edit checks were not implemented as expected, (3) the database was not designed for optimal use, and (4) good practices and procedures were not developed and/or followed. As a result of the above, the data cleaning process is typically the largest bottleneck within the entire DM production process. This often results in the most resource-intensive and costly area within DM.

By following the integrated approach, the data cleaning process can be a very efficient and streamlined process. Since this approach ensures that the study is designed according to the analysis plan and study requirements, it ensures that both the database and edit checks are implemented for optimal use. In addition, this approach ensures that the proper procedures and practices as well as open communication channels are in place within the entire study team supporting an efficient data processing/cleaning process. As a result, immediate benefits are seen through a significant reduction in all DM processing cycle times, from last CRF in house to last DCF resolved as well as last DCF resolved to database freeze. Not only does this approach result in a reduction in cycle times and cost, but also ensures the quality and integrity of the data supporting a submission.

Analysis and Final Reporting Typically, the analysis and final reporting is another area that can delay a final submission. This is often a result of not planning and working from the end goal with a clearly defined analysis plan and standard data presentations. Typically, a study will start without ever having an analysis plan defined, resulting in unclear study requirements and goals.

By following the integrated approach, it is the analysis plan that drives the study requirements throughout the DM process, analysis and final reporting. From the start of the study, the analysis plan, standard data presentations and final report are defined and drafted. Prior to the start of the DM production phase, the templates for the standard data presentations and final report are finalized. This approach ensures that the on-going access and view of the data within the clinical database is available and accurate throughout the clinical trial process. This then provides the statistician and medical writer with the ability to access the data once the production process begins, therefore avoiding the typical scenario in which these individuals must wait until the database is locked before programming and report writing can begin. With this approach, the majority of the standard data presentation programming is completed well in advance of database lock. Once the programming is completed for the standard data presentations, it can then be applied to all studies, therefore reducing the need for additional programming for future studies. The programming for the standard presentations need be performed only once, after which it can then be applied to all subsequent reports.

In addition, since the template for the final report is developed well in advance, when the study is over and the analyses are complete, writing the final report will only be a matter of filling in the blanks of the template with the information generated during the study.

CHAPTER 24

Evaluation of Safety During Clinical Drug Development

By Walker A. Long, MD

The final judgments on whether potential new drugs should be marketed are made by regulatory authorities such as the US FDA and the European Agency for the Evaluation of Medicinal Products (EMEA) in Europe. These judgments are rendered after careful risk/benefit assessments of manufacturing, nonclinical, and clinical data. These risk/benefit assessments are conducted by in-house experts within the regulatory authorities. Regulatory authorities also often utilize external experts to assist in these evaluations; the FDA's advisory committee system is one such formalized example.

The data that regulatory authorities use to make these judgments are generated by "sponsors" who are willing to invest heavily in the high-risk world of pharmaceutical development. The "sponsors" behind the vast majority of new drug approvals are large pharmaceutical companies. The large pharmaceutical companies are essentially large merchant banks that put enormous amounts of their own capital at risk every year in pursuit of new drugs.

The regulations in the United States, Europe, and most other countries require demonstrations that new drugs are both safe and effective at the dose recommended in the disease to be treated. It is important to recognize that evaluations of safety and efficacy are two different requirements. Although it is not always the case, more often than one might expect, evaluations of safety can require far more patients than are required for evaluations of efficacy.

The purpose of this chapter is to outline an approach to the clinical evaluation of safety for new pharmaceuticals. The approach outlined is largely restricted to the development of new pharmaceuticals intended for use in adults rather than children.

Background Drug development is a highly competitive field in which time is the scarcest resource. Successful drug development requires: a) repetitive if not continuous integration of progressively accumulating information from a variety of fields, b) quick and effective decision-making in response to this new information, and c) impeccable execution of the decisions made. Without impeccable execution, delivery of new medicines that could potentially save lives (many diseases remain without effective treatment) will be delayed. Without impeccable execution, even great new drug discoveries will often be overtaken by competing products that are not as safe or not as effective, and be beaten to approval and marketing.

In designing a clinical program to evaluate the safety of a potential new drug, it is of fundamental importance to recognize the following facts. First, "modern" medicine is in its infancy, and although many amazing and beautiful medical advances have taken place in the last 50 years, the great majority of people who die do so prematurely because our medical treatments for our most common diseases are not good enough. Second, as people age and develop disease, the great majority go through debilitating loss of function (physical and mental) and increasing suffering. Loss of function and suffering associated with aging and disease can at least be ameliorated if not prevented with new safe and effective pharmaceuticals.

Third, every new drug candidate should be considered a potential breakthrough that could save the life of one's own child, one's own life, the lives of others one loves, the lives of friends, or the lives of strangers.

Fourth, even if not life-saving, every new drug candidate should be considered a potential breakthrough in the alleviation, if not the prevention, of the consequences of aging and disease (suffering and loss of function).

For these reasons, developing new drugs is an honorable endeavor that is at least as important as any other human activity. Those developing new drugs must always put the safety of the patients in their clinical trials first, but at the same time those developing new drugs must never forget that the potential new drug on which they are working may be another medical miracle that prevents death and human suffering.

Expediting Drug and Biologics Development

With these considerations in mind, it is safe to say that plans for evaluation of clinical safety often require adjustment and/or revision as development of a particular new drug unfolds. For many drugs, unanticipated issues affecting clinical safety end up dictating, in order of increasing delays to development of the new drug, a) revision of the clinical safety plan, b) reformulation of the new drug, c) pursuit of an alternative route of administration, d) pursuit of a different indication, or d) abandonment of development. The earlier it is discovered that a development of a new drug should be altered or abandoned, the better.

Consistently early redirection of scarce human and financial resources to the development of other potential new drugs when a given candidate compound can be demonstrated to be unsafe or impractical is not only a key competitive advantage in major pharmaceutical companies, but is also the right thing to do from a societal and ethical perspective. The poorly treated and untreatable diseases afflicting the human family are exacting an enormous price, a price that can be eliminated with continued medical discovery and drug development. One key to rapid progress will be rapid redeployment of available resources to more promising compounds when deficiencies in a given compound are noted.

STRATEGY FOR THE EVALUATION OF CLINICAL SAFETY The first step in the clinical evaluation of safety of a new compound is to develop an overall strategy for the endeavor. The strategy for clinical evaluation of safety is best developed as part of an integrated clinical drug development plan, a plan that outlines in sequential order all clinical trials needed for the evaluation of both safety and efficacy. An important point to understand is that the clinical drug development plan is a living document that must be adjusted rapidly in response to new information that can come from a variety of sources.

Factors that determine the original plan for evaluation of clinical safety, and factors that also necessitate the frequent modification of the clinical safety plan as new data and information accumulate include: compound structure/source; formulation; route of administration; duration of administration; pharmacology; toxicology; regulatory expectations/requirements/standards; clinical effects; Phase 1 findings; Phase 2a findings; Phase 2b findings; Phase 3a findings; Phase 3b findings; and Phase 4 findings. Differences in the clinical safety plan that can be dictated by each of these factors are summarized below.

Compound Source/Structure The chemical structure and source of the potential new drug (hereafter referred to as the "compound") are of fundamental importance to its overall development (including pharmacology, manufacturing and toxicology) and to its clinical development. The most important distinction is whether a new compound is a biologic agent or a new chemical entity. Biologic agents, such as therapeutic (rather than preventive) vaccines, proteins, peptides, genes, antisense technologies, antibodies, or stem cells, are physically far larger than new chemical entities, carry greater manufacturing challenges, often have specific toxicology requirements that are unique to each type of biologic agent, and usually are studied differently in the clinic (because normal volunteers are infrequently used). In contrast, new chemical entities are classically relatively easy to manufacture, have uniform toxicology requirements, and are usually studied first in normal volunteers (unless the new chemical entity is a cytotoxic compound intended for cancer patients). For the purposes of this chapter, the rest of the discussion of evaluation of clinical safety will apply to new chemical entities rather than biologic agents, although the principles are generally the same (specifics may vary, however).

Any compound that is not already approved for marketing is considered to be a new chemical entity, no matter how close the compound's structure is to an already approved drug. From both a scientific and a regulatory perspective, this position makes sense, as very minor changes in chemical structure can result in dramatically different clinical effects. For example, removing a single hydrogen atom from the 15 position of prostaglandin D2 (thereby changing the hydroxyl group at that position to a ketone group) changes the compound from a pulmonary vasodilator in the neonate to a pulmonary vasoconstrictor, a complete inversion of the compound's pharmacologic effect on neonatal lung vasculature (1).

On the other hand, many times, compounds closely related in structure have similar (although not identical) biologic effects; these similar profiles of efficacy and safety for drugs of similar structure are often termed "class effects." A recent example has been the concern over increased cardiovascular risks associated with Cox-2 inhibitors (2). The chemical structures of the Cox-2 inhibitors are remarkably similar, but excess risk for myocardial infarction and for stroke varies substantially with compound. For some Cox-2 inhibitors, long-term treatment (> 2 years) at high doses is required for increased cardiovascular risk to become manifest. For others, increased cardiovascular risk is apparently manifest at low doses during short-term use.

However, a better term from a safety perspective for such observations is "class risks" rather than "class effects," as no two compounds have identical safety profiles, and minor differences in structure can result in quite different safety (and also efficacy) profiles.

If a compound is a new chemical entity from a known class of drugs (such as beta blockers or ACE inhibitors), typically the safety effects of the class are already well-characterized, and what one might expect from a safety perspective in the clinic is already known-with the caveat that any new drug in the class may have a higher or lower incidence of known clinical effects, or heretofore unrecognized effects.

If the potential new drug has a new chemical structure dissimilar from all known drugs, the roadmaps to predicting clinical toxicity are: 1) toxicological findings in animals, and 2) thought experiments during which the known pharmacology of the compound in animals is exaggerated for each organ system in man (nervous, cardiovascular, respiratory, gastroenterological, genitourinary, musculoskeletal, and dermatological).

Formulation If one is fortunate, the formulations of new compounds studied in the clinic are dictated by the disease target and the planned duration of therapy (obviously compounds intended for long-term use are much more easily administered orally rather than intravenously). However, not infrequently the pharmacology, pharmacokinetics, or chemistry of a new compound dictates a formulation that inherently restricts clinical use and thereby informs the clinical evaluation of safety. For example, prostacyclin is a useful and powerful pulmonary vasodilator that is unstable a physiologic pH and has a two-minute half life. As a result, prostacyclin is provided as a sterile lyophilized powder, is reconstituted at the time of use with sterile glycine buffer (pH = 10), and is only approved for continuous intravenous infusions (3).

However a potential new drug is formulated (whether a solid such as a tablet, capsule, ointment, powder, or liquid [such as an oral solution or suspension, inhaled solution or suspension, or an injectible solution or suspension]), the formulation itself dictates to some extent both overall development and clinical development. For example, any compound formulated as a sterile solution (such as prostacyclin above) immediately raises safety questions about injection site irritation and pulmonary irritation as a result of the fact that sterile drug solutions usually end up being both injected into the blood and also inhaled into the lungs by accident, or on purpose, or both, no matter what the originally intended route of administration of the original formulation. Similarly, any new drug formulated as an ointment immediately raises safety questions about both local (topical) irritation and possible systemic absorption with distant effects. Also, any tablet or capsule immediately raises questions about local gastrointestinal effects, as well as first-pass hepatic metabolism that could alter safety, efficacy, or both.

Some formulations (such as sustained-release oral formulations, time-dependent release formulations (typically targeting small bowel), or pH-dependent release formulations (again typically targeting small bowel)) permit enhancement of desirable pharmacokinetic profiles, minimization of local toxic effects, or both.

For some compounds, multiple formulations have been proven to be useful in man; for example, corticosteroids are administered as ointments, tablets, injectibles, and as aerosols. For other compounds, only a single formulation is available; prostacyclin is an example (3).

Late Discoveries In Chemistry, Manufacturing & Controls For The Formulation Sometimes, a potential new drug is well into clinical development when, during scale-up of manufacturing of either the drug substance (the compound itself) or drug product (the final formulation), new impurities or contaminants are identified that were not present in the drug manufactured and administered during the toxicology studies. This problem presents manufacturing, toxicologic and clinical challenges, and can entirely derail some drug development programs. The ultimate solution has to balance manufacturing realities for the compound against money and more importantly against time lost for new toxicology and repeat clinical studies, versus the potentials of other new drugs coming along in the pipeline after the drug with manufacturing problems.

Route Of Administration The route by which a new drug is administered usually not only dictates the type of formulation but also has a strong influence on the overall development plan and on the clinical evaluation of safety. The toxicology studies must be done using the same route of administration intended in man. On occasion, when no toxicity is identifiable in animals using the intended route of administration (in man) and the highest possible doses achievable in animals (because of ethical limitations in dosing of animals, solubility issues, or other issues), toxicology studies exaggerating doses by a route of administration different from the one intended in man may also be required. This problem most commonly occurs for drugs intended for pulmonary deposition via aerosols; sometimes, intravenous toxicity studies prove to be required to demonstrate the true toxic effects of the compound in animals. Another example occurs with new compounds intended for transdermal use; intravenous toxicology studies can prove to be required if systemic toxicity is not demonstrated during dermal applications of the new drug in animals.

Whatever the non-clinical requirements for a given formulation of a given compound, and whatever the non-clinical findings of toxicity prove to be, simply knowing the route of administration informs certain decisions about evaluation of clinical safety. The primary principle dictated by the route of administration is to look carefully for clinical toxicity at the site of administration. For example, in developing a rectal suppository, careful screening of the rectum itself during clinical development with sigmoidoscopy would be at least prudent for the drug developer if not frankly required by the regulatory authorities. Similarly, gastroscopy should be used to look for gastric irritation of tablets or capsules, nasopharyngoscopy should be used to look for nasal irritation of nasal sprays or drops, and opthalmoscopy/slit lamp exams should be used to look for corneal or ocular irritation from eye drops.

Duration Of Administration The timeframe required for efficacy determines the minimum timeframe over which safety must be evaluated; obviously, shorter durations of treatment are inherently safer. How long a new potential drug must be given to be effective is a function of whether the disease is acute or chronic, and of how long it takes for the drug to achieve its therapeutic effect in that disease. Sometimes, follow up for safety must continue for long periods after a drug has done its work and can be discontinued. The latter is particularly true in new medications intended for use in infants or children.

In the best case from an effectiveness point of view, a single dose of a new drug may prove to be life-saving, as was shown with the introductions of synthetic surfactant for the prevention and treatment of hyaline membrane disease in premature infants (4-7). However, such dramatic life-saving effects from single doses are not common in drug development. Further, in the pivotal trials of surfactant, infants who received single doses at or shortly after birth were still followed for safety (and also for efficacy) for a minimum of one year (for all infants) (8-16) and up to two years for some infants after dosing (17).

How long a potential new drug must be administered for demonstration of reduction in mortality (or in other deleterious outcomes) is a function of both the effectiveness of the drug, and of the baseline event rate per unit of time. For example, 12-week infusions of prostacyclin were proven to reduce mortality in patients with NYHA Class III/IV primary pulmonary hypertension (3); the 20% mortality over 12 weeks in the control group made proof of reduction in mortality on prostacyclin fairly easy in that timeframe, as prostacyclin is highly effective in primary pulmonary hypertension. However, since prostacyclin does not cure the disease, but instead either halts its progression or causes regression, patients with primary pulmonary hypertension who are treated with prostacyclin typically go on drug for the rest of their lives. Thus, it should not be surprising that safety data from extremely long-term infusions (up to ten years) were included in the marketing application, although efficacy was proven in only 12 weeks.

In any case, the reduction in mortality provided by prostacyclin in patients with NYHA Class III/IV primary pulmonary hypertension over 12 weeks is supported by similar evidence from earlier eight-week trials (18,19), and confirmed by longer-term follow up of the original randomized cohorts (3) for other purposes (20-23). The survival benefit from original randomization to prostacyclin was still present three years later (20-23).

Far more commonly, long-term-to-permanent dosing is required for proof of reduction in mortality or other deleterious outcomes. For example, a double-blind, pivotal trial designed to evaluate atorvastatin's efficacy was planned for a five-year observation period, but halted prematurely after a median of 3.3 years observation because of overwhelming evidence of efficacy (24). During the trial, the incidence of non-fatal myocardial infarction + fatal coronary disease was 3.0 % in the control group and 1.9 % in the treated group, p<0.008 (24). Again, safety data on dosing periods much longer than 3.3 years were contained in the marketing application, as treatment with atorvastatin is typically permanent.

Thus, the bottom line is that the period of observation required for evaluation of safety of a potential new drug will always exceed that required for evaluation of efficacy.

Pharmacology The primary pharmacology of the new compound also informs decisions about how to look in the clinic for toxicity. If the pharmacology is well-known, the simple operative principle is to exaggerate the primary pharmacology mentally (as in a potential overdose), and design clinical trials to detect evidence of "too much" effect from the primary pharmacology. For example, in developing a new ACE inhibitor, the drug developer might prudently look for signs and symptoms of too much blood pressure reduction, but not just in the vital signs measurements. Clinical effects of "too much ACE" would include such things as weakness, tiredness, dizziness on standing, syncope, confusion, car wrecks (from fainting spells), and broken bones (from falls).

If the primary pharmacology is new and therefore unknown (i.e., the compound is a blocker or an agonist for a new and previously unknown receptor), one has to depend on observed pharmacologic effects in nonclinical experiments, exaggerate those as best one can mentally in the clinical setting, and design the clinical trials to look for those changes.

Late Discoveries From Pharmacology Sometimes, late discoveries from pharmacology (once one is already well into the clinic) have important effects on not only the plan for the clinical evaluation of safety, but also on the overall drug development plan. For example, when, during the clinical development phase a new potential drug is discovered to be a significant inhibitor of CYP3A4 (the mitochondrial enzyme responsible for the metabolism of 50% of the drugs administered to man), the whole drug development program has to be re-evaluated and either redesigned or abandoned. Once significant CYP3A4 inhibition is identified, scrutiny of drug safety must expand to include careful searches for possible drug interactions (in previously collected clinical data and in planned clinical data). Further, the concept of long-term oral use probably has to be abandoned, and the route of administration probably has to change from oral to intravenous (short-term, in-hospital) administration because of the risk of fatal drug-drug interactions during long-term outpatient treatment.

Toxicology The toxicological findings in animals using the same route of administration planned for the clinic are of great importance in designing the safety assessments during clinical development. The greatest utility of the initial toxicology studies is the fairly reliable identification of what organ systems are likely to evidence drug toxicity in man. For example, toxicology experiments (in animals) are surprisingly accurate in identifying what toxicities are likely to occur in man (i.e., bone marrow toxicity or hepatic toxicity versus renal toxicity or pulmonary toxicity). Less reliably predicted from toxicology studies is the actual form the toxicity in the affected organ system will take in man. Least reliably predicted from the toxicology studies are the doses at which toxicity in that organ system will become manifest in man.

One important issue when toxicity is identified in non-clinical experiments is whether that toxicity is reversible once drug is stopped. Having toxicities in animals that are reversible upon cessation of dosing provides a good measure of reassurance that any toxic effects seen in the same organ systems in man will also be reversible.

With the clue(s) provided by the non-clinical toxicology studies as to what organ system(s) is likely to be affected in man, it is fairly straightforward to tailor a series of clinical and laboratory measurements in each clinical trial to determine whether toxicity in that organ system also occurs in man, and if it does, at what doses/durations of treatment that toxicity occurs, what form that toxicity takes, and whether that toxicity is reversible or not. For example, if a potential new drug causes cardiac toxicity in animals, serial non-invasive and invasive measurements of cardiac function have to be built into the clinical evaluation of safety.

Late Discoveries In Toxicology In recent years, the toxicology requirements to enter clinical trials have been escalating in the developed world. At present, not only are repeated-dose studies in two species for 14 days required for first doses in man, but genotoxic and mutagenicity studies are also required even for compounds that occur naturally in man (in which cases reason would clearly dictate that such studies are virtually useless).

However, for drugs intended for long-term human use, not only are long-term toxicity studies required, but carcinogenicity studies are also required. These later studies are both expensive and time-consuming, easily costing millions of dollars and lasting for up to three years. In the United States, the protocols for carcinogenicity studies must be reviewed and approved by a special committee at FDA.

In any case, findings appearing late during long-term toxicity studies and/or in carcinogenicity studies may dictate amendments to ongoing clinical trials, entirely new clinical trials, or abandonment of clinical development, depending upon the nature of the findings and the severity of the disease under study. Such late deleterious findings in animals are not particularly common, but when present frequently prove challenging to, if not disastrous for, continued development of the drug.

Regulatory Expectations/Requirements/Standards The regulatory authorities are the repositories of huge amounts of proprietary information not available elsewhere. From exposure to proprietary information on similar compounds, regulators often suspect that a given compound under investigation will have certain effects that the sponsor of the compound may not have considered. In such situations, and without of course revealing why, regulators often ask for/require specialized non-clinical and/or clinical measurements and/or studies. Perceptive drug developers recognize these requests as coming from prior experience at the regulatory authority, and use these requests to expand their thinking about the compound and their searches for toxicity.

ALERT REPORTING

The FDA requires a sponsor to submit a written IND safety report each time the company receives or otherwise obtains information about a serious and unexpected AE that is associated with the use of the drug.

Serious To help achieve the goal of timely notification of potentially critical safety data, Title 21 of the Code of Federal Regulations Part 312.32 (21 CFR 312.32) dictates criteria for determining whether or not an adverse event qualifies for alert reporting. According to 21 CFR 312.32, an adverse event that meets one of the criteria specified below is to be considered "serious" from a regulatory perspective (it is important to note that "serious" from a regulatory perspective does not necessarily mean "serious" from a clinical perspective, and vice versa.) A "serious" adverse event from a regulatory perspective is defined as an event occurring after any dose of investigational drug that results in any of the following outcomes:
- death;
- a life-threatening event (places the subject, in the view of the investigator, at immediate risk of

death from the reaction as it occurred. This definition does not include a reaction that might have caused death had it occurred in a more severe form);

- inpatient hospitalization or prolongation of existing hospitalization (hospitalization would be considered "prolonged" even in the situation where the hospitalization was not actually prolonged, since the patient would have been in the hospital anyway from a separate injury. In that case, the patient would have been hospitalized if he/she had not already been in the hospital);
- a persistent or significant disability/incapacity (a substantial disruption of a person's ability to conduct normal life functions); or
- a congenital anomaly/birth defect (depending on circumstances, this could involve both male and female parents as test subjects)

Unexpected An AE is unexpected if the specificity or the severity of the AE is not consistent with what is described in the current investigator brochure (IB) or other written materials provided to the investigators. If an IB is not required or available, this statement refers to the risk information described in the general investigational plan or elsewhere in the current application (IND), as amended. Generally speaking, if the AE is not described in the IB or other written materials provided to the investigators (such as prior safety letters sent to investigators describing the same event) at all, or is not described with the same specificity or severity, the AE is unexpected. It is generally best if the company makes the final determination of expectedness with respect to alert reports, because the company is generally much more familiar with exactly what is and what is not already present in the IB and in other written materials.

Related Because so little information about the compound's true effects is available in the early stages of clinical development, an investigator's assessment of whether a given adverse event is "related" to study medication or not can have some importance (even when the blind is not broken in double-blind, placebo-controlled studies). An investigator's opinion that a given serious adverse event is likely related to an investigational drug (because the adverse event is not consistent with the patient's underlying disease and prior disease course) can be a useful red flag to instigate both further searches of existing data and more intense scrutiny of ongoing trials for similar events.

In later stages of clinical development, determination of what adverse events are truly related to the compound is clearly best accomplished by comparison of safety data from large-scale, double-blind, randomized trials. Adverse events that occur more frequently on drug than on placebo or active control in double-blind trials are those that are related to the drug, no matter what the investigators may think. Consistent with this statement, the safety sections of package inserts (product labels) never include investigator attributions of relatedness, but instead present comparisons of the incidence of each adverse event for the new drug versus control from randomized clinical trials.

For regulatory reporting purposes, as stated in 21 CFR 312.32, an AE should be considered related (associated) if there is a reasonable possibility that the event might have been caused by the drug. In practical terms, most sponsors consider an event to be at least possibly related unless a relationship can be ruled out. An example of an unrelated AE would be an AE whose relationship to the drug would be biologically implausible. The investigator should make the initial call on whether the AE is related to the investigational agent. The company should never reverse an investigator's decision that an AE is related, but can and sometimes should overrule a decision by the investigator that an adverse event is not related when, in fact, from what the company knows the adverse event in question is likely related.

Reporting Requirements Written reports must be received by the FDA within 15 days of the date on which the sponsor (including affiliates and subsidiaries) becomes aware of the event. In addition, the FDA requires sponsors to communicate the subset of serious AEs that are fatal or life threatening within 7 days through telephone safety reports, followed-up by a written IND safety report in 15 days. This requirement is consistent with the ICH's E2A guideline. If sponsors are to comply with these requirements, they must understand the minimum reporting requirements and the definitions applied to each of the reportable items.

In the United States, the regulations require that important new safety findings from non-clinical studies be reported promptly to 1) the FDA, 2) the investigators participating in clinical studies, and 3) the institutional review boards (IRBs) that authorized the ongoing clinical studies. In the United States, the regulations similarly require the prompt reporting, to the same recipients, of adverse events that are deemed serious, unexpected, and related. Similar alert reporting requirements exist in the national regulations in most developed countries and in ICH, although language and specifics differ slightly. These regulations make clinical sense, as investigators and patients should be informed as quickly as possible when potentially important new safety information comes to light.

Breaking Blinds Practices surrounding breaking of blinding for patients who are participating in double-blind trials and who develop serious adverse events that are considered related and unexpected vary by country. One statement that might get unanimous endorsement would be that the blind should be broken if knowledge of the treatment assignment (investigational drug versus placebo or active control) could improve the patient's outcome (i.e., that a specific antidote for the investigational drug's (or active control's) toxic effects is available and could be utilized). However, such antidotes are a great exception rather than the rule.

In the United States, the blind for patients who develop serious adverse events that are judged related and unexpected would very seldom be broken, and the event would be reported to FDA, the investigators, and the IRBs without knowing what the patient received. In contrast, in Germany, the regulatory authorities refuse to accept alert serious adverse event reports for serious adverse events that are judged related and unexpected unless the blind has been broken.

Clinical Effects The safety-related clinical effects of a potential new drug can only be determined in man. As the clinical drug development program proceeds, safety data accumulate in an almost exponential fashion as a series of progressively larger clinical trials of longer dosing duration are conducted.

The earliest possible detection of a potential new drug's clinical safety effects (also known as clinical safety problems) is to everyone's advantage, including most importantly volunteers or patients participating in ongoing clinical trials, but also future participants in planned clinical trials, the principal investigators conducting the trials, the clinical drug development team running the trials, the sponsor, and of course the potential new drug itself. Identification of the existence of a clinical safety problem is the first step in characterizing its frequency, severity, natural history, precipitating factors, ameliorating factors, and best treatment—all of which must be carefully characterized in ongoing and subsequent clinical trials if the adverse event is medically important and related to drug, and the drug is going to make it to approval and marketing.

Potential new safety findings discovered in a given clinical trial can include a) occurrence of a previously unrecognized adverse event, b) occurrence of a previously recognized adverse event in a more severe form than previously encountered, and c) occurrence of a previously recognized adverse event at a higher rate (higher incidence) than previously encountered. All three of these findings can have important implications for ongoing and for planned clinical trials, depending upon the nature of the adverse event and the disease or condition under study. For example, the occurrence of aplastic anemia in a clinical trial of an investigational drug is likely to end the development of the compound completely, even if the compound is being developed for a fatal disease. In contrast, detection of an increase in the incidence of gastric ulcers may do little to impede the process when the new drug is intended for the treatment of a life-threatening condition such as ARDS (but would still end development of a new drug targeted for allergic rhinitis). Such risk/potential benefit assessments have to be made repeatedly during the development of each new drug.

The most important principles in correctly identifying safety problems early in clinical development are as follows. First, the protocols under which safety is being studied must be sound, with clearly specified safety measurements (safety measurements chosen based on preclinical findings and on prior clinical findings) at clearly specified time points. Second, the investigators conducting the clinical studies must be competent, honest, experienced, and energetic. Third, the drug development staffs monitoring the studies must also be competent, honest, experienced, and energetic. Fourth, the medical monitor responsible for the safety of the patients in the trial must know the drug, the disease, and the protocol under study very well, so that he or she can recognize when something new is observed.

For convenience, the clinical development program generally is divided into four phases: Phase 1, Phase 2, Phase 3 and Phase 4. Each phase has its unique purpose and its unique safety objectives and constraints. However, the most important factor in characterizing the safety of the new compound in all phases of development is the inclusion of concurrent blinded placebo control arms. Blinded placebo control arms are essential to discerning the new compound's true safety effects. At all stages of development, every additional placebo patient can be considered to be "money in the bank" from a drug development perspective; data from placebo patients are the only protection from false perceptions of a potential new drug's toxicity.

Phase 1 The first trial conducted in man is termed a Phase 1 trial, although other Phase 1 trials, such as drug-drug interaction studies, mass balance studies, special population studies (such as hepatic or renal dysfunction populations) or QTc studies, are often conducted later in the drug development process—after there is accumulating evidence that the drug may work and may have an acceptable safety profile. These latter Phase 1 studies, required for full understanding of a new drug's potential for harm and for safe use, are obviously staged later in the drug development process to minimize investment in compounds that are destined to prove unsafe in Phase 1 or Phase 2 studies or ineffective in Phase 2 or 3 studies.

First-in-man Phase 1 trials are typically escalating single dose/pharmacokinetic studies in which higher doses are studied in successive cohorts. The typical goals of a first-in-man Phase 1 study are to identify doses at which toxicity becomes evident clinically, to characterize the clinical toxicity observed (what organ system(s) are affected, and what form(s) does toxicity assume in that organ system), to determine how reversible that clinical toxicity is, and to determine the blood concentrations at which the clinical toxicity occurs.

First-in-man Phase 1 studies can be conducted in either normal volunteers or in patients. If the target disease is rare, normal volunteers are virtually always used. If the target disease is common, patients are sometimes used for first-in-man Phase 1 studies. Patients with cancer are virtually always used in Phase 1 trials of cytotoxic agents intended for treatment of cancer.

The advantages of using normal volunteers include the following: a) only one clinical site is needed; b) more rapid subject accrual is possible; and c) minor side effects are more easily identified in volunteers than in diseased patients. The disadvantages of using normal volunteers include the following: a) a narrow age range is usually studied; b) typically only males are enrolled; and c) a similar escalating single dose/pharmacokinetic study in successive cohorts will have to be conducted in patients eventually. However, in most cases, the key advantage of using normal volunteers—speed to completion, and as a result, more rapid entry into Phase 2—outweighs the disadvantages. Typically, it is not possible to detect preliminary evidence of efficacy prior to Phase 2, the phase in which patients with the targeted disease are first treated.

Starting Dose In Phase 1 The starting dose in Phase 1 is typically 1/10 of the NOAEL dose identified in the toxicology in the most sensitive species. Each cohort has its own concurrent placebo-control subjects in order to reliably identify which adverse events are related to the new compound. The ratio of placebo to active drug in each cohort is typically 1:3. A typical cohort size is eight subjects, resulting in two subjects on placebo and six subjects on drug at each dose.

Dose increments in Phase 1 are typically two-to-three fold at each step, although slower or more rapid steps in dosing can be required, depending upon the nature and reversibility of the toxicity findings in animals.

Multiple Doses In Phase 1 For many potential new drugs, multiple dosing is not explored in early Phase 1 trials in normal volunteers, but instead is explored in early Phase 2 trials in patients with the targeted disease. However, exploring the toxicity and pharmacokinetics of multiple doses of a new compound in normal volunteers can be a good idea when a compound appears to have little toxicity in animal testing, because toxic effects are more easily detected in normal, healthy subjects. Knowing what clinical toxicities to look for in patients in Phase 2 is a key goal of the Phase 1 program; if escalating single doses in volunteers do not identify toxicity, multiple dose studies in volunteers can be very useful, as volunteers are typically more sensitive to the adverse effects of drugs than are patients.

Use Of Phase 1 Data The safety and pharmacokinetic data from Phase 1 are critical to the decision of whether to proceed to Phase 2, what doses should be explored in Phase 2, and what clinical toxicities should be searched for. For example, if important clinical toxicities occur in Phase 1 at doses/blood levels below those at which efficacy is projected to be seen in Phase 2, the test drug should be abandoned because risks are occurring at doses below those projected to be necessary for efficacy. If clinical toxicities occur in Phase 1 at doses/blood levels well above those at which efficacy is projected to be seen in Phase 2, but those toxicities are either serious or are not readily reversible, the potential new drug should again be abandoned—unless the target disease has no proven treatments and is fatal. Typically, a potential new drug should be carried into Phase 2 only when the toxicities observed in Phase 1 occur at much higher doses/blood levels than those expected to be required for efficacy in Phase 2, are easily identifiable clinically, are not serious, and are quickly reversible when drug is stopped.

The maximum tolerated single dose in Phase 1 is typically the ceiling for single doses in later phases of drug development. All organ systems affected by toxicity in Phase 1 are carefully monitored for toxicity in Phase 2, and specialized testing of the affected organ systems is often utilized. For example, if the new compound caused pulmonary irritation in animals at high doses, and was found to cause cough, chest congestion or wheezing in Phase 1 at high doses, chest radiographs and pulmonary function tests to examine pulmonary irritation at lower doses in Phase 2 would be indicated.

Phase 2a Dose exploration in patients is the hallmark of Phase 2a. Serial escalations of increasing single doses in patients are the first step. The starting dose and the size of the dose increase for each subsequent cohort are determined by the findings in Phase 1. Each cohort has its own concurrent placebo-control patients in order to reliably identify which adverse events are related to the new compound rather than the underlying disease or its treatment. Randomization to placebo versus drug within each cohort can range from 1:3 to 1:1. Equal numbers of patients on drug and placebo (1:1 randomizations) are critical to protect the new compound from false perceptions of toxicity when the patients enrolled have serious diseases.

Multiple doses are also explored in patients in Phase 2a. Most Phase 2a explorations of multiple dosing have "cohort" designs with serial escalations in dose to protect patients from being exposed to toxic doses of drug before the threshold of toxicity with multiple dosing in patients is identified. Again, each cohort has its own concurrent placebo-control patients in order to reliably identify which adverse events are related to the new compound rather than the underlying disease or its treatment.

Occasionally, parallel designs for comparisons of dose safety are utilized in Phase 2a during the exploration of multiple dosing, but in such cases the projected safety margin between therapeutic effects and toxic effects for the compound generally is large, and the toxic effects in animals and in man in Phase 1 are readily identifiable and reversible upon cessation of drug. Again, a concurrent placebo-control arm is critical in order to reliably identify which adverse events are related to the new compound rather than the underlying disease or its treatment.

Use Of Phase 2a Data The data from Phase 2a are used to decide whether the compound should advance to Phase 2b studies. For the compound to advance to Phase 2b, the toxicities identified in Phase 2a should occur only at higher doses, the toxicities identified should occur only at low frequencies, and the toxicities identified should be fully reversible upon cessation of dosing. If preliminary evidence that the drug is effective is also obtained in Phase 2a, and that effectiveness was observed at doses lower than those that caused toxicity, it is far easier to generate support for advancing the compound to Phase 2b.

Phase 2b The hallmark of Phase 2b is dose selection for design of the far larger Phase 3 trials. The typical Phase 2b trial has four arms, one of which is placebo, and the other three of which are low, medium and high doses of the new compound. The randomization is 1:1:1:1. Such a design is not only useful in detecting dose-related changes in efficacy, but also in characterizing safety. Adverse events detected in such a design that occur more frequently on drug and increase with increasing dose are clearly drug-related. In contrast, adverse events that occur less frequently on drug and decrease with increasing dose are clearly a reflection of efficacy, not safety. Adverse events that appear to occur more frequently on drug than on placebo on lower doses of drug, but that occur less frequently on drug than on placebo at higher doses, are not related to drug at all; the findings at the lower doses are noise.

Use Of Phase 2b Data The data from Phase 2b are critical in designing the Phase 3 program, including choices of dose, sample size, and efficacy endpoints, and safety endpoints. The safety effects of the drug identified in Phase 2b are fully characterized in Phase 3, using far larger sample sizes and also specialized testing where needed. Sometimes, sub-studies in which several but not all participating sites run specialized tests such as cardiac MRIs or maximal exercise tests are useful in characterizing the compound's safety findings.

Phase 3a The two classic "adequate and well-controlled" trials that are typically required for proof of efficacy under FDA requirements are Phase 3a trials. The two exceptions to the "repeat it" rule for demonstrations of efficacy in the US are: a) convincing demonstrations of reductions in mortality in the first trial (3, 20-23), in which case it would be unethical to repeat the trial; and b) compounds awarded "fast track" status because they have the potential to address unmet medical needs in the treatment of serious or life-threatening conditions. Under the fast track program, demonstration of efficacy (other than mortality) from a single trial can suffice for marketing approval, in combination with "other confirmatory evidence".

Sometimes, more than one dose of active drug is used in Phase 3a trials; if so, more conclusive evidence on subtle safety effects can be generated. For example, a slightly higher incidence of a given adverse effect in a trial with only one dose of active drug might be presumed to be due to chance. However, a still higher incidence of that same adverse event in a second arm of the trial utilizing a higher dose would constitute solid evidence that the adverse event was in fact drug-related. Usually, when more than one dose is utilized in a Phase 3a trial, the purpose is better characterization of efficacy rather than better characterization of safety, although the latter is accomplished as well.

It is important to recognize that the samples sizes of Phase 3a trials are driven by efficacy, not safety. Typically, enough safety data are generated in the Phase 3a trials for a reasonable risk/benefit assessment to be possible. However, regulators rightly insist on seeing the safety data on all subjects exposed to a new drug in marketing applications, as each subject exposed to the potential new drug contributes to the safety database and betters the chance of detecting rare events.

ICH guidance specifies that 1,500 patients is the minimal total subject exposure for marketing applications, but this number is impractical for very rare diseases, and woefully low when the new compound is for benign or self-limited conditions that are commonplace. It is not too uncommon for additional patient exposures to be required after Phase 3a trials have proven that a new drug is effective and reasonable safety. These additional exposures, often in open, uncontrolled studies, are necessary to obtain adequate safety data for the detection of rare events.

Use Of Phase 3a Data The efficacy and safety data from the Phase 3a trials comprise the centerpiece of a marketing application. The safety data from the Phase 3a trials appear directly in the package inserts of approved compounds as adverse event frequency tables that compare placebo and/or active control to the new drug.

Expediting Drug and Biologics Development

Identifying what remains unknown or insufficiently known (i.e., what else one would like to know about the new drug) in the Phase 3a data is equally important, as continued research and investigation in Phase 3b and Phase 4 are key to refining and implementing the new drug's safety and effectiveness profile. (28)

Phase 3b Trials The term "3b" applies to trials that are conducted after completion of what the sponsor believes constitute successful Phase 3a trials, but before marketing approval. Typically, placebo is abandoned in Phase 3b, particularly when the diseases being treated are serious or life-threatening. Generally, data collection in Phase 3b is streamlined and simplified in comparison to earlier phases.

In the United States, unapproved drugs for serious conditions can be made available for more widespread use as part of trials under a so-called "treatment IND." For example, during the development of synthetic surfactant, a life-saving breakthrough in the prevention and treatment of hyaline membrane disease (respiratory distress syndrome) in premature infants (4-6), an increase in the frequency of pulmonary hemorrhage (from 1% to 2% it turned out) was not recognized in some 17 double-blind trials involving about 3500 patients (25, 26). This failure in detection was purely a function of the combination of the low incidence of pulmonary hemorrhage in the control group and the relatively small effect of synthetic surfactant on that rate (i.e., synthetic surfactant doubled the rate of pulmonary hemorrhage, but did not quadruple it or quintuple it).

The increase in pulmonary hemorrhage caused by synthetic surfactant only came to light during a 10,500-patient study under a treatment IND that went into effect while the NDA NDA was being prepared (27). Identification of this safety problem prior to initial marketing permitted its characterization in the package insert at the time of initial marketing, and led to the insertion of guidance on both reducing its incidence and managing its occurrence in the package insert (25-26). For every 200 babies treated, 40 fewer babies died from hyaline membrane disease or its complications, and one extra baby died from pulmonary hemorrhage.

Randomized comparisons against other drugs approved for the same disease are sometimes conducted during 3b, but more often such comparisons are conducted in Phase 4.

Use Of Phase 3b Data Data from Phase 3b can have many uses, including revisions of package inserts (as above), refinements of designs of new trials in Phase 4, explorations in other indications, and marketing.

Phase 4 Phase 4 trials are trials conducted after marketing approval using the approved dose and approved dosing regime in the approved indication. Such trials can have a variety of designs, depending upon their purposes. Randomized comparisons against other drugs approved for the same disease are often conducted in Phase 4. Open, uncontrolled "physician use" and "patient use" trials are also common.

Use Of Phase 4 Data Similar to data from Phase 3b studies, data from Phase 4 studies can have many uses, including revisions of package inserts, refinements of designs of new trials in Phase 4, explorations in other indications, and marketing. One truism is that continued investment in new clinical trials in Phase 4 is critical to the new drug's widespread adoption in the market and safe use (28).

Conclusion New drug development must be as efficient as possible to maximize the substantial improvements in health and well-being that are possible from ongoing medical discoveries, available capital, and available expertise. Safety problems that limit or prevent developments of potential new drugs should be identified as early as possible during drug development. Doing so will permit redesign or termination of drug development programs at earlier stages, and enable more efficient re-allocation of scarce resources.

References

1. Long WA. Developmental pulmonary circulatory physiology. In Long WA (ed), Fetal and Neonatal Cardiology, WB Saunders, Philadelphia, 1990, pp. 76-96.

2. Solomon SD, McMurray JJ, Pfeffer MA, et al. Cardiovascular risk associated with celecoxib in a clinical trial for colorectal adenoma prevention. N Engl J Med. 352(11):1071-80, 2005.

3. Barst RJ, Rubin LJ, Long WA et al. A comparison of continuous intravenous epoprostenol (prostacyclin) with conventional therapy for primary pulmonary hypertension. N Engl J Med 334:296-301, 1996.

4. Long WA, Thompson T, Sundell H, Schumacher R, Volberg F, Guthrie R. Effects of two rescue doses of a synthetic surfactant on mortality in 700-1300 gram infants with RDS. J Pediatr 118:595-605, 1991.

5. Corbet AJ, Bucciarelli R, Goldman SA, Mammel MA, Wold D, Long WA. Decreased mortality rate among small premature infants treated at birth with a single dose of synthetic surfactant: a multicenter controlled trial. *J Pediatr* 118:277-284, 1991.

6. Long WA, Corbet AJ, Cotton R et al. A controlled trial of synthetic surfactant in infants weighing 1250g or more with respiratory distress syndrome. *NEJM* 325:1696-1703, 1991.

7. Corbet A, Gerdes J, Long W et al. Double blind randomized trial of one versus three prophylactic doses of synthetic surfactant in 826 700-1100 gram infants: effects on mortality. *J Pediatr* 126:969-978, 1995.

8. Courtney SE, Long W, McMillan D et al. Double blind follow up in 1540 infants with respiratory distress randomized to rescue treatment with two doses of synthetic surfactant or air in four clinical trials. *J Pediatr* 126:S43-S52, 1995.

9. Walther FJ, Mullett M, Schumacher R, Sundell H, Easa D, Long W. One year follow up of 66 premature infants weighing 500-699 grams treated with a single dose of synthetic surfactant for air placebo: results of a double blind trial. *J Pediatr* 126:S13-S19, 1995.

10. Sell M, Cotton R, Hirata T, Guthrie R, LeBlanc M, Mammel M, Long W. One year follow up of 273 infants with birth weights of 700-1100 grams after prophylactic treatment of respiratory distress syndrome with synthetic surfactant or air placebo. *J Pediatr* 126:S20-S25, 1995.

11. Casiro O, Bingham W, MacMurray B, Whitfield M, Saigal S, Vincer M, Long W. One year follow up of 89 infants with birth weights of 500-749 grams and respiratory distress syndrome randomized to two rescue doses of synthetic surfactant or air placebo. *J Pediatr* 126:S53-S60, 1995.

12. Gong A, Andalay E, Boros S, Bucciarelli R, Burchfield D, Zucker J, Long W. One year follow up evaluation of 260 premature infants with respiratory distress syndrome and birth weights of 700-1350 gm randomized to two rescue doses of synthetic surfactant or air placebo. *J Pediatr* 126:S68-S74, 1995.

13. Sauve R, Long W, Vincer M et al. Outcome at 1 year adjusted age of 957 infants weighing more than 1250 gm with respiratory distress syndrome randomized to receive synthetic surfactant or air placebo. *J Pediatr*, 126:S75-S80, 1995.

14. Saigal S, Robertson C, Sankaran S, Bingham W, Casiro O, MacMurray B, Whitfield M, Long W. One year outcome in 232 premature infants with birth weights of 750-1249 grams and respiratory distress syndrome randomized to receive two doses of synthetic surfactant or air placebo. *J Pediatr* 126:S61-S67, 1995.

15. Gerdes J, Gerdes M, Beaumont E, Cook L, Dhanireddy R, Kopelman A, Jarrett R, Long W. Health and neurodevelopmental outcome at 1 year of age in 508 infants weighing 700-1100 gm who received prophylaxis with one versus three doses of synthetic surfactant. *J Pediatr* 126:S26-S33, 1995.

16. Corbet A, Bose C, Long W et al. Double blind developmental evaluation at 1 year corrected age of 597 premature infants with birth weights from 500 to 1350 grams enrolled in three placebo-controlled trials of prophylactic synthetic surfactant. *J Pediatr* 126:S5-S12, 1995.

17. Kraybill EN, Bose C, Corbet A, Garcia Prats J, Asbill D, Edwards K, Long W. Double blind evaluations of developmental outcome and health status to age 2 years of infants weighing 700-1350 grams treated prophylactically at birth with a single dose of synthetic surfactant or air placebo. *J Pediatr* 126:S33-S42, 1995.

18. Barst RJ, Rubin LJ, McGoon MD, Caldwell EJ, Long WA, Levy PS. Survival in primary pulmonary hypertension with long term continuous prostacyclin. *Ann Int Med* 121:409-415, 1994.

19. Rubin LJ, Mendoza J, Hood M, McGoon M, Barst R, Williams WB, Diehl JH, Crow J, Long W. Treatment of primary pulmonary hypertension with continuous intravenous prostacyclin: results of a randomized trial. *Ann Intern Med* 112:485-491, 1990.

20. Hinderliter AL, Willis PW, Barst RJ, Rubin LJ, Badesch DB, Groves BM, McGoon MD, Tapson VF, Bourge, RC, Brundage BH, Koerner SK, Lanleben D, Keller CA, Murali S, Urestky BF, Koch G, Lis S, Clayton LM, Jobsis, MM, Blackburn SDJr, Crow, JW, Long W. Effects of long-term continuous infusion of prostacyclin (epoprostenol) on echocardiographic measures of right ventricular structure and function in primary pulmonary hypertension. *Circulation* 95:1479-1486, 1997.

21. Hinderliter AL, Willis PW 4th, Long W et al. Frequency and prognostic significance of pericardial effusion in primary pulmonary hypertension. PPH Study Group. Primary Pulmonary Hypertension. *Am J Cardiol* 84:481-484, 1999.

22. Raymond JK, Hinderliter AL, Willis PW 4th, Clark WR, Ralph D, Caldwell EJ, Williams W, Ettinger NA, Hill NS, Summer WR, de Boisblanc B, Schwartz T, Koch G, Clayton LM, Jobsis MM, Crow JW, Long W. Echocardiographic predictors of adverse outcomes in primary pulmonary hypertension. *JACC* 39:1214-1219, 2002.

23. Hinderliter AL, Willis PW IV, Long WA et al. Frequency and severity of tricuspid regurgitation determined by doppler echocardiography in primary pulmonary hypertension. *Am J Cardiol* 91:1033-1037, 2003.

24. Sever PS, Dahlof B, Poulter NR, et al. Prevention of coronary and stroke events with atorvastatin in hypertensive patients who have average or lower-than-average cholesterol concentrations, in the Anglo-Scandinavian Cardiac Outcomes Trial—Lipid Lowering Arm (ASCOT-LLA): a multicentre randomised controlled trial. *Drugs* 64 Suppl 2:43-60, 2004.

25. Van Houten J, Long W, Mullett M et al.: Pulmonary hemorrhage in premature infants following treatment with exogenous surfactant: an autopsy evaluation. *J Pediatr* 120:S40-S44, 1992.

26. Long W, Corbet A, Allen A et al. Retrospective search for bleeding diathesis among premature newborn infants with pulmonary hemorrhage after treatment with synthetic surfactant. *J Pediatr* 120:S40-S44, 1992.

27. Andrews E, Marucci G, White A, Long W. Associations between antenatal corticosteroids and neonatal outcomes within the Exosurf Neonatal Treatment IND. *Am J Ob Gyn* 173:286-289, 1995.

28. Long WA, Zeng G, Henry GW. New drugs for perinatal practice: the role of industry-sponsored clinical trials. In Sinclair JC (ed), Evidence-Based Perinatal Practice, *Semin Perinatol* 19:132-143, 1995.

CHAPTER 25

Developing a Risk Minimization Action Plan

Louis A. Morris, Ph.D.

The Food and Drug Administration (FDA) recently published a series of guidances that described the agency's best thinking about discovering, managing and evaluating the risks of pharmaceutical products. One of these documents described a new mandate for the pharmaceutical industry—the development of a risk minimization action plan (RiskMAP) for certain drugs. This RiskMAP will need to be submitted to FDA with the new drug application. These guidances explain how companies may comply with FDA regulations.

A RiskMAP is a strategic safety program designed to minimize known product risks while preserving benefits. RiskMAPs target one or more safety goals and use one or more interventions or "tools." These "tools" extend beyond the package insert and routine post marketing surveillance. They are categorized into three areas: education and outreach, reminder systems, and performance-linked access systems. The FDA guidance also describes the conditions triggering the need for a RiskMAP, the selection of tools, the format for RiskMAPs, and the evaluation processes necessary to develop and monitor the success of a risk minimization plan. The RiskMAP describes the background, research, rationale and logic necessary to develop and implement the strategy and tactics for the risk management program.

Some companies have already begun to develop RiskMAPs in anticipation of FDA's request. Others have begun to explore the requirements necessary to create such a plan and still others have not addressed the issue. The development of a RiskMAP requires pharmaceutical companies to "think through" not only how a drug is supposed to be used (the indications, contraindications, precautions, warnings, etc.) but also how it will be used or misused by prescribers, dispensers and patients using of the medication. The role of the RiskMAP is to minimize risks throughout the lifecycle of the drug. For the most part, the plan deals with the control of known or suspected risks, while other risk management activities concentrate on the discovery and quantification of suspected risks. FDA also expresses concerns about overly burdensome risk minimization processes that might interfere with the use of the medication, thereby decreasing the likelihood or magnitude of benefits derived from use of the product.

To fulfill the obligations of developing a competent RiskMAP, drafters must seek to influence the behavior of the parties responsible for drug safety, particularly patients, physicians, pharmacists and allied medical staff. This is not as easy task, as we have seen in evaluations of current risk management programs, such as for Accutane. Therefore, a reasonable RiskMAP must demonstrate that the company understands the "system" of drug prescribing, dispensing, monitoring and use for their particular product. The company must also understand the impact (positive and negative) and limits of various "tools" or combinations of tools selected for implementation, how to test tools before implementation and evaluate the implemented RiskMAP with sufficient specificity to understand the impact of the selected interventions, and how to improve outcomes if the original program does not reach reasonable effectiveness targets. In addition, the implemented RiskMAP must not detract from product sales. Developing risk minimization action programs that assure safe use while simultaneously maintaining sales presents an added difficulty and series of concerns.

While the FDA risk minimization guidance provides pharmaceutical companies with a clear set of directions on the format for RiskMAP submissions, to comply with the guidance, drafters need to apply an appropriate analytical framework, along with insights from original research:

- to conceive of a rational approach for controlling risks,
- to justify the selection of tools or the development new tools,
- to justify why other tools that may be more "potent" (but cause patients or prescribers to reject the medication) are not selected,
- to evaluate the tools prior to implementation and the program after implementation, and
- to plan for quality improvements in the plan as it evolves and to plan for the ultimate withdrawal of the risk management program.

Expediting Drug and Biologics Development

The purpose of this chapter is to provide drafters not only with advice for meeting FDA requirements, but also suggestions on how they may approach the development of a RiskMAP in a manner specific for their drug, select the most appropriate tools and meet FDA requirements without mitigating sales potential.

When is a RiskMAP Needed? To determine if a new drug will need a RiskMAP, the company must consider the risks posed by the product in light of its benefits. For drugs designed to treat serious or life-threatening illnesses, such as cancer and AIDS, there is a great deal more tolerance for personal risk than for drugs used for cosmetic purposes, such as acne or head lice. However, even for serious drugs, when the risk posed may be prevented, a RiskMAP will need to be seriously considered.

The starting point for any RiskMAP is as complete knowledge as possible of the product's safety hazards. Some hazards may be suspected and subjected to continuing post marketing surveillance. There is always debate regarding which signals denote real risks and which denote false positives. Following the precautionary principle, it is likely that even suspected risks will be the subject of some risk intervention, even if it means only notifying prescribers of its possibility. The proposed package insert is likely to serve as the best source of information about the known or suspected risks of the product and the best basis for risk minimization planning.

The FDA suggests three considerations for determining if a RiskMAP is needed: the nature of risks verses benefits (risk tolerance issues such as population affected, alternative therapy available and reversibility of adverse events); preventability of the adverse event, and probability of benefit or success of the risk minimization intervention. Drugs that have serious or life-threatening contraindications, warnings, precautions or adverse effects are the most likely candidates for a RiskMAP. Patient behaviors that can mitigate risks, such as pregnancy prevention, blood tests, overdose/misuse avoidance, awareness and action related to specific safety signals (e.g., a hypersensitivity reaction, depression and suicide), make a RiskMAP more appealing. When people other than the patient may be at risk (e.g., a child may use the product inadvertently), a RiskMAP may also be required. FDA singles out Schedule II controlled drugs, with concerns for misuse, abuse, addiction, diversion and overdose as likely candidates for a RiskMAP.

Rationale and Justification The most important aspect of developing a RiskMAP is to understand the risks involved in using the product in question and the factors that might increase or mitigate those risks. The sections of the drug label where the risk information is provided may provide a clue as to the overarching goals or objectives for the RiskMAP. Contraindications may be related to patient selection or testing that must occur before the drug is prescribed, precautions may relate to advice about how to use (or not use) the product, and adverse reactions may be related to warning signs that must be monitored by the patient and physician or risk/benefit decisions underlying the use of the medication.

Companies must provide a logical rationale for the implementation of a risk management program. The RiskMAP developed must specify this rationale in the background section. Here, the company must enumerate each of the risks to be managed by the program. For each risk, the company must fully characterize the risk severity, the population (or subpopulation) at greatest risk, the extent to which the risk is predictable, preventable or reversible, as well as the time course of the risk (if the risk is time-limited, continuous or cumulative).

The questions imposed for the development of a Medication Guide can be used to help identify/summarize the risks to be managed in a RiskMAP. The exhibit below (Worksheet 1: Determining the Risks to be Managed) can be used to help identify these risks.

Goals, Objectives and Tools The guidance mandates that each plan must specify the overall goals of the risk minimization plan. These goals are the desired endpoints for safe product use. For example, if a drug causes birth defects, a reasonable goal would be that no women who are pregnant should be given the drug. A second goal might be that no women should become pregnant while taking the drug. It should be noted that some goals may never be fully met. However, making progress toward meeting the goal, rather that actually achieving the goal, may be an acceptable outcome.

Once the goals have been enumerated, the FDA calls for companies to identify a series of objectives for each goal. The objectives must be specific and measurable. They specify the behaviors and processes necessary for the stated goals to be achieved. For example, if our goal is to prevent pregnancy, then we may specify an objective that all women must have a negative pregnancy test performed within seven days of initiating therapy. Objectives often identify the particular individual (i.e., patient, pharmacist, physician, allied health professional) responsible for the desired behavior. This aids in the development of a communications plan directed to that individual, which will likely be a core element of the risk management program.

Once goals and objectives are specified, the company must select a series of tools designed to intervene and mitigate risks. The FDA specifies three categories of tools. The first category is "targeted education or outreach." These tools concen-

---

Worksheet 1

What are the Risks to be Managed?

Use the following checklist to determine what, if any, risks need to be managed. After listing, highlight those that are of highest priority. These may serve as the basis of selecting goals, developing communication objectives, and developing systems for mitigating negative effects or outcomes.

I. Who Should Not Take this Medicine?

Demographics (e.g., gender, age,) _____

Medical Conditions (e.g., existing illnesses, poor functioning (e.g., liver, kidney), pregnancy/nursing status) _____

Current Therapy (e.g., medical, pharmaceutical) _____

Previous Therapy (e.g., unless previous therapies are tried) _____

Activities commonly undertaken (e.g., sexual, athletic) _____

Other _____

II. How to Take the Medicine?

Timing _____

Delivery (e.g., injection, inhaler) _____

How to Take (e.g., standing, after meals) _____

Other _____

III. What to Avoid While Taking?

Other Medication _____

Activities (e.g., sexual, physical) _____

Dietary (e.g., certain foods, dieting restrictions) _____

Other _____

IV. What Reactions are the Important Adverse Effects?

Signals or Serious Side Effects

Side Effects that may be Unavoidable:

Physical or Mental (e.g., side effects denoting a serious reaction) _____

Common and frequent side effects _____

Rare but serious side effects _____

Other _____

---

trate on the communication of information intended to minimize risk. They include a variety of media that carry messages to health care professionals (e.g., letters; training programs, (including continuing education (CE) programs, courses or materials; public notifications (such as letters to the editor)). In addition, promotional techniques can be used to publicize risk management concerns, including advertisements and sales representatives' distribution of risk minimization information. Similarly, communications to consumers such as medication guides and patient package inserts may be used. Interestingly, FDA includes limitations on the use of promotional techniques, such as product sampling or direct-to-consumer advertising, as a risk minimization tool. However, these latter tools may do more to limit demand for the medication than directly communicate information on how to minimize product risks.

The second category of risk minimization tools is characterized by FDA as "reminder systems." This is a broad category of tools that go beyond mere information dissemination. Often, reminder systems solicit a commitment to engage in the dictates of the risk minimization program. For example, these tools include training or certification programs or physician attestation of capabilities to use the medication safely. They also include patient agreements or acknowledgment forms that seek the patient's commitment to follow dictates for safe drug use. They include specialized product packaging to enhance safety by influencing who may take a medication or providing reminder information at the point of product use. This category also includes distribution channel controls, such as limiting the amount of medication in any single prescription or refill of a product, as well as specialized systems or records that limit dispensing unless certain measures have been satisfied (e.g., prescription stickers).

The third category of tools is characterized as "Performance-Linked Access Systems." These are tools intended to limit access to the medication based on the fulfillment of certain criteria. For example, the product may not be made available unless there is an acknowledgment, certification, enrollment, or appropriate test records made available. This category of tools would also include limiting prescribing to specially certified health care practitioners, limiting dispensing to specially certified pharmacies or practitioners, or limiting the product to patients with evidence of fulfilling certain conditions (e.g., negative laboratory test results).

The FDA tool characterization is helpful in providing a wide range of options for RiskMAP designers. However, it does not provide a mechanism for determining which tools (or combinations of tools) would be most appropriate in which circumstances. To be fair, although there have been some evaluations of risk management interventions (cf., Goldman, 2004) there is an inadequate knowledge base for objectively determining how these tools should be applied. However, there is a broad set of theoretical models that may be applied to characterize the behavioral aspects of product prescribing, dispensing and utilization. These models may be applied to help determine what mix of tools makes the most sense in terms of influencing safe-use behavior. Acceptance of the tools must also be considered. It is clear, even at this early stage, that risk management tool implementation may have unintended consequences. Prescribers may find certain tools overly burdensome, offensive or adverse and avoid use of the drug not only in spite of, but because of the risk minimization tools selected. Therefore, acceptance as well as effectiveness of any risk minimization plan must be considered when designing the RiskMAP.

Designing the RiskMAP The FDA guidance asks companies to select and justify their choice of tools. In doing so, it behooves a company to develop a conceptual model for how their drugs are used and what "system failures" may lead to product misuse. In addition to relying on a systems analysis, using a behavioral model of product use (i.e., how beliefs, motives, and situational constraints influence how a drug is used) can help a company select a coordinated set of tools and specify core messages that must be communicated or systems implemented to define the elements of their risk management program.

A good starting point for developing a model of drug use is to identify the various steps necessary to use a drug properly. Failure Mode and Effects Analysis (FMEA) is a systematic analysis of how failures in any "system" may occur. An FMEA delineates the steps in a "system," and identifies where mistakes may occur (i.e., potential failure modes) before the system is implemented. It is a complement to root cause analysis, which is aimed at identifying the source of a system's failure once a mistake is identified. If a drug is already marketed, a root cause analysis should be used to identify problems or concerns based on existing information. If the drug has not been marketed, an FMEA is the best alternative. In addition to listing the steps in using a drug effectively, an effective FMEA identifies corrective actions required to prevent failures and to assure the highest possible system quality.

To undertake a FMEA, the system steps and potential failure modes are identified. Each step may be broken down into subprocesses with each "sub-step" in the "system" being considered as a separate element with the potential for failure. Each of the postulated steps where failure might occur is assigned a severity value, a probability that a given effect might occur, and a likelihood value that the user may detect (and correct) the problem. Recommended actions (i.e., tool interventions) are developed to reduce the probability and (most importantly) severity of harm, with priority given to the highest.

While developed as a method to improve product quality, FMEA can only be as good as the quality of the system description. Specifying steps at too broad a level of specificity can miss important elements. For example, we performed a system analysis for a medications error problem, where pharmacists were dispensing the incorrect medication of patients. We found that many physicians correctly wrote the drug name on the prescription and the pharmacist dispensed what the physician had identified. The problem was that some physicians recalled the incorrect drug name from memory when they wrote the prescription. If we would have used a FMEA that did not specify the need for the physician to recall the correct drug name from memory, we would have missed an important source of error.

In addition to specifying the subprocesses, it is necessary to understand the "system" from the perspective of the individuals performing the tasks involved. It is well established that the relationship between knowledge and behavior is not direct or simple. We often know what we should do but fail to behave in a fashion consistent with our knowledge. To develop a predictive model, it is necessary to understand: (1) the full set of beliefs underlying behavioral intentions, (2) the motivations that support or stand in the way of exhibiting desired behavior, and (3) the environmental conditions that facilitate or place barriers to compliance.

There are a variety of psychological and health behavior models that can be used to organize these influences. Some models may help to improve the processing of presented information—for example, by improving participants' involvement (personal relevance) or competency (self-efficacy) with the information or advocated behavior. Some models may help to understand the processes underlying choice among alternative courses of behavior (behavioral decision making). Some models may help to structure advocated behavior into a series of stages, permitting a series of messages that seek to "move" respondents through a necessary series of stages in order to attain behavioral compliance (stage models or precaution adoption). Some models seek to motivate compliance through emotion (fear appeals or positive affect) or through highlighting desired outcomes (approach or avoidance goals).

Worksheet 2

What should people do to use the drug properly?

Developing a FMEA

1. Use the general steps listed below to begin your work. Delete, add or adapt steps in the primary system (main headers) and subsystem (secondary headers) that are peculiar to the drug in question.

2. List the possible sources of system failure (note: while only one is listed, there may be several for each step).

3. For each source of failure, using a ten-point scale (1-10), rate the probability that the failure will occur, the severity of harm if it does occur and the likelihood that the failure may be detected and corrected under the current system (for the later item, 1= high likelihood of detection and 10=low likelihood of detection).

4. Multiply the three ratings to obtain a Sum Score (ranging from 1 to 1000). Using a cutoff, highlight those items that have the highest index. Selected cutoffs ranging from 500 to 900 is possible corresponding to a 50% to 90% index. Also highlight those items with high severity scores, regardless of probability or detection scores.

5. The highlighted items represent those steps that are in most of need of some intervention or set of interventions to prevent failure. Select an intervention for that item. Note that one intervention may apply to several steps (e.g., a Medication Guide can inform patients about several possible failure modes).

System/Subsystem	Sources of Failure	Probability	Severity	Likelihood Of Detection	Sum	Intervention
I. Diagnosis	MD Skill is poor					
A. History Taken	Patient memory is poor					
B. Lab Test Taken	Patient had no time to get lab tests					
C. Other...						
II. Drug Prescribed	Patient is Contraindicated					
A. Concomitant Medications Assessed	Patient does not know previous medications taken (never knew names)					
B. Laboratory Findings Reviewed	No Lab Test available					
C. Patient Consent Obtained	Patient does not understand risks/benefits					
D. Other						
III. Counsel Patient	Poor Communications					
A. Review Safe Use Instructions	Time Pressures on Doctor					
B. Provide Written/Audiovisual Information	Not Easily Available					
C. Assign Testing/Revisit Instructions	Scheduling for patient or doctor difficult					
IV. Materials Reviewed/Obligations Fulfilled by Patient	Patient does not understand information provided					
A. Read all Patient Materials	Low Literacy					
B. Ask Questions/Seek Clarifications	Patient does not want to "question" doctor					
C. Sign any Agreements, Consents, etc	None available					
D. Other						
V. Obtain Rx at Pharmacy	Patient does not receive correct medication or instructions					
A. Accuracy of SIG verified	Pharmacist misreads Rx MD writes wrong name/SIG					
B. Obtain Counseling / Information	Pharmacist too busy to counsel					
C. RPh Checks for Prescription/ Dispensing Adequacy (i.e., Drug Utilization Review System)	System to check accuracy is turned off					
Other...						
VI. Patient Takes Medication	Patient does not comply with instructions					
A. Number/Timing of Medication Taking	Patient Forgets Dose					
B. Concurrent Activities/ Conditions Modified as Required	Patient forgets contraindications and precautions					
C. Other...						
VII. Patient Monitors Therapy	Patient is unaware of monitoring requirements					
A. Patient asks for advice when needed	Patient uncertain when to ask for help					
B. Patient is aware of/actively monitors for warning signals	Patient does not understand what constitutes condition for a warning signal					
C. Laboratory Tests/Revisits as required	Patient cannot get to test facility					
D. Other						

Expediting Drug and Biologics Development

The selection of a model depends on the particular problem (objective) addressed. If we advocate complex behaviors, such as avoiding drug dependency, it may be necessary to "move" respondents through a series of stages in order to overcome situational barriers. If we advocate simpler behaviors, such as standing upright when taking tablets, providing a strong, even emotional, rationale for compliance and a reminder system might provide the best model to influence behavior. "Diagnosing" the behavioral problem and selecting (or custom building) the correct behavioral model can provide a clear method for the design of the risk management plan.

Because we are dealing with programs that are expected to reach and influence the vast majority of participants, it may be difficult to anticipate the full range of issues influencing the behavior of all of the patients and healthcare professionals. Research studies that provide insights into these issues are invaluable. Identifying particular at-risk segments can also help to design program interventions targeted at particular failure modes for a specified group of individuals.

To design a RiskMAP, it is important to understand the "system" that underlies correct use of the product...and the points in the system where "failure" may occur. The "generic" system in the exhibit below (Worksheet 2: Developing a FMEA) can be used to to delineate the steps necessary for correct use.

Developing Interventions Once a system has been specified, we can identify the needed interventions. Although the FDA specifies three categories of tools, we find it helpful to use a two-class categorization. The first class of tools are those that rely on information dissemination to foster adaptation of behavior. This class may be further divided in terms of the specific objectives sought (see below). The second class of tools relies on distribution channel controls to limit access to the medication to certain prescribers, pharmacies or patients. Additional classes of tools are also conceivable, such as a redesign of the medication itself (e.g., reformulating a product, such as adding a difficult-to-defeat timed release form of the product to permit safe use of extended release pain relievers) or economic incentives for compliance with safe use mandates (e.g., decreasing the cost of the product through rebates or coupons if certain procedures are followed). This categorization follows the classic lines of marketing positioning, where we seek to influence perception (and use) of a product by design of the four "Ps": product, place (distribution), promotion (communications) and price.

Whether information and/or distribution controls are necessary will depend on the nature of the risk to be minimized. For contraindications, where proper diagnosis or patient selection is an issue, where certain conditions must be met before the drug may be issued or, where certain commitments are desired, some form of distribution control may be helpful. For risk/benefit decision making, where proper monitoring for reactions to the drug is essential or where certain precautions must be followed, information dissemination is likely the indicated class of tools. Information dissemination is likely to be important for any RiskMAP, because even if distribution controls are the tools of choice, participants must be able to understand the program's requirements. Distribution controls may be more likely to be perceived as undesirable by patients and providers because of the additional hurdles needed to prescribe, dispense or obtain the medication.

It is likely that multiple interventions will be necessary, if for no other reason than the need for redundancy to assure exposure to the key messages. For patient information, there are a number of communication vehicles, each with a slightly different purpose (see exhibit below). The tool or combination of tools selected should be based on the purpose of the document. If patient commitment to a long-term behavior is an issue, a patient agreement or contract may be advised. If situational cues are needed, packaging reminders or telephone calls may be advised. The selected tool should match the particular need for particular impact.

Message Development and Tool Designation A broad process model may be helpful in selecting communication tools. The process model specifies that, in order for communications to influence behavior, several steps must occur. Specifically, participants must: be exposed to the information; pay attention to the communication; understand what is advocated; accept the persuasive intent; remember the message; incorporate the message in their decision making process; and display the advocated behavior over the time period as needed.

Designing a set of communications to influence all of these steps requires some thought and some trade-offs. For example, having patients exposed to the message may be better accomplished if the information is delivered in the medication package. However, patients may not pay attention to a long document written in small type on thin paper. Thus, a smaller document that provides key messages may be more likely to be noticed. This may be augmented by a longer brochure provided by the physician or pharmacist that explains the rationale for advocated behaviors. Adding a reminder program, such as warning symbols on the package, could also help stimulate memory for the advocated behaviors and provide a more complete communications program. A certain amount of repetition and redundancy in message delivery can increase the likelihood that desired communications are delivered and a higher order of information processing is undertaken by the patient. However, too much repetition can "wear out" the reader, causing a lack of willingness to read and process the presented communication.

Patient Communications Vehicles

Tool	Distribution	Purpose
Brochure	Physician	General Information
Patient Package Insert	Package or Pharmacist	Risk Communication
Medication Guide	Package	Risk Communication and Methods of avoidance
Informed Consent	Physician	Acknowledgement of Risks
Warning Stickers	Package	Risk "signal"
Wallet Card	Starter Kit	Reminder
Stickers for Medication Vial	Pharmacist on Medication Vial	Reminder
Patient Agreement or Contract	Physician	Behavioral Commitment
Decision Aid	Physician	Choice of Therapy
Video Tape or CD	Physician or Starter Kit	Persuasion or Choice of Therapy
Recurring Interventions (telephone calls)	Telephone	Behavioral Maintenance

Drafting risk management communications requires attention to both the content and the style/format of communication. The content of the message needs to be clearly specified. Developing a list of communication objectives (COs) can help to identify key messages for any document. These COs may also be used to assess the impact of the communication and the risk management plan in general. To develop this list, it is important to rely on the FEMA system, the behavioral model developed or adapted for this product, and the base beliefs of the target audience.

A simple, but helpful model for selecting content is to use the "Philou Window" (designed by Philip Ley and Lou Morris) (see exhibit below), which identifies the nature and degree of explanation needed for describing risk minimization directions. It is based on the idea that people must be willing and able to comply with each risk minimization direction. Thus, people must know what to do, and depending on the behavior advocated, they may also need to know how and/or why to do it. Thus, for some messages, it will be sufficient to tell people what to do (i.e., how to comply with the risk minimization procedures). For other messages, the advocated behavior may require certain skills (e.g., long-term behavioral maintenance, difficult to identify warning signals). For certain behaviors, we may request that people refrain from desired actions (e.g., avoiding alcoholic beverages or sexual intercourse). To convince people that such advocated behavior is worthwhile, we may need to provide a persuasive rationale for the risk minimization procedure.

Designing Risk Message Content

Risk Message Content	Patient is Able to Perform	Patient is Unable to Perform
Patient is Willing to Perform	What to do (Necessary Risk Minimization Actions)	How to do it (Skills Necessary)
Patient is Unwilling to Perform	Why to do it (Persuasion)	All

Some risk communication experts advocate a "mental models" approach to specifying content. In this instance, the base beliefs of health experts are compared to those of recipients of the communication. Areas where the belief systems vary are highlighted to assure that the risk communication focuses on areas where information is most needed. However, this approach has the potential to expand the information content base for patient information. To the fullest extent possible, the COs should be "trim" and focused. Too many COs can reduce the likelihood of communicating any single CO. For complex messages, specifying primary and secondary COs can help to organize the information.

The style of communication also needs to match the CO's intent. Primary messages need to be emphasized by "signals" such as placement, graphics and language. There are a number of "document design principles" that may help to make the communications clear and comprehensible. For example, short sentences, vivid and understandable terminology and avoiding extraneous information can help to reduce the "cognitive load" of any communication and aid in achieving high levels of comprehension (Morris and Aikin 2001).

Patients store information in memory in the form of a "schema." This is a network of associations that, when "activated" causes patients to remember key information. The content and design of the schema dictates how warning messages are understood and remembered. By organizing the content of patient information tools in a particular fashion, we can help patients construct a schema that is consistent with our risk minimization goals. See exhibit below (Worksheet 3: Designing Patient Schema).

System Enhancements Most of the tools discussed above involve the one-way transfer of information. With well-designed documents and repeated interventions, the probability that key messages will be communicated increases. However, developing an education program that tests an individual respondent's understanding of these messages can go a long way to improving communication. Rather than rely on individual "tools," we may develop an integrated "system" for educating patients of prescribers. Using an interactive voice response (IVR) system, the web, or even a paper-based format, patients may enroll in a system that surveys knowledge (based on the COs). Tests are scored and a "feedback" message can be delivered to the physician and/or the patient. The feedback message reinforces areas where key messages were understood and provides tailored feedback in areas where the key messages were not understood. This focus on the patient's knowledge, as opposed to the content and format of the message, can improve the likelihood that core messages are comprehended. By testing for beliefs, motivations, decision making ability and behavioral intent, feedback forms can provide a variety of messages intended to influence behavior beyond mere knowledge transfer. By applying the test prior

---

Worksheet 3

How to Say It: Designing a Patient Schema

Schemas may be described as a series of nodes with connectors. The central nodes are the primary messages, with secondary and tertiary messages "fanning" out. Memory activation starts with the central nodes and "activation spreads" to adjoining nodes. The further out from the central node, the least likely the information is to have sufficient "activation" to be retrieved in memory. The best message organization, therefore, is one where most important messages are centrally stored, with additional rationale or explanation as supporting information. What are the most important messages...see your communication objectives. Remember, the purpose of the document is of modify or reinforce certain behaviors.

Exercise A: Review Example Messages 1 and 2 below. Which Message is better? Explain why by reviewing the resulting schema.

Exercise B: Based on the message presented, draw the resulting schema. Review the schema and then redraw it by placing the most important information (actions to be undertaken) in the central node position and secondary messages radiating outwards. Revise the message to improve the likelihood of behavioral compliance. (Remember, we can emphasize key messages with the use of graphic signals as well as rewriting content).

Example Message 1: This drug may cause birth defects if taken while pregnant. Patients taking this drug have had children with clef palates. Use both a primary form and a secondary form of birth control to prevent pregnancy. Birth control pills are a primary form and condoms and barrier methods are secondary forms.

Example Schema 1:

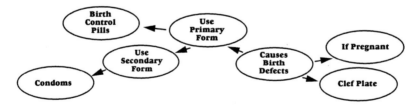

Example Message 2: Do not get pregnant while taking this medicine. If taken while pregnant, it may cause birth defects in the unborn child, such as clef palate. To prevent pregnancy, use two forms of birth control simultaneously. One form should be a primary form, such as birth control pills, and the other form should be a secondary form, such as condom or barrier method.

Example Schema 2:

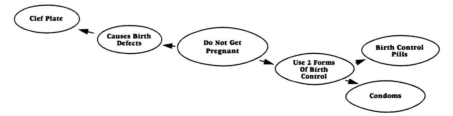

Example Message: If you have ever had liver problems, you should not take this product. People with liver or kidney problems may have difficulty getting rid of the drug. The drug may build up in your system and may cause an overdose. This may cause more permanent problems, such as difficulty taking other medicines or digesting certain foods.

Draw the sample Schema.

---

to the prescribing of the drug product, minimum test scores can be set, assuring that only competent patients are certified to receive the prescription.

Risk minimization programs may also be designed to help discover or quantify risks. These programs may involve some form of patient registry. A registry is defined as a systematic collection of defined events or product exposures, in a defined patient population, for a defined period of time. Thus, all patients (or all patients from selected sites) may be enrolled in a registry so that their experience using the medication may be followed. In this instance, measured experience is likely to be focused on selected adverse outcomes. Alternatively, all patients with selected outcomes (e.g., pregnancy) may be enrolled in a registry to determine the outcome of the precipitating event.

In the process of enrolling patients into the registry, it is possible to also implement certain risk minimization interventions. For example, for the Tracleer(r) (bosentan) registry, patients are telephoned monthly. Outcomes data are obtained and patients are reminded of liver and pregnancy testing requirements. If the patient states "no test done," the prescriber is contacted. Because there are only three distributors, there is thorough control over drug distribution.

Testing and Evaluation Finally, the FDA concept paper guidance implores companies to test their risk management interventions and to evaluate the risk management program. Individual tools can be tested to assure that they meet their intended purposes. For example, it is important that patients be able to comprehend key warnings and be convinced that advocated behaviors be undertaken to prevent harm. Using mall intercept or small patient studies, draft communications tools can be assessed to determine if core communication objectives are understood. Messages that are not communicated can be analyzed and redrafted. Comprehension testing has become routine in the development of OTC labels. These labels are often redrafted several times in order to develop a comprehensible label (changing language, placement, graphic emphasis for particular communication objectives). Not only may comprehension testing assess the communication of core messages, but other outcomes may be measured, such as assessing: (1) belief change and persuasion, (2) ability to problem solve and influence decisions, and (3) the impact of the communication on behavioral intentions. Testing of communication tools before implementation (including tools directed at healthcare professionals) may help not only to improve the utility of the tool, but also to protect the company from product liability in failure to warn cases.

FDA specified the need for two methods to assess the overall impact of the risk management program. The use of an administrative database (such as those maintained by several health plans) may serve to assess the overall impact of the risk management program. For example, if a program is designed to assure that all of the individuals taking a certain medication have a blood test prior to each refill, the percentage of patients obtaining a blood test within the health care system may be assessed. Each database has specific limitations, and expert epidemiologists can attest to the strengths and limitations of each database. Even without strong confidence that the majority of patients are captured in a database, comparisons of pre-to-post risk management program implementation can provide a reasonable estimate of the program's impact. Repeating the analysis in a second database would help to provide confidence in the reliability of the estimate. However, if a program is found to perform at less-than-hoped-for levels of effectiveness, use of an administrative database may not be capable of determining the reason for lack of success. Therefore, a second method of assessment, such as a survey of patients or providers, can assess the "intermediate impacts" of a program (e.g., awareness of the protective behavior, understanding the need to engage in the behavior, persuaded to engage in the advocated behavior, ability to overcome situational barriers to compliance, being able to repeat and maintain the behavior over time), which can help a risk management planner revise the program where it is most needed.

Rather than advocate the need to achieve a specified level of performance, as an evaluation goal, each RiskMAP should advocate continuous quality improvement. Planned evaluation periods are essential. Prior to program implantation, it may not be possible to understand the degree of noncompliance with a risk-minimization program. It also may not be possible to understand the cause of system failures. Overly burdensome programs may inhibit product use by making prescribers unwilling to try the product or by making it difficult for patients to obtain the product. While "unintended consequences" may be assessed in a survey evaluation of the product, they may not be fully understood in terms of their actual impact. By performing evaluations that assess the broad outcomes and the intermediate impacts of the program, we can institute modifications to shore up these weaknesses. Thus, it may be possible to continuously improve the program. In this manner, we may ascertain the continued need for the individual tools and for the coordinated program. Further assessment of the presented risks may reveal that they are not as severe, that they are not as likely, or that they may be easier to prevent than originally feared. Thus, the need for or the type of risk minimization interventions may be modified as new information is accumulated.

A reasonable and competent program must be initially proposed for the drug to be accepted for marketing. However, risk management, by its very nature, seeks a high degree of impact and compliance to assure the safety of the product's users.

Expediting Drug and Biologics Development

The FDA cannot accept programs that are shown to be ineffective. Nor is it reasonable for a program to be fully effective without some trial. Thus, companies must make a commitment toward developing and achieving effective risk management programs. The alternative-withdrawing the drug from the market—offers little solace to either the pharmaceutical company marketing the product or the patients who need access to the medication.

Conclusion Risk management provides both a challenge and an opportunity for pharmaceutical companies. It forces companies to understand not only how a drug treats disease, but how it is used. It also forces companies to develop a coherent set of interventions intended to influence use. Developing the informational tools and system controls should benefit patients and providers by improving the safe use of medicines. However, it should also benefit the drug company, not only by improving drug safety, but also by building trust and support,, and by increasing personal responsibility for safe drug use.

References

Morris, L. A. and Aikin, K. J. The "pharmacokinetics" of patient communications. Drug Information Journal, 2001, 36(2), 509-527.

Stamatis, D. H. Failure Mode and Effects Analysis. ASQ Quality Press: Milwaukee, Wisconsin, 1995.

* An earlier version of this paper was published in Pharmaceutical Executive, June, 2004.

CHAPTER 26

Assembling and Filing the Common Technical Document

By Diana Fordyce, PhD, RAC, Stephen P. Truocchio, MS, RAC, and Karl Whitney, PhD, RAC

Compiling a CTD: Paper or Electronic?

Now that the common technical document (CTD) format has emerged as the standard format for marketing applications in the ICH (International Conference on Harmonisation of Technical Requirements for Registration of Pharmaceuticals for Human Use) regions, industry sponsors are faced with deciding whether to submit the application in paper or electronic form. While paper-based submissions have been the standard for many years, some of the more prominent worldwide regulatory agencies have started allowing-and increasingly encouraging—sponsors to submit electronic applications. Initially, this movement was fragmented, with different regions adopting different standards for electronic applications. The ICH's development of the electronic common technical document (eCTD) format represented an attempt to standardize the way in which the pharmaceutical industry can transmit electronic applications to regulatory agencies, much the same way the CTD format attempted to standardize the way in which information is organized in a marketing application.

Paper submissions have one major advantage over electronic: paper will never be obsolete. If stored under appropriate conditions, paper can survive for centuries. In contrast, there is uncertainty regarding the long-term storage of electronic documents. The electronic storage of data is only in its infancy; CD-ROMs were invented barely two decades ago. Although testing has been done, it has not been conclusively proven that electronic media will stand the test of time as well as paper. Furthermore, assuming electronic media can survive the test of time, will we be able to read the media in the future? Technology is rapidly advancing, so much so that programs and operating systems less than a decade old are already obsolete. In the end, we may be in a situation in which we saved the information properly, but are not able to read or process it.

Another advantage of paper in this context is its familiarity. Most seasoned agency reviewers have been using paper, and not advanced electronic review tools, their entire careers. For some, it is more intuitive to reach for a binder on a shelf and thumb to a particular page or section than to have to point-and-click through hyperlinks and read large documents on a computer screen. Over time, as these reviewers retire and are replaced by others who grew up with computers much or all of there lives, this phenomenon should be far less significant. In recognition of the current reality, however, eCTD specifications do not prevent reviewers from printing portions of electronic applications on-demand when paper review would be more beneficial.

These advantages of paper aside, electronic submissions are the future of regulatory applications. Electronic documents, coupled with the eCTD's use of lifecycle management attributes, will allow regulatory reviewers to improve their review speed and efficiency in ways that could never be realized with paper-based submissions. The principle advantage is the concept of the lifecycle management concept inherent in the XML (eXtensible Markup Language) backbone of the eCTD. This allows an application to grow over time, so that reviewers can always see the most current information. This concept is sometimes referred to as the so-called "cumulative table of contents." Although the CTD and eCTD were developed initially for marketing applications, the FDA has long maintained that the true value of the eCTD's lifecycle management/cumulative table of contents approach would be unlocked once industry also began to apply the format to earlier submissions, particularly IND submissions, to which separate submissions (e.g., safety reports, protocol changes) are provided over many years.

When an electronic application is submitted, agency reviewers have tools through which they can view the application as a whole and drill-down to the information necessary for the review quickly and easily. Outdated information that has been updated or replaced can be marked as such by the XML backbone, which will notify reviewers and prevent them from wasting time on information that is no longer current. Review tools will also provide agency reviewers with an opportunity to "customize" their views of an application so that they can readily start and stop their reviews as time permits. In addition, the ability to transmit clinical and nonclinical data in electronic format affords the reviewer the opportunity to reproduce the sponsor's data displays quickly and easily, without having to manually recreate them. Reviewers can also manipulate the data displays to validate the sponsor's conclusions regarding the product's is safety and effectiveness.

Electronic submissions can shave time off both sponsor submission and agency review times. In the end, however, the decision over whether to develop and submit an application in paper or electronic format is ultimately the sponsor's, since regulatory agencies continue to accept paper-based submissions. This chapter is designed to help sponsors in developing marketing applications in both the paper-based CTD format and the eCTD format.

Reference Tools for CTD and eCTD Submissions

The following discusses highlight the ICH and FDA guidances that should be consulted when constructing a CTD or eCTD.

M4 CTD Organization Specification

While the contents of this guidance, entitled "Common Technical Document for the Registration of Pharmaceuticals for Human Use (2001), are discussed in another chapter, a company should consider the granularity options presented in this document when preparing for the CTD/eCTD's compilation. This document also provides information on document pagination and formatting (applicable to electronic and paper), and formatting the module-level tables of contents (paper only).

CTD General Questions and Answers Documents

These useful "Q and A" documents are compilations of the questions that were submitted by industry and agency sources and that were then addressed at semi-annual ICH meetings. There are now more than half a dozen of these Q&A documents that address specific sections of the CTD/eCTD (overall organization, quality section, efficacy section, safety section). These documents are updated periodically, and should be consulted when a particular guidance does address a topic of concern to the sponsor.

M2 eCTD Specification

This guidance, entitled "eCTD: Electronic Common Technical Document Specification," is the cornerstone for submissions in the eCTD format. The body of this document is brief and places in context the background, scope, requirements, and change control procedures for the eCTD. The bulk of the information is contained in the nine appendices outlined below. Much of the information in this guidance is discussed in more detail throughout this chapter.

1. Overall Architecture: This contains a discussion of the business model and reasoning behind the eCTD. The eCTD was designed as a way for industry to transmit data to regulatory agencies in an electronic fashion that can be used over the entire lifecycle of a product-from initial application through amendments, eventual approval, and future supplements/variations. This is accomplished through the use of a computer language called XML, or eXtensible Markup Language. While the eCTD requires the respective regulatory authorities to create and establish specifications for the eCTD's Module 1 (Administrative and Prescribing Information), the specifications for Modules 2 thorough 5 are identical across the three ICH regions. The FDA established the specifications for Module 1 in the September 2001 draft guidance entitled, "Submitting Marketing Applications According to the ICH/CTD Format: General Considerations."

2. The eCTD Submission: In the most basic terms, the eCTD is merely a collection of folders and files, with a single file (the XML backbone) containing information about all the files comprising the submission. The submitted files contain data and reports necessary for the agency review. This appendix contains a general overview of the presentation of the eCTD and how regulatory authorities will see and use the eCTD submission.

3. General considerations for CTD modules: This appendix provides detailed information on folder and filename conventions as well as sample screenshots of the eCTD folder hierarchy.

4. File organization for the eCTD: This appendix provides a large table that shows the organization of the eCTD files, including the section number, title, XML element name, the directory name (i.e. pathname), filename, and any applicable comments. This information should be coupled with the

information provided in Appendix 3 to flesh out the eCTD structure. The file names are not mandatory, but are highly recommended.

5. Region-specific information: This section recommends that applicants consult the applicable regulatory agencies on issues such as how the region-specific forms should be transmitted, methods of transport, security (especially if the eCTD will be transmitted over the Internet). The section also provides an outline of what information should be provided in the cover letters, regardless of region.

6. XML submission: This appendix contains information on the use of XML metadata to accomplish the lifecycle management, including the use of the operation attribute (discussed in more detail in the section on document lifecycle).

7. Specification for submission formats: This appendix contains detailed information on how the submission's PDF content files should look, including such information as font size, page size and orientation, bookmarking, hypertext linking, and page numbering. The formats for XML files and other types of files are also discussed.

8. XML DTD: The line-level code of the eCTD XML DTD (document type definition) is provided in this appendix. The XML DTD defines the hierarchical structure of the CTD and the allowable metadata. As such, the DTD is used to validate the index.xml file to ensure that the proper conventions outlined throughout the eCTD spec were followed. The DTD is versioned whenever the specs are changed—a history of the changes to the DTD as a result of changes to the spec are outlined near the beginning of the file in plain text. A copy of the DTD must be provided in the util folder of every submission.

9. Glossary: This appendix provides terms associated with the eCTD. A more complete explanation of some of these terms is found in the Glossary of Terms section at the end of this chapter.

FDA Guidance for Industry: Providing Regulatory Submissions in Electronic Format - Human Pharmaceutical Product Applications and Related Submissions Using the eCTD Format (October 2005)

This guidance provides general information on how sponsors should organize information within eCTD-formatted submissions to be filed with the FDA. This document makes reference to several other guidance documents and attachments that contain more specific technical information on the different modules, including the study tagging files specification for the submission of study reports and the submission of clinical trial data in electronic format. Since the eCTD can accommodate "lifecycle management," the FDA permits not only NDA/BLAs, but also INDs, drug master files (DMF), and other related applications to be submitted in the eCTD format. The guidance also discusses the FDA's willingness to permit the conversion of paper submissions to eCTD format without requiring the resubmission of previous paper-based information.

Paper Compilation

When a sponsor is planning for a paper application, it must consider the issue of volume separation. To further organize the submission, the company should consult the granularity guidance (the M4 Granularity Annex, October 2005) when determining where tabs should divide individual granular documents. These granular documents should be page numbered from 1-n, where n is the number of pages within a document. The tabs should include the section number and the name; however, abbreviated titles may be used. These abbreviated titles can also be used in the document headers. For example, the title "3.2.S.7.2 Post-approval Stability Protocol and Stability Commitment (name, manufacturer)" can be shortened to "3.2.S.7.2 Postapproval Stability (name, manufacturer)."

According to CTD guidance, modules should be separated into separate volumes according to the following schema:

Module 1	Single volume (e.g., Volume 1 of 1) With tabs for each individual document
Module 2	
• Sections 2.1-2.5	Volume 1 of 3 With tabs for each granularity section (e.g., 2.1, 2.2, etc.)

–continued–

–continued–

Section 2.6	Volume 2 of 3* With tabs for each granularity sub section (e.g., 2.6.1, 2.6.2, etc.)
Section 2.7	Volume 3 of 3* With tabs for each granularity sub section (e.g., 2.7.1, 2.7.2, etc.)
Module 3	Volumes as necessary (1 to X) With tabs for each granularity section (e.g., 3.2.S.1.1, 3.2.S.1.2, etc.) and literature reference
Module 4	Volumes as necessary (1 to X) Study reports (1 tab each or tabs within as necessary) Literature references (1 tab each)
Module 5	Volumes as necessary (1 to X) Study reports (1 tab each or tabs within as necessary) Literature references (1 tab each)

*more than 1 volume is possible for Section 2.6 and 2.7

Paper CTD Tables of Contents and Cross-References

Since there is no overall page stamping in the CTD, the module-level paper Table of Contents (TOC) should refer to the volume in which a document can be found (e.g., Module 3, Volume 2). The depth of the module-level TOC is dependent on the granularity chosen for that particular module (e.g., 2.3.S vs. 2.3.S.1), and should point the reviewer to a document that is delineated by a tab. The TOC should not provide any detailed sections beyond the given CTD headings, since those are best expressed in a document-level TOC. For Modules 4 and 5, the depth of the TOC should go down at least to the level of the study reports, but can go beyond to delineate the individual items within a study report if desired.

When providing cross-references in a paper CTD in the text, authors should include the CTD section number, title (abbreviations are acceptable), and page as well as the module/volume number where the document can be found. As an example: for a comprehensive discussion of the analysis methods, see Section 2.6.4.2 Methods of Analysis (Mod 2 Vol 2; 2.6.4 PK Written Summary; Page 7)

Document Formatting for Paper and Electronic Submissions

If a sponsor is submitting the application to multiple ICH regions, the company should employ margins that allow the application to be printed on both standard 8.5" x 11" (US) and A4 paper (EU and Japan) without obscuring information in the binding margin. Margins of less than 1" should be avoided. For font selection, the CTD guidance recommends 12-point, Times New Roman font for narrative text. The corresponding size for Japanese font is 10.5-point MS Mincho. No recommendations are offered regarding tables, although the text should be large enough to be legible and to be photocopied with minimal loss of quality. In most instances, using less than a 10-point font should be avoided.

Section Numbering

Sponsors have two choices for section numbering. The first is to use complete CTD numbering for headings within a document. For example, a section numbered 2.6.2.3.3.1.1 is permissible. As an alternative, sponsors may choose to abbreviate the numbering within a document. Using the same example, the section could also be numbered 3.3.1.1, provided that the document number and name (2.6.2 Pharmacology Written Summary) are clearly marked in the header or footer of the document. Regardless of the numbering system chosen, it is wise to use the built-in automatic numbering functions within popular word processing software to keep section numbering issues to a minimum.

Pagination

Pagination for individual granular documents should always begin at number 1 and continue consecutively until the next document. Exceptions to this rule can be made for literature references (for which the journal page numbering will suffice) and for appendices that may have their own internal pagination.

Electronic Compilation

PDF (portable document format) is the most commonly accepted format for electronic files, and should be used whenever possible. In some instances, it is permissible to use other types of files (e.g., graphics files for building layouts). Under a December 2003 regulation, the FDA requires that the elements of product labeling be submitted in electronic format in

NDAs, and the agency used an April 2005 guidance document to describe how sponsors could submit the so-called "content of labeling" section using a standard based on XML.

According to the M2 eCTD guidance, the files should be named properly. Allowable characters include lower case letters, numbers, and hyphens. Spaces, colons, periods (except to separate the filename from the extension), underscores, and uppercase letters are not permitted. The maximum allowable filename length is 64 characters, and the maximum pathname is 230 characters

When possible, documents should be created electronically from their inception to permit reviewers to conduct full-text searches. Scanned documents cannot be searched in this way, and should only be used for legacy documents or for pages on which signatures are required.

Bookmarks and Hyperlinks

When documents are provided in PDF format, they should be bookmarked and hyperlinked to promote ease of navigation. Bookmarks should be provided for at least each major section within a document. Hyperlinks in the body text should link reviewers to all references, related sections, publications, appendices, tables, and figures not located on the same page. In general, hyperlinks should be used whenever a cross-reference would have been used in a paper submissions. Also, lists of references should be hyperlinked to the appropriate publications.

There are computer programs that facilitate the linking of documents, although these programs require consistency in how the reference is expressed in the text if their auto-linking capabilities are to prove beneficial. Before authoring begins, these conventions should be outlined and explained for authors to reduce the amount of time spent hyperlinking once the sections are complete.

Although quality control of created bookmarks and hyperlinks can be a tedious and time-consuming task, it is crucial to ensure that navigation within the application goes smoothly for the reviewer. First, plan ahead in timelines for this task. Similar to the creation of links, there are programs available that can be used to check the validity of the links; however, these programs only indicate whether or not a link is broken. They cannot be used to confirm that a link goes to the correct target when clicked (e.g., the link might go to the wrong page). Sponsors should use such programs to quickly find broken links, but should also plan for a human check of all links before the final submission.

Document Lifecycle

The eCTD embraces the concept of document lifecycle for regulatory submissions. Since lifecycle management has no relevance to the paper submissions of the past, it can be difficult to grasp at first. Lifecycle management is accomplished technically by making use of the operation attribute in the XML backbone along with the modified file attribute. The operation attribute is a "meta datum" that tells the reviewing agency how the files within a submission are to be treated. In conjunction with the operation attribute, the modified file attribute signifies which previously submitted file is affected by the operation. Only append, replace, and delete operators require a value for a modified file.

The allowable values for the operation attributes are as follows:

Operation Attribute Value	Meaning	This file is:	The previous file is:
• New	The file has no relationship with files submitted previously.	Current	NA-there is no previous file
• Append	This means there is an existing file to which this new file should be associated (e.g., providing missing or new information to that file). It is recommended that append not be used to associate two files in the same submission (e.g., splitting a file due to size restrictions).	Current	Current-Appended
• Replace	This means there is an existing file that this new file replaces.	Current	Replaced
• Delete	There is no new file submitted in this case. Instead, the leaf has the operation of "delete" and the "modified file" attribute identifies the file in a previous submission that is to be considered no longer relevant to the review.	NA-no file is submitted when using the delete operation	No longer relevant to the review

NA = not applicable

Expediting Drug and Biologics Development

The exhibit below provides an example of how the operation attribute can be used and how the agency reviewers will see the submission in their review tools. In this example, the document (manufacturer1.pdf) describing "Manufacturer 1" was submitted in the original application with a "new" operator.

Sequence Number	Filename	Operation Attribute	Modified File	What Agency sees
0000	0000\...\manufacturer1.pdf	New		manufacturer1.pdf (current)

In the next submission (0001), the sponsor has changed manufacturers and submits a replacement document with information on the new manufacturer. The agency reviewer will see that Manufacturer 1 has been replaced and that Manufacturer 2 is the current manufacturer of the product.

Sequence Number	Filename	Operation Attribute	Modified File	What Agency sees
0000	0000\...\manufacturer1.pdf	New		manufacturer1.pdf (current)
0001	0001\...\manufacturer2.pdf	Replace	0000\...\manufacturer1.pdf	manufacturer1.pdf (no longer current) manufacturer2.pdf (current)

Here, we see the delete operator using an analytical method document (Method 1) as an example.

In a subsequent submission (0015), the sponsor is no longer using that analytical method and notifies the agency using a delete operator. Note that no new file is submitted here; the information regarding the deletion is only contained in the XML backbone.

Sequence Number	Filename	Attribute	Operation Modified File	What Agency sees
0000	0000\...\ method-1.pdf	New		method-1.pdf (current)
0015		Delete	0000\...\method-1.pdf	method-1.pdf (no longer current)

Study Tagging Files

The Study Tagging File (STF) specification was created to provide additional information about nonclinical and clinical studies, such as the species, route, duration, and controls used in the study. The eCTD backbone files do not contain information on the subject matter of the study report documents. Hence, this additional information is provided in the STF.

It is helpful to think of the STF as a mini-XML backbone that provides information about a particular study. In terms of lifecycle, the STF can be treated in the same way as any other eCTD file. When a sponsor makes the first submission for a study, the STF gets a "new" operation attribute. Subsequent submissions can make use of the "replace" operation when new study information is being submitted. This allows STFs to be used at the IND stage, whereby a clinical study report is built "from the inside out"—first with the submission of the protocol and investigator information, and eventually the full report and associated data as it becomes available.

The reason it is called a study tagging file is that the information that comprises a study report can be "tagged" using the values specified in the exhibit below to signify what is contained in a particular file. Each of the element names in the following table need not be in a separate file. The "info-type-value" is used to signify the agency (e.g., FDA) for a particular tag. While there are only values for ICH and FDA currently, it is reasonable to believe that other agencies will create tags for region-specific documents. The STF spec is versatile, and allows more than one tag to be assigned to a particular document within a study. For example, the study protocol and list of investigators could be contained in the same file with two tags in the STF (protocol-or-amendment and list-description-investigator-site) for the one combined file.

Study Tag Element Name	info-type-value	Contents (ich-e3 references)
legacy-clinical-study-report	ich-e3	Complete study report.
synopsis	ich-e3	Study Report Synopsis (e.g., E3 2)
study-report-body	ich-e3	Study Report Body (e.g., E3 1, 3 to 15)
protocol-or-amendment	ich-e3	Protocol and/amendments (e.g., E3 16.1.1)
sample-case-report-form	ich-e3	Sample CRF (e.g., E3 16.1.2)

–continued–

Study Tag Element Name	info-type-value	Contents (ich-e3 references)
iec-erb-consent-form-list	ich-e3	IEC and IRB and Consent Form Listings (e.g., E3 16.1.3)
list-description-investigator-site	ich-e3	Description of Investigators (e.g., E3 16.1.4) and Sites
signatures-investigators cer (e.g., E3 16.1.5)	ich-e3	Signatures of principal or coordinating investigator(s) or sponsor's responsible offi-
list-patients-with-batches	ich-e3	Listing of patients receiving test drug(s) from specified batch (e.g., E3 16.1.6)
randomisations-scheme	ich-e3	Randomisations Scheme (e.g., E3 16.1.7)
audit-certificates-report	ich-e3	Audit Certificates (e.g., E3 16.1.8) or similar documentation
statistical-methods-interimanalysis-plan	ich-e3	Documentation of statistical methods and interim analysis plans (e.g., E3 16.1.9)
inter-laboratory-standardisation-methods-quality-assurance	ich-e3	Documentation of Inter-laboratory Standardization Methods and Quality Assurance (e.g., E3 16.1.10) or similar documentation
publications-based-on-study	ich-e3	Publications Based on the Study (e.g., E3 16.1.11)
publications-referenced-inreport	ich-e3	Publications Referenced in the Study Report (e.g., E3 16.1.12)
discontinued-patients	ich-e3	Discontinued Patients Listing (e.g., E3 16.2.1)
protocol-deviations	ich-e3	Protocol Deviation Listing (e.g., e.g., E3 16.2.2)
patients-excluded-from-efficacy-analysis	ich-e3	Patients Excluded from Efficacy Analysis Listing (e.g., E316.2.3)
demographic-data	ich-e3	Demographic Data Listing (e.g., E3 16.2.4)
compliance-and-drug-concentration-data	ich-e3	Compliance and/or Drug Concentration Data Listing (e.g., E3 16.2.5)
individual-efficacy-response-data	ich-e3	Individual Efficacy Response Data Listing (e.g., E3 16.2.6)
adverse-event-listings	ich-e3	File contains Adverse Event Listings (E3 16.2.7)
listing-individual-laboratory-measurements-by-patient	ich-e3	Individual Laboratory Measurements Listed by Patient (e.g., E3 16.2.8)
case-report-forms	ich-e3	CRF for an individual subject (e.g., E3 16.3). You should also provide a "property" element, described below, with its "name" attribute = "site-identifier" and its value the site identification where the study was performed.
available on request	ich	A file that lists documents available on request. Consult regional guidance for use.
data-tabulation-dataset	us	Data tabulation dataset
data-tabulation-data-definition	us	Data definitions for data tabulation datasets
data-listing-dataset	us	Data listing dataset
data-listing-data-definition	us	Data definitions for data listing datasets
analysis-dataset	us	Analysis datasets
analysis-program	us	Program file for analysis dataset
analysis-data-definition	us	Data definition for analysis datasets
annotated-crf	us	Annotated CRF for datasets
ecg	us	Annotated ECG waveform dataset
image	us	Image files
subject-profiles	us	Subject profile. You should also provide a "property" element, described below, with its "name" attribute = "siteidentifier" and its value the site identification where the study was performed.
safety-report	us	IND safety report
antibacterial	us	Antibacterial microbiology report
special-pathogen	us	Special pathogens (e.g., fungi, parasites, mycobacteria) and immune modulator microbiology report
antiviral	us	Antiviral microbiology report
iss	us	Integrated analysis of safety - integrated summary of safety report
ise	us	Integrated analysis of efficacy - integrated summary of efficacy report
pm-description	us	Postmarketing periodic adverse event drug experience report description
individual-subject-data-listing	us	Individual subject data listing
nonclinical data	us	Data developed prior to module 5 clinical studies

Expediting Drug and Biologics Development

The figure below is a representation of an STF for fictional Study 201. At the top, we can see a display of the metadata describing this study. After the metadata, we see the study report contents on the left side of the screen (synopsis, protocol-or-amendment, etc.), and on the right is the metadata for each file for the study. Looking closer at the study report body, we see the property containing the Leaf ID of the study report body file in the XML backbone. Because of the leaf ID, the STF can be used to co-locate files from across different folders (when data are provided in a different folder) and across multiple submissions, allowing the study report to be put together over time.

Study Files' Content Infomation

Category	Category Value
Study Title:	A double-blind placebo controlled study of therapy X versus therapy Y
Doc ID:	Study Report 98765
type-of-control(ich) placebo	

File Content Labels		Study Tagging File Extract
study-report-body	Document title=	
	Relative Filename=	
	Property= leaf-id(fda) : ./././././/0001/index.xml#id_91_0001	
protocol-or-amendment	Document title=	
	Relative Filename=	

Submission of Data

The recommended format for the submission of data to reviewers is SAS Transport format. The submission of data in this format allows reviewers to process data collected by the sponsor to validate the sponsor's conclusions regarding a drug's safety and effectiveness. All SAS datasets should be accompanied by a data definition file (define.pdf) that explains the variable names used as well as any coded values (e.g., 1 = related, 2 = not related). In addition to the data definition, the annotated case report form (CRF) should be provided in PDF format to allow reviewers to see how the data were collected.

The recently released Study Data Tabulation Model (SDTM), which was developed in conjunction with CDISC (Clinical Data Interchange Standards Consortium, an independent standards organization), should be consulted for variable naming conventions as well as details regarding the collection, processing, and analysis of data for regulatory submission. The data itself should be placed in the "datasets" folder of Module 5 as in the following diagram:

⊟ 📁 [folder name]	Replace with folder name, e.g., m5
⊟ 📁 Datasets	
⊟ 📁 [study]	Replace with study identifier, e.g., 123-070
⊟ 📁 analysis	Contains analysis datasets and associated files
📁 programs	Contains program files
📁 ecgs	Contains annotated ECG waveform datasets
📁 listings	Contains data listing datasets and associated files
📁 profiles	Contains subject profiles
📁 tabulations	Contains data tabulation datasets and associated files

If the above convention is followed, all study data files should be appropriately tagged and linked from the STF. This allows reviewers to start at the STF and get to both text and data, depending on their preference, and mitigates having to navigate to data differently than the text.

eCTD Glossary of Terms

Checksum: An alphanumeric character string that is calculated for each file contained in a particular submission. The checksum is calculated using an algorithm known as MD5 (message digest 5), and corresponds to a particular file's size and the date/time last modified. If a file is modified, then its checksum will change. The checksum for each file is added to the XML backbone metadata. When a submission arrives at the reviewing agency, the checksum is verified to ensure that none of the transmitted files have been altered since the submission was finalized. The checksum can also be used by the regulatory agency to verify that a document was not altered over time while at the agency (e.g., when an upgrade or migration occurs).

Document Type Definition (DTD): The ICH eCTD XML DTD contains the rules for how the XML tags should be formed and organized for a regulatory submission, and is used to validate the XML backbone when it arrives at the agency. The contents of this file are dictated by the eCTD M2 specifications. The ICH DTD should be included in the util folder of every submission.

Granularity: A granular document is defined by the granularity guidance. In a paper submission, a granular document is separated from another with a tab. In an electronic document, a granular document is contained within a single file (i.e., one PDF file).

Leaf ID: A unique identifier that is part of the metadata for a document in the eCTD submission. The leaf ID should start with a letter (e.g., ID_00001) and be unique within an XML Instance. The Leaf ID is used to identify a particular document when, during its lifecycle, the operation attribute is used to append, replace, or delete the document. It is also used in the STF to identify the document for a particular study.

Operation attribute: The operation attribute of the eCTD permits "lifecycle management" to occur. The operation attributes for the eCTD are: new, append, replace, and delete. In the initial application, all files are marked "new." As subsequent amendments are made, the attributes can be used to notify the regulatory agency of changes to the application so that the reviewer can see which information is current and which information is out-of-date.

Metadata: Metadata are data that describe data; therefore, they are data about data. The XML backbone contains metadata for the entire submission and for every file in the submission. Metadata on the submission level include information about the submitting and receiving organization, the manufacturer, the type of submission (e.g., NDA, IND, DMF), and the submission number. Examples of metadata on the document level are versioning information, operation attributes, language, and descriptive information, such as document names and checksums.

Portable Document Format (PDF): PDF is an open file format that preserves the appearance of a document regardless of the application in which it was created.

Study Data Tabulation Model (SDTM): A set of specifications for the collection, processing, and analysis of data devised by the Submission Data Standard working group of the Clinical Data Interchange Standard Consortium (CDISC). More information on the SDTM is available from the CDISC web site at www.cdisc.org.

Study tagging file (STF): The STF is an XML file that contains metadata for a particular nonclinical or clinical study. One STF is submitted for each nonclinical and clinical study in an eCTD application. The STF contains information about each study, such as the species, route, duration, and type of control used, and allows reviewers to easily navigate to and within a particular study. The STF also contains links to the individual files that make up the study report, including data files.

eXtensible Markup Language (XML): A computer language that facilitates the transfer of data and associated metadata (see metadata) from one point to another by marking the data with tags. The language is "extensible" because the tags that identify data are not defined inherently by the computer language, but rather are defined externally using an XML DTD (an XML schema may also be used) (see DTD). ICH has developed an XML DTD to define the content of regulatory submissions capable of lifecycle management.

XML Instance: An XML instance is defined by a single XML file. For example, the XML backbone of an Initial IND submission could be considered an XML Instance. The backbone of each subsequent IND amendment is an individual XML instance. An STF is an example of another XML instance.

XML stylesheet: An XML stylesheet is used to display the contents of a submission (i.e., the index.xml file) in a standard web browser (e.g., Internet explorer, Netscape) with hyperlinks to each individual document. A simple XML stylesheet is provided by ICH, and should be included with each submission in the util folder.

CHAPTER 27

The FDA Marketing Application Review Process

By Craig Ostroff, Pharm.D., R.Ph.

Many pharmaceutical industry professionals frequently joke that submitting their newly completed marketing application (new drug application, or NDA) to the FDA for review is akin to placing the NDA in the slot of a "black box" and watching to see if an approval comes out the other side. This is unfortunate. The review of a marketing application at the FDA is a rigorous, multi-disciplinary, and deadline-oriented process that requires that the applicant's development program be carefully evaluated within a strict, agency-mandated timeframe. The final result of this review is the FDA's determination regarding whether the applicant has adequately evaluated the product and whether the safety and efficacy of the product have been adequately demonstrated for its intended use and target population.

Organization of the Review Process The review of a marketing application is a complex process that requires the input of a number of different scientific disciplines as part of a core review team. This core team, ultimately led by either the respective office[1] or review division director or his/her appointed designee, works toward assimilating the many points of input into an overview perception of the product's safety and efficacy and will also formulate the product labeling based upon this perception. In order to assure that this process occurs in an orderly and timely fashion, a project manager (sometimes known as a consumer safety officer (CSO)) is assigned to manage the application's review by the respective reviewers upon its arrival at the appropriate review division. (CDER's Office of New Drugs (OND) is composed of a number of review divisions, each with specific therapeutic areas of expertise.)

The reviewers first assigned to a marketing application represent the three key review disciplines that make up a review division: project manager (review management and labeling); medical officer (clinical); and pharmacology/toxicology.

The initial review assignments then continue into the standard review disciplines that are "co-located," or are assigned to a review division but that actually report through a separate line authority: review chemist (e.g., chemistry, manufacturing, and controls (CMC)); clinical pharmacology reviewer (e.g., pharmacokinetics/pharmacodynamics (PK/PD)); biostatistician (e.g., for clinical efficacy or safety review; CMC stability study data). Other scientific or administrative disciplines are brought into the review as "consults" on an as-needed basis.

How the separate disciplines form a review team A core review team of the three key review disciplines is formed from members of the IND review team that was responsible for the original and/or ongoing review of the IND, when relevant, and as personnel workload allows. The respective office, review division director or appointed designee then leads this team and is also designated the "signatory authority" for the eventual action letter issued at the conclusion of the review. The team works towards assimilating the many points of input from the extended review team into an overall perception of the safety and efficacy of the product, and will formulate the product labeling based upon this perception.

FDA review philosophy The review division must determine if the application contains "substantial evidence" of the safety and efficacy of the new product or use.[2] The evidence is then described as appropriate in the different sections and types of the labeling for the product.

In order to do this, the agency also considers all past meetings, correspondence, information requests, and outstanding issues in arriving at the final evaluation. The FDA generally assumes that, when an original application (NDA, or abbreviated NDA (ANDA)), supplement to an approved application (SNDA), or resubmission of an application or supplement is submitted to the agency for review, the applicant believes that the agency can approve the application with the as-submitted data. This means that applications should be as complete as possible at the time of submission, and that applicants should not plan, as a rule, to amend their applications with significant additional information during the review cycle.

Determination of Product Jurisdiction When a marketing application arrives at the FDA, either: (1) the NDA will be forwarded to the division that was responsible for the product's IND; or (2) the center's ombudsman will determine intercenter product jurisdiction if the product is a drug/device and drug/biological combination product. This determination of jurisdiction for combination products is made in accordance with memoranda of understanding that have been set up between the respective Centers.[3]

Application Receipt and Processing The physical receipt and processing of an application has been streamlined since the full implementation of the electronic document room. Electronic versions of complete marketing applications are received by the central document room (CDR) and placed onto an internal website within 3-5 days of receipt. Prior to electronic submissions, the NDA volumes would arrive in cartons at the CDR. Considering that a large NDA can number at greater than 1,500 volumes, it could take three to five days for the CDR to barcode and process the volumes for delivery to the appropriate review division.[4] A key issue with the paper submission is where to store the hundreds of volumes, as it is each reviewer's responsibility to do so either in his/her office or by negotiating with colleagues for the limited shelf space lining the corridors of his/her floor.

Assignment of Reviewers Once the marketing application arrives, the project manager must determine who will comprise the review team. This is done by cursorily reviewing the application and determining the review disciplines initially needed. The team leaders for the key review disciplines are contacted and provided with the first volume of the submission in paper or the EDR link, as appropriate. The team leaders review the document and, in consideration of current and expected workload, resources, and timelines, will assign a reviewer. The premise is to maintain continuity of review by assigning the same reviewer who had handled the IND submissions, if possible.

Prescription Drug User Fees and the Review Clock Under the Prescription Drug User Fee Act (PDUFA),[5] FDA committed to meeting certain goals for reviewing and acting on marketing applications for human drugs.[6] The underlying assumption of the user fee goals is that the agency will commit to reviewing the marketing application within a set timeframe after the applicant has submitted a complete application. "Complete" is used here in the sense that the applicant is not planning to submit for consideration major portions of additional data later on during the review cycle.

PDUFA II arose from revisions to the user fee provisions as included in the enactment of the Food and Drug Administration Modernization Act of 1997[7] (FDAMA). The goals were further revised in conjunction with the enactment of the Prescription Drug User Fee Amendments of 2002 (PDUFA III).[8] PDUFA III specifically states that user fees will be dedicated to expediting the drug development process and the process for the review of human drug applications in accordance with the new performance goals.[9] Further information, including current fee schedules, can be located on the FDA website.[10]

The project manager must determine if a submission is subject to user fees. PDUFA provides for different user fees for original applications depending upon whether they are accompanied by clinical data on safety and efficacy (other than bioavailability or bioequivalence studies). PDUFA also levies fees on supplements to human drug applications that contain clinical data.[11]

A determination then takes place as to whether or not proper payment of the user fees has been rendered. If the payment is not rendered within five days of receipt of the marketing application, or the company is considered to be in "arrears" (i.e., the applicant has not paid any and all outstanding fees by the payment due date to the satisfaction of the FDA Office of Financial Management), FDA will refuse to accept the application for filing and therefore delay the start of the review clock until the situation is resolved. [12]

Determination of Review Clock The agency's activities are ruled by deadlines, and those deadlines for marketing applications are taken quite seriously. According to the U.S. Code of Federal Regulations (CFR), technically within 180 days of receipt of an NDA, FDA will review it and send the applicant either an "approval letter," an "approvable letter," or a "not approvable letter."[13] This 180-day period is called the initial review cycle or clock. For marketing applications that are affected by PDUFA[14], the initial review cycle will be adjusted to be consistent with the agency's user fee performance goals for reviewing such applications and supplements. It is important to note that at any time prior to approval, an applicant may withdraw an application and later submit it again for consideration.[15]

Additionally, it is determined if the review clock will be set as a Priority or Standard review. A priority review is typically a 6-month review clock. The product must provide a significant improvement compared to a marketed product in treatment, diagnosis, or prevention of a disease (the disease does not have to be serious or life-threatening). Examples of how the improvement can be shown include a documented improvement in patient compliance, elimination or significant reduction of a treatment-limiting drug reaction or by demonstration of safety or effectiveness in a new subpopulation of patients.

Applicants will typically try and secure an agreement with the agency prior to actual submission that a marketing application will be reviewed a particular way. Although a reviewer may believe that an application might be a priority or standard review after the pre-NDA meeting, not until the complete application is finally submitted can the true assessment take place. Otherwise, any commitment would be made on an assumption of what may be submitted as part of the application versus what actually is listed in the volumes.

Determination of Chemical Classification Type Determination of chemical class type is an administrative activity little known outside of the agency, but it is worth mentioning. The application has to be classified into one of a number of categories for tracking purposes:

- Type 1 = New Molecular / Chemical Entity or where the active ingredient has not been approved in US
- Type 2 = New Ester, Salt or Other Non-covalent Derivative (Active ingredient is not new, but derivative is)
- Type 3 = New Form, Formulation or Strength
- Type 4 = New Combination of drug products that have not previously been combined
- Type 5 = New Manufacturer (of a duplicate drug as already approved)
- Type 6 = New Indication (that uses identical drug product as already approved)
- Type 7 = Drug already marketed but done so without an NDA (Products marketed before 1938, or on the DESI list from 1938-1962)[16]

The Administrative Filing Review of the Application While the industry may use the term "filing" as a synonym for submitting an application, within the agency this term has a specific meaning. Sponsors submit; the FDA files. Within 60 days of receipt of the marketing application, the agency has to determine if it is "filable." The agency must then "report substantive deficiencies identified in the initial filing review to the applicant" in a single communication, which will include the agency's expectations for applicant responses, if any.[17] A filing review issue is defined as:

> Substantive deficiencies or concerns identified by the review team during the initial filing review for an NDA or efficacy supplement that appear to have been inadequately addressed in the application and merit particular attention during the review process. These issues may have a significant impact on the agency's ability to complete the review of the application or approve the application or parts of the application. Filing review issues are distinct from application deficiencies that serve as the basis for a refusal to file action.

The filing review philosophy considers the question, "Is the NDA sufficiently complete on its face to permit a substantive review?" This means that, when each of the reviewers looks at the submission, he/she must determine if it appears to contain what is likely to be necessary in order to render an opinion on the application. The fact that a reviewer may conclude that an application will not obtain approval during this review cycle has no bearing on the outcome of this review of the initial "filability."

Each review discipline has its own requirements for the filing review. An example for a medical officer could be a review of the application's table of contents to confirm that the studies listed are in fact present in their entirety. The medical officer could then create an overview of the application, set up a review plan, and perform a data analysis in order to identify the investigators who had the most impact on the key studies, for example, by either having the most patients or generating particular results that overly influenced a key safety or efficacy measure. The project manager, meanwhile, would have more administrative concerns to review, such as assuring that all of the filing requirements are met as outlined later in this section and filing the appropriate internal paperwork attesting to the fact. The project managers also help to ensure that each of the review disciplines have what they may need as they perform their own review.

A pharmacology reviewer would review the application's table of contents to confirm that the studies listed for that section are in fact present in their entirety. Then an overview of the nonclinical section would be created and a review plan set up.

The chemistry reviewer and the clinical pharmacology reviewer would perform a similar review for their respective sections.

The biostatistician, in addition to performing the above, has to also work with cross-cutting multiple review disciplines depending on the discipline's needs. Analyses of the medical safety and efficacy data, chemistry stability tables and clinical pharmacology studies also need to be performed.

Additionally, each of the disciplines can have specific guidelines for the review that are individualized.

Expediting Drug and Biologics Development

A filing review meeting is usually combined with a project-planning meeting, and traditionally takes place near Day 45 of the review clock. The meeting aims to address the following topics:

- Decision to File, or Refuse to File, based upon 21 CFR 314.101(d)

  Refusals to file are rare, and mostly occur in extreme cases where the application is frustratingly incomplete or vastly disorganized. The reviewers are counseled by agency management to work as diligently as possible to resolve the deficiencies with the applicant and not refuse-to-file an application. If the application is missing some documents or the index is poorly constructed, the reviewers should advise the applicant and afford them the opportunity to amend the application accordingly.

- Determine Level of Sign-off

  If the application is a new molecular entity (NME) or the first in a new class of compounds, then the responsible Office of Drug Evaluation director will sign the action letter and retain ultimate oversight of the review. For all other non-CMC related applications, the review division director will assume this role.

- Application Integrity Policy

  The Application Integrity Policy (AIP) describes "the actions FDA takes when it finds that an NDA/ANDA applicant has compromised the government's product application review process. The AIP policy is invoked for applications pending for the affected facility or company when the agency's findings reveal: (1) a pattern or practice of submission of false or misrepresented data, which is material to approval in applications; or, (2) bribery or paying of illegal gratuities to agency employees. The Agency will then ordinarily defer scientific review of all pending applications and supplements until it conducts a satisfactory evaluation of the accuracy and reliability of the information submitted in those applications.[18] The FDA checks to see if the applicant has previously been subject to the application of this policy and if it is currently on the list of concern.

- Debarment Certification[19]

  A check is also performed to determine if the required certification is present concerning the disassociation of the application with any debarred person or site. The required statutory language of the certification statement states that the "applicant did not and will not use in any capacity the services of any person debarred in connection with the application."

- Financial Disclosure by Clinical Investigators[20]

  A confirmation is made that a financial disclosure statement (Form FDA 3454) and the relevant follow-up information (Form FDA 3455) is present and in order, when relevant. The agency may choose to refuse to file any marketing application that does not contain either "a certification that no specified financial arrangement exists or a disclosure statement identifying the specified arrangements or a statement that the applicant has acted with due diligence to obtain the required information, and an explanation of why it was unable to do so." The agency has issued a detailed industry guidance on this issue.[21]

- Patent Information and Certification[22]

  The submission of patent information and the appropriate certifications is confirmed.

- Trade Name Review

  The proprietary name of the product is sent out for review by the time of the filing meeting, so members of the Office of Drug Safety can evaluate the proprietary name aside from the review division. The office performs an analysis of the name to see if there are any approved drugs with look-alike or sound-alike names that could potentially cause a medication error once out on the market. This analysis often involves focus-groups, verbal and handwritten analysis, along with computerized testing. A trade name can be pre-reviewed at any time, but any clearance previously provided must be rechecked just prior to approval in case new products have been approved that could cause problems.

- Environmental Assessment[23]

  A determination is made regarding whether the requirements for an assessment of any potential environmental impact caused by the manufacture, etc., of the drug product, as set forth in 21 CFR 25, have been met. If the impact is calculated to be within acceptable limits, then a "Categorical Exemption" is allowed and no further action is necessary. If the requirements were not met, then an Environmental Assessment would need to take place with a resultant outcome of a Finding of No Significant Impact, (FONSI) in order to proceed with the application's approval.

- Is there a Need for a Site Audit?

  As mentioned previously, the medical officer will perform a data analysis in order to identify the investigators who had the largest impact on the key studies, had the most patients, generated particular results that overly influenced a key safety or efficacy measure, or disclosed that they had significant financial arrangements with the applicant. Depending on the degree of influence a site has on the overall results, a site audit (to be performed by the Division of Scientific Investigations (DSI)) may be requested. The DSI auditors would review the data at the site to assure that it was in compliance with Good Clinical Practice (GCP) or Good Laboratory Practice (GLP), as relevant. Although more rare, site audits can also be requested for a key toxicology study if its outcome is at the center of a challenging review and the data look questionable.

  In addition to the clinical site audit, a site audit of the manufacturing site(s) (i.e., a pre-approval inspection) by the Office of Compliance is also requested at this time.

- The Need for Clinical Pharmacology input is assessed.

  If the application contains bioequivalence studies or assessments of the PK or PD of the product in varying situations (e.g., a food-effect study), a clinical pharmacology review will be necessary.

- Is the Index sufficient?

  The Index/Table of Contents is checked to assure that it is complete and accurate.

- Do the electronic portions of the application all work as described/intended?

  Hypertext links are checked to assure that they are valid and work as expected.

- Are the paper portions present? Are they legible?

  Paper or electronic portions are checked to make sure that they are legible, interpretable, and not otherwise clearly inadequate (e.g., a Table of Contents should have hypertext links and bookmarks).

- Internal review schedule planning

  Each discipline, and the review team as a whole, considers its workload and sets milestones for the review. At the beginning of a 10-month review, project team meetings might be every other month. Within 90 days of the action date, the project team begins to meet more frequently. Usually, when just two disciplines such as the medical officer and the statistician have to work out study details, this will be done informally (e.g., in someone's office). There is a lot of interaction with the review team members during the review period. This is assisted by the fact that the majority of the team is also working together on other projects—therefore, the opportunity for team members to ask questions of one another is often available.

- Content of the Filing Review Issue letter is Discussed

  Once the filing meeting is complete and a decision is made to file or to refuse to file the application, a Filing Review letter is created and sent to the applicant within 14 days of the close of the filing period. At the conclusion of the filing meeting or immediately thereafter, the issues to be included in that letter are reviewed.

Once the application is filed, the full review of the application begins.

FDA Application Review Philosophy In addition to assuring that all regulations and statutory requirements were met, reviewers also consider the balance of the data for the drug product between its safety and its efficacy. The safety of the patient is always paramount in the reviewer's mind, and that is viewed in consideration of how a drug will be indicated for use. A product that is used for 10 days requires a distinctly different scientific judgment of its unique benefit:risk ratio compared to that of a chronic, maintenance medication. The same is true for products intended to treat more serious diseases where a little more risk might be permitted compared to the potential benefit (e.g., oncology treatments). The opposite is true in products intended to treat milder diseases (e.g., seasonal allergy medication) where the tolerance for risk of an adverse effect (e.g., high liver enzymes) is lower.

120 day Safety Update The applicant is expected to update its application by Day 120 of the review with any new safety information that has been gathered since submission of the marketing application. Typically, this is a short submission consisting of ongoing adverse event counts or similar reports. Applicants sometimes try to use this update to incorporate major or additional information that was not available at the time of the original submission into the review cycle. The review division has the discretion to either review any amendments during the initial review cycle or defer review until the subsequent review cycle. Typically, if an amendment is received more than three months before the end of the initial review cycle, its submission will not trigger an extended cycle. Submission of a major amendment to an application within three months of the end of the initial review cycle constitutes an agreement by the applicant to extend the initial review cycle by three months.[24] A major amendment is defined as "containing significant new data from a previously unreported study or a detailed new analysis of previously submitted data."

Inter-review occurrences & communications with the company During the review, the ultimate approvability of the product is unclear and unofficial until the action letter is actually signed. Up until that point, internal opinions can change and issues on the ultimate action can teeter back and forth until clarity is gained from internal discussions. Therefore, reviewers and others cannot clearly tell the applicant what the final decision/outcome will be because it's only an educated but unofficial guess at that time. In the U.S., any material information about the action of the review may be reportable under SEC regulations for a publicly held company, which could force interim comments about the application to be released that may ultimately turn out to be untrue. For these reasons, preliminary information regarding a final decision is not released.

When any questions arise during the review that were not already covered in the filing review letter, an information request letter will be sent to the applicant requesting either information or clarification on a specific point. If any review discipline (traditionally, the chemistry reviewers) completes its review significantly early in the review cycle, a discipline review letter can be issued. This letter is a courtesy to inform the applicant of the deficiencies that were found in their application, and allows the applicant an early opportunity to begin resolving the issues. Sometimes, the issues in the letter can be resolved rather quickly and the applicant will amend its application with the response. It will be up to the discretion of the chemistry reviewer to determine if the new information will be compiled in the initial cycle's review. This discretion is directly based upon the reviewer's current workload and the work that would be generated by the amendment.

Obtaining advice/Input for the Review Division During the review process, a consult can provide a mechanism for input from other groups in the agency that have a particular expertise in (at least) the drug review process, marketing and advertising, compliance issues, legal/congressional proceedings, etc. Consults are considered recommendations, where the received outcome is reviewed by review team, as appropriate, and the ultimate determination to "agree" or "disagree" with conclusions received lies with the requestor (e.g., review division). A well-known consult group is the review division's advisory committee, which the division can ask for an opinion on specific questions. See related chapter on advisory committees elsewhere in this text.

End of Review Activities Toward the conclusion of the review cycle, the team meetings become more frequent and an opinion becomes apparent from each of the review disciples concerning its survey of the data. Usually within 30 days of an action date, via a "wrap-up" meeting, the review team comes to agreement on the approvability of the product. The remainder of the time is spent on finalizing reviews and working on the labeling for the product. A division may also work on product labeling if the action is not going to be an approval and if the reasons for the non-approval are simple or straightforward (such as inadequate chemistry stability data) and will likely be resolved by the applicant in a reasonable manner. The reason for this is so that the review team does not have to revisit the entire application and try to refresh its memory later on when the straightforward data (here, the example is chemistry information) come in and are found to be acceptable. The possible necessity for a risk-management plan may also be brought up at this time, as the reviews are near completion and the review team has a rather good handle on the issues of concern that a product may have once it is on the mass market.

Once an opinion has been generated by the review team, it sometimes becomes important to brief the center's or agency's senior management on a new first-in-class product, a controversial application in which the action will draw considerable public and media interest, or a review in which it is preferable to obtain management input on interpreting the data.

Wrap-Up Meeting This meeting traditionally takes place when there are approximately three to four weeks left in the review cycle. There is complete team and even office-level participation at times. Each review discipline presents a concise presentation of the studies it reviewed, presents its major review recommendations, notes any deficiencies in the package, and draws final conclusions. Each discipline's presentation is discussed among the team members and overall final conclusions are drawn, with the office or division director making the final decision on the outcome of the application.

Proposed labeling comments are also considered by the review team, with the Division of Drug Marketing, Advertising and Communication (DDMAC) providing input on promotional words, phrases or statements that may be present in the labeling and that could potentially mislead or misrepresent the qualities of the product. The labeling issues are internally resolved at this time or at a subsequent meeting.

Labeling An application approval has two outcomes: permission to market in the U.S. and to provide labeling for use of the product as approved. Types of labeling that may be part of a product's labeling package can include the Package Insert, Patient's Instructions for Use, a MedGuide, Patient Package Insert, packaging carton design, and immediate container labeling. A key philosophy in preparing labeling is considering what is in the best interests of keeping the patient safe, the prescriber well-informed, and providing the clearest directions on how to safely use the product to its greatest effect.

The applicant, as part of the application, submits proposed labeling for the product. The agency reviews the labeling and revises it based upon its assessment of the data submitted in the application. The revised labeling is then sent back to the applicant for concurrence and this process continues until both sides arrive at the agreed-upon labeling text.

Traditionally, labeling negotiations/discussions are held starting approximately two weeks prior to the action date and potentially up until the latest hour of the due date. These meetings can be held as applicant/FDA group teleconferences in which each of the revised lines is discussed, accepted or challenged. It may seem as if FDA has the upper hand in this circumstance, but the playing field is rather level. Not granting an applicant an approval letter solely due to unresolved labeling issues is looked upon poorly by agency management and, therefore, the review divisions are under significant pressure to resolve all labeling issues prior to approval. According to the regulations, the agency can only send an approval letter if either it has agreed-upon labeling or it has only minor/editorial changes to the draft labeling text that was proposed by the applicant.[25] Therefore, this can make the negotiations work toward a reasonable and timely resolution. It is generally felt that if an applicant has not heard from the FDA regarding labeling issues in the days immediately prior to an expected action, the applicant might assume that an approval letter is not likely to be sent, unless the review division has chosen to accept the proposed labeling with only minor grammatical or editorial changes (e.g., not content).

Final Action After the wrap-up meeting, the reviews of the primary reviewers (e.g., medical officer's review) will then incorporate the agreed-upon labeling text, and will subsequently be finalized. The summary reviews by the secondary reviewers for each discipline (usually the team leaders) either supporting or refuting the review of the primary reviewer are also written and finalized at this time.

A final decision on the action for the application is rendered and the action letter is then drafted and circulated. Given the complexity of some action letters (as detailed in the following section), the letter could circulate multiple times and take more than a week to sort out and finalize. The finalized action letter is then signed by the designated signatory authority, and then shared with the applicant on the same day.

The FDA press office is also notified of any approval action along with the Freedom of Information Office that will place the approval letter on the FDA website within a few days of approval.

Possible FDA actions on a pending marketing application The Agency can take a number of actions on a marketing application at the conclusion of the review:

- Approval[26] - An approval is sent after the FDA has determined, via exercise of scientific judgment, that the drug meets statutory standards for safety and efficacy, manufacturing and controls and labeling or when none of the reasons listed in 21 CFR 314.125 for refusing to approve an application apply.
- Tentative Approval[27] - This type of letter is sent when a marketing application meets the scientific and technical requirements for approval under section 505(b) or (j) of the Food Drug and Cosmetic Act, but marketing exclusivity (e.g., pediatric exclusivity, orphan drug exclusivity) or patent rights preclude a final and effective approval of the drug product.
- Approvable[28] - Indicates that the NDA substantially meets requirements of part 314 (21 CFR part 314) and FDA can approve it if the applicant submits additional information or agrees to specific conditions (e.g., labeling changes).
- Not approvable[29] - This letter is issued when deficiencies with the marketing application are major (e.g., no adequate and well-controlled studies, failure to demonstrate effectiveness, and a major safety concern). Rather than provide specific, focused remedies, these letters might speak more on the guiding philosophy for the required resolution.
- Complete response[30] - FDA has proposed regulatory changes that would replace approvable and not approvable letters with complete response letters because the distinction between the two former letters has become blurred. Both approvable and not approvable letters indicate that a marketing application is not approvable in its current form, and that changes are necessary or that the agency requires additional information. A single complete response letter would describe the deficiencies in a marketing application and, where appropriate, the actions necessary to place the application in condition for approval.
- Refuse to Approve[31] - This letter is intended to cover a variety of circumstances, but is rarely used. Examples of such circumstances include if the development program was not conducted under

GMP, GLP, and GCP guidelines. If this letter is sent, the applicant is also advised that it has an opportunity for a hearing (under 21 CFR 314.200).

Working towards a good review cycle Many activities are taking place inside the review division during the review of a marketing application, although on the outside it might seem the opposite. Aside from an applicant's marketing application, the division is working on a myriad of other applications, policies and assignments. Communication between the applicant and the review division can be a key factor in this process as well as throughout the course of the drug's development. If a complete application has been submitted and the agency understands ahead of time what it is actually receiving for review, this will facilitate the process and build a strong working relationship between the applicant and the agency. It is vital that the review division understands that the applicant is available to quickly and completely respond to information requests—and actually does so. It is also important that the review division appreciates the urgent reaction to an FDA information request that occurs within an applicant's firm, and therefore bundles the requests together into groups and is also very specific with its needs. The working relationship during a review cycle between the two parties is an important two-way relationship although it may look at times rather one-sided from the applicant's point of view.

References

[1] OND is actually composed of a number of Offices of Drug Evaluation, each of which houses roughly three Review Divisions

[2] 21 CFR 314.126(a)

[3] http://www.fda.gov/cder/ombud/

[4] The FDA treats every submission volume (no matter how large or small) in a manner similar to a library. Each volume is bar-coded, as is every reviewer's office. The physical location of every volume can be looked up in a database.

[5] Public Law 102-571

[6] As noted in FR Vol. 69, Number 138, July 20, 2004, page 43351, "For example, we [FDA] promised that by September 30, 1997, we would review and act on at least 90 percent of standard NDAs within 12 months after the submission date (H. Rep. No. 895, 102d Cong., 2d. sess. 32 (1992) (letter from David A. Kessler, M.D., Commissioner of Food and Drugs, to Representatives John Dingell and Norman Lent, House Committee on Energy and Commerce (September 14, 1992))).

[7] Public Law 105-115

[8] Public Law 107-188

[9] Set forth in an enclosure to letters from Tommy Thompson, Secretary of Health and Human Services, to the Chairman of the House Committee on Energy and Commerce and the Ranking Member of the Senate Committee on Health, Education, Labor and Pensions (June 4, 2002)

[10] http://www.fda.gov/cder/pdufa/

[11] FDA Draft Guidance for Industry entitled, "Submitting Separate Marketing Applications and Clinical Data for Purposes of Assessing User Fees" December 2000, Revision 1.

[12] CDER Manual of Policies and Procedures (MAPP) 6050.1 entitled, "Refusal To Accept Application For Filing From Applicants In Arrears."

[13] 21 CFR 314.100; For more information, also see section in this chapter entitled "Possible FDA actions on a pending marketing application."

[14] As defined in section 735(1)(A) and (B) of the Food Drug and Cosmetic Act, or supplements to such applications, as defined in section 735(2).

[15] 21 CFR 314.65

[16] Drug Efficacy Study Implementation list. When FDA was required via the 1962 Kefauver-Harris Amendments to ensure that the efficacy of a drug product also had to be adequately demonstrated in addition to it's safety with, the Agency undertook a program that reviewed pre-1962 products for efficacy.

[17] MAPP 6010.5, entitled, "NDAs: Filing review issues."

[18] Human Drug CGMP Notes, Vol. 2, No. 1, March 1994.

[19] Draft Guidance for Industry entitled " Submitting Debarment Certification Statements."; September 1998.

[20] 21 CFR 54

[21] Guidance for Industry entitled, "Financial Disclosure by Clinical Investigators"; March 2001.

[22] 21 CFR 314.50(h) - (i)

[23] Guidance for Industry entitled, "Environmental Assessment of Human Drug and Biologics Applications." July 1998, revision 1.

[24] 21 CFR 314.60

[25] 21 CFR 314.105

[26] 21 CFR 314.105

[27] 21 CFR 314.107

[28] 21 CFR 314.110

[29] 21 CFR 314.120

[30] FR Vol. 69, Number 138, July 20, 2004, pp 43351-43366

[31] 21 CFR 314.125

CHAPTER 28

Preparing for FDA Inspection

By Hugh N. Tucker, Ph.D.

The FDA's Division of Scientific Investigations will conduct surveillance inspections in response to the acceptance for filing of a new drug application (NDA). Directed or for cause inspections will be in response to information regarding serious or persistent noncompliance of an investigator, sponsor, or contract research organization (CRO). The negative observations during the surveillance inspection of the clinical study site may also cause the FDA to initiate a directed inspection of the drug development sponsor and the CRO. Preparation for the visit by the FDA inspector must begin at the time the clinical phase of the development starts and continue until the final study report of the last trial is finalized and the final FDA inspection has been completed.

Prepare Early and Often All of us are painfully familiar with the college class that appeared unbelievably easy at the beginning. We were told that there would be no graded class work, no pop quizzes, and no interim tests. No class attendance record would be made. At the time, it seemed like a very good thing. Then came the end of the semester and the final exam loomed that would constitute the entire grade for the class. Horror and panic ensued. Having had no opportunity for feed-back regarding the instructor's expectation or on the important learning aspects to be tested, the risk of failure became unacceptably high. When the end of the semester inevitably came we wished futilely for previous exam grades or other quantitative guidance from which to judge our progress before the final challenge.

Procedures that require internal, external, and independent third party audits must be incorporated into the developmental program to provide the guidance with which to judge the adequacy of the program. Early and frequent audits provide the same security as graded class work, pop quizzes, and interim exams. No one can afford to risk the results of a clinical trial in the long and expensive realm of drug and biologics development. There is little assurance that your carefully designed, implemented development program will succeed without the quantitative information derived from well-done audits, audit reports, and implemented corrective action plans.

The tasks of a clinical monitor have different intent from those of an auditor. Excellent clinical monitoring does not in any way lessen the requirement for early and frequent audits. The clinical monitor is focused on the verification of the clinical data and on the observation and reporting of compliance issues at the clinical trial site. Most monitoring plans, especially for late phase clinical trials, dictate 100% source verification of data on the subject's case report form. On the other hand, auditors frequently use a data sampling protocol to verify that the processes are controlled and sufficiently robust to ensure that the resulting data listings will represent the individual subject records and supporting documents. The auditor's view extends over the entire process to include clinical trial sites, contract research organizations, clinical data management, and the sponsor. Any process deficiencies must be detected early. It is impossible to rectify process deficiencies after the trial has been completed.

Internal Audit Waiting until all of the data are collected to conduct a third-party independent audit or other investigator site review in preparation of an FDA inspection is courting disaster. Resources from the sponsor's organization or CRO should be identified, usually in a separate quality system function, to review all of the documentation routinely to ensure that it is current and that each of the standards is met. It is good practice to set up internal audits on a regular schedule throughout the development program. These internal audits should follow the same format and rigor as would be expected from third party auditors or FDA inspectors. Timely periodic internal audits are indispensable to successful research and development processes.

External "Third Party" Audit The third-party audit provides the sponsor or the CRO with the opportunity for an independent, unbiased, and systematic examination of the processes, tasks, and deliverables of a development program. Most drug and biologic development programs include the use of third party auditors after the trial is completed to verify the integrity of the data. While these final audits are one method to prepare for FDA inspections and can provide an opportunity to practice discussion of compliance issues with individuals that have not been previously involved in the study, it is too late in the process to take meaningful corrective action. It is a better practice to enlist third party auditors periodically through out the clinical phase of the program in addition to a final audit. Selection of specific clinical study sites or monitor coverage areas where there have been issues of compliance provides the sponsor and the investigator opportunity to adjust deficient processes or practices and to implement corrective and preventive action.

Both the internal and external audit programs must be viewed by the project team as excellent opportunities for ensuring a robust and compliant drug and biologic development program. Each team member should be made comfortable that it is the process that is being audited, not the individual. Audits can be welcomed as good things with the right management attitude in a collaborative work environment.

The FDA Inspector's Frame of Reference One thought and one phrase from the regulations summarizes the purpose of the regulatory environment and focuses attention on the things that will be of utmost importance to FDA inspectors. The charge of the regulatory bodies worldwide is "to ensure that the rights, safety, and well-being of human subjects are protected." As long as that objective is foremost in the thinking of the project team, the answers to hard questions regarding compliance become easier to find. This central thought is the basis for diligence in protocol design and good clinical practice. A poorly devised and poorly executed protocol puts the study subject at risk without the assurance that the data generated will be usable. In that sense, preparation for FDA inspection begins during the early drafting stages of the protocol.

Elements of the clinical study that ensure study subject rights are IRB processes and oversight and the consent process. It can be expected that these will be prime areas for FDA inspector attention. Additionally, all patients, including the study subjects, have the right to confidentiality and the protection of their individually identifiable health information. The project team must be sensitive to these strict requirements. The FDA inspector will review all of the documentation to verify that processes, procedures, and documentation all guarantee that those subject rights are protected.

The primary objective of the investigational new drug process and the associated regulations is to ensure the safety of the clinical study population. Sponsor oversight of the clinical study and of the investigator is a prime concern of the FDA. The inspector will require evidence that the sponsor has trained the study staff in the intricacies of the protocol, provided clinical monitoring, and taken action when there were any observations of noncompliance. If there are instances of serious or persistent investigator noncompliance, the FDA will require evidence of repeated attempts to correct the noncompliance and the sound reasoning for not terminating the investigator. The study subjects' safety is dependent upon investigator compliance with the protocol. The most common observations cited by the FDA inspectors are protocol deviations. It is also reasonable that serious adverse event reporting will be extremely important to the inspector. Discrepancies, errors, or omissions in safety reporting will not be overlooked and will jeopardize the usefulness of the study for support of the new drug application.

FDA Inspectors Frame of Mind The mind set of the inspectors must be taken into account to understand their expectations. There are five basic conceptual rules that describe the thought processes at the time of an FDA inspection - Mulder's Law, the Genesis Factor, Stephen's Legacy, the Hoover Hypothesis, and Murphy's Correlate.

Mulder's Law

> Trust no one. The truth is out there.
>
> - Fox Mulder, The X-files

Much like the paranoid Fox Mulder, some in the industry are paranoid and believe that inspectors and auditors are certain that a clinical trial cannot be conducted without fraud, bias, lies, subterfuge, and obfuscation. They feel that the goal of the inspection is to discover where the project team has hidden the facts that will lead to the discovery of this truth. Whether or not you are paranoid, no data point or file will be overlooked. One error will be considered the tip of the rest of the iceberg that must be found. Obvious data changes without attribute, discrepancies in handwriting between signature and date, missing pages, SOPs that were all approved on one day, training records that suspiciously appear and are dated the day before the audit, and many other incriminating bits of evidence are all supportive of Mulder's Law. For these types of issues, it they do exist, there is no corrective action that can be taken. If the deficiencies are numerous and cast doubt on the integrity of the data, the entire drug development program will be placed in jeopardy.

Genesis Factor

> In the beginning there was truth . . . , or was there?

With sufficient inspection of the clinical trial subject medical record, medical history, and original laboratory reports, inconsistencies will be found. For instance, the FDA inspection training information instructs the inspector to review the original radiology films for consistency with the radiology report. The inspector must be mindful at the outset that the subject may not exist and the medical records may be falsified. It would not be the first time. It is the FDA inspector's job to discover the trail that leads to confirmation of any irregularities.

Stephens' Legacy

If it's not written down, it didn't happen.

- Inky Stephens, 19th Century

In 1832, Dr. Henry Stephens invented "Blue-Black Writing Fluid." The family firm that manufactured ink and various accessories established the foundations for an auditing empire. His son, Henry Charles Stephens, continued the development of the family business. His nickname, "Inky" Stephens, has since remained familiar to regulatory inspectors worldwide. Only those things that are documented adequately in ink are relevant to the drug development program. Numbers, dates, signatures, or other writings that are not written in ink or that appear with visible changes without attribution are simply unacceptable. The action or result that was meant to be recorded by that notation did not happen. There must be an established, non-refutable ink trail for all data and accountabilities from the generation of the information to the final study report. Failure of Stephens' Legacy is a prime indicator of Mulder's Law.

Hoover Hypothesis

You are not who you say you are.

- J. Edgar Hoover, FBI

The inspector will check to see that individual accountability for action is properly documented. Signatures that are not in consistent handwriting, shared passwords to allow approval of electronic records, and other identity thefts are investigated. Systems and procedures that guarantee non-refutability of identity are mandatory for the Hoover Hypothesis to be disproved.

Murphy's Correlate

Something has gone wrong. Find it.

- Murphy's Law Correlate

Protocol deviations, consent process deficiency, data inconsistency, and regulatory violations are all common findings of FDA inspectors. Why, with repeated experience, do the same deviations continue to be found? All of us are well aware of the requirement, but somehow in the fray of encouraging enrollment, case report form collection, and hectic clinical schedules each clinical site continues to repeat the same mistakes. It is very simple for FDA inspectors to find quickly that Murphy's Correlate is well founded.

Preparing the Clinical Study Site Diligent preparation of the clinical study site with the FDA inspector's frame of reference and mindset is mandatory for successful FDA inspections. For clinical investigations, the standards are clear and have been enumerated by Federal Food, Drug, and Cosmetic Act (Chapter V - Drugs and Devices); the Code of Federal Regulations (Title 21 Food and Drugs); and the International Conference on the Harmonisation of Technical Requirements for the Registration of Pharmaceuticals for Human Use (ICH) (Q1-Q7, S1-S7, E1-E12, M1-M4). All clinical trial sites involved in late-phase trials should expect an FDA surveillance inspection. However, those sites that have the highest enrollment, have visible and vocal clinical investigators, or have had repeated compliance issues documented in monitoring reports require special and dedicated attention. The exhibit below provides a minimum listing of those items that require special attention and organization prior to an FDA inspection. These are areas that are frequently cited in deficiency observations by FDA inspectors. ICH E6 provides a more complete listing of all documents and indicates where the documents should be housed.

Attention should be given to the appearance and organization of all of the documentation at the study site. Disorganized and unattractive study files are an indication that the study staff and investigator have provided insufficient priority and concern for the study. A well-organized study file is a good reflection of adequate sponsor or CRO oversight, and makes the inspector more comfortable that the study subjects have been handled with care,

The clinical site study staff and investigator should be provided with training on FDA inspections. This training should include what they should expect from the investigator and how they will be expected to respond. It is a good practice to conduct a mock FDA inspection after training and organizing the study site. Mock inspections are an excellent mechanism to have the clinical study staff and investigator feel confident and practice the type of interaction that will be important in a successful FDA inspection.

Critical clinical study site documents

Documentation	Verification
Clinical source documents	Available and easily retrievable for each study subject. Information and data are consistent with data listings and original case report forms. All data queries are documented and consistent.
Drug accountability	It is critical that clear documentation is available to demonstrate that the correct drug was provided to the study subject and that all clinical trial material, active and placebo, has been counted.
Financial Certifications	Indication in the study file that certification of no financial interest on the part of investigators exists. If there has been disclosure of financial interest, absolute proof by protocol design or other method must exist to exclude bias.
Informed consent	Process was adequate, signatures and dates consistent and appropriate for the enrollment date, no subject was treated in any way prior to the completion and documentation of the consent process.
IRB documents	IRB approvals exist for protocol and all protocol amendments. There is documentation that the investigator provided all required communication to the IRB as the trial progressed, e.g., safety reports, study termination, etc.
Laboratory certifications	Verify that all laboratory certifications are current for the period of the clinical study.
Monitoring log	Monitoring visits are consistent with follow-up letters to the investigator and that adequate monitoring has occurred to ensure sponsor oversight.
Responsibility and Signature Log	Verification that the initial and signatures required for attribution of changes, review, and approval of data are consistent with the Responsibility and Signature Log listed on the log.
Review monitors reports paying special attention to protocol compliance	Ensure that all compliance issues identified in the monitoring report have been addressed where possible and notes to file have explained complicated resolutions.
Study personnel qualifications	FDA Form 1571 should be current and all previous forms should have investigator names should be consistent with the signature at the time of the approval. The documented education, training, and experience should be appropriate for all study staff based on their role in the study as described in the Responsibility and Signature Log.
Subject study eligibility	Clinical source documents must be consistent with the protocol description and case report form inclusion and exclusion criteria. Subject ineligibility is a frequent finding.

Preparing the Sponsor or CRO In addition to the applicable regulatory requirements and legal standards, it is essential that there be complete, written, and enforceable policies, standard operating procedures, and employee guidance documents that describe the expected performance of each of the individuals involved in the drug and biologic development process. The sponsor or CRO must be equally as diligent with its documentation as is required at the clinical study site. Documentation that all standards have been met will be expected by the inspector. In all cases, documents must be easily retrievable and found in the quality system files, employee training records, or in the trial master file.

An inspector must never be kept waiting for documents to be retrieved. After any request, no more than 15 minutes should pass before the document is provided. FDA inspections will always focus on the same documents regardless of the reason for the audit. Because the same information is always requested, it is amazing that project teams continue to receive deficiency reports that require corrective and preventive action. The exhibit below lists the common categories of compliance documentation that must be kept correct and current at the drug development sponsor or CRO.

An FDA inspection in the US or its territories may occur at any time, with or without notice, in addition to the surveillance inspection that is certain after the submission of the NDA. The only way to be prepared for inspection is to ensure that a standard of 100% compliance is maintained and documented throughout the development program. All foreign inspections by the FDA are pre-announced as a matter of policy, although US inspections are not.

The FDA Inspection

Having completed many internal and several external audits, implemented the corrective actions indicated in each of the audit reports, and having reviewed the clinical study site and sponsor or CRO documents, you are feeling pretty comfortable. It is surprising how quickly that comfort evaporates when the receptionist calls with the message, "There are FDA inspectors at the front desk. Who should they see?"

In some instances, there is pre-notification of an FDA inspection. Announced inspections are typical for surveillance inspection of clinical study sites in response to the filing of an NDA. The time from notification to inspection is kept intentionally short. In most instances, approximately a week notice is given. It is possible, but not advisable, to request

Compliance documentation

Documents	Description	Audit Purpose
Organizational Chart	Listing of responsible individuals by function	Accountability for results
Controlled documents	Policies Standard Operating Procedures Employee Guidance	Completeness and adequacy that ensure compliance with all applicable regulations. Approval authority and date. Document of management commitment and revision history.
Employee Files	Curriculum Vitae Training Records	Document clinical trial monitor and project team training and experience SOP training Protocol and project specific training
Trial Master File	All documents relevant to the conduct of the trial - protocol, protocol, revisions, investigator information, monitoring reports, regulatory correspondence, investigator correspondence, safety reports, clinical trial material distribution, etc.	Physical evidence of adequate trial oversight by the sponsor
Data Listings	Listing of all data collected and entered from monitored study case report forms.	Consistency, accuracy and integrity of data.
Team Member	One-on-one interviews with the team members, clinical trial managers, and clinical monitors.	Verification of education, training and experience and individual understanding of responsibility, accountability, and role in the clinical investigation

that the FDA inspector change the proposed date for the visit. Any request for change should be completely justified and explained in detail. Unjustified delays cast doubt on the preparedness of the organization being inspected and, even worse, may be interpreted by the inspector as a refusal to permit the inspection. Any request for a delay heightens the sensitivity of the inspector and serves to reinforce the mindset that fraud, deception, and bias are present.

Directed or for cause inspections that are the result of suspected noncompliance and subsequent inspection of the CRO and sponsor will be unannounced. Each day in the drug development process should be considered the day before an FDA inspection, and everyone involved should be prepared to execute his/her part during that inevitable inspection. Maintaining a professional and calm demeanor under the stress of an inspection requires written procedures, employee guidance, training, and practice.

Long Before the Visit The preparation for a visit by an inspector or auditor requires the development of specific thought regarding each step that will be required and an action strategy that will ensure a positive outcome.

Procedure A standard operating procedure must be constructed and enforced that details each required step during the inspection process. Every employee should have extensive training on the execution of the procedure and be provided with helpful guides that can be referenced during the inspection. These should include a communication plan for the notification of the organization that an auditor or investigator is on site, a prioritized listing of the name, title, and telephone number for the highest ranking responsible party who will receive the inspector, the name and contact information for the audit coordinator and back-ups, and any specific instructions relating to the facilities, such as use of conference rooms, paging systems, or conversation in public spaces. The procedures and guidances should be kept simple and easy to implement with minimal staff and with no additional preparation. The standard operating procedure for handling audits and inspections is always of interest and will be reviewed by the inspector to determine if the organization maintains compliance.

Personnel Each of the individuals who interacts with the FDA inspector is the face of the development program. An attitude of cooperation and professionalism from all participants must be evident to the inspector if the inspection is to be successful. Establishing clear roles and responsibilities prior to any interaction will provide the infrastructure that will give the team confidence.

Inspection Coordinator The most critical resource to the successful implementation of an FDA inspection is the individual responsible for hosting the inspector and orchestrating the interactions. The Inspection Coordinator is responsible for making sure that the facilities are available and set up appropriately, and that all documents and interviews are controlled and orderly. The Inspection Coordinator never leaves the side of the inspector, takes notes on all comments and interactions, and may electronically communicate the progress of the investigation to others outside of the inspection location. The Inspection Coordinator arranges and conducts daily debriefings, organizes the response to requests, and ensures that all follow-up items are handled by the assigned staff member. This individual should be permanently assigned, extensively trained, and exhibit the appropriate demeanor and temperament. There should be assigned backup for the coordinator in the event that the inspection takes place during the permanent Inspection Coordinator's absence.

Responsible Parties The individuals identified as responsible parties are generally the most senior officers of the organization or, if at a clinical study site, the investigator. There should be a prioritized listing of the responsible parties. For instance, the potential responsible parties for a sponsor could be the Sr. Vice Presidents of Regulatory, Quality Assurance, Compliance, or Medical. The listing would detail the order in which the contacts should be made, based on the organizational hierarchy, role within the organization, experience, and training. Each Responsible Party must be thoroughly trained in the procedures and strategies used during an investigation. Role-playing practice will help to make the real experience less intimidating.

Reception Frequently overlooked resources are those important individuals who will be the initial contact for any inspector or auditor. Receptionists must be specifically instructed regarding their critical role in a FDA inspection. They should have written guidance that describes what questions they should ask, who they should notify, and in what order all of the tasks should proceed. There should be some method for the receptionist to notify the entire organization that an FDA inspector is on site. Internal audits, external audits, and mock FDA inspections are good opportunities to verify that the communication system is workable and that the receptionist has adequate information for smooth implementation.

Study Staff or Project Team The individuals who have been the most involved in the development program need to be aware of their anticipated roles in the inspection process. Each should receive training and practice in audit interview techniques and be provided with guidance on why and how to respond. Each team member should be familiar with the organizational structure, all of the elements of their written job description, and the contents of their education and training files. Each should be able to verbalize precisely the responsibilities and accountabilities associated with their job function. Mock FDA audits, again, are excellent practice venues to hone the skills required to be an effective interviewee.

Facilities The appearance of organization and professionalism is an important psychological advantage. The facilities to be made available to the FDA inspector will play a large role in creating that perception. A large, bright conference room located in an area that will have limited traffic and noise should be identified and permanently assigned to house the inspector and the materials requested for review. Ideally, there should be a computer and LAN access from that room to allow the Inspection Coordinator to communicate actively during the inspection process. Staff should be notified that noise and conversation that can be heard inside the conference room must be avoided. It is good practice to have a second conference room dedicated to the project team for triage of requests and quick review of all documents to be provided to the inspector. All functions of the team should be represented in the conference room so that any request can be handled rapidly and efficiently without having to track down team members if they are required for information. A copier that is close to the triage conference room should be dedicated for use to provide copies of documents immediately when requested by the inspector.

Just Before the Visit An announced visit will begin with the FDA investigator's notification, by telephone, of the inspection date. Several questions should be asked to gain as much information as possible prior to the visit. The exhibit below provides some questions that might provide hints of what the Investigator is expecting.

The Visit When the FDA inspectors arrive, they should present their official FDA credentials and a Form FDA 482, Notice of Inspection. If, for some reason, those documents are not presented, they should be requested by the receptionist or initial contact. A request for credentials and inspection documentation will not offend the inspector. In fact, the organization may be cited for lack of procedures if they are not requested. The FDA inspector should be asked to sign in based on the organizational procedures, and should be issued a badge that clearly indicates his/her status as a visitor or an FDA inspector.

The receptionist or initial contact should immediately contact the Inspection Coordinator to take charge of the FDA inspector. Then, going down the Responsible Party list, he/she should notify the first available contact. The Inspection Coordinator's first job is to ensure that the FDA inspector is guided to the pre-arranged conference room and that everything that the inspector initially requires is available. The first contact that the Inspection Coordinator arranges must be with the Responsible Party. The roles of the Inspection Coordinator and Responsible Party should remain consistent throughout the rest of the inspection if possible. The Responsible Party should receive the Form FDA 482 from the inspector and discuss how the inspector wishes to proceed.

Questions for Announced Visits

Question	Rationale
What are the dates of the inspection? How many days should be blocked for the inspection?	It is important to determine how long the investigator is estimating the task to take. The length anticipated may provide some hint at to the depth and breadth of the information to be reviewed.
What size working space will be required? Do you need to accommodate more than one investigator?	This information is needed to determine if the selected conference room is adequate. Also, if several inspectors are coming, there is an indication of greater concern and an anticipation of greater review.
Who will need to be available to meet with the FDA investigator?	Everyone's schedule is likely to change with notification. The investigation coordinator, Responsible Party, project team will all need to be available regardless of the answer. However, if certain individuals are specifically requested (e.g., clinical trial monitors, study coordinator) it will provide some indication of the motivation for the inspection.
What records or documents does the inspector wish to review?	While you should know the answer already, in some instances, there will be a specific clinical study site or investigator that is of interest. An indication from the inspector can provide you the opportunity to ensure that those documents are reviewed and are immediately accessible.
Will facilities for copying be required?	You will have that available in any case, but a positive response from the Investigator will verify the intent to remove documents from the premises.
Any additional requirements or requests?	The inspector may provide additional information with an open-ended question that could be of assistance in preparing.

The inspector will generally wish to interview key members of the project team to establish the degree of oversight and diligence directed to the study. The inspector's interest will be to ascertain the quality, integrity, and validity of the data and to determine the adequacy of the protection of the rights, safety, and well being of study subjects. The inspector will review the documents listed in the exhibits above. The scope and length of the inspection process is extremely variable, and will depend upon the inspector's comfort with the control of the processes and the completeness of the documentation.

During the inspection, it is important to maintain composure and to never become defensive. Ensure that each request is understood and responded to without elaboration or editorializing. Documents should be presented in a neat, easily reviewed manner. When the inspector requests copies of any documents, always make two—one for the inspector and one for the Inspection Coordinator that will indicate which of the documents had copies that are removed from the site.

Each day of the inspection should end with an exit interview that involves the FDA inspector, the Inspection Coordinator, and Responsible Party. These discussions are essential to the process, and allow the opportunity to resolve issues that have arisen during the day. It is advisable to take immediate action on any of the inspector's observations that can be corrected while the inspection is proceeding. This action may avoid the observation listing on the final day.

After the Visit At the close of the inspection, the FDA inspector will review the results of the inspection at a close-out meeting that will involve, at a minimum, the Inspection Coordinator and the Responsible Party. The FDA inspector may leave a Form FDA 483, Inspectional Observations, describing any deficiencies and discuss required FDA follow-up actions. If corrections have already been made, the FDA inspector should be reminded. It is possible to request a note of the correction on the Form FDA 483, but the inspector is under no obligation to do so. Any misunderstandings regarding the facts of an observation must be discussed and resolved at this point. A good Inspection Coordinator should have resolved these issues prior to the close-out meeting and avoids risking these discussions at the last minute.

Immediately after the FDA inspector leaves, a detailed inspection report should be constructed while all events are still fresh in memory. The report should include the date, times, and perceived purpose of the inspection with attached Form FDA 482, the questions asked by the inspector and the responses given, the documents viewed and copies removed, and the FDA inspector's verbal comments. There should be a table of all corrective actions taken during the course of the inspection. A copy of any Form FDA 483 should be included, if left by the inspector.

The entire project team should gather to discuss the inspection results, the FDA inspector's comments, and to provide a critique of the team's performance during the inspection. This meeting is not only an opportunity to begin to develop the critical corrective or preventive action plan, but also to provide the organization an opportunity to improve compliance status and the handling of inspections and audits.

The stated purpose of an FDA inspection is to secure the correction of deficiencies. A formal response must be made to the FDA on all observations listed on any Form FDA 483. The response must include corrective actions for each observation. A request can be made that the response be filed with the Form FDA 483. The request can include that the response be released if a Freedom of Information (FOI) request is made for the Form FDA 483. Prompt response to a Form FDA 483, while not legally required, can help convince the FDA of the organization's good intentions and reduce the chance of further regulatory action.

With successful preparation, practice, and diligence, no Form FDA 483 will be left by the FDA inspector. However, if deficiencies are noted and a Form FDA 483 is issued, the FDA may also prepare a detailed establishment inspection report (EIR). This report is also available for release under FOI regulations. An immediate request for an EIR is not recommended. The FDA does not always prepare an EIR, especially if no deficiencies were found, if the deficiencies were minor, and if observations did not suggest that the integrity of the data or the safety of the study subjects were compromised. Requesting a copy may increase the likelihood that an EIR will be prepared. After a reasonable period of time, a request may be made through a third party to determine if an EIR has been issued and, if so, its contents. If there is an indication that an EIR has issued, a copy should be obtained to determine the exact content.

Conclusion This chapter has presented, in a very abbreviated form, a few of the important processes that should be included to consider a drug development program complete and robust. Individual plans for preparing for FDA inspections can be developed with assistance from a variety of sources. Quality assurance and regulatory compliance functions from other organizations are almost always willing to discuss their policies, procedures, and experiences.

Continual preparation, the development of written policies and procedures governing the handling of FDA inspections, and careful preparation of the project team are the keys to a successful outcome from an FDA inspection. With the procedures and personnel in place, early and frequent audits provide verification of success and practice in execution. The impetus for today's dedication is the certain knowledge that tomorrow the FDA inspector will arrive.

CHAPTER 29

Preparing for an FDA Advisory Committee Meeting

Steven Biedenbach, M.S., Michael J. Vivion, Ph.D., Bao-Van Tran, M.S., and Steven C. Cohen

For many new drugs, advisory committee meetings are critical milestones in the FDA's regulatory process. Given that companies spend hundreds of millions of dollars developing drugs and biologics and that an advisory committee meeting is often one of the final hurdles for product approval, it only stands to reason that a sponsor's commitment to preparing for such a meeting must have full support from top management.

Although they are seen as harbingers of FDA decisions regarding new drugs, it is important to understand that advisory committee recommendations are not binding on the agency. History, however, has shown that FDA review divisions generally follow the opinions rendered by advisory committees. Experience has also shown, sometimes in harsh ways, that inadequate sponsor preparation for advisory committee meetings most often results in unfavorable committee recommendations. For this reason alone, companies cannot place too much emphasis on managing the meeting preparation process, or on the importance of making a well-rehearsed, concise, and professional presentation before an advisory committee.

History of Advisory Committees The executive branch of the federal government has historically benefited from the advice and recommendations of various committees, boards, commissions, and councils when evaluating issues and making decisions. Recognizing the value of the advice offered by such groups, Congress passed the Federal Advisory Committee Act in 1972. The act set forth a system to govern the creation, operation, and duration of advisory committees to the executive branch. Primarily, the goals of the act were to dictate uniform procedural standards for all federal advisory committees (to include also committees outside of the executive branch), promote openness and transparency in the process, and to reduce the number of ad hoc advisory committees convened.

Subsequently, an amendment to the Act, called the Government in Sunshine Act, emphasized the importance of citizens in the federal government's decision-making process by stating that the rights of citizens to participate in, and obtain information on, the process is balanced with protecting the rights of the individual. By definition, as stated by the Act, a federal advisory board "is not composed entirely of full-time officers or employees of the Federal Government."

There are three types of advisory committees: presidential, discretionary or non-statutory, and statutory. Presidential advisory committees are established by an executive order. Discretionary or non-statutory advisory committees are established at the discretion of a Secretary, agency head, or other official with establishment authority. Statutory advisory committees (which include those in the Center for Drug Evaluation and Research, or CDER) are established by Congress, and the authority for their creation must be included within the language of an Act. With the exception of the statutory type, advisory committees are chartered for two years and must be re-evaluated for renewal at the end of each charter term. Due to the high costs of conducting each FDA committee meeting, a regular review serves to benefit taxpayers, to eliminate committee redundancy and to keep committee objectives focused.[1]

The FDA initiated the advisory committee system in the 1960s and early 1970s. It was after the thalidomide developments in the 1960s that the Commissioner created the Advisory Committee on Teratology. Throughout the 1960s, numerous advisory committees were created, suspended, and re-enacted by the various FDA commissioners. Finally, in the late 1960s, several advisory committees were established that remain in place today. Today, the centers of the FDA have approximately 30 standing technical advisory committees.

Roles of Advisory Committee Meeting Participants Advisory committee members typically are pre-eminent researchers and scientists in specialty fields, or are academic physicians. Prior to 1991, members were appointed by the Secretary of the Department of Health and Human Services. Since 1991, members have been appointed by the FDA Commissioner. Committees are typically composed of 10-13 members who, with the exception of those representing industry, are appointed as "Special Government Employees" (SGEs). During their four-year terms, these SGEs provide expert, independent scientific and technical non-binding advice to the agency. The Food and Drug Administration Modernization Act (FDAMA) provided that each committee include at least two specialists in the disease or conditions being discussed.

Among FDA staff that attend committee meetings is the consumer safety officer (CSO) or project manager, who is the sponsor's primary contact at the FDA throughout the drug development process. The project manager is assigned by, and represents, the review division responsible for the company's drug product.

Another important FDA staff member in the committee process is the executive secretary, who organizes and coordinates the logistics of the meeting, including scheduling meetings, working with review divisions and committee chairpersons to set meeting agendas, distributing meeting materials to sponsors and advisory committee members, and conducting due diligence investigations for conflicts of interest. Sponsors should establish contact with the executive secretary early in the advisory committee meeting preparation process, and maintain regular communication thereafter for updates.

Controlling the meeting is the advisory committee chairperson, whose roles are to keep to the agenda topics and times, protect committee discussion time, and ensure that committee deliberations are brought to closure by providing clear advice to the agency regarding questions posed.

Other non-FDA participants at advisory committee meetings include consumer representatives and patient representatives, who speak on behalf of potential users of the product being discussed. Often, patients who have used a particular drug or biologic, relatives of such individuals, or even representatives of organizations that represent patients with particular illnesses take this opportunity to voice their views on the benefits of a particular therapy. The presence of various industry representatives at these meetings is increasing as well. Additional SGE representatives or guest speakers can attend advisory committee meetings, although they cannot vote or sit with the committee.

Typically, the sponsor's team comprises the following individuals: regulatory affairs personnel, the lead clinical investigator, a second principal clinical investigator, the program's toxicologist/pharmacologist, the principal biostatistician, and additional scientists familiar with issues such as the product's mechanism of action, metabolism, efficacy studies in cell and animal models, stability, and environmental factors. Product launch experts are also helpful at committee meetings for addressing potential market issues. Typically, the company is also represented by a senior management officer, sometimes the president or CEO. This is often well advised, since there may be issues requiring a decision with respect to company resources.

The Briefing Package The preparation of the sponsor briefing package for an advisory committee meeting is a process that requires careful planning and detail. It is the document that summarizes the safety and efficacy analysis presented in the NDA or BLA, and is typically between 50 and 100 pages in length, depending on the particular drug or biologic. The information in the briefing package must be consistent with the data in the company's application, and should follow the order of the information in the advisory committee meeting presentation. Any new information that is not already in the NDA or BLA should not be presented in this document. In all cases, sponsors should keep in mind that the advisory committee members have limited time to prepare for the meeting, so the briefing package should be a well-organized and easily readable summary of the data.

Invaluable resources capable of providing input and support to the content, organization, and clarity of the briefing package include key opinion leaders and past advisory committee members. Sponsors should utilize the experience offered by such experts as much as possible. Key opinion leaders should also be considered as presenters at the advisory committee meeting, as they can bring a great deal of credibility to a company's presentation.

The sponsor's regulatory liaison should contact the committee's executive secretary early in the process to obtain specific instructions on the preparation of the briefing package. If time permits, the briefing package should also be shared with the FDA reviewing division for input. In many cases, the NDA/BLA's reviewing medical officer can offer valuable comments that can enhance the overall document. The reviewing division responsible for an NDA also prepares its own briefing package for the advisory committee. This critical document can also be obtained from the executive secretary prior to the meeting. The divisional briefing package will likely provide the company with additional insights into the agency's positions and views on a particular product, as well as its interpretation of the data submitted by the sponsor.

What to Expect at an Advisory Committee Meeting The FDA conducts advisory committee meetings for several reasons, all with the best interests of the public in mind. Primarily, advisory committees provide independent advice to FDA regarding its evaluation of a drug, biologic or device, as well as on broad regulatory issues not related to a specific product. Advisory committee meetings serve to enhance, complement, and speed the decision-making process. They increase the credibility of FDA's decisions in the eyes of the public and medical community, and increase awareness of public health issues by giving them visibility. Most importantly, advisory committee meetings provide an open forum for the public to provide input into FDA's decisions by way of an open public hearing segment, which is held at the beginning of each meeting. In the open public hearing, members of the public can address the committee on their views, both positive and negative, regarding the product or issue at hand.

Typical issues discussed at advisory committee meetings include the following: the safety and/or efficacy and/or dosing concerns regarding new molecular entities (NMEs) and new indications (when first in class), prescription to over-the-counter switches, risk vs. benefit questions, post-marketing assessments and safety issues, draft guidances, study and protocol design issues, target population and labeling issues, novel scientific or public controversies, and appeals of FDA decisions.

The order of events for advisory committee meetings can vary considerably. Most meetings begin with a call to order by the chairperson, followed by an introduction of the panel and its members. A statement regarding the conflicts of interest of committee members is read. The chairperson will welcome attendees on behalf of the FDA and focus the issues in terms of the meeting agenda. The opening events are then followed by the open public hearing (minimum of one hour), followed by presentations by the sponsor and the FDA, as listed in the meeting agenda. Committee discussion and a question and answer session ensue, followed by a committee vote, and finally, adjournment of the meeting. "Affected persons" are then informed of the agency's decision (i.e., in light of the committee recommendation) within 90 days of the advisory committee meeting.

Under the Federal Advisory Committee Act, a part of every advisory committee meeting must be open to the public. Examples of "open sessions" are those in which NDAs, supplements, post-approval safety, and risk vs. benefit issues are discussed. Sessions that are not open to the public, the so-called "closed sessions," include those in which trade secrets or commercial confidential information (e.g., INDs and review division updates to the committee) are discussed. Only SGEs, FDA employees, and invited sponsor representatives are allowed to attend closed sessions of advisory committee meetings.

The Conflict of Interest Dilemma Conflict of interest is a recurring obstacle whenever one attempts to make informed decisions and form opinions without bias. The FDA, empowered with making decisions about the public health, seeks consultants with the most knowledge and the most relevant experience on specific issues. As noted previously, those appointed to serve on FDA advisory committees are noted experts, pre-eminent researchers and scientists in specialty fields. Industry uses the same pool of scientific experts during the drug development process as well. There is, therefore, a challenge in balancing the agency's need for the most qualified experts against the reality that that these experts are likely to be highly involved in the development of either the drug under committee evaluation or competing products (i.e., a potential conflict of interest). Would committee members stand to benefit from the success or failure of either product(s)? If it is determined that a committee member has an interest in any of the affected parties, a waiver must be granted for that individual to participate in the advisory committee's discussion of the relevant topic. However, after evaluating the potential conflict of interest, the FDA is entitled to deny a waiver, such as one to allow an advisory committee member to review his or her own work.

Evaluating potential conflicts of interest is an extremely complex and controversial process that requires very specific criteria. In a 2002 draft guidance, the FDA proposed that more information regarding the nature and magnitude of an advisory committee member's conflict of interest be made publicly available whenever that member is granted a waiver for those conflicts of interest.

Before the Advisory Committee Meeting Before initiating major preparations for an advisory committee meeting, a company should take steps to gain an adequate background on the advisory committee itself. It is worth the company's time to research the advisory committee and attend other advisory committee meetings, as well as to hand-pick an experienced team capable of taking on the challenge of meeting planning and execution.

The first and most important step in researching an advisory committee is to learn about its members. The current committee rosters are available on the FDA website and via the advisory committee's executive secretary. The members' curricula vitae are available via the FDA's freedom of information process and, since many of the members are likely to be well-known and widely published, their research and published articles can be found through Internet searches. Knowing whether a member has specific expertise in a particular disease or specific views on relevant issues is important, since sponsors can identify deficiencies in their own data and are able to request that committees be supplemented with experts that can add to the collective experience. This allows the sponsor to better focus the presentation and anticipate the types of questions and issues that might be raised. Further, sponsors should not seek to make contact with committee members after they have been identified. All committee-related issues must be communicated through the committee's executive secretary.

Expediting Drug and Biologics Development

The best way to assess the current approaches, tendencies, and workings of a particular committee is to attend its meetings. In this way, a company can quickly learn what types of issues and information each committee member tends to emphasize. Often, a company may be able to determine that certain individuals will dominate the panel and focus discussions on particular issues. An alternative to attending meetings is to obtain and review videotapes of past meetings. By observing meetings, whether in person or by videotape, a company can observe members' behavior and their responses to sponsor tactics and issues.

Strategies for Advisory Committee Meetings In a world of best practices, an advisory committee meeting is one of the final events in a series of communication events beginning early in drug development. Although only some of these events are regulatory in nature, proper strategic focus in all communication from the beginning will contribute to quality meeting preparation and planning. For those teams that did not recognize early communication activities as essential preparation for a possible advisory committee meeting, the preparation process will be more intense, more stressful, and more complicated. For these teams, the preparation directly preceding the meeting must be designed carefully and well-executed with a full understanding of the nuances of the advisory committee meeting process. A rigorous, professionally designed process can still protect them and reduce the negative impact of their lack of early focus.

Managing Messages in Early Drug Development Preparation for an advisory committee meeting should begin in the early stages of a development project, even before the company knows that it will face such a meeting. A company should prepare and implement an integrated communication plan directed to a variety of forums and audiences to articulate its proposed "product messages." This communication plan should include both internal and external events, such as presentations to internal boards, planned publications, press releases based on completed and ongoing studies, and also regulatory milestones like end-of-phase 2 meetings, filings, and advisory committee meetings.

The integrated communication plan should establish a product's central scientific, medical, regulatory, and marketing messages and claims. The sponsor should show the ability to anticipate potential regulatory and professional objections and obstacles during the product's development. The sponsor should be able to take feedback from internal and external sources to develop insightful ideas and contingency plans to respond to these issues. The integrated communication plan should also enable the sponsor to identify current or potential sources of evidence to support the company's positions.

To prospectively reach the disparate stakeholders and attain the dual goals of registration and successful marketing, a company must develop a strategic approach that results in a process and an end product—a process that helps manage the rigorous intellectual inquiry that challenges the development plan, and an end product that captures the messages and issues as they develop over time. This approach enables a dynamic connection between the product in development and the external marketplace that begins early enough to test product messages and to actively shape perceptions of the drug while it is still in development. In addition to forming the foundation for future regulatory interactions like the advisory committee meeting, this early control of messages and issues can have a significant positive effect on such subsequent steps as advocacy, acceptance, and uptake in the market.

Managing Issues in Early Drug Development Managing messages, of course, is only part of the process. Because of the inherent complexity of drug development, multiple issues will arise and will have the potential to become obstacles to the successful delivery of product messages. It is easy to think of drug development as a process of resolving these issues in order to attain registration and a potent marketing platform. The advisory committee meeting, by its very nature, is an interaction oriented toward such issues, including those issues that the FDA has identified and those that the members of the committee are likely to identify.

The very fact that a product has been scheduled for an advisory committee meeting may mean that the company has significant issues to address before the product can be marketed. If sponsors are successful in defining and considering these issues prospectively, then the reality of an advisory committee meeting will be no more than another anticipated step in the drug development process.

In general, issue management is part of a larger interactive knowledge management process that helps a company obtain the maximum possible benefit from its products in early development. The system triggers a collaborative process through which a company can thoroughly characterize a product in early development and identify the essential content for the development of an ongoing communication strategy.

One key to this process is the creation of a management document—a structured, dynamic "database" tool—that captures both the company's messages and the potential issues associated with each individual message. This living document should serve as a snapshot of a product's message development at a given point in time and as a seed document for all of a team's communications during that time period. The team should update it whenever new information (e.g., study results) is received. As new milestones are reached, new data are generated, or the market shifts, the document should be revisited to reflect the changes and to adapt the company's communications. Such a tool will be an invaluable resource for the company throughout the advisory committee meeting strategy process.

Just-In-Time Preparation for the Advisory Committee Meeting No matter what communication management process a company has used to get to this point or whether it has started early or late, the advisory committee meeting generates a set of specific needs that must be met successfully to establish a company's messages and to respond to its issues.

Every company knows that data do not always speak for themselves; they often need some help. To succeed in front of an advisory committee, a drug development team must bring its data to life through the quality of its communication efforts. The team must come across as capable, credible, and compelling as it performs two critical functions. First, the team must be able to present a clear, data-supported argument supporting its efficacy and safety claims and establishing a positive benefit/risk ratio for drug approval. Second, the team must show that it can respond effectively to questions reflecting the committee's concerns and issues.

The rigorous process of preparing for an advisory committee meeting should be implemented to ensure optimal communication between the team and the committee. The first step should be to map out key messages, both those created in response to FDA concerns and those the company wants to make in the advisory committee meeting forum, and to cascade those messages into the presentation, the briefing document, and the question and answer (Q&A) sessions. Simultaneously, the team should perform a detailed analysis of its audience and develop a plan to shape the communication strategy around audience needs. Based on the proposed messages and the audience's likely responses to them, the team should assess the current issues and the lines of questions that are likely to arise from them. As the database of likely questions evolves, the team should formulate focused responses that use data to advance its arguments in the face of the questions, knowing when and how to shut down entire lines of questioning with strategically crafted responses.

The purpose of coordinating the development of the briefing document, presentation, and responses to questions is to reveal gaps which, when identified, will prompt changes to the team's evolving approach to the committee. Rehearsals and mock advisory meetings will add to this process by testing the arguments, their delivery, and the slide support system. To achieve such a well-planned, practiced, and precise delivery of strategically focused messages and responses to questions, it is imperative that an experienced team of highly trained and skilled communicators be assembled.

Advisory Committee Audiences The advisory committee meeting presents a challenging audience analysis. The members of the committee comprise the primary audience not only because their vote influences the FDA, but also because their vote influences all the public stakeholders who will know the exact nature of the vote, including how many voted for and against a recommendation. Further, many of these public stakeholders are clinical practice leaders who would be influential in the drug's acceptance should it enter the market.

Since the meeting is public, the press will be present and able to report on the entire meeting. Additionally, their reports would likely include quotes from individual committee members. This open access means that public stakeholders, including competitors, health practitioners, financial analysts, researchers, and the general public, will be privy to the results of this public hearing. What they hear can have a dramatic impact on a variety of influences on the drug's future, ranging from participation in future trials, uptake of the drug once launched, reimbursement, and even overall perceptions of the company. Because of the public nature of the advisory committee meeting, companies should consider such a forum an excellent opportunity to place its key messages before various audiences, but should remember that, in reaching the members of the committee, the team does nothing to jeopardize its relationship with the FDA reviewers who hold the ultimate power of approval.

Preparing the Team for the Advisory Committee Meeting The overall preparation process for an advisory committee meeting can be long and tense, requiring tremendous effort, focus, patience and resources. Each team facing an advisory committee must design a process that respects the scientific integrity of the drug development program and that contends with the business realities of the company without neglecting the humanity of the people involved. This highly structured process must effectively engage all of the people on the team and enable them to achieve their objectives, scientifically and professionally, collectively and individually.

Since, in addition to understanding the issues facing it, the team must maintain awareness that the messages delivered during the meeting will be heard by the FDA and the public, time must be spent at the beginning of the preparation process harmonizing the messages that will be presented to the advisory committee meeting with those that have been developed preparing for registration and marketing. A three-step message and issue workshop is an effective way for a team to focus its approach.

Expediting Drug and Biologics Development

The facilitator should begin the workshop by interviewing team members. These interviews allow the facilitator to gain insight into how the individual members of the team position the product's messages and issues surrounding the advisory committee meeting. Most frequently, the facilitator discovers the nuances of agreement and disagreement within the team. This information helps transform the subsequent workshop into an active exercise that prepares the intellectual framework for the upcoming meeting.

Next in the workshop should be a brainstorming session. The facilitator begins the brainstorming session by establishing consensus among the team members on the core messages that the team wants to emerge from the meeting. After the messages have been established, the team should face its issues, identifying those raised by the FDA and exploring other issues the advisory committee meeting is likely to raise.

The final step in the workshop should be to begin planning how the team proposes to respond to the identified issues and where support for the messages and responses can be found. For the workshop to be most effective, the team should capture its work in a "message matrix." After team review and approval, the matrix will become the content plan for both the advisory committee meeting presentation and the Q&A preparation.

Designing the Briefing Package and Presentation Using the material from the message matrix, the team now determines the argument that will be elucidated in the briefing document and the core presentations necessary to make its case. It can then create presentation prototypes defending the company's position on the risk/benefit of its product and its responses to the FDA questions and concerns. The briefing package and presentation should evolve in tandem. Failure to develop them together can create end products that are not only out of sync but also potentially in conflict. By starting both simultaneously from the message matrix, both can be developed coherently. Still, it will require ongoing effort to keep them aligned. Very often, the internal feedback that each receives can pull them in different directions. A process must be in place to harness team members' activities and keep them moving along parallel but harmonious paths.

Ultimately, there needs to be a clear and consistent communication strategy. The strategy should be apparent not just in the briefing document and presentation, but also in the responses to questions. Above all, neither the briefing document nor the presentation can afford to step around potential issues or dismiss them too lightly. The company's communication must not only *be honest*, it must also be constructed so that it *conveys honesty*. The company's credibility can be enhanced or diminished by the quality and focus of its communication.

The Issue Book as a Critical Tool The message matrix also serves as the source for the "Issue Book" and the responses to the anticipated questions. The message matrix, which ideally has been updated rather than created anew, contains the collective team thoughts on issues and their priority as well as issue-by-issue responses with annotated support.

The Issue Book is the focus of the Q&A preparation process. It should anticipate every likely or critical question and provide a strategically focused response with complete data support. A successful Issue Book will anticipate 90% to 100% of the questions the committee will ask. It also provides strategically focused responses that the team will be able to develop, review, and evolve throughout the preparation process.

The team should develop the Issue Book throughout the preparation process because it should be the only source of back-up slide generation. Every back-up slide should be created to respond to a specific question. The Issue Book helps teams focus their efforts on the back-up slide process, avoiding the wasted effort of creating back-up slides in a vacuum. Slides that do not respond to a specific question usually end up generating more questions than they answer and can cause the advisory committee meeting to lose focus. Again, the team's responses must be honest and convey honesty. Responses to questions must be carefully constructed to answer questions without creating new questions, to deal with a question directly without creating animosity, and to establish a clear company position without appearing arrogant. The Issue Book is key to the team's success.

Rehearsal, Drilling, and Mock Advisory Committee Meeting Sessions Rehearsal is central to every successful advisory committee meeting. Presentations must be tested by experts outside the team, sharpened, and tested again. Q&As must undergo the same rigorous testing and retesting. Participants need to be coached in delivery techniques, in various techniques for answering difficult questions, and in seamless slide retrieval.

Effective preparation is an iterative process. Each iteration of content should bring the team closer to its final product by incorporating feedback and building effectiveness. The practice of rehearsal and coaching should result in a gradual refinement of message and delivery. Each segment of the primary presentation and every response to a question needs to be clear, compelling, and concise. Rehearsal not only develops the necessary muscle memory but also allows for coaching and guidance from experts on the scientific content and on the communication process.

In addition, the team needs to develop a rapid and reliable ability to call up the right slides to support the speaker during Q&A. This requires a nearly telepathic link between the speaker and the slide team that can only come from the combination of an effective process and rigorous drilling and rehearsal. The team needs to be able call up the right slide every time, and to be able to do so within seconds (not minutes) of the question. It is not unusual for a well-practiced team to have the appropriate slide located before the question is fully asked.

The highest level of rehearsal occurs in the mock advisory committee meeting sessions. These sessions begin months ahead of the actual meeting to test messages with people who are not on the team, both internally and with external experts. These sessions are essential to the effective evolution of the argument and responses to questions. The mock sessions force the team to take into account perspectives that they may not reach on their own. The early mock sessions may generate feedback that requires dramatic changes to the structure of the arguments, and contents of the presentation, briefing document, and responses to questions. With each subsequent mock session, the changes should be smaller, until the final mock session, which ideally will only serve to unearth a few small issues and mostly serve as a polishing rehearsal. However, the final mock session may still end up requiring significant changes to content, so it is important to allow time to adjust and then to rehearse the changed presentation before the actual meeting.

Effective Advisory Committee Meeting Execution FDA advisory committee meetings have been called the Super Bowl of FDA meetings. The importance of an advisory committee meeting demands that the sponsor commits maximum effort to assure a positive outcome. And, like the Super Bowl, the commitment to excellence demands a team effort. The stakes are high and everyone seems to be watching. The concluding task of the advisory committee, after presentations, question-and-answer sessions, and deliberations, is a public committee vote on issues of safety and efficacy. The sponsor's hope is that the hard work and rigorous preparation that have been focused on influencing the meeting outcome culminate in a conclusive vote in support of approval.

Three primary elements can contribute to the desired outcome: good data, honesty, and the ability to answer questions with convincing and effective skill. These elements are interesting because sponsors are often scheduled for advisory committee meetings due to marginal, or at least questionable, data. In these cases, honesty and the ability to answer questions gain even more importance.

The Importance of Practicing Slide Management The production and management of presentation slides should be assigned to an individual or group with experience in technical graphics and knowledge of the dynamics of an advisory committee project. A gatekeeper should be assigned to manage activity relating to slide production. The gatekeeper is a liaison between the content providers and the slide production and management team.

Slide design templates should be established and respected for the duration of the project. Legibility, simplicity, and rapid comprehension are the goals of good slide design. Slides produced for an advisory committee meeting can be divided into two groups: presentation or "core" slides and backup slides. The sponsor should prepare a presentation that is generally one hour long and contains about 100 slides. Very often, the production of these two kinds of slides takes different paths early in the project. As the slide files evolve, there tends to be more and more crossover between core and backup slides. As more slides become part of the "deck," the task of managing becomes more complex. The process is very dynamic and must be appreciated and managed properly. Failure to keep the process focused within acceptable parameters can be disastrous. Management of file ownership is critical to maintaining focus. It is helpful to establish a rule such that only the owner of a file should be authorized to make electronic changes to the slides. Failure to adhere to this rule can result in multiple versions, which will require time and effort to reconcile.

Consultants have stated that a sponsor cannot have too many backup slides. A sponsor presenter during an advisory committee meeting once stated that, "I thought putting an NDA together was a big job until I started dealing with backup slides." In typical advisory meeting presentations, the number of backup slides produced can range from 300 to 3,000. A sponsor needs as many back-up slides as there are potential questions about the approvability of its product. The message here is to appreciate the scope and have processes to manage the complexities.

Backup slide production has no hard deadline and consequently takes a back seat to core slide production, briefing document production, and presentation rehearsals. Nevertheless, it is wise to have the discipline to maintain a continuous schedule for backup slide production, and preferably a schedule that begins early in the meeting preparation process.

This chapter has emphasized that sponsor honesty and the resulting trust established between the sponsor and both the advisory committee and others in the meeting are of paramount importance. The nature of questions and discussion, and even the outcome of the vote at the end of the day, may be affected by the amount of trust developed during the meeting. This honesty should be demonstrated in the content of every slide presented during the meeting.

Types of Backup Slides There are several types of backup slides, each of which is unique in terms of its content and style. Such slides include replica slides, surgical and shotgun slides, prompt slides, and module or vignette slides, as will be described below. Sponsors might also have slides to address more sensitive or difficult issues, and prefer to sequester them in a different file to prevent accidental projection. There are also preview techniques that provide fail-safe handling of sensitive material slides, which will be discussed in detail later in this section.

Replica slides have the appearance of the original data. Examples would be figures and tables from the briefing document. They should be produced exactly as they appear in the document. Trust is built and maintained between the sponsor and the advisory committee if there is no suspicion that the sponsor is trying to conceal or alter information. A renowned statistician who frequently serves on advisory committees has mentioned that he "gets aggressive" when he perceives that a sponsor is overstating data.

Surgical slides have content designed to answer one specific question. Shotgun slides have large amounts of data (whether good or bad), and can be troublesome for several reasons. The volume of information diverts attention from the speaker's message, and prompts more questions that the sponsor may not want to answer. Decisions to show shotgun slides should be made carefully. One approach is to display shotgun slides to only the speaker as an aid or prompt.

Prompt slides are intended for the speaker's eyes only and serve as talking points during the delivery of the answer to a given question. As mentioned previously, shotgun slides can serve as prompt slides, and only if absolutely necessary should they be projected for the audience. One technique to distinguish prompt slides from other backups is to have a different background color, which alerts the team not to project them.

Finally, there are module or vignette slides. These are sequential groupings of slides that tell a story in the course of answering a question. Experienced teams plan ahead for these sets of slides even to the extent of having placeholder title slides in the deck in anticipation of the need before the slides are produced.

Creating such a diverse deck of slides demands adequate production capacity and management. Compressed timelines and the volume of slide additions/revisions frequently require heroic effort to keep the schedule on track. Multiple revision cycles are inevitable and a challenge to the sanity of the graphics team. In addition, consultants' time is precious and must be used wisely. Getting all the right minds in a room at once is difficult, so when achieved, it may be prudent to have a real-time slide revision session with them present. Such sessions are grueling and require strong meeting facilitation as well as expert level graphics production and support.

The Importance of Effective Indexing Imagine that you are a slide in an advisory committee meeting project. You could be a core slide or a backup slide. You could be moved from one status to the other. You could be a slightly modified version of an existing slide. You could be discarded and subsequently recalled at the next rehearsal. You could be the victim of endless revisions. You could be moved around in the deck many times or exist as a stand-alone, but also be needed as part of a vignette.

How can all this information be tracked and organized so as to be useful to the team when needed? The answer is indexing. Metadata about each slide can be entered into a relational database and supplemented with cataloging information that can then be sorted in logical content order. A printout of these records can serve as a useful tool to identify slides that help answer questions during the Q&A period of an advisory committee meeting. The dynamic nature of slide development dictates that two-number sets be employed to identify and track slides. One number set is the position of the slide in the file. The other is a unique serial number that identifies the content of the slide. Core slides are forever being moved around in the presentation, or from core to backup and vice versa. This movement changes the slide position in the deck and possibly many other slides as well. However, the content may not change at all. When the content does change, then version control is used to track and manage revisions. This can be accomplished by an extension on the serial number, such as "1.0, 1.1," and so on.

High Performance Q&A Session Execution Perhaps the most feared segment of an FDA advisory committee meeting from the perspective of the meeting participant is the Q&A session. There can be one or two Q&A sessions during the committee meeting. One occurs immediately after the sponsor presentation and consists of clarification questions only. The other might be consecutive with the first or occur after all other presentations are made. The duration of the Q&A sessions may vary from 15 minutes to several hours.

For the typical advisory committee meeting, the sponsor is given 30 seats in a location, called the "bullpen," to one side of the U-shaped table occupied by the advisory committee. The bullpen is a place for contributors to the sponsor presentation, and not for employee spectators or seat-fillers. Bullpen occupants consist of core presenters, consultants, content experts, and slide retrieval teams. Employment of a seating plan facilitates communication during the meeting. Audience seating is available for other sponsor associates, and early arrival, 75 minutes prior to the meeting start, usually guarantees a good location.

The key to successful Q&A session execution, as with the rest of the advisory committee meeting segments, is preparation and rehearsal. This includes practicing verbal answers and slide retrieval. The bullpen captain acts as liaison between the slide identifiers and the projection team. It is common for the slide production gatekeeper to also be the bullpen captain. Many successful sponsors use monitors positioned at the podium, floor microphone, and bullpen to preview slides before they might be sent to the screen. This technique provides the podium responder with options to use the previewed slide as a prompt, reject it and ask for another slide, or signal the projection team to send the slide image to the projector.

A typical scenario for the bullpen during Q&A might be as follows:
- A committee member asks a question
- The sponsor representative at the podium and the bullpen support team listen intently to make sure the question is understood
- The podium responder starts answering the question
- Bullpen slide identifiers give slide cues to retrieval/projection team
- The bullpen captain triages the selected slides and gives the command to send the slide to the preview monitors
- The podium responder decides whether to accept the slide as a hidden prompt, reject it, or project it
- If the decision is to project, the slide image is sent to projector
- The preview system is cleared for the next slide
- The podium responder or bullpen captain gives the "slide off" signal

A well-rehearsed team can perform the aforementioned activities with few if any audible signals. The audience can then be aware of only the podium responder and the projected slide. Bullpen body language is also an important factor in the audience perception of sponsor control. A calm demeanor at all times and minimal shuffling of paper is the goal. The best performing bullpens attract no attention. Further, the best tool for successful bullpen support is a photographic memory. For those less fortunate, there are other tools: thumbnail images of slides, index printouts sorted by category or issue, and key question pages containing scripted answers and supporting slides.

Advisory Committee Meeting Details and Logistics Advisory committee meeting preparation is complex, time consuming, expensive, and stressful for any sponsor. The best way to address these challenges is to take advantage of experienced professional services when possible. An integral part of using experienced professionals is the employment of a professional meeting planner, whose business is to make sure all the details are addressed. A good meeting planner can make everything happen in a seamless fashion and resolve problems quickly and efficiently. It can be a mistake to assign this function to a company administrative assistant who is inexperienced in orchestrating support for an advisory committee project team.

In terms of facilities management, hotel selection in the Washington, D.C. area for the sponsor team requires advance planning and consideration. If there are multiple sponsors presenting at your advisory committee meeting, it is important to consider whether to stay at the panel meeting hotel, the same hotel as another sponsor, or a different hotel to avoid interference. Decision-making is complicated sometimes because the actual meeting location is unknown early on. Early booking allows better property selection as well as internal proximity of meeting rooms. It is prudent to develop a good working relationship with the hotel audiovisual manager and the conference sales representative. Leave nothing to chance. Follow up on everything. The hotel staff you make arrangements with on a weekday may not be on duty on weekends. It is easy for details to get lost. The professional meeting planner can be of great value when reconciling these details.

In terms of meeting materials, the administrative logistics of preparing handouts are time-sensitive. Production of handouts of the core slides is a task that can only be started after the core slides are locked from further changes, a milestone that is often not achieved until just prior to the meeting. Therefore, once the core slides are locked from changes, the administrative logistics must be fluid and well executed. Seventy sets of two-per-page images are needed for the committee, FDA, and bullpen combined. Audience handouts may also be needed, and are six-per-page and usually black and white. Copying all of these materials is time consuming, so the process must be scheduled appropriately. Sponsors either rent high-capacity equipment to be used in their hotel, or they contract with a local copy service. Be aware that you may not get quick turnaround as a walk-in customer at a 24-hour retail copy center. An alternative is to purchase dedicated service from an independent vendor. Again, the professional meeting planner can secure these resources so that the sponsor can concentrate on producing effective slides for the meeting. After the handouts are produced, the sponsor will be responsible for forwarding all documents and slides that are to be presented to the committee on to the executive secretary.

Editor's Note: Portions of this chapter were developed from a lecture on this topic by Jayne Peterson, R.Ph., J.D., Deputy Director, CDER Advisory Committee Staff, FDA.

[1] Sherman, L., Looking Through a Window of the Food and Drug Administration: FDA's Advisory Committee System, *Preclinica* 2(2), 99-102 (March/April 2004). http://www.preclinica.com/pdf/articles/sherman_2-2.pdf

CHAPTER 30

Post-Marketing Safety Assessment

By Wei Dong, M.D., Ph.D.

Introduction

Post-marketing safety assessment (or risk assessment) is part of an iterative process of risk management. Its goal is to identify opportunities to minimize any potential risks of a medicine so that its benefit/risk profile is maximized. Specifically, safety assessment in this setting encompasses all post-approval scientific and data-gathering activities relating to the detection, assessment and understanding of adverse events.

As evidenced by recent issues regarding the Cox-2 inhibitors, a new product's safety profile developed for marketing/licensure applications may be considered as "provisionally" established at the time of NDA/BLA submission. A product's effects in routine clinical practice, however, would require continued evaluation in a less-closely monitored environment and among patients who have not been represented in highly refined pre-approval studies.

On a practical note, post-marketing safety assessment should focus on the following questions:
- How can the most informative and accurate benefit-risk assessment be performed?
- What is the size of the risk (numerically speaking)?
- How likely is the product responsible for the problem?
- Who is at risk? Is the risk manageable or modifiable?
- What should be the company's plan for action?

Given these considerations, this chapter will provide an overview of the major types of safety information that a product sponsor might encounter or generate in a post-approval setting, and will discuss relevant issues regarding the utility of the information that they may produce.

Sources of Safety Data Whether one is reviewing a product's existing safety information or planning to collect additional information, data sources must be considered first. This is because the "meaning" of the information is largely influenced by the nature and quality of the data sources. Safety data may derive from a variety of sources, ranging from spontaneous reporting of safety events and observational studies of patients "at-large" to randomized controlled clinical studies (see exhibit below).

The sections below discuss two major types of information commonly encountered in post-marketing settings—namely, spontaneous reports and epidemiological studies. Phase 4 clinical trials, especially those involving the randomization of patients into treatment arms, are less commonly used, in part because of concerns over ethics and/or feasibility.

Principal sources of information for safety assessment

1. Spontaneous adverse reaction reporting
2. Epidemiological studies
   Cohort
   Case-control
   Cross-sectional
   Data collected for other purposes
   　　Routine official statistics
   　　Databases of prescriptions and outcomes
3. Clinical trials

Modified from: Waller and Lee. 1999. Responding to Drug safety issues. PDS.

Expediting Drug and Biologics Development

Spontaneous reports The evaluation of spontaneous reports may serve dual roles: the need for regulatory reporting as well as for signal detection. Spontaneous reports are adverse drug events/reactions that are voluntarily reported either to pharmaceutical manufacturers, to national or regional pharmacovigilance centers, or to national regulatory authorities by healthcare professionals, other professionals or consumers. Spontaneous reporting is the historical cornerstone of pharmacovigilance and signal detection. It may be the only source of information available, especially in the immediate period after approval. These reports are particularly useful to identify rare, serious, unusual or unexpected adverse drug reactions.

Questions commonly asked at this stage of safety review evaluation may include the following: Does this event represent a "signal"? Is it important enough to warrant a signal work-up? What additional data should be acquired in order to verify the signal? Can quantitative measures of the signal be generated? Does it meet the criteria for a serous adverse event (SAE) and, therefore, require more stringent or speedy reporting to regulatory agencies?

In answering these questions, the sponsor must acquire as much data as possible from the cases deemed to be important. Such data may include the time of onset of signs and symptoms, the use of suspected and concomitant product therapy (i.e., dose, schedule, dates, duration), patient characteristics, baseline medical history, co-morbid conditions, the clinical course of the event and patient outcomes (hospitalization or death) and any laboratory results. Other information, such as the patient's response to de-challenge and re-challenge (though rarely available), should be documented whenever possible. For more information, please see FDA's 2001 guidance entitled, "Postmarketing Safety Reporting for Human Drug and Biological Products Including Vaccines."

If necessary, case series may be developed to facilitate any issue work-up. Additional cases may be identified from the company's global safety databases, the published literature, and other available databases, such as the FDA's Adverse Event Reporting System (AERS). The successful identification of these cases would require the development of a clear case definition. This can be complicated when a given event consists of a cluster of syndromes or when it does not have a corresponding "term" within ICD or MedDRA terminologies.

Reports of a subset of adverse events may warrant more emphasis. These events are certain distinct medical events known to be associated more frequently with drug therapy than not. This may include agranulocytosis, anaphylaxis, anaphylactoid reactions, toxic epidermal necrolysis, torsade de pointes, aplastic anaemia, and Guillain-Barré syndrome. Serious adverse events (SAEs) are those events that have one or more of the following outcomes: death, life-threatening adverse experience, initial inpatient hospitalization or prolongation of hospitalization, significant or persistent disability/incapacity, congenital anomaly/birth defect (including that occurring in a fetus), and important medical events based upon appropriate medical judgment that may jeopardize the patient or subject and may require medical or surgical intervention to prevent one of the other outcomes listed in the definition of serious (FDA 2001). It is prudent to notify the regulatory agencies in a timely manner (e.g., 15-day reports of serious and unexpected events) as specified by appropriate regulations.

The question as to whether or not a product is responsible for the event can rarely be addressed with a high level of confidence based on individual cases alone. Because of this uncertainty, the FDA has not recommended any specific categorization of causality; nevertheless, sponsors may describe causality as *probable, possible, or unlikely*. The WHO has used the following categories of causality: *certain, probably/likely, possible, unlikely, conditional/unclassified, and unassessable/unclassifiable* to describe causality.

It is worth noting that information, albeit limited, generated from spontaneous reports can be published in peer-reviewed journals. For example, Bonnel RA and Graham DJ (2004) studied 80 case reports of peripheral neuropathy among patients treated with leflunomide therapy. They argued that "leflunomide use is associated with peripheral neuropahy in some patients" and that "patients who stopped leflunomide use within 30 days of symptom onset were more likely to have improvements of symptoms or complete recovery than were patients who continued to use the drug for longer periods of time."

Limitations of data from spontaneous reports, apart from being limited and sometimes confounding, may also result in over- but more likely under-reporting of true underlying risk interests. In addition, the frequency of reported cases may be influenced by many external factors, such as the time elapsed since launch, pharmacovigilance-related regulatory activity and media attention. With this caveat, crude reporting rate has been used to help quantify the signal. This reporting rate is simply calculated as the number of known cases of events divided by the number of patients estimated to be exposed to the product. The latter may be estimated based on sales figures from IMS (a company that provides these figures) or the sponsor itself. Caution should be used when interpreting this "reporting rate," since not all cases of relevant safety events might have been reported.

Pharmacoepidemiology Studies Several recent regulatory guidance documents—for example, the ICH's E2E guidance entitled, "Pharmacovigilance Planning" (2005) and the FDA guidance entitled, "Good Pharmacovigilance Practices and Pharmacoepidemiologic Assessment" (2005)—provide a comprehensive overview of the rationale and utility of these observational studies in a post-marketing setting. Additional guidance is also available in the International Society for Pharmacoepidemiology's "Guidelines for Good Pharmacoepidemiology" (ISPE 2004) and the 2000 text entitled, "Pharmacoepidemiology" (edited by Strom).

As discussed earlier, it is rarely possible to know with a high degree of certainty whether or not there was a causal association between a product and a particular safety event when no data other than those from individual case reports are available. To address this challenge, well-planned pharmacoepidemiologic studies, such as case-control studies and cohort studies with longer-term follow-up, have been recommended. Data collection can be either prospective or retrospective. These studies are also known as "observational studies," primarily because they do not require patients to be treated per a study protocol. Instead, patients usually receive the standard of care at their treating physicians' discretion, and observations are then made about their treatment and outcomes. These studies can be either descriptive or analytical in nature. Descriptive studies simply describe the frequency (e.g., expressed as incidence, prevalence, or absolute risk) of an event of interest in a patient population. Analytical studies take this one step further by comparing the frequency in one patient group to another, with a group being defined based on factors of interest (e.g., treatment regimen, presence of co-morbidity, etc.). In this case, statistical measures of association, such as the relative risk or odds ratio (which are particularly useful for examining causality), will be reported. Different study approaches may be used in sequence or in parallel, depending on the nature of research objectives and considerations of feasibility. Other aspects of risk measures may also be considered, such as trend in risk over time; the goal is to gather evidence to ensure that SAEs are rare and that this remains true in the long-term (Waller and Evans, 2003 PDS).

A common question involves how one should weigh the evidence of safety (or risk) from observational studies in order to decide if a product remains sufficiently safe to remain on the market. This can be illustrated by the recent FDA Advisory Committee discussions regarding the safety of the Cox-2 inhibitors. The FDA asked the committee to comment on the following: "Please discuss the contributions and limitations of the currently available observational studies to the assessment of cardiovascular risk for the non-selective and COX-2 selective NSAIDs. In particular, please discuss the role of such observational studies in informing regulatory decisions about post-marketing safety issues" (FDA 2005).

This question arises for a number of reasons. Different study approaches possess varying degrees of (un)certainty with respect to the evidence. In theory, certainty is the highest (and uncertainty the lowest) for randomized controlled clinical trials, with certainty decreasing for observational studies, and reaching its low for case reports. As a result, there is a disadvantage, at least in theory, in moving away from clinical trials. There have been situations in which results from observational studies were inconsistent with those from randomized studies, even though such discrepancies might result, in part, from differences in study population (e.g., severity of disease), use of therapies, and study measurement.

To minimize bias in observational studies, one should evaluate and act on potential biases through all stages of design, conduct and implementation. This may include strategies such as selecting the right patients for the right endpoint, collecting prognostic and risk factors at baseline, designing clear case report forms (CRFs) with a validated questionnaire, and maintaining patient follow-up over time.

More recently, safety epidemiology has extensively used databases that are collected for other purposes, such as those known as claims databases or automated databases. As its name suggests, a claims database consists of records of medical, pharmacy and/or other claims for a large number of patients with very diverse characteristics in terms of demographics and therapeutic interventions. Many databases have been used for safety studies, including the HMO Research Network, United Health Care (UHC), General Practice Research Database (GPRD), and the Prescription-Event Monitoring (PEM) database. Databases are most useful for treatments and clinical events that can be readily identified through pharmacy and medical claims records. The validity of information contained in the databases may vary by internal factors (e.g., sample size and availability of certain data), as well as external factors (e.g., research objectives). Before embarking on any studies, it is prudent to examine these issues to ensure that the database's capacity meets the need of a particular safety question. Garnering much recent attention in this field was a study regarding the risk of acute myocardial infarction and sudden cardiac death in patients treated with cyclo-oxygenase 2 selective and non-selective non-steroidal anti-inflammatory drugs (Graham DJ 2005). This nested case-control study was conducted in the California Kaiser Permanente population.

Another example of claims data analysis illustrated its utility to examine treatment patterns (as opposed to safety outcomes). In the United States, cisapride was indicated for the symptomatic treatment of nocturnal heartburn due to gastroesophageal reflux disease. Post-marketing safety reports revealed a potential risk of serious cardiac arrhythmias during cisapride's administration, mostly involving concomitant exposure to another drug. This led to a series of label changes and warnings between 1995 and 1999, and the product was eventually removed from general distribution in July 2000. Jones JK et al., (2003) identified all the patients that had cisapride prescriptions between July 1993 and December 1998 and that were under a managed care organization. They found that among 131,485 cisapride prescriptions dispensed after the warnings began, 4,414 (3.4%) overlapped with at least one drug contraindicated in the labeling at the time of the prescription. Of all overlapping prescription pairs, about half of them were by the same physicians, and 90% of them were dispensed by the same pharmacies. This study was useful in identifying the critical importance of both the pharmacy and the physician in preventing contraindicated drugs from being used together.

Finally, there appears to be an increased demand for large, observational safety studies (also known as "registries") for post-marketing commitments (PMCs). Such commitments and studies generally are sought when additional safety information (beyond that in the NDA/BLA) is required in order to confirm existing data, raise or answer questions, or provide new data following approval. Other circumstances under which the FDA requires PMCs are generally related to the so-called "accelerated approval" program for fast track products or for those products for which safety/efficacy data in children is considered necessary. PMC safety studies can be resource intensive, as evidenced by FDA data showing the number of "pending" (i.e., open or uncompleted) PMCs. However, given the value of the results that these studies provide, efforts should be made to ensure their timely execution and completion, and to design study protocols that employ the best available epidemiology data on the target population size and background rate of events of interest.

Safety Information Submission and Benefit-Risk Assessment In conveying safety information that are synthesized from multiple sources in an effort to communicate potential product-related concerns, a submission ideally should include as much information as possible to facilitate a causality assessment. In its "Guidance Regarding Pharmacovigilance and Pharmacoepidemiology Practices" (March 2005), the FDA's recommendations for these submissions include the following:

- Spontaneously reported and published case reports, with denominator or exposures information to aid interpretation;
- Background rate for the event in general and specific patient population, if available;
- Relative risk, odds ratio, or other measures of association derived from pharmacoepidemiologic studies;
- Biologic effects observed in preclinical studies and pharmacokinetic or pharmacodynamic effects;
- Safety findings from controlled clinical trials; and
- General marketing experience with similar products in the class.

There are no standard formulas, in a numeric sense, that would describe a product's benefit-risk profile. Nevertheless, many factors should be taken into account, including an unmet medical need, the existence of any safer or more efficacious alternative therapies, a causality possibility, the estimated number of patients that could be treated, and the magnitude of the risk (in the context of benefit).

Conclusions Many lessons can be learned from the recent market withdrawals of several products. Safety evaluation is a complex process. This is especially true when large numbers of patients are quickly exposed to a newly approved product, and when an event of interest is a common co-morbid condition in the target population (e.g., cardiovascular disease in elderly patients potentially eligible for Cox-2 inhibitors). A few other contextual factors may also present themselves as unique challenges and opportunities. The list may include increasing consumer expectations for safer products, the wide use of technology (e.g., Web-based medicine, computer-based prescription refill), broader collaboration among regulatory agencies internationally, and advances in pharmacogenomics and diagnostics. In conclusion, the ultimate goal of effective safety assessment is to maximize the benefit/risk profile. This may be accomplished by keeping updated with regulatory developments and scientific advances, leveraging multidisciplinary expertise, and using the best tools and methods in early signal detection.

References

Bonnel RA. Graham DJ. Peripheral neuropathy in patients treated with leflunomide. *Clinica Pharmacology & Therapeutics.* 75(6):580-5, 2004.

Current challenges in Pharmacovigialnce; Pragmatic Approaches. Report of CIOMS Working Group V. CIOMS. Genenva 2001.

Discussion Points. Joint Meeting of the Arthritis Advisory Committee and the Drug Safety and Risk Management Advisory Committee Hilton, 620 Perry Parkway, Gaithersburg, MD February 16, 17, and 18, 2005.

Guidance for Industry. "Good Pharmacovigilance practice and Pharmacoepidemiologic Assessment." FDA 2005.

Guidance for Industry. "Postmarketing Safety Reporting for Human Drug and Biological Products Including Vaccines" (draft guidance). FDA 2001.

Guidelines for Good Pharmacoepidemiology. The International Society for Pharmacoepidemiology has published (ISPE 2004).

Graham DJ. Campen D. Hui R. Spence M. Cheetham C. Levy G. Shoor S. Ray WA. Risk of acute myocardial infarction and sudden cardiac death in patients treated with cyclo-oxygenase 2 selective and non-selective non-steroidal anti-inflammatory drugs: nested case-control study. *Lancet.* 365(9458):475-81, 2005.

ICH E2E. Pharmacovigilance Planning (PVP).December 2004.

Jones JK. Fife D. Curkendall S. Goehring E Jr. Guo JJ. Shannon M. Coprescribing and codispensing of cisapride and con-traindicated drugs. JAMA. 286(13):1607-9, 2001.

ICH "Post Approval Safety Data Management: Definitions and Standards for Expediting Reporting" (E2D). 2003.

Pharmacovigilance. Edited by Mann RD & Andrews EB. John Willey & Sons, Ltd. 2002.

"Report on the Performance of Drug and Biologics Firms in Conducting Postmarketing Commitment Studies." Federal Register: February 18, 2005 (Volume 70, Number 33). FDA.

Strom BL (ed), 2000. Pharmacoepidemiology, 3rd edition, Chichester: John Wiley and Sons, Ltd.

"Managing The Risks From Medical Product Use — Creating A Risk Management Framework. Report To The FDA Commissioner." From The Task Force On Risk Management. FDA 1999.

Waller PC. Evans SJ. A model for the future conduct of pharmacovigilance. *Pharmacoepidemiology & Drug Safety.* 12(1):17-29, 2003.

Waller PC. Lee EH. Responding to Drug Safety Issues. *Pharmacoepidemiology & Drug Safety.* 8:525-552, 1999.